USMLE STEP 3

SECRETS

USMLE STEP 3

SECRETS

THEODORE X. O'CONNELL, MD
Program Director
Family Medicine Residency Program
Kaiser Permanente Napa-Solano
Napa, California
Assistant Clinical Professor
Department of Community and Family Medicine
University of California, San Francisco, School of Medicine
San Francisco, California
Assistant Clinical Professor
Department of Family Medicine
David Geffen School of Medicine at UCLA
Los Angeles, California

THOMAS E. BLAIR, MD
Resident Physician Emergency Medicine
Harbor-UCLA Medical Center
Los Angeles, California

RYAN A. PEDIGO, MD
Chief Resident Physician Emergency Medicine
Harbor-UCLA Medical Center
Los Angeles, California

ELSEVIER
SAUNDERS

ELSEVIER
SAUNDERS

1600 John F. Kennedy Blvd.
Ste 1800
Philadelphia, PA 19103-2899

USMLE STEP 3 SECRETS   ISBN: 978-1-4557-5399-4
Copyright © 2015 by Saunders, an imprint of Elsevier Inc.

Notices

Library of Congress Cataloging-in-Publication Data
O'Connell, Theodore X., author.
  USMLE step 3 / Theodore X. O'Connell, Thomas E. Blair, Ryan A. Pedigo.
    p. ; cm. -- (Secrets)
  Includes bibliographical references and index.
  ISBN 978-1-4557-5399-4 (pbk. : alk. paper)
  I. Blair, Thomas, 1984- , author. II. Pedigo, Ryan, author. III. Title. IV. Series: Secrets series.
  [DNLM: 1. Clinical Medicine--Examination Questions. WB 18.2]
  RC58
  616.0076--dc23

                                                                        2014042526

Senior Content Strategist: James Merritt
Content Development Specialist: Julia Rose Roberts
Publishing Services Manager: Anne Altepeter
Senior Project Manager: Doug Turner
Design Manager: Steven Stave

Working together
to grow libraries in
developing countries

Printed in the United States of America

www.elsevier.com • www.bookaid.org

Last digit is the print number: 9 8 7 6 5 4 3 2 1

To Nichole, Ryan, Sean, and Claire. I love you.
THEODORE X. O'CONNELL

To my wife, Jenny Blair, and my parents, Robert and Linda Blair.
Thank you for your limitless love, support, and encouragement.
THOMAS E. BLAIR

To my beautiful wife, Tiffany, for her unconditional love and support,
and to my father for making me the man I am today.
RYAN A. PEDIGO

CONTENTS

CHAPTER 1   GENERAL PRINCIPLES   1

CHAPTER 2   DISORDERS OF THE NERVOUS SYSTEM AND SPECIAL SENSES   22

CHAPTER 3   DISORDERS OF THE RESPIRATORY SYSTEM   47

CHAPTER 4   CARDIOVASCULAR DISORDERS   63

CHAPTER 5   NUTRITIONAL AND DIGESTIVE SYSTEM DISORDERS   88

CHAPTER 6   BEHAVIORAL AND EMOTIONAL DISORDERS   111

CHAPTER 7   DISORDERS OF THE MUSCULOSKELETAL SYSTEM   124

CHAPTER 8   DISORDERS OF THE SKIN AND SUBCUTANEOUS TISSUE   135

CHAPTER 9   DISORDERS OF THE ENDOCRINE SYSTEM   154

CHAPTER 10   RENAL AND URINARY DISORDERS   166

CHAPTER 11   DISEASES AND DISORDERS OF THE FEMALE REPRODUCTIVE SYSTEM   175

CHAPTER 12   PREGNANCY, LABOR AND DELIVERY, THE FETUS, AND THE NEWBORN   189

CHAPTER 13   DISORDERS OF BLOOD   215

CHAPTER 14   DISORDERS OF THE MALE REPRODUCTIVE SYSTEM   234

CHAPTER 15   DISORDERS OF THE IMMUNE SYSTEM   239

CHAPTER 16   CLINICAL CASE SCENARIOS   253

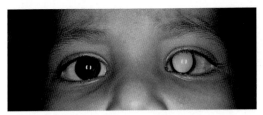

Plate 1. Leukocoria (white pupillary reflex) is the most common presenting feature of retinoblastoma and may be first noticed in family photographs. See Figure 1-1, p. 3. (*Courtesy of U. Raina.*)

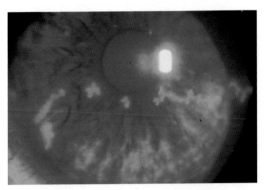

Plate 2. Varicella dendritic keratitis. Numerous dendrites are seen in this slit-lamp photograph with fluorescein staining of the dendritic lesions from active viral growth in the corneal epithelium. See Figure 2-6, p. 42. (*From Krachmer JH et al. Cornea. 3rd ed. Philadelphia: Mosby, 2010, Figure 80.2.*)

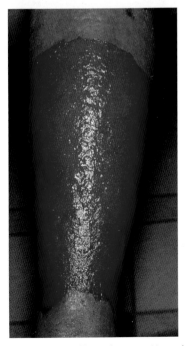

Plate 3. Allergic contact dermatitis of the leg caused by an elastic wrap. Notice the well-marginated distribution that differentiates it from cellulitis. See Figure 8-1, p. 136. (*From Auerbach PS: Wilderness medicine, 6th ed. Philadelphia: Mosby, 2011, Fig. 82-46.*)

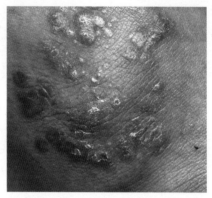

Plate 4. Lichen planus. Flat-topped, purple polygonal papules of lichen planus. See Figure 8-2, p. 137. (*From Kliegman RM: Nelson textbook of pediatrics, 19th ed. Philadelphia: Saunders, 2011, Fig. 649-10.*)

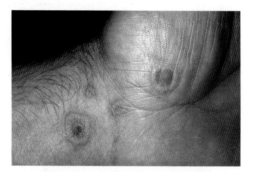

Plate 5. Erythema multiforme. Bull's-eye annular lesions with central vesicles and bullae. See Figure 8-3, p. 137. (*From Goldman L, Schafer AI: Goldman's Cecil medicine, 24th ed. Philadelphia: Saunders, 2011, Fig. 447-10*)

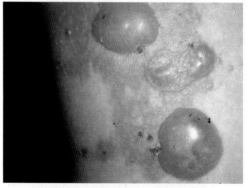

Plate 6. Bullous pemphigoid. Tense subepidermal bullae on an erythematous base. See Figure 8-4, p. 138. (*From Goldman L, Schafer AI: Goldman's Cecil medicine, 24th ed. Philadelphia: Saunders, 2011, Fig. 447-6.*)

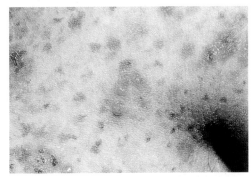

Plate 7. Dermatitis herpetiformis is characterized by pruritis, urticarial papules, and small vesicles. See Figure 8-5, p. 138. *(From Feldman M, Friedman LS, Brandt LJ: Sleisenger and Fordtran's gastrointestinal and liver disease, 9th ed. Philadelphia: Saunders, 2010, Fig. 22-26. Courtesy of Dr. Timothy Berger, San Francisco, CA.)*

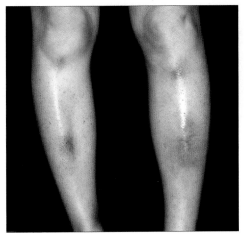

Plate 8. Erythema nodosum on the legs of a young woman. See Figure 8-6, p. 140. *(From Hochberg MA, Silman AJ, Smolen JS, Weinblatt ME: Rheumatology, 5th ed. Philadelphia: Mosby, 2010, Fig. 159.13.)*

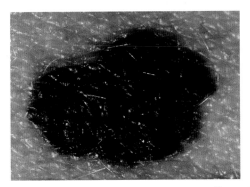

Plate 9. Melanoma (superficial spreading type). See Figure 8-7, p. 141. *(From Goldman L, Schafer AI: Goldman's Cecil medicine, 24th ed. Philadelphia: Saunders, 2011, Fig. 210-3.)*

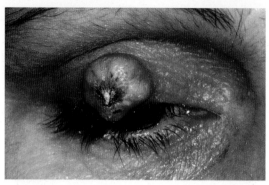

Plate 10. Keratoacanthoma on the right upper lid. Lesions are solitary, smooth, dome-shaped red papules or nodules with a central keratin plug. See Figure 8-8, p. 141. *(From Albert DM, Miller JW: Albert & Jakobiec's principles and practice of ophthalmology, 3rd ed. Philadelphia: Saunders, 2008, Fig. 250.3.)*

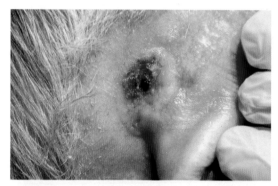

Plate 11. An ulcerated basal cell carcinoma with rolled borders on the posterior ear. See Figure 8-9, p. 142. *(From Abeloff MD, Armitage JO, Niederhuber JE, Kastan MB, McKenna WG: Abeloff's clinical oncology, 4th ed. Philadelphia: Churchill Livingstone, 2008, Fig. 74-2.)*

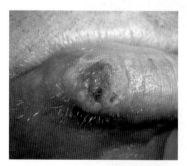

Plate 12. Squamous cell carcinoma on the lower lip. See Figure 8-10, p. 142. *(From Rakel D, Rakel RE: Textbook of family medicine, 8th ed. Philadelphia: Saunders, 2011, Fig. 33-85. Copyright Richard P. Usatine.)*

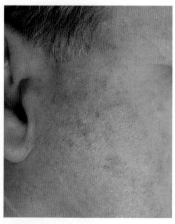

Plate 13. Multiple actinic keratoses visible as thin, red, scaly lesions. See Figure 8-11, p. 143. *(From Goldberg D: Procedures in cosmetic dermatology—Lasers and lights: Vol. 1, 2nd ed. Philadelphia: Saunders, 2008, Fig. 5.2.)*

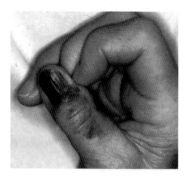

Plate 14. Nailbed melanoma. See Figure 8-12, p. 143. (*From Dartmouth University and Dermnet Weekly Clinic, July 30, 2001.*)

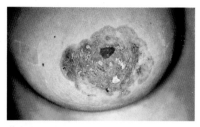

Plate 15. Paget disease of the nipple. Note the erythematous plaques around the nipple. See Figure 8-13, p. 143. (*From Bolognia JL, Jorizzo JL, Rapini RP: Dermatology, 1st ed. Edinburgh: Mosby, 2003, Fig. 53.8.*)

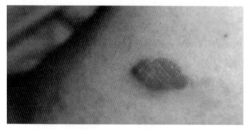

Plate 16. Kaposi sarcoma. See Figure 8-14, p. 144. (*From Hoffman: Hematology: Basic Principles and Practice, 5th ed. Philadelphia: Churchill Livingstone, 2008, Fig. 121-35.*)

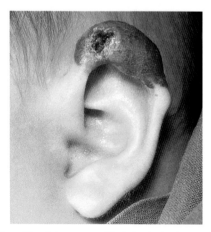

Plate 17. Infantile hemangioma. These lesions grow rapidly during the first few months of life once they appear (20% at birth), but they are asymptomatic unless they bleed, become infected, or obstruct a vital structure. Complete resolution is typical before the age of 7 years, and no treatment is usually required. See Figure 8-15, p. 145. (*From du Vivier A: Atlas of clinical dermatology, 3rd ed. New York: Churchill Livingstone, 2002, Fig. 8.28, with permission.*)

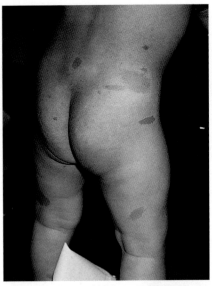

Plate 18. Multiple café-au-lait macules on a child with neurofibromatosis type 1. See Figure 8-16, p. 145. (*From Eichenfield LF Frieden IJ, Esterly NB: Neonatal dermatology, 2nd ed. Philadelphia: Saunders, 2007, Fig. 22-2.*)

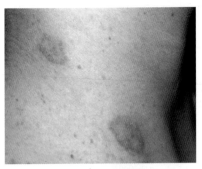

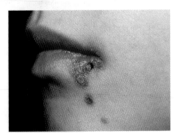

Plate 20. Impetigo. Multiple crusted and oozing lesions. See Figure 8-19, p. 147. (*From: Kliegman RM: Nelson textbook of pediatrics, 19th ed. Philadelphia: Saunders, 2011, Fig. 657-1.*)

Plate 19. Tinea corporis. Red ring-shaped lesions with scaling and some central clearing. See Figure 8-18, p. 146. (*From Kliegman RM: Nelson textbook of pediatrics, 19th ed. Philadelphia: Saunders, 2011, Fig. 658-8.*)

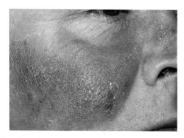

Plate 21. Sharply defined erythema and edema characteristic of erysipelas. See Figure 8-20, p. 147. (*From Zaoutis LB, Chiang VW: Comprehensive pediatric hospital medicine, 1st ed. Philadelphia: Mosby, 2007, Fig. 156-2.*)

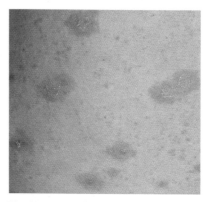

Plate 22. Pityriasis rosea. Both small oval plaques and multiple small papules are present. See Figure 8-21, p. 150. (*From Habif TP: Clinical dermatology, 5th ed. Philadelphia: Mosby, 2009, Fig. 8-44.*)

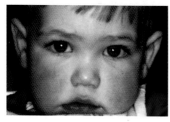

Plate 23. Slapped cheek appearance of erythema infectiosum. See Figure 8-22, p. 151. (*From Baren JM, Rothrock SG, Brennan J, Brown L: Pediatric emergency medicine, 1st ed. Philadelphia: Saunders, 2007, Fig. 123-5.*)

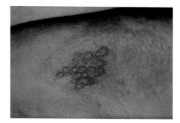

Plate 24. Herpes zoster. Grouped vesicopustules on an erythematous base. See Figure 8-23, p. 151. (*From Marx J, Hockberger R, Walls R. Rosen's emergency medicine: concepts and clinical practice, 7th ed. Philadelphia: Mosby, 2009, Fig. 118-28. Courtesy of David Effron, MD*).

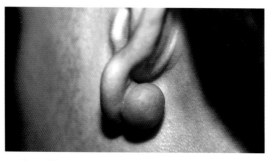

Plate 25. Keloid scar on the ear lobe after piercing. See Figure 8-24, p. 152. (*From Kliegman RM: Nelson textbook of pediatrics, 19th ed. Philadelphia: Saunders, 2011, Fig. 651-1.*)

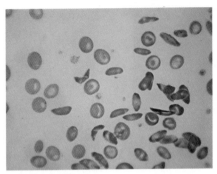

Plate 26. Sickle cells show a sickle or crescent shape resulting from polymerization of hemoglobin S. This smear also shows target cells and boat-shaped cells with a lesser degree of polymerization of hemoglobin S than in a classic sickle cell. See Figure 13-1, p. 216. *(From Goldman L, Schafer AI: Goldman's Cecil medicine, 24th ed. Philadelphia: Saunders, 2011, Fig. 160-7).*

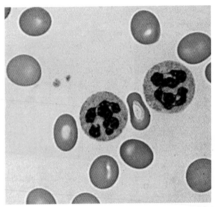

Plate 27. Megaloblastic changes of macrocytosis and a hypersegmented neutrophil. See Figure 13-2, p. 216. *(From Goldman L, Schafer AI: Goldman's Cecil medicine, 24th ed. Philadelphia: Saunders, 2011, Fig. 170-6).*

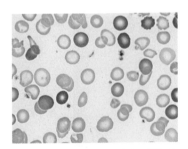

Plate 28. Iron-deficiency anemia. Pale red blood cells with an enlarged central area of pallor. See Figure 13-3, p. 217. *(From McPherson R, Pincus M: Henry's clinical diagnosis and management by laboratory methods, 21st ed. Philadelphia: Saunders, 2006, Fig. 31-2.)*

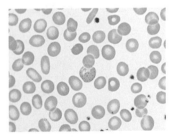

Plate 29. Basophilic stippling. Irregular basophilic granules in red blood cells; often associated with lead poisoning and thalassemia. See Figure 13-4, p. 217. *(From McPherson R, Pincus M: Henry's clinical diagnosis and management by laboratory methods, 21st ed. Philadelphia: Saunders, 2006, Fig. 29-23.)*

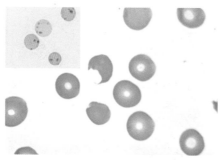

Plate 30. Bite cells with Heinz bodies. See Figure 13-5, p. 217. (Courtesy of Dr. Robert W. McKenna, Department of Pathology, University of Texas Southwestern Medical School, Dallas, TX.).

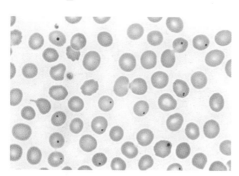

Plate 31. Howell-Jolly bodies in peripheral blood erythrocytes. These nuclear remnants indicate a lack of splenic filtrative function. See Figure 13-6, p. 218. (*From Orkin SH, et al.: Nathan and Oski's hematology of infancy and childhood, 7th ed. Philadelphia: Saunders, 2009, Fig. 14-4.*)

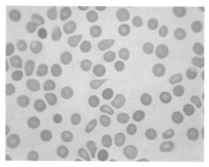

Plate 32. Teardrop red blood cells, usually seen in myelofibrosis. See Figure 13-7, p. 218. (*From Goldman L, Ausiello D: Cecil Medicine, 23rd ed. Philadelphia: Saunders, 2008, Fig. 161-13.*)

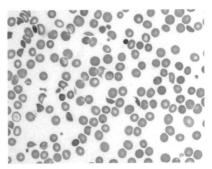

Plate 33. Schistocytes and helmet cells. Red blood cell fragments seen in microangiopathic hemolytic anemia and disseminated intravascular coagulation. See Figure 13-8, p. 218. *(From McPherson R, Pincus M: Henry's clinical diagnosis and management by laboratory methods, 21st ed. Philadelphia: Saunders, 2006, Fig. 29-19.)*

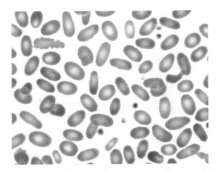

Plate 34. Hereditary elliptocytosis. A blood film reveals characteristic elliptical red blood cells. See Figure 13-9, p. 219. *(From McPherson R, Pincus M: Henry's clinical diagnosis and management by laboratory methods, 22nd ed. Philadelphia: Saunders, 2011, Fig. 30-16.)*

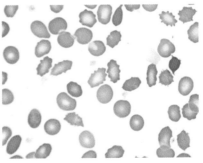

Plate 35. Acanthocytes. Irregularly spiculated red blood cells, frequently seen in abetalipoproteinemia or liver disease. See Figure 13-10, p. 219. *(From McPherson R, Pincus M: Henry's clinical diagnosis and management by laboratory methods, 21st ed. Philadelphia: Saunders, 2006, Fig. 29-20.)*

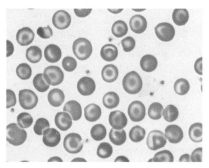

Plate 36. Target cells are frequently seen in hemoglobin C disease and liver disease. See Figure 13-11, p. 219. (*From McPherson R, Pincus M: Henry's clinical diagnosis and management by laboratory methods, 21st ed. Philadelphia: Saunders, 2006, Fig. 29-18.*)

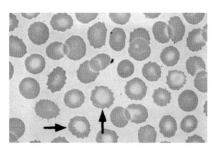

Plate 37. Echinocytes, or burr cells (*arrows*), are the hallmark of uremia. See Figure 13-12, p. 220. (*From Hoffman R, et al.: Hematology: basic principles and practice, 5th ed. Philadelphia: Churchill Livingstone, 2008, Fig. 156-1.*)

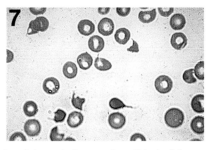

Plate 38. Microangiopathic hemolytic anemia demonstrating red blood cell fragments, anisocytosis, polychromasia, and decreased platelets. See Figure 13-13, p. 220. (*From Tschudy MM, Arcara KM: The Harriet Lane handbook, 19th ed. Philadelphia: Mosby, 2011, Plate 7.*)

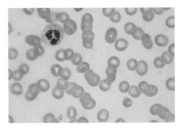

Plate 39. Rouleaux formation of stacked red blood cells seen in multiple myeloma. See Figure 13-14, p. 220. *(From Goldman L, Ausiello D: Cecil medicine, 23rd ed. Philadelphia: Saunders, 2008, Fig. 161-19.)*

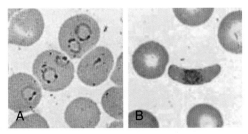

Plate 40. Malaria. Peripheral blood film examples of various stages of *Plasmodium falciparum.* **A,** Small ring forms. **B,** A crescentic gametocyte with centrally placed chromatin. See Figure 13-15, p. 221. *(From Hoffman R, et al.: Hematology: basic principles and practice, 5th ed. Philadelphia: Churchill Livingstone, 2008, Fig. 159-5).*

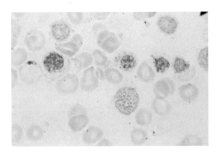

Plate 41. Ringed sideroblasts seen in sideroblastic anemia. See Figure 13-16, p. 221. *(From Goldman L, Ausiello D: Cecil medicine, 23rd ed. Philadelphia: Saunders, 2008, Fig. 163-5.)*

GENERAL PRINCIPLES

CHAPTER 1

NORMAL DEVELOPMENT

INFANCY/CHILDHOOD

1. Give the average ages at which the following commonly tested milestones are achieved.

MILESTONE	AGE*
Social smile	1-2 mo
Cooing	2-4 mo
While prone, lifts head up 90°	3-4 mo
Rolls front to back	4-5 mo
Voluntary grasp (no release)	5 mo
Stranger anxiety	6-9 mo
Sits with no support	7 mo
Pulls to stand	9 mo
Waves "bye-bye"	10 mo
Voluntary grasp with voluntary release	10 mo
Plays pat-a-cake	9-10 mo
First words	9-12 mo
Imitates others' sounds	9-12 mo
Separation anxiety	12-15 mo
Walks without help	13 mo
Can build tower of 2 cubes	13-15 mo
Understands 1-step commands (no gesture)	15 mo
Good use of cup and spoon	15-18 mo
Can build tower of 6 cubes	2 yr
Runs well	2 yr
Ties shoelaces	5 yr

*Reduce the age of premature infants in the first 2 years for assessing development. For example, for children born after 6 months of gestation, subtract 3 months from their chronologic age. Therefore they should be expected to perform only at the 6-month-old level when they are 9 months old.

2. True or false: The overall pattern of development is more important than the age at which individual milestones are reached.
True. The exact age is not as important as the overall pattern in looking for dysfunctional development. When in doubt, use a formal developmental test.

3. What screening and preventive care measures should be performed at every pediatric visit?
Height, weight, blood pressure, developmental/behavioral assessment, and anticipatory guidance (counseling/discussion about age-appropriate concerns) should be part of every pediatric visit.

4. **True or false: Screening and preventive care are important mainly during a well check-up.**
False. Screening and preventive care are an important part of every encounter with a patient (adult or child). USMLE questions may try to fool you on this point. For example, a mother complains that her 4-year-old child sleeps 11 hours every night. This is normal behavior. The answer to the question, "What should you do next?" may be to give an objective hearing examination, which is a routine screening procedure in a 4-year-old child.

5. **What items are frequently tested under the umbrella of primary prevention using anticipatory guidance?**
Parents should be told the following:
- Keep the water heater at less than 120° F (48.9° C).
- Use proper car restraints (e.g., child safety seat, booster seat).
- Put the infant to sleep on his or her side or back to help prevent sudden infant death syndrome (SIDS), the most common cause of death in children aged 1 to 12 months.
- Do not use infant walkers because they cause injuries.
- Watch out for small objects, which may be aspirated.
- Do not give honey before 1 year of age.
- Do not give cow's milk before 1 year of age.
- Introduce solid foods gradually, starting at 6 months.
- Supervise children in bathtubs and swimming pools.

6. **How often should height, weight, and head circumference be measured? What do they signify?**
Head circumference should be measured at every visit in the first 2 years; height and weight should be measured routinely until adulthood. All three parameters are markers of general well-being; abnormal values may suggest disease.

7. **What if a child has low height, weight, or head circumference compared with peers?**
The pattern of growth along growth curves plotted over time (which you may be asked to interpret) tells more than any single measurement. If a child has always been low or high compared with peers, the pattern is generally benign. A patient who goes from a normal to an abnormal curve is much more worrisome. Parents commonly bring in a child with delayed physical growth or delayed puberty. You need to know when to reassure and when to do further testing and questioning.

8. **Define failure to thrive. What causes it?**
There is no consensus on the definition of failure to thrive, but commonly used definitions include a head circumference, height, or weight less than the 5th percentile for age; a weight less than 80% of the ideal weight for age; or a weight loss that causes a decrease by two or more major percentage lines on the growth curve. Failure to thrive is most commonly due to psychosocial or functional problems. Vigilance is required for signs of neglect and child abuse. Organic causes usually have specific clues to trigger your suspicion.

9. **What conditions are suggested by obesity in children?**
Obesity is usually is due to overeating and too little activity (>95% of cases). Fewer than 5% of cases are due to organic causes (e.g., Cushing syndrome, Prader-Willi syndrome).

10. **What conditions should you consider in a child with an abnormal head circumference?**
Increased head circumference may suggest hydrocephalus or tumor, whereas decreased head circumference may suggest microcephaly (e.g., from congenital TORCH* infection). Again, the pattern of head circumference over time (plotted on a growth curve) is most helpful in defining pathology.

11. **How are hearing and vision screened?**
Hearing and vision should be measured objectively at least once by 4 years of age. After the initial screen, these parameters should be measured every few years until adulthood or more often if the history so dictates.

---

*TORCH, *Toxoplasmosis*, other, rubella, cytomegalovirus, and hepatitis infections.

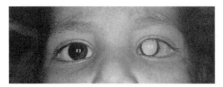

Figure 1-1. Leukocoria (white pupillary reflex) is the most common presenting feature of retinoblastoma and may be first noticed in family photographs. See Plate 1. *(Courtesy of U. Raina.)*

12. **What is the red reflex? What should an abnormal reflex suggest?**
    Loss of the red reflex should be checked at birth and routinely thereafter to detect congenital cataracts or ocular tumors. On shining a penlight at the pupil, red is usually seen because of the underlying fundus. If a cataract (or tumor) is present in the eye, the red reflex disappears and white is observed (known as *leukocoria* and classically caused by retinoblastoma; Fig. 1-1).

13. **True or false: Intermittent strabismus is normal before a certain age.**
    True. It is normal for infants to have occasional ocular misalignment (strabismus) until 3 months of age. After 3 months (or with constant eye deviation), strabismus should be evaluated and managed by an ophthalmologist to prevent possible blindness in the affected eye.

14. **How is screening for anemia performed?**
    Recommendations for routine screening for anemia (with a complete blood count or hemoglobin/hematocrit) vary and are changing. Hemoglobin or hematocrit measurement is recommended at 12 months of age but may be required at other times as dictated by history and risk assessment. Recommendations for screening during adolescence vary, but adolescents should be screened at least once. If any risk factors for iron deficiency are present during infancy (prematurity, low birth weight, ingestion of cow's milk before 1 year of age, low dietary intake, low socioeconomic status), screen with a complete blood count or hemoglobin and hematocrit if given the option.

15. **True or false: All children should be given prophylactic iron supplements.**
    False. Exclusively breastfed infants do not require supplementation. All other children should receive supplementation via fortified formula, cereal, or an iron supplement. Start supplementation in full-term infants at 4 to 6 months of age and in preterm infants at 2 months of age. Most infant formulas and cereals contain iron, so separate supplements are usually not required.

16. **How and when do you screen for lead exposure?**
    Screening for lead toxicity is controversial. Routine screening is no longer recommended. However, all Medicaid-eligible children must be screened. Consider screening high-risk children (those who live in old buildings, have a sibling or playmate with lead toxicity, eat paint chips, live near a battery recycling plant, or have a parent who works at a battery recycling plant). Screen for lead exposure by measuring the serum lead level. If the initial lead level is abnormally high, closer follow-up and intervention are needed. The best first step is to stop the exposure.

17. **True or false: Most children need fluoride supplementation.**
    False. Because most water is fluoridated, supplementation is not needed. However, if a child lives in an area where the water is inadequately fluoridated (rare) or the child is fed exclusively from premixed, ready-to-eat formulas (which use nonfluoridated water), fluoride supplements should be given.

18. **True or false: Breastfed infants are more likely to require vitamin D supplements than formula-fed infants.**
    True. The American Academy of Pediatrics recommends that exclusively and partially breastfed infants receive vitamin D supplements shortly after birth and continue until they are weaned and consume formula or whole milk. Formula-fed infants do not require supplements in the United States because all formulas contain vitamin D supplements.

19. **When should children be screened for tuberculosis?**
    Universal screening for tuberculosis is not recommended. There is no need to screen children who have no risk factors. Risk assessment should occur regularly until 2 years of age and then annually. Test those at high risk (family member with tuberculosis, family member with a positive tuberculosis test, a child born in a high-risk country, a child who has traveled to a high-risk country, or a child who has consumed unpasteurized milk or cheese).

20. **True or false: Screening children for renal disease via urinalysis is not recommended.**
    True. However, screening is required for congenital/anatomic abnormalities (e.g., vesico-ureteral reflux) after a febrile urinary tract infection in children 2 months to 2 years of age, which should involve an ultrasound scan and either a voiding cystourethrogram (VCUG) or a radionuclide cystogram (RNC). Screening after the age of 2 years is more controversial and likely will not be asked in the USMLE.

21. **True or false: Current vaccine recommendations and schedules are always provided in the USMLE.**
    False. However, because the timing of normal immunizations is constantly being updated, the administration schedule for common vaccines may be provided in the Step 3 exam. Higher-yield information relates to special patient populations (e.g., give pneumococcal vaccine to patients with sickle cell disease or splenectomy) and vaccine contraindications (no measles-mumps-rubella or influenza vaccines for egg-allergic patients, no live vaccines for immuno-compromised patients). Live vaccines include measles-mumps-rubella, varicella-zoster, and the intranasal influenza vaccine (the intramuscular formulation is inactivated).

22. **When should you recommend that a child see a dentist for the first time?**
    Around 2 to 3 years of age.

23. **When does the anterior fontanelle usually close? What disorder should you suspect if it fails to close?**
    The anterior fontanelle usually is closed by 18 months of age. Delayed closure or an unusually large anterior fontanelle may indicate hypothyroidism, hydrocephalus, rickets, or intrauterine growth retardation.

24. **True or false: Milky-white and possibly blood-tinged vaginal discharge is usually abnormal in the first week of life for a female newborn.**
    False. This discharge is usually physiologic and due to maternal hormone withdrawal.

25. **True or false: Children have the same range of normal vital signs as adults do.**
    False. Children have lower blood pressure and higher heart and respiratory rates than adults. In addition, children often have different laboratory values. For example, a child's hemoglobin/hematocrit value is normally higher at birth and lower throughout childhood compared with that of an adult. Normal laboratory value ranges should be provided in the USMLE. In addition, the renal, pulmonary, hepatic, and central nervous systems (CNS) are not fully mature or functional at birth.

26. **When should the Moro reflex and palmar grasp reflex disappear?**
    By 6 months of age.

27. **True or false: A diagnosis of encopresis or enuresis cannot be made before a certain age.**
    True. Encopresis is normal until age 4 years and enuresis is normal until age 5 years. This diagnostic point is obviously important when the parent complains, because both are normal findings in a 3-year-old child. Physical problems (e.g., Hirschsprung disease, urinary tract infection) should be ruled out and then treatment should involve behavioral therapy ("gold star for being good" charts, alarms, biofeedback). Desmopressin and imipramine may be used for refractory cases of enuresis.

ADOLESCENCE

1. **What are the Tanner stages? When do they occur?**
   The Tanner stages measure the stages of puberty. Stage 1 is preadolescence and stage 5 is adulthood. Advancing stages are assigned for testicular and penile growth in boys and breast

growth in girls. Both male and female stages also apply pubic hair development as a criterion. The average age of puberty (when a patient first has changes from preadolescent stage 1) is 10.5 years in girls and 11.5 years in boys. The classic first events of puberty are testicular enlargement in boys and breast development in girls.

2. **Define precocious puberty and pseudoprecocious puberty.**
   True precocious puberty is defined as activation of the hypothalamic-pituitary axis with sexual maturation before the age of 8 years in females and before the age of 9 years in males. In **pseudoprecocious puberty**, secondary sex characteristics develop prematurely because of high circulating levels of androgen or estrogen.

3. **How does precocious puberty differ from pseudoprecocious puberty?**
   A general rule of thumb is that true precocious puberty causes testicular or ovarian enlargement, which does not occur with pseudoprecocious puberty (ovarian cysts are not considered true ovarian enlargement). All patients with suspected precocious puberty should have a gonadotropin-releasing hormone (GnRH) stimulation test. If a dose of GnRH produces the typical pubertal response of increased follicle-stimulating hormone (FSH) and luteinizing hormone (LH), true precocious puberty is diagnosed. Magnetic resonance imaging (MRI) of the brain should be performed to rule out CNS disease (e.g., hamartomas, tumors, cysts, trauma) as the cause.

4. **What causes pseudoprecocious puberty?**
   Pseudoprecocious puberty may be caused by exogenous hormones, adrenal tumors, congenital adrenal hyperplasia (e.g., 21-hydroxylase deficiency), hormone-secreting tumors, or **McCune-Albright syndrome** in females (ovarian cysts, pseudoprecocious puberty, polyostotic fibrous dysplasia of bone, and café au lait spots).

5. **What causes precocious puberty?**
   Precocious puberty is usually idiopathic but may be caused by **McCune-Albright syndrome** (in girls), ovarian tumors (granulosa, theca cell, or gonadoblastoma), testicular tumors (Leydig cell tumors), CNS disease or trauma, adrenal neoplasm, or congenital adrenal hyperplasia. Congenital adrenal hyperplasia presents in boys as precocious puberty or salt-wasting crisis. In girls it presents at birth as ambiguous genitalia. It is due to 21-hydroxylase deficiency more than 95% of the time.

6. **True or false: If the underlying cause for precocious puberty is uncorrectable or idiopathic after diagnostic workup, patients should receive treatment.**
   True. Most patients are given long-acting GnRH agonists to suppress the progression of puberty. This approach helps to prevent premature epiphyseal closure with short stature.

7. **How is precocious puberty treated?**
   Because premature puberty causes premature fusion of growth plates in bone and can cause serious social problems for affected children, treatment is indicated. Treatment of any underlying disorders is indicated for pseudoprecocious puberty. For true idiopathic precocious puberty, treatment with long-acting GnRH agonists is indicated to suppress the pituitary-hypothalamic axis and to delay the onset of puberty until an appropriate age.

8. **Define delayed puberty. What is the most common cause?**
   Delayed puberty is defined as a lack of testicular enlargement in boys by age 14 years or a lack of breast development or pubic hair in girls by age 12 years. The most common cause is **constitutional delay**, a normal variant. Watch for parents with a similar history of being "late bloomers." The child's growth curve consistently lags behind that of peers, but the line representing the child's growth curve is parallel to the normal growth curve. Treatment is reassurance only.

9. **What are other causes of delayed puberty?**
   Rarely, delayed puberty is due to primary testicular failure (Klinefelter syndrome, cryptorchidism, history of chemotherapy, gonadal dysgenesis) or ovarian failure (Turner syndrome, gonadal dysgenesis). Even more rarely, delayed puberty is caused by a hypothalamic or pituitary defect, such as Kallmann syndrome or tumor.

10. **What are the three leading causes of death in adolescents?**
    Accidents, homicide, and suicide together cause about 75% of teenage deaths.

ADULTHOOD

1. Cover the right-hand column in the following table and give the indications for each of the vaccines in adults.

VACCINE	ADULTS WHO SHOULD RECEIVE THE VACCINE AND OTHER INFORMATION
Hepatitis B	Persons at increased risk of hepatitis B virus infection (children are vaccinated as well)
Influenza	Anyone who wants to reduce the chances of getting the flu can get vaccinated. Vaccination is recommended for people at high risk of having serious flu complications or those who live with or care for people at high risk of serious complications. People who should get vaccinated each year are children aged 6 mo to 18 yr, women who will be pregnant during the flu season, individuals who are immunosuppressed, adults aged ≥50 yr, people with chronic medical conditions (pulmonary, cardiovascular, renal, hepatic, hematologic, or metabolic disorders including diabetes), people who live in nursing homes and other long-term care facilities, health care personnel, household contacts and caregivers of children <5 yr and adults ≥50 yr, and household contacts and caregivers for those at high risk of serious flu complications.
Pneumococcus	All adults ≥65 yr; people aged 2 to 64 yr with chronic cardiovascular disease, chronic pulmonary disease, chronic liver disease or diabetes mellitus; people aged ≥2 yr with functional or anatomic asplenia; people aged ≥2 yr living in environments in which the risk of disease is high; and immunocompromised persons ≥2 yr at high risk of infection.
Rubella	All women of child-bearing age who lack immunity or history of immunization. Do not give to pregnant women. Women should avoid pregnancy for 4 wk after receiving the vaccine. Also give to health-care workers (to protect the unborn children of pregnant women). Give to susceptible adolescents and adults without evidence of rubella immunity. Do not give to immunocompromised patients (except HIV-positive patients).
Tetanus	All people should be given a tetanus booster every 10 yr. Give tetanus prophylaxis for any wound if vaccination history is unknown or the patient has received less than 3 doses in total. Give a tetanus booster in people with full vaccination history if more than 5 years have passed since the last dose for all wounds other than clean, minor wounds (including burns). Give tetanus immunoglobulin with vaccine for patients with unknown/incomplete vaccination and unclean or major wounds. Adults (aged ≥11 yr) should receive a single dose of Tdap to replace a single dose of Td if they received their last dose of Td 10 or more years earlier (this is a new recommendation from the CDC in June 2012 that now includes adults ≥65 yr). Adults who have or anticipate having close contact with an infant younger than 12 mo should receive a single dose of Tdap. Health care workers should receive Tdap. Tdap is preferred to Td if prophylaxis is indicated for a wound. It is now recommended that Tdap be given to women with every pregnancy regardless of their prior immunization history, preferably in the late 2nd or the 3rd trimester (recommended by the CDC in October 2012).

CDC, Centers for Disease Control.

2. Cover all but the left-hand column in the following table and give the appropriate screening recommendations. Although other guidelines for cancer screening are in clinical use, the recommendations of the American Cancer Society are a good guideline to use for the USMLE.

CANCER	PROCEDURE	AGE	FREQUENCY
Colorectal	Colonoscopy or	>50 yr for all studies; if there is a family history of colorectal cancer, perform colonoscopy beginning 10 yr younger than the age at which the relative was diagnosed	Every 10 yr
	Flexible sigmoidoscopy or		Every 5 yr
	Double contrast barium enema or		Every 5 yr
	CT colonography or		Every 5 yr
	Fecal occult blood test or		Annually
	Fecal immunochemical test or		Annually
	Stool DNA test		Interval uncertain
Colon, prostate	Digital rectal exam	>40 yr	Annually
Prostate	Prostate-specific antigen test	>50 yr	Controversial and now generally not recommended, but should be discussed with patient
Cervical	Pap smear	Begin at age 21 yr regardless of sexual activity	If conventional Pap test is used, test annually, then every 2-3 yr for women ≥30 yr who have had three negative cytology test results; if Pap and HPV tests are used, test every 3 yr if both HPV and cytology results are negative
Gynecologic	Pelvic exam	Controversial with different recommendations from different societies. Unlikely to be tested on the USMLE	Annually; every 2-3 yr after 3 normal exams
		≥65 yr	Annually; when to stop is not clearly established

Continued

CANCER	PROCEDURE	AGE	FREQUENCY
Endometrial	Endometrial biopsy	Menopause	No recommendation for routine screening in the absence of symptoms
Breast	Breast self-examination	>20 yr	Benefits and limitations should be discussed, but breast self-examination is no longer recommended by the American Cancer Society
Breast	Physical exam by doctor	20-40 yr	Every 3 yr
		>40 yr	Annually
Breast	Mammography	>40 yr	Annually
Lung	Sputum, chest x-ray		Testing is not recommended for asymptomatic individuals, even if they are at high risk
	CT scan		Annual CT scan has been controversial, but in Dec. 2013 the USPSTF recommended an annual low-dose CT scan for asymptomatic adults aged 55-80 yr who have a 30 pack-year smoking history and currently smoke or have quit smoking within the past 15 yr; discontinue screening when the patient has not smoked for 15 yr

CT, Computed tomography; HPV, human papilloma virus; USPSTF, United States Preventive Services Task Force.

This table is for the screening of asymptomatic, healthy patients. Other guidelines exist, but these recommendations will serve well for the USMLE.

3. **True or false: Tumor markers are generally not used for cancer screening.**
   True. Prostate-specific antigen is the exception to this rule. Alpha-fetoprotein (liver and testicular cancer), carcinoembryonic antigen (CEA), CA-125, and other serum markers are not appropriate for screening the general population. However, abnormal laboratory values in questions can provide a clue to diagnosis.

4. **True or false: Urinalysis should not be used to screen the general population for bladder cancer.**
   True. Screening with urinalysis for urinary tract cancer (which causes hematuria) is not recommended. However, persistent, painless hematuria can provide a clue that urinary tract cancer may be present.

5. **What specific problems are caused by obesity?**
   Obesity causes an increase in overall mortality (at any age) and increases the risk of insulin resistance and diabetes, hypertension, hypertriglyceridemia, coronary artery disease, gallstones, sleep apnea and hypoventilation, osteoarthritis, thromboembolism, varicose veins, and cancer (especially endometrial cancer).

SENESCENCE

1. **What age group constitutes the most rapidly growing segment of the population?**
   Persons older than 85 years.

2. **True or false: An 80-year-old person needs more calories than a 30-year-old person.**
   False. An 80-year-old person has half the lean body mass of a 30-year-old person and thus needs fewer calories. The basal metabolic rate is based on lean body mass. Older patients, however, need more sodium, vitamin B_{12}, vitamin D (and/or calcium), folate, and nonheme iron than younger patients do.

3. **True or false: Hearing and vision changes are a normal part of aging.**
   True. **Presbyopia** (hardening of the lens that decreases the ability to accommodate) becomes almost universal after the age of 50 years, so there is a common need for reading glasses after this age. **Presbyacusis,** the loss of ability to discriminate sounds, is also part of the normal process of aging.

4. **True or false: Brain atrophy is a normal part of aging.**
   True. Decreased brain weight, enlarged ventricles and sulci, and a slightly decreased ability to learn new material are normal parts of aging.

5. **Describe the normal changes in male sexual function that occur with aging.**
   - Increased refractory period (after ejaculation, it takes longer before another erection is possible)
   - Increased amount of time to achieve an erection
   - Delayed ejaculation (an older man may ejaculate only 1 of every 3 times that he has sex)

6. **Describe the normal changes in female sexual function that occur with aging.**
   - Decreased vaginal lubrication (women not on hormone replacement therapy may use estrogen cream or water-soluble lubricants)
   - Dyspareunia due to atrophy of clitoral, labial, and vaginal tissues (treated with estrogen cream)
   - Delayed orgasm

7. **True or false: Impotence and lack of sexual desire are normal in older people.**
   False. Impotence in men and a lack of sexual desire in either sex are not normal and should be investigated. Causes include psychiatric disorders (e.g., depression) as well as physical causes, such as medications (selective serotonin reuptake inhibitors and antihypertensives are notorious culprits), vascular disease (watch for atherosclerosis risk factors), and neurologic disease (especially in diabetics).

8. **Describe the normal changes in sleep habits in older people.**
   Older persons require less sleep, sleep less deeply, wake up more frequently during the night, and awaken earlier in the morning. It also takes longer for older persons to fall asleep (longer sleep latency) and they have less stage 3 and 4 and rapid eye movement sleep.

9. **Define pseudodementia. How do you recognize it in the Step 3 exam?**
   Depression in older individuals can resemble dementia. Look for a history that would trigger depression (e.g., loss of a spouse, terminal or debilitating disease) and other symptoms of depression (e.g., frequent crying, suicidal thoughts).

10. **True or false: Almost 50% of patients over the age of 65 suffer from some type of dementia.**
    False. Roughly 15% of people over the age of 65 suffer from dementia. The most common types of dementia are Alzheimer dementia, dementia with Lewy bodies, vascular dementia, Parkinson dementia, and frontotemporal dementia. Other disorders that can cause dementia include HIV and Pick disease (a subtype of frontotemporal dementia). Test for reversible causes of dementia such as hypothyroidism, depression, and vitamin B_{12} deficiency.

11. **What else do you need to know about dementia?**
    The various types of dementia are discussed in detail in Chapter 2.

12. **What is the best prophylaxis for pressure ulcers in an immobilized patient?**
    Frequent turning and the use of special air mattresses.

MEDICAL ETHICS AND JURISPRUDENCE

CONSENT AND INFORMED CONSENT TO TREATMENT

1. **What are the components of informed consent?**
   Informed consent involves giving the patient information about the following:
   - Diagnosis (his or her condition and what it means)
   - Prognosis (the natural course of the condition without treatment)
   - Proposed treatment (description of the procedure and what the patient will experience)
   - Risks and benefits of the treatment
   - Alternative treatments

   The patient then must be allowed to make his or her own choice. The consent forms that patients are asked to sign are not technically required or sufficient for informed consent. They are used for medicolegal purposes (i.e., lawsuit paranoia).

2. **What should you do if a patient is in critical condition or in a coma and has made no advance directive or living will?**
   The wishes of the family, next of kin, or healthcare power of attorney should be followed. In cases of disagreement among family members, suspicion of ulterior motives, or uncertainty, the ethics committee of the hospital should be involved. As a last resort, the courts can provide help.

3. **True or false: A living will should not be respected if the next of kin asks you not to follow it.**
   False. Such situations are tricky, but technically (and for the USMLE) living wills or patient-mandated "do not resuscitate" orders should be respected and followed if properly documented. The classic boards question involves a patient who says in a living will that if he or she is unable to breathe independently, a ventilator should not be used. Do not put the patient on a ventilator, even if the husband, wife, son, or daughter tells you to do so.

4. **What should you do if a patient is incompetent to make decisions?**
   The family and/or courts should be asked to appoint a guardian (surrogate decision maker or healthcare power of attorney).

5. **What should you do if a child has a medical emergency and the parents are unavailable for decision making?**
   Treat the child as you see fit; that is, act in the child's best interest.

6. **What should you do if a patient requires emergency care but the patient cannot communicate and no family members are available?**
   Treat the patient as you see fit unless you know that the patient wishes otherwise.

7. **What should you do if a child has a life-threatening condition and the parents refuse a simple, curative treatment (e.g., antibiotics for meningitis)?**
   First try to persuade the parents to change their mind; if this fails, attempt to get a court order to give the treatment. Do not treat until you have talked to the courts unless it is an emergency. Even for Jehovah's Witnesses who do not want their children to receive a blood transfusion, the court's assistance should be sought in getting the transfusion if it is the only treatment option available.

8. **True or false: Adult patients of sound mind are allowed to refuse life-saving treatments.**
   True. You should not force blood products, antibiotics, or any other treatments on a patient who does not want them.

9. **What about depression in the context of end-of-life decisions?**
   Depression should always be evaluated as a reason for "incompetence." Patients who are suicidal may refuse all treatment, but their refusal should not be respected until the depression is treated.

10. **True or false: In some circumstances, patients can be hospitalized against their will.**
    True. Psychiatric patients are frequently hospitalized against their will if they are deemed to be a danger to themselves or others. For example, in California a patient can be held only for a limited time (a section 5150 order is an involuntary 72-hour hold) before a hearing before a court official is required to determine whether a patient must remain in custody (a section 5250 order is an involuntary 14-day hold but a hearing must be held to determine if it is justified).

These decisions are based on the principle of **beneficence** (the principle of doing good for the patient and avoiding harm).

11. **True or false: Restraints can be used on patients against their will.**
True. Restraints can be used on an incompetent or violent (e.g., delirious, psychotic) patient if needed, but their use should be brief and reevaluated often (at least once every 24 hours). Be aware that the use of restraints in delirious or demented patients rarely helps to prevent falls and may cause injury.

12. **When do patients under the age of 18 years not require parental consent for a medical decision?**
In general, individuals under the age of 18 years do not require parental consent if they are emancipated (married, living on their own and financially independent, raising children, or serving in the armed forces); have a sexually transmitted disease, want contraception, or are pregnant; want illicit drug treatment or counseling; or have a psychiatric illness. Some states have exceptions to these rules, but for Step 3 purposes, in such situations minors should be allowed to make their own decisions.

PHYSICIAN–PATIENT RELATIONSHIP

1. **With whom can you discuss your patient's condition?**
Only with people who need to know because they are directly involved in the patient's care and with people authorized by the patient (e.g., authorized family members). Do not tell a medical colleague who is uninvolved with the patient's care how that patient is doing, even if the colleague is a friend of yours or of the patient.

2. **In what situations are you allowed to breach patient confidentiality?**
Break confidentiality only in the following situations:
- The patient asks you to do so.
- Child abuse is suspected.
- The courts mandate you to do so.
- You must fulfill the duty to warn or protect (if a patient says that he is going to kill himself or someone else, you have to tell that person, the authorities, or both).
- The patient has a reportable disease.
- The patient is a danger to others (e.g., if a patient is blind or has seizures, let the proper authorities know so that they can revoke the patient's license to drive; if the patient is an airplane pilot and is a paranoid, hallucinating schizophrenic, then the authorities need to know).

3. **True or false: It is acceptable to hide a diagnosis from a patient if the family asks you to do so.**
False. Do not hide a diagnosis from a patient (including a child) if the patient wants to know (even if the family asks you to do so). Do not lie to any patient because the family asks you to do so. Conversely, you should not force patients to receive information against their will; if they do not want to know the diagnosis, do not tell them.

4. **What findings should make you suspect child abuse?**
- Failure to thrive
- Multiple fractures, bruises, or injuries in different stages of healing
- Metaphyseal "bucket handle" or "corner" fractures (Fig. 1-2)
- Shaken baby syndrome (retinal hemorrhages or subdural hematomas with no external signs of trauma)
- Behavioral, emotional, or interactional problems
- Sexually transmitted diseases
- Multiple personality disorder (classically caused by sexual abuse)
- Whenever a parent's story does not fit the child's injury

5. **True or false: You do not need proof to report child abuse.**
True. In fact, reporting any suspicion of child abuse is mandatory. You do not need proof and cannot be sued for reporting a suspicion. The job of the physician is to report suspicion, even if definitive proof is not present; the job of the agency that investigates the report is to determine whether or not abuse occurred and what should be done about it.

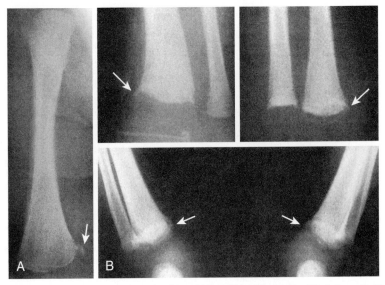

Figure 1-2. Metaphyseal fractures. Radiographs of the right femur (**A**) and both ankles (**B**) of a 2-month-old abused infant demonstrating metaphyseal corner fractures of the distal femur and both distal tibia (*arrows*). The angled tangential view reveals the "bucket handle" appearance of the fracture. (*From Adam A, et al. Grainger & Allison's diagnostic radiology. 5th ed. Edinburgh: Churchill Livingstone, 2008, Fig. 68-24.*)

DEATH AND DYING

1. True or false: People with terminal illnesses can choose to die.
   True. This is the rationale behind hospice care. Let competent people die if they want to do so. Do not commit active euthanasia, but respect a patient's wishes for passive euthanasia.

2. What is the difference between active and passive euthanasia?
   Active euthanasia is the intentional hastening of death, whereas passive euthanasia is withholding treatments and letting nature take its course.

3. True or false: Withdrawing care and withholding care are the same in the eyes of the law.
   True. It is important to communicate this principle to family members who feel guilty. The simple fact that a patient is on a respirator does not mean that you cannot turn the respirator off.

4. True or false: In terminally ill, noncurable patients, one of the primary goals is to relieve pain.
   True. Opioids are commonly used, even though they may cause respiratory depression. It is more important to make patients comfortable and pain free than to worry about respiratory depression in this setting. Of note, although it is illegal to actively euthanize a patient, it is legal and ethical to ensure relief of the terminally ill patient's pain and suffering (e.g., with morphine or sedative agents) even if it causes the patient to die sooner than they otherwise would.

APPLIED BIOSTATISTICS AND CLINICAL EPIDEMIOLOGY

UNDERSTANDING STATISTICAL CONCEPTS

1. How is the sensitivity of a test defined? What are highly sensitive tests used for clinically?
   Sensitivity is defined as the ability of a test to detect disease, and mathematically as the number of true positives divided by the number of people with the disease. Tests with high sensitivity are used for disease screening. False positives occur, but the test does not miss many people with the disease (low false-negative rate). One way to remember this is the word *snout*, written "Sn-N-out," meaning with high **sen**sitivity (Sn) a **n**egative (N) test rules **out** (out) the disease.

2. **How is the specificity of a test defined? What are highly specific tests used for clinically?**
   Specificity is defined as the ability of a test to detect health (or nondisease), and mathematically as the number of true negatives divided by the number of people without the disease. Tests with high specificity are used for disease confirmation. False negatives occur, but the test does not identify anyone who is actually healthy as sick (low false-positive rate). The ideal confirmatory test must have high sensitivity and high specificity; otherwise, people with the disease may be identified as healthy. One way to remember this is the word *spin*, written "Sp-P-in," meaning that with high **sp**ecificity (Sp) a **p**ositive (P) test rules **in** (in) the disease.

3. **Explain the concept of a trade-off between sensitivity and specificity.**
   The trade-off between sensitivity and specificity is a classic statistics question. For example, you should understand how changing the cutoff glucose value in screening for diabetes (or changing the value of any of several screening tests) will change the number of true- and false-negative and true- and false-positive results. If the cutoff glucose value is raised, fewer people will be identified as diabetic (more false negatives, fewer false positives), whereas if the cutoff glucose value is lowered, more people will be identified as diabetic (fewer false negatives, more false positives). As an example, if the diagnostic threshold for a fasting blood sugar for diabetes were raised from ≥125 mg/dL to ≥300 mg/dL, most people with diabetes would be missed (low sensitivity because a patient with blood sugar of 285 mg/dL would be negative for diabetes according to this criterion). In addition, the test would be very specific for patients with blood sugar ≥300 mg/dL (a patient would certainly have diabetes if he had a positive test).

4. **Define positive predictive value (PPV). On what does it depend?**
   When a test is positive for disease, the PPV measures how likely it is that the patient has the disease (probability of having a condition given a positive test). PPV is calculated mathematically by dividing the number of true positives by the total number of people with a positive test. PPV depends on the prevalence of a disease (the higher the prevalence, the higher the PPV) and the sensitivity and specificity of the test (e.g., an overly sensitive test that gives more false positives has a lower PPV).

5. **Define negative predictive value (NPV). On what does it depend?**
   When a test is negative for disease, the NPV measures how likely it is that the patient is healthy and does not have the disease (probability of not having a condition given a negative test). It is calculated mathematically by dividing the number of true negatives by the total number of people with a negative test. NPV also depends on the prevalence of the disease and the sensitivity and specificity of the test (the higher the prevalence, the lower the NPV). In addition, an overly sensitive test with many false positives leads to a higher NPV.

6. **Define attributable risk. How is it measured?**
   Attributable risk is the number of cases of a disease attributable to one risk factor (in other words, the amount by which the incidence of a condition is expected to decrease if the risk factor in question is removed). For example, if the incidence rate of lung cancer is 1:100 in the general population and 10:100 in smokers, the attributable risk for smoking in causing lung cancer is 9:100 (assuming a properly matched control group).

7. **Given the 2 × 2 table in the following table, define the formulas for calculating the test values indicated.**

	DISEASE			TEST NAME	FORMULA
Test or exposure		(+)	(−)	Sensitivity	$A/(A + C)$
	(+)	A	B	Specificity	$D/(B + D)$
				PPV	$A/(A + B)$
	(−)	C	D	NPV	$D/(C + D)$
				Odds ratio	$(A \times D)/(B \times C)$
				Relative risk	$[A/(A + B)]/[C/(C + D)]$
				Attributable risk	$[A/(A + B)]-[C/(C + D)]$

NPV, Negative predictive value; *PPV*, positive predictive value.

8. **Define relative risk. From what type of studies can it be calculated?**
   Relative risk compares the disease risk in people exposed to a certain factor with the disease risk in people who have not been exposed to the factor in question. Relative risk can be calculated only after prospective or experimental studies; it cannot be calculated from retrospective data. If a Step 3 question asks you to calculate the relative risk from retrospective data, the answer is "cannot be calculated" or "none of the above."

9. **What is a clinically significant value for relative risk?**
   Any value for relative risk other than 1 is clinically significant. For example, if the relative risk is 1.5, a person is 1.5 times more likely to develop the condition if exposed to the factor in question. If the relative risk is 0.5, the person is only half as likely to develop the condition when exposed to the factor; in other words, the factor protects the person from developing the disease.

10. **Define odds ratio. From what type of studies is it calculated?**
    The odds ratio attempts to estimate relative risk with retrospective studies (e.g., case-control). An odds ratio compares two factors—(1) the incidence of disease in persons exposed to the factor and the incidence of nondisease in persons not exposed to the factor and (2) the incidence of disease in persons unexposed to the factor and the incidence of nondisease in persons exposed to the factor—to see whether there is a difference between the two. As with relative risk, values other than 1 are significant. The odds ratio is a less than perfect way to estimate relative risk (which can be calculated only from prospective or experimental studies).

11. **What do you need to know about standard deviation (SD) for the USMLE?**
    You need to know that for a normal or bell-shaped distribution, the mean ± 1 SD contains 68% of the values, the mean ± 2 SD contains 95% of the values, and the mean ± 3 SD contains 99.7% of the values. A classic question gives the mean and SD and asks what percentage of values will be above a given value. For example, if the mean score on a test is 80 and the SD is 5, 68% of the scores will be within 5 points of 80 (scores of 75 to 85) and 95% of the scores will be within 10 points of 80 (scores of 70 to 90). The question may ask what percentage of scores are over 90. The answer is 2.5% because 2.5% of the scores fall below 70 and 2.5% of the scores are over 90. Variations of this question are common.

12. **Define mean, median, and mode.**
    The mean is the average value, the median is the middle value, and the mode is the most common value. A question may give several numbers and ask for their mean, median, and mode. For example, if the question gives the numbers 2, 2, 4, and 8:
    The mean is the average of the four numbers: $(2 + 2 + 4 + 8)/4 = 16/4 = 4$.
    The median is the middle value. Because there are four numbers, there is no true middle value. Therefore take the average between the two middle numbers (2 and 4), so the median = 3.
    The mode is 2, because the number 2 appears twice (more times than any other value).
    Remember that in a normal distribution, mean = median = mode.

13. **What is a skewed distribution? How does it affect the mean, median, and mode?**
    A skewed distribution implies that the distribution is not normal; in other words, the data do not conform to a perfect bell-shaped curve. **Positive skew** is an asymmetric distribution with an excess of high values; in other words, the tail of the curve is on the right (mean > median > mode) (Fig. 1-3). **Negative skew** is an asymmetric distribution with an excess of low values; in other words, the tail of the curve is on the left (mean < median < mode). Because such distributions are not normal, the SD and mean are less meaningful values.

14. **Define test reliability. How is it related to precision? What reduces reliability?**
    From a practical perspective, the reliability of a test is synonymous with its precision. Reliability measures the reproducibility and consistency of a test. For example, if the test has good interrater reliability, the person taking the test will get the same score if two different people administer the same test. Random error reduces reliability and precision (e.g., limitation in significant figures).

15. **Define test validity. How is it related to accuracy? What reduces validity?**
    From a practical perspective, the validity of a test is synonymous with its accuracy. Validity measures the trueness of measurement; in other words, whether the test measures what it

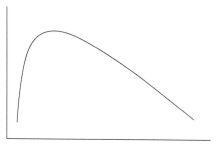

Figure 1-3. Positive skew. An excess of higher values makes this a nonnormal distribution. (*From O'Connell T. USMLE Step 2 secrets. 4th ed. Philadelphia: Elsevier, 2014, Fig. 3-2.*)

claims to measure. For example, if a valid IQ test is administered to a genius, the test should not indicate that he or she has an intellectual disability. Systematic error reduces validity and accuracy (e.g., when the equipment is miscalibrated).

16. **Define correlation coefficient. What is the range of its values?**
A correlation coefficient measures to what degree two variables are related. The value of the correlation coefficient ranges from −1 to +1.

17. **True or false: A correlation coefficient of −0.6 is stronger than a correlation coefficient of +0.4.**
True. The important factor in determining the strength of the relationship between two variables is the distance of the value from zero. A correlation coefficient of 0 equates to no association whatsoever; the two variables are totally unrelated. A correlation coefficient of +1 equates to perfect positive correlation (when one variable increases, so does the other), whereas −1 corresponds to perfect negative correlation (when one variable increases, the other decreases). Therefore the absolute value indicates the strength of the correlation (e.g., the strength of −0.3 is the same as that of +0.3).

18. **Define confidence interval. Why is it used?**
When you take a set of data from a subset of the population and calculate the mean, you may want to say that this is equivalent to the mean for the whole population. In fact, the two means are usually not exactly equal. A confidence interval of 95% (the value used in most medical literature before data are accepted by the medical community) indicates that there is 95% certainty that the mean for the entire population is within a certain range (usually 2 SD of the experimental or derived mean calculated for the subset of the population examined). For example, if the heart rate of 100 people is sampled and the mean is calculated as 80 beats per minute with an SD of 2, the confidence interval (also known as *confidence limits*) is written as $76 < X < 84 = 0.95$. In other words, there is 95% certainty that the mean heart rate of the whole population (X) is between 76 and 84 (within 2 SD of the mean).

19. **When are a chi-squared test, *t*-test, and analysis of variance test used?**
All of these tests are used to compare different sets of data.
Chi-squared test: used to compare percentages or proportions (nonnumeric or nominal data)
***t*-Test:** used to compare two means
Analysis of variance (ANOVA): used to compare three or more means

20. **What is the difference between nominal, ordinal, and continuous types of data?**
Nominal data have no numeric value—for example, the day of the week. Ordinal data give a ranking but no quantification— for example, class rank, which does not specify how far number 1 is ahead of number 2. Most numerical measurements are continuous data— for example, weight, blood pressure, and age. This distinction is important because of question 19: chi-squared tests must be used to compare nominal or ordinal data, whereas a *t*-test or ANOVA test is used to compare continuous data.

21. Define the following rates commonly seen on the USMLE.

RATE	DEFINITION
Birth rate	Live births/1000 population
Fertility rate	Live births/1000 population
Death rate	Deaths/1000 population
Neonatal mortality rate	Neonatal deaths (first 28 days of life)/1000 live births
Perinatal mortality rate	Neonatal deaths + stillbirths/1000 total births
Infant mortality rate	Deaths (from 0 to 1 yr old)/1000 live births
Maternal mortality rate	Maternal pregnancy-related deaths (deaths while pregnant or in the first 42 days after delivery)/100,000 live births

22. **What five types of studies should you know for the Step 3 exam?**
From highest to lowest quality and desirability: (1) experimental studies, (2) prospective studies, (3) retrospective studies, (4) case series, and (5) prevalence surveys.

23. **What are experimental studies?**
Experimental studies are the gold standard. They compare two equal groups in which one variable is manipulated and its effect is measured. Experimental studies use double blinding (or at least single blinding) and well-matched controls to ensure accurate data. It is not always possible to perform experimental studies because of ethical concerns.

24. **What are prospective studies? Why are they important?**
Prospective studies (also known as *observational, longitudinal, cohort, incidence,* or *follow-up studies*) involve choosing a sample and dividing it into two groups based on the presence or absence of a risk factor and following the groups over time to see what diseases they develop. For example, individuals with and without asymptomatic hypercholesterolemia may be followed to determine if those with hypercholesterolemia have a higher incidence of myocardial infarction later in life. The relative risk and incidence can be calculated from this type of study. Prospective studies are time consuming and expensive but practical for common diseases.

25. **What are retrospective studies? Discuss their advantages and disadvantages.**
Retrospective (case-control) studies choose population samples after the fact according to the presence (cases) or absence (controls) of disease. Information can be collected about risk factors. For example, you can compare individuals with lung cancer and individuals without lung cancer to determine if those with lung cancer smoked more before they developed lung cancer. In a retrospective study an odds ratio can be calculated, but true relative risk cannot be calculated and incidence cannot be measured. Compared with prospective studies, retrospective studies are less expensive, less time consuming, and more practical for rare diseases.

26. **What is a case series study? How is it used?**
A case series study simply describes the clinical presentation of people with a certain disease. This type of study is good for extremely rare diseases (as are retrospective studies) and may suggest a need for a retrospective or prospective study.

27. **What is a prevalence survey? How is it used?**
A prevalence (cross-sectional) survey looks at the prevalence of a disease and of risk factors. When used to compare two different cultures or populations, a prevalence survey may suggest a possible cause of a disease. The hypothesis then can be tested in a prospective study. For example, researchers have found a higher prevalence of colon cancer and a diet higher in fat in the United States versus a lower prevalence of colon cancer and a diet lower in fat in Japan.

28. **What is the difference between incidence and prevalence?**
Incidence is the number of new cases of a disease in a unit of time (generally 1 year, but any time frame can be used). The incidence of a disease is equal to the absolute (or total) risk of developing a condition (as distinguished from relative or attributable risk).
Prevalence is the total number of cases of a disease (new or old) at a certain point in time.

29. **If a disease can be treated only to the point that patients can be kept alive for longer without being cured, what happens to the incidence and prevalence of the disease?**
This is the classic question about incidence and prevalence on the Step 3 exam. Nothing happens to the incidence (the same number of people contract the disease every year), but the prevalence will increase because individuals with the disease live longer. For short-term diseases (e.g., influenza) the incidence may be higher than the prevalence, whereas for chronic diseases (e.g., diabetes or hypertension) the prevalence is greater than the incidence.

30. **Define *P*-value.**
The significance of the *P*-value is high yield in the Step 3 exam. If $P < 0.05$ for a set of data, there is a less than 5% chance ($0.05 = 5\%$) that the data were obtained by random error or chance. If $P < 0.01$, the chance is less than 1%. For example, if the blood pressure in a control group is 180/100 mmHg but falls to 120/70 mmHg after drug X is given, $P < 0.10$ means that the chance that this difference is due to random error or chance is less than 10%. It also means, however, that the chance that the result is random and unrelated to the drug may be as high as 9.99%. A value of $P < 0.05$ is generally used as the cutoff for statistical significance in the medical literature.

31. **What three points about the *P*-value should be remembered for the Step 3 exam?**
    1. A study with a value of $P < 0.05$ may still have serious flaws.
    2. A low *P*-value does not imply causation.
    3. A study that has statistical significance does not necessarily have clinical significance. For example, if drug X can lower blood pressure from 130/80 to 129/80 mmHg with $P < 0.0001$, drug X is unlikely to be used because the result is not clinically important given the minimal blood pressure reduction, the costs, and probable side effects.

32. **Explain the relationship of the *P*-value to the null hypothesis.**
The *P*-value also is related to the null hypothesis (the hypothesis of no difference). For example, in a study of hypertension, the null hypothesis is that the drug under investigation does not work; therefore any difference in blood pressure is due to random error or chance. If the drug works well and lowers blood pressure by 60 points, the null hypothesis must be rejected because clearly the drug works. For $P < 0.05$, the null hypothesis can be rejected with confidence because the p value indicates that there is less than a 5% chance that the null hypothesis is correct. If the null hypothesis is wrong, the difference in blood pressure is not due to chance; therefore it must be due to the drug.
  In other words, the p value represents the chance of making a type I error that is, claiming an effect or difference when none exists or rejecting the null hypothesis when it is true. If $P < 0.07$, there is a less than 7% chance of a type I error if a true difference (not due to random error) in blood pressure between the control and experimental groups is claimed.

33. **What is a type II error?**
In a type II error the null hypothesis is accepted when in fact it is false. In the previous example, this would mean that the antihypertensive drug works but the experimenter says that it does not.

34. **What is the power of a study? How do you increase the power of a study?**
Power measures the probability of rejecting the null hypothesis when it is false (a good thing). The best way to increase power is to **increase the sample size.**

35. **What are confounding variables?**
Confounding variables are unmeasured variables that affect both the independent (manipulated, experimental) variable and dependent (outcome) variables. For example, an experimenter measures the number of ashtrays owned and the incidence of lung cancer and finds that people with lung cancer have more ashtrays. He concludes that ashtrays cause lung cancer. Smoking tobacco is the confounding variable, because it causes the increase in ashtrays and lung cancer.

36. **Discuss nonrandom or nonstratified sampling.**
City A and city B can be compared, but they may not be equivalent. For example, if city A is a retirement community and city B is a college town, of course city A will have higher rates of mortality and heart disease if the groups are not stratified into appropriate age-specific comparisons.

37. **What is nonresponse bias?**
Nonresponse bias occurs when people do not return printed surveys or answer the phone in a phone survey. If nonresponse accounts for a significant percentage of the results, the experiment will suffer. The first strategy in this situation is to visit or call the nonresponders repeatedly. If this strategy is unsuccessful, list the nonresponders as unknown in the data analysis and determine if any results can be salvaged. *Never* make up or assume responses.

38. **Explain lead-time bias.**
Lead-time bias is due to time differentials. The classic example is a cancer screening test that claims to prolong survival compared with older survival data, when in fact the difference is due only to earlier detection and *not* to improved treatment or prolonged survival.

39. **Explain admission rate bias.**
The classic admission rate bias occurs when an experimenter compares the mortality rates for myocardial infarction (or some other disease) in hospitals A and B and concludes that hospital A has a higher mortality rate. But the higher rate may be due to tougher admission criteria at hospital A, which admits only the sickest patients with myocardial infarction. Hence hospital A has higher mortality rates, although the care may be superior. The same bias can apply to mortality and morbidity rates for a surgeon if he or she takes on only difficult cases.

40. **Explain recall bias.**
Recall bias is a risk in all retrospective studies. When people cannot remember exactly, they may inadvertently overestimate or underestimate risk factors. For example, John died of lung cancer and his angry widow remembers him as smoking "like a chimney," whereas Mike died of causes not related to smoking and his loving wife denies that he smoked "much." In fact, both men smoked one pack per day.

41. **Explain interviewer bias.**
Interviewer bias occurs in the absence of blinding. A scientist receives a large amount of money to perform a study and wants to find a difference between cases and controls. Thus he or she may inadvertently call the same patient comment or outcome "not significant" in the control group and "significant" in the treatment group.

42. **What is unacceptability bias?**
Unacceptability bias occurs when people do not wish to admit to embarrassing behavior. For example, they may claim to exercise more than they do to please the interviewer, or they may claim to have taken experimental medications when they actually spat them out.

GENERAL EMERGENCY MEDICINE PRINCIPLES

1. **Explain the ABCDEs of trauma. How are they used?**
The ABCDEs of trauma are **a**irway, **b**reathing, **c**irculation, **d**isability, and **e**xposure. They are the keys to initial management of trauma patients. Follow them in order if simultaneous management is not possible. For example, if a patient is bleeding to death and has a blocked airway, address airway management first.

2. **What is the difference between airway and breathing in trauma protocol?**
Airway means provision, protection, and maintenance of an adequate airway at all times. If the patient can answer questions, the airway is fine. You can use an oropharyngeal airway in uncomplicated cases and give supplemental oxygen. When you are in doubt or the patient's airway is blocked, intubate. If intubation fails, perform a cricothyroidotomy.
   Breathing is similar to airway, but even patients with an open airway may not be breathing spontaneously. The end result is the same. When you are in doubt or the patient is not breathing, intubate. If intubation fails, perform a cricothyroidotomy.

3. **Explain circulation, disability, and exposure.**
Circulation refers to circulating blood volume. For practical purposes, if the patient seems hypovolemic (tachycardic, bleeding, weak pulse, pale, diaphoretic, capillary refill more than 2 seconds), give intravenous fluids and/or blood products. Initially you should start two large-bore intravenous lines and give a bolus of 10 to 20 mL/kg (roughly 1 L) of lactated Ringer

solution or normal saline. Then reassess the patient after the bolus for improvement. Repeat the bolus if needed.

Disability refers to the need to check neurologic function. In practical terms, this translates into performing a Glasgow coma scale assessment.

Exposure reminds you to expose and examine the entire body. In other words, remove all of the patient's clothes and put "a finger in every orifice" so that you do not miss any occult injuries.

4. **What imaging films are routinely ordered for most patients with at least moderately severe trauma?**
   Chest and pelvic radiographs.

5. **What is the imaging study of choice for head trauma?**
   Noncontrast CT (better than MRI for acute trauma).

6. **What are the three zones of the neck? How is trauma in each of the different zones managed?**
   Zone I is the base of the neck from 2 cm above the clavicles to the level of the clavicles.
   Zone II is the midcervical region from 2 cm above the clavicle to the angle of the mandible.
   Zone III is the top of the neck from the angle of the mandible to the base of the skull.
   For zone I and III injuries, you should generally order an arteriogram before going to the operating room. Classical teaching states that zone II injuries should proceed to the operating room for surgical exploration without an arteriogram. In patients with obvious bleeding or a rapidly expanding hematoma in the neck, proceed directly to the operating room, no matter where the injury is. These prior classifications were assigned because zone II was the most amenable to surgical exploration. However, with the availability of CT angiography of the neck and other advanced imaging techniques, these zones are becoming less clinically relevant.

7. **What are toxidromes? Describe the toxidromes associated with cholinergic crisis, anticholinergic crisis, sympathomimetics, and opiates.**
   Toxidromes are syndromes caused by dangerously high levels of toxic substances in the body.
   - Cholinergic crisis classically presents with SLUDGE (excessive salivation, lacrimation, urination, defecation, and gastrointestinal activity with emesis). Also look for pinpoint pupils and a decreased heart rate.
   - Anticholinergic crisis presents with a patient who is "blind as a bat" (eye muscles unable to focus), "hot as a hare" (temperature dysregulation), "mad as a hatter" (CNS disturbances), "dry as a bone" (decreased secretion of bodily fluids), and "red as a beet" (flushing). Also look for dilated pupils and an increased heart rate.
   - Sympathomimetics can cause hypertension, tachycardia, increased activity, anxiety, dilated pupils, diaphoresis, and possibly altered mental status. Note that anticholingergic crisis has many overlapping features. Look for the presence or absence of diaphoresis to distinguish the two.
   - Opiates cause coma, pinpoint pupils, and respiratory depression. Also look for bradycardia and hypotension.

8. **On the USMLE, bizarre, unique, and fatal side effects are tested, as well as common side effects of common drugs. Cover the right-hand column in the following table and name the side effects of the drugs listed.**

DRUG	SIDE EFFECT
Trazodone	Priapism
Aspirin	Gastrointestinal bleeding, hypersensitivity
Bleomycin	Pulmonary fibrosis
Cyclophosphamide	Hemorrhagic cystitis
Bupropion	Seizures
Isoniazid	Vitamin B_6 deficiency, lupus-like syndrome, liver toxicity, peripheral neuropathy, seizures

Continued

DRUG	SIDE EFFECT
Cyclosporine	Renal toxicity
Penicillins	Anaphylaxis; rash with Epstein-Barr virus
Angiotensin-converting enzyme inhibitors	Cough, angioedema
Demeclocycline	Diabetes insipidus
Lithium	Diabetes insipidus, thyroid dysfunction
Sulfa drugs	Allergies, kernicterus in neonates
Halothane	Liver necrosis
Local anesthetic	Seizures
Phenytoin	Folate deficiency, teratogenesis, hirsutism
Vincristine	Peripheral neuropathy
Amiodarone	Thyroid dysfunction, pulmonary toxicity
Valproic acid	Neural tube defects in offspring
Isotretinoin	Major teratogenesis
Thioridazine	Retinal deposits, cardiac toxicity
Heparin	Thrombocytopenia, thrombosis
Vancomycin	Red man syndrome
Clofibrate	Increased gastrointestinal neoplasms
Tetracyclines	Photosensitivity, teeth staining in children
Quinolones	Teratogens (cartilage damage)
Quinine	Cinchonism (tinnitus, vertigo), thrombocytopenia, QT prolongation
Morphine	Sphincter of Oddi spasm
Clindamycin	Pseudomembranous colitis (can be caused by any broad-spectrum antibiotic)
Chloramphenicol	Aplastic anemia, gray baby syndrome
Doxorubicin	Cardiomyopathy
Busulfan	Pulmonary fibrosis
Monoamine oxidase inhibitors	Tyramine crisis (after eating cheese or wine)
Hydralazine	Lupus-like syndrome
Procainamide	Lupus-like syndrome
Minoxidil	Hirsutism
Aminoglycoside	Hearing loss, renal toxicity
Acetaminophen	Liver toxicity (at doses high than those recommended)
Chlorpropamide	Syndrome of inappropriate antidiuretic hormone (SIADH)
Oxytocin	SIADH
Opiates	SIADH
Didanosine (ddI)	Pancreatitis, peripheral neuropathy
Halogen anesthesia	Malignant hyperthermia
Succinylcholine	Malignant hyperthermia
Zidovudine (AZT)	Bone marrow suppression
Digitalis	Gastrointestinal disorders, vision changes, arrhythmias

DRUG	SIDE EFFECT
Acetazolamide	Metabolic acidosis
Clozapine	Agranulocytosis
Selective serotonin reuptake inhibitors (e.g., fluoxetine)	Anxiety, agitation, insomnia, sexual dysfunction
Warfarin	Necrosis, teratogen
Niacin	Skin flushing, pruritus
HMG-CoA reductase inhibitors (e.g., simvastatin)	Liver and muscle toxicity
Ethambutol	Optic neuritis
Metronidazole	Disulfiram-like reaction with alcohol
Cisplatin	Nephrotoxicity
Methyldopa	Hemolytic anemia (Coombs test-positive)

9. Name the antidote for each of the poisons or overdoses listed in the following table.

POISON OR OVERDOSE	ANTIDOTE
Acetaminophen	Acetylcysteine
Benzodiazepines	Flumazenil (rarely used because it may precipitate seizures)
Beta-blockers	Glucagon
Carbon monoxide	Oxygen (hyperbaric if severe)
Cholinesterase inhibitors	Atropine, pralidoxime
Copper or gold	Penicillamine
Digoxin	Normalize potassium and other electrolytes, digoxin antibodies
Iron	Deferoxamine
Lead	Edetate (EDTA)
Methanol or ethylene glycol	Fomepizole, ethanol
Muscarinic receptor blockers	Physostigmine
Opioids	Naloxone
Quinidine or tricyclic antidepressants	Sodium bicarbonate (cardioprotective)

10. If the following medications are given at the same time, what may happen?

MEDICATION	POSSIBLE EFFECT
MAO inhibitor plus meperidine	Coma
Aminoglycoside plus loop diuretic	Increased ototoxicity
Thiazide plus lithium	Lithium toxicity
MAO inhibitor plus SSRI	Serotonin syndrome (hyperthermia, rigidity, myoclonus, and autonomic instability)

MAO, Monoamine oxidase; SSRI, selective serotonin reuptake inhibitor.

CHAPTER 2

DISORDERS OF THE NERVOUS SYSTEM AND SPECIAL SENSES

1. Cover all but the left-hand column in the following table and describe the classic findings of cerebrospinal fluid (CSF) analysis in the conditions listed.

CONDITION	CELLS* (cells/mL)	GLUCOSE (mg/dL)	PROTEIN (mg/dL)	PRESSURE (mm H₂O)
Normal CSF	0-3 (L)	50-100	20-45	100-200
Bacterial meningitis†	>1000 (PMN)	<50	~100	>200
Viral/aseptic meningitis	>100 (L)	Normal	Normal/ slightly increased	Normal/ slightly increased
Pseudotumor cerebri	Normal	Normal	Normal	>200
Guillain-Barré syndrome	0-100 (L)	Normal	>100	Normal
Cerebral hemorrhage‡	Bloody (RBC)	Normal	>45	>200
Multiple sclerosis§	Normal/slightly increased (L)	Normal	Normal/ slightly increased	Normal

CSF, Cerebrospinal fluid; L, lymphocyte; PMN, neutrophil; RBC, red blood cell.
*Main cell type in parentheses.
†Tuberculous and fungal meningitis have low glucose (<50 mg/dL) with higher cell counts (>100 cell/mL), predominantly lymphocytes. In patients with fungal meningitis, a positive India ink preparation indicates *Cryptococcus neoformans*.
‡Think of subarachnoid hemorrhage, but this pattern may also occur after an intracerebral bleed.
§On electrophoresis of CSF look for oligoclonal bands caused by increased IgG production and an increased level of myelin basic protein in CSF during active demyelination.

2. Cover the right-hand column in the following table and localize the neurologic lesion for each of the symptoms and signs listed.

SYMPTOM/SIGN	AREA
Fasciculations, atrophy, decreased or no reflexes	Lower motor neuron disease (or possibly muscle problem)
Hyperreflexia, clonus, increased muscle tone	Upper motor neuron lesion (cord or brain)
Apathy, inattention, disinhibition, labile affect	Frontal lobes
Broca (motor) aphasia	Dominant frontal lobe*
Wernicke (sensory) aphasia	Dominant temporal lobe*
Memory impairment, hyperaggression, hypersexuality	Temporal lobes
Inability to read, write, name, or do math	Dominant parietal lobe*
Ignoring one side of the body, trouble with dressing	Nondominant parietal lobe*
Visual hallucinations/illusions	Occipital lobes
Cranial nerves 3 and 4	Midbrain

SYMPTOM/SIGN	AREA
Cranial nerves 5, 6, 7, and 8	Pons
Cranial nerves 9, 10, 11, and 12	Medulla
Ataxia, dysarthria, nystagmus, intention tremor, dysmetria, scanning speech	Cerebellum

*The left side is dominant in more than 95% of the population (99% of right-handed people and 60% to 70% of left-handed people).

3. **For delirious or unconscious patients in the emergency department with no history of trauma, for what three common causes should you think about giving empiric treatment?**
   1. Hypoglycemia (give glucose)
   2. Opioid overdose (give naloxone)
   3. Thiamine deficiency (give thiamine before giving glucose in a suspected alcoholic)
   Other common causes are alcohol, illicit drugs, prescription drugs, diabetic ketoacidosis, stroke, and epilepsy or postictal state. Remember the mnemonic **DON'T** for altered mental status: **d**extrose, **o**xygen, **n**aloxone, **t**hiamine.

4. **Define spina bifida. How can it be prevented?**
   Spina bifida is a congenital abnormality in which lack of fusion of the spinal column, specifically the posterior vertebral arches, allows protrusion of the spinal membranes, with or without the spinal cord. Spina bifida occulta, the mildest form of the disease (bone deficiency without dural membrane or cord protrusion), is often asymptomatic and should be suspected in patients with a triangular patch of hair over the lumbar spine. More serious defects are usually obvious and occur most often in the lumbosacral region. A **meningocele** is protrusion of the meninges outside the spinal canal, whereas a **myelomeningocele** is protrusion of the meninges plus central nervous system (CNS) tissue outside the spinal canal. Patients with a myelomeningocele almost always have an associated Arnold-Chiari malformation. Giving folate supplementation to potential mothers reduces the incidence of spina bifida and other neural tube defects, but the neural tube closes early in development (gestational age of 4 weeks), so ensuring that folate supplementation is started before pregnancy is the most effective strategy.

5. **Define hydrocephalus. How is it recognized in children?**
   Hydrocephalus is excessive accumulation of CSF in the cerebral ventricles. In children, look for increasing head circumference, increased intracranial pressure, a bulging fontanelle, scalp vein engorgement, and paralysis of upward gaze. The most common causes include congenital malformations, tumors, and inflammation (e.g., hemorrhage, meningitis). Treat the underlying cause, if possible; otherwise a surgical shunt is created to decompress the ventricles.

6. **Define subclavian steal syndrome. What symptoms does it cause? How is it treated?**
   Subclavian steal syndrome is usually due to left subclavian artery obstruction proximal to the vertebral artery origin. To perfuse an exercising arm, blood is "stolen" from the vertebrobasilar system; that is, it flows backward into the distal subclavian artery instead of forward into the brainstem. The typical presentation includes CNS symptoms (e.g., syncope, vertigo, confusion, ataxia, dysarthria) and upper extremity claudication during exercise. Treat with surgical bypass.

DEGENERATIVE/DEVELOPMENTAL DISORDERS

1. **What treatable causes of dementia must always be ruled out?**
   The American Academy of Neurology recommends screening for vitamin B_{12} deficiency and hypothyroidism. Other treatable causes of dementia that might be considered screening for but that do not have clear data to support or refute screening in all patients with dementia include hyperhomocysteinemia, endocrine disorders (parathyroid), uremia, liver disease, hypercalcemia, syphilis, Lyme disease, brain tumors, and normal-pressure hydrocephalus. Treatment of Parkinson disease may reverse dementia if it is present.

2. **Define pseudodementia.**

Depression can cause some clinical symptoms and signs of dementia, classically in the elderly. This type of "dementia" is reversible with treatment. Step 3 questions will give other signs and symptoms of depression (e.g., sadness, loss of a loved one, weight or appetite loss, suicidal ideation, poor sleep, feelings of worthlessness).

3. **What are the classic differential points between delirium and dementia?**

	DELIRIUM	**DEMENTIA**
Onset	Acute and dramatic	Chronic and insidious
Common causes	Illness, toxin, withdrawal	Alzheimer disease, multiinfarct dementia, HIV/AIDS
Reversible	Usually	Usually not
Attention	Poor	Usually unaffected
Arousal level	Fluctuates	Normal

4. **What symptoms and signs do delirium and dementia have in common?**

Both may have hallucinations, illusions, delusions, memory impairment (usually global in delirium, whereas remote memory is spared in early dementia), orientation difficulties (unawareness of time, place, person), and "sundowning" (worse at night).

5. **Describe the characteristics of Alzheimer dementia.**

Alzheimer dementia is a neurodegenerative disorder primarily affecting older adults and characterized by memory impairment, particularly memory for facts and events. Memory loss develops insidiously and progresses slowly over time. Language function, visuospatial skills, and executive function tend to be affected early in the disease process.

6. **Describe the characteristics of dementia with Lewy bodies.**

Dementia with Lewy bodies is an increasingly recognized clinical entity characterized by dementia plus two of the three following distinctive clinical features: visual hallucinations, parkinsonism (bradykinesia, limb rigidity, and gait disorders), and cognitive fluctuations. In contrast to Alzheimer dementia, the memory loss in dementia with Lewy bodies presents later in the course of the disease. Early symptoms include driving difficulties (e.g., getting lost) and impaired job performance. Sleep disorders such as acting out dreams are common in patients with dementia with Lewy bodies.

7. **Describe a scenario that would make you suspect vascular dementia.**

A patient with vascular risk factors (e.g., hypertension, diabetes, dyslipidemia, coronary artery disease) whose symptoms include dementia with abrupt onset and a stepwise deterioration should make you suspect vascular dementia.

8. **Describe the characteristics of frontotemporal dementia.**

Frontotemporal dementia is characterized by focal deterioration of the frontal and/or temporal lobes, leading to changes in personality or social behavior, with eventual progression to dementia. The age of onset is typically in the 50s or 60s.

9. **Define Parkinson disease. How do you recognize it on the Step 3 exam?**

Parkinson disease has a classic tetrad of (1) slowness or poverty of movement, (2) muscular ("lead pipe" and "cog-wheel") rigidity, (3) "pill-rolling" tremor at rest (which disappears with movement and sleep), and (4) postural instability (manifests as the classic shuffling gait and festination). Patients may also have dementia and depression. The mean age of onset is around 60 years.

10. **Describe the pathophysiology of Parkinson disease. How is it treated pharmacologically?**

The cause is thought to be a loss of dopaminergic neurons, especially in the **substantia nigra**, that project to the basal ganglia. The result is decreased dopamine in the basal ganglia. Drug therapy, for which the aim is to increase dopamine, includes dopamine precursors (levodopa with carbidopa), dopamine agonists (bromocriptine, apomorphine, pergolide, pramipexole, and ropinirole), monoamine oxidase-B inhibitors (selegiline), catechol-O-methyl transferase inhibitors (entacapone and tolcapone), anticholinergics (trihexyphenidyl and benztropine), and amantadine.

11. **What is the classic iatrogenic cause of parkinsonian signs and symptoms?**
Antipsychotics (which have dopamine antagonist activity) may cause parkinsonian symptoms in schizophrenics. Treat this side effect of antipsychotic medication with anticholinergics (benztropine, trihexyphenidyl) or antihistamines (diphenhydramine).

12. **True or false: Dementia is common in patients with Parkinson disease.**
True. Dementia is a common feature of Parkinson disease. Factors that influence the incidence of dementia include older age, age ≥60 years at onset of Parkinson disease, longer duration of Parkinson disease, and severity of parkinsonism.

13. **Give a classic case description of multiple sclerosis.**
Multiple sclerosis classically presents with an insidious onset of neurologic symptoms in white women aged 20 to 40 years, with exacerbations and remissions. Common presentations include paresthesias and numbness, weakness and clumsiness, visual disturbances (decreased vision and pain caused by optic neuritis, diplopia caused by cranial nerve involvement), gait disturbances, incontinence and urgency, and vertigo. Also look for emotional lability or other mental status changes. Internuclear ophthalmoplegia (a disorder of conjugate gaze in which the affected eye shows impairment of adduction) and scanning speech (spoken words are broken up into separate syllables separated by a noticeable pause and sometimes with stress on the wrong syllable) are classic; the patient may have a positive Babinski sign.

14. **What is the most sensitive test for diagnosis of multiple sclerosis? How is it treated?**
Magnetic resonance imaging (MRI) is the most sensitive diagnostic tool and reveals demyelination plaques. Also look for increased immunoglobulin G (IgG)/oligoclonal bands and possibly myelin basic protein in CSF. Treatment is not highly effective but includes interferon, glatiramer, mitoxantrone, natalizumab, cyclophosphamide, and methotrexate. Acute exacerbations are treated with glucocorticoids.

15. **How do you recognize amyotrophic lateral sclerosis (ALS) on the Step 3 exam?**
ALS (Lou Gehrig disease) is the only condition likely to be asked about that causes both upper and lower motor neuron lesion signs and symptoms. This idiopathic neurodegenerative disease is more common in men, and the mean age at onset is 55 years. The key is to notice a combination of upper motor neuron lesion signs (spasticity, hyperreflexia, positive Babinski sign) and lower motor neuron lesion signs (fasciculations, atrophy, flaccidity) present at the same time. Treatment is supportive. Fifty percent of patients die within 3 years of disease onset.

NEUROMUSCULAR/DEGENERATIVE DISORDERS

1. **Define Guillain-Barré syndrome.**
Guillain-Barré syndrome is a postinfectious polyneuropathy. Look for a history of mild infection (especially of the upper respiratory tract) or immunization roughly 1 week before the onset of symmetric distal weakness or paralysis with mild paresthesias that starts in the feet and legs with loss of deep tendon reflexes in affected areas. The hallmark of the disease is that motor function is often affected with intact or only minimally impaired sensation. As the ascending paralysis or weakness progresses, respiratory paralysis may occur. Watch carefully; spirometry is usually performed to follow inspiratory ability. Intubation may be required. Diagnosis is by clinical presentation. CSF is usually normal except for markedly increased protein. Nerve conduction velocities are slowed. The disease usually resolves spontaneously. Plasmapheresis (for adults) and intravenous immune globulin (for children) reduce the severity and length of disease. Do *not* use steroids; they no longer have a role in the treatment of Guillain-Barré syndrome.

2. **What causes nerve conduction velocity to slow?**
   Demyelination. Watch for Guillain-Barré syndrome and multiple sclerosis as causes.

3. **What causes an electromyography (EMG) study to show fasciculations or fibrillations at rest?**
   A lower motor neuron lesion (i.e., a peripheral nerve problem).

4. **What causes an EMG study with no muscle activity at rest and decreased amplitude of muscle contraction on stimulation?**
   Intrinsic muscle disease such as the muscular dystrophies or inflammatory myopathies (e.g., polymyositis). You now know enough about EMG for the USMLE.

5. **Describe the signs and symptoms of Huntington disease. How is it acquired? What is the classic computed tomography (CT) finding?**
   Huntington disease is an autosomal dominant condition that usually presents between the ages of 35 and 50 years. Look for choreiform movements (irregular, spasmodic, involuntary movements of the limbs or facial muscles) and progressive intellectual deterioration, dementia, or psychiatric disturbances. **Atrophy of the caudate nuclei** may be seen on CT or MRI scans. Treatment is supportive; tetrabenazine or atypical neuroleptics (olanzapine, risperidone, or aripiprazole) may help with the chorea and agitation/psychosis.

6. **Describe the pathophysiology of myasthenia gravis (MG). Who is affected? What are the classic physical findings?**
   MG is an autoimmune disease that destroys acetylcholine receptors. Most patients have antibodies to acetylcholine receptors in their serum. The disease usually presents in women between the ages of 20 and 40 years. Look for ptosis, diplopia, and general muscle fatigability, especially toward the end of the day or with repetitive use.

7. **How is MG diagnosed? What tumor is associated with it?**
   Diagnosis is made with the Tensilon test. After injection of edrophonium (Tensilon), a short-acting anticholinesterase inhibitor, muscle weakness improves. Nerve stimulation studies can also be used. Watch for associated **thymomas** (tumors of the thymus). Thymectomy is generally recommended for patients aged less than 60 years with or without thymoma. Chronic medical treatment consists of long-acting anticholinesterase inhibitors (pyridostigmine) and immunotherapy (glucocorticoids, mycophenolate, azathioprine, and cyclosporine).

8. **What three conditions may cause an MG-like clinical picture?**
   1. **Eaton-Lambert syndrome** is a paraneoplastic syndrome (classically seen with small-cell lung cancer) associated with muscle weakness. The extraocular muscles are spared, whereas MG is almost always characterized by prominent involvement of the extraocular muscles. Eaton-Lambert syndrome has a different mechanism of action (impaired release of acetylcholine from nerves because of antibodies against voltage-gated calcium channels that facilitate acetylcholine release into the synaptic cleft) and a differential response to repetitive nerve stimulation. The weakness in MG worsens with repetitive use or stimulation, whereas the weakness in Eaton-Lambert syndrome improves because increased stimulation leads to increased calcium influx and therefore increased acetylcholine release.
   2. **Organophosphate poisoning** also causes MG-like muscle weakness via inhibition of acetylcholine esterase and overstimulation of postsynaptic receptors by acetylcholine. Poisoning usually occurs as a result of agricultural exposure. Look for symptoms of parasympathetic excess (e.g., miosis, excessive bronchial secretions, urinary urgency, and diarrhea). Edrophonium causes worsening of the muscular weakness. Treat with atropine and pralidoxime. Pralidoxime is only effective early before a process called *aging* occurs, which happens when the bond becomes permanent and can no longer be displaced by pralidoxime. Exceedingly high levels of atropine may be required to treat severe cases (often using the entire hospital supply!).
   3. **Aminoglycosides in high doses** may cause MG-like muscular weakness and/or prolong the effects of muscular blockade after anesthesia.

CEREBROVASCULAR DISEASES

1. **In what common situation is a lumbar puncture contraindicated?**
   In the setting of acute head trauma, a lumbar puncture is contraindicated in the case of
   signs of intracranial hypertension (e.g., papilledema) or suspicion of a subarachnoid hemorrhage. You should do a lumbar tap only after you have obtained a negative CT or MRI
   scan of the head in these settings. Otherwise, a lumbar tap may cause uncal herniation and
   death.

2. **List the four major types of intracranial hemorrhage.**
   1. Subdural hematoma
   2. Epidural hematoma
   3. Subarachnoid hemorrhage
   4. Intracerebral hemorrhage

3. **What causes a subdural hematoma? How do you recognize and treat it?**
   Subdural hematomas are due to bleeding from veins that bridge the cortex and dural sinuses.
   On a CT scan the hematoma is crescent shaped (Fig. 2-1). Subdural hematomas are common
   in alcoholics and victims of head trauma. They may present immediately after trauma or as
   long as 1 to 2 months later. If the patient has a history of head trauma, always consider the
   diagnosis of subdural hematoma. If the hematoma is large, expanding, or accompanied by
   neurologic deficits, treat with surgical evacuation.

4. **What causes an epidural hematoma? How do you recognize and treat it?**
   Epidural hematomas are due to bleeding from meningeal arteries (classically, the middle
   meningeal artery). On a CT scan the hematoma is lenticular in shape (Fig. 2-2). At least
   85% of epidural hematomas are associated with a skull fracture (classically, a temporal
   bone fracture), and many patients have an ipsilateral "blown" pupil (dilated, fixed, nonreactive pupil on the same side as the hematoma because of uncal herniation). The classic
   history comprises head trauma with loss of consciousness, followed by a lucid interval of
   minutes to hours, and then neurologic deterioration. Treatment usually includes surgical
   evacuation.

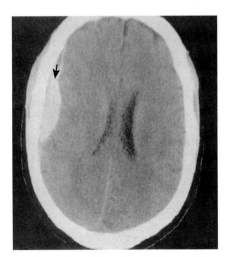

Figure 2-1. Subdural hematoma. An axial, nonenhanced computed tomography scan of the brain demonstrates an acute extraaxial hematoma. There is hyperdense blood *(arrow)* layered along the lateral aspect
of the right brain margin separating the brain from the inner table of the skull, consistent with an acute
subdural hematoma. *(From Layon AJ et al. Textbook of neurointensive care. 1st ed. Philadelphia: Saunders, 2003,
Fig. 2-38.)*

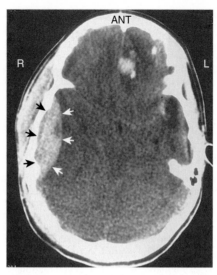

Figure 2-2. Epidural hematoma. In this patient, who was in a motor vehicle accident, a lenticular area of increased density is seen on a noncontrast axial computed tomography scan in the right parietal region. Areas of hemorrhage are also seen in the left frontal lobe. The *black* and *white arrows* mark the edges of the hematoma. (*From Mettler FA Jr. Essentials of radiology. 2nd ed. Philadelphia: Saunders, 2004, Fig. 2-14.*)

5. **Define subarachnoid hemorrhage. What causes it? How is it treated?**

   A subarachnoid hemorrhage is bleeding between the arachnoid and pia mater. The most common cause is trauma, followed by ruptured berry aneurysms. Blood can be seen in the cerebral ventricles and surrounding the brain or brainstem on a CT scan. The classic patient describes the "worst headache of my life," although many die or are unconscious before they reach the hospital. Patients who are awake have signs of meningitis (positive Kernig sign and Brudzinski sign). Remember the association between polycystic kidney disease and berry aneurysms. CT is the test of choice and should be performed before a lumbar puncture. A lumbar puncture shows grossly bloody CSF or xanthochromia. Xanthochromia is a yellow discoloration of CSF that represents products of hemoglobin degradation.

   Treat with support of vital functions, anticonvulsants, and observation. Once the patient is stable, perform a CT or MRI angiogram to look for aneurysms or arteriovenous malformations, which may be treatable with surgical clipping or catheter-directed angiographic procedures.

6. **What causes an intracerebral hemorrhage? How do you recognize and treat it?**

   Intracerebral hemorrhage is bleeding into the brain parenchyma (Fig. 2-3). The most common cause is hypertension, but it also may be caused by other forms of stroke, trauma, arteriovenous malformations, coagulopathies, or tumors. Two thirds of intracerebral hemorrhages occur in the basal ganglia (especially with hypertension). The patient may present with coma or, if awake, contralateral hemiplegia and hemisensory deficits. Blood (which appears white on a CT scan) can be seen in the brain parenchyma and may extend into the ventricles. Surgery is reserved for large, accessible hemorrhages, although it is usually not helpful.

7. **What causes strokes? How common are they?**

   Cerebrovascular disease (stroke) is the most common cause of neurologic disability in the United States and the third leading cause of death. Ischemia due to atherosclerosis (atherothrombotic ischemia) is by far the most common type of stroke (>85% of cases). Hypertension is another cause of stroke, typically hemorrhagic stroke, most commonly in the basal

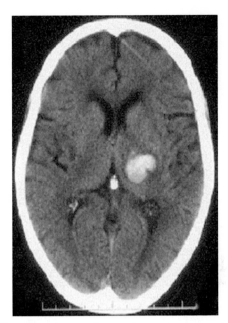

Figure 2-3. Intracerebral hemorrhage. A computed tomographic scan shows a parenchymal hemorrhage involving the left thalamus and posterior internal capsule. *(Courtesy of Gregory W. Albers, Stanford University, Stanford, CA.)*

ganglia, thalamus, or cerebellum. Nevertheless, be aware of more exotic causes of stroke, such as atrial fibrillation with resultant clot formation and emboli to the brain, septic emboli from endocarditis, and sickle cell disease.

8. **How is an acute stroke treated?**
Treatment for an acute stroke in evolution is supportive (e.g., airway, oxygen, intravenous fluids). The first step is to obtain a CT scan of the head without contrast to evaluate for bleeding or a mass (Fig. 2-4). If no blood is seen on the CT scan, aspirin is usually the medication of choice. Heparin is not recommended for treatment of acute ischemic stroke and should be avoided on the USMLE. Thrombolysis with tissue plasminogen activator (t-PA) can be attempted if patients come to the hospital within 3 hours (up to 4.5 hours in certain circumstances) and meet strict criteria for its use.

9. **Define transient ischemic attack (TIA). How is it managed?**
TIA is a brief episode of neurologic dysfunction resulting from temporary cerebral ischemia not associated with cerebral infarction. This newer definition is tissue based rather than time based. TIA is often a precursor to stroke and is due to ischemia. The classic presentation is ipsilateral blindness (amaurosis fugax) and/or unilateral hemiplegia, hemiparesis, weakness, or clumsiness that lasts for less than 5 minutes.
   Order a carotid duplex scan to look for carotid stenosis. The correct choice for long-term therapy is aspirin and antiplatelet medications. Choose carotid endarterectomy (CEA) over aspirin if the degree of carotid stenosis is 70% to 99%.

10. **Discuss the relationship between aspirin and strokes.**
Low-dose aspirin is of proven benefit in reducing strokes in patients with TIAs and/or known carotid artery stenosis. Nevertheless, the risks may outweigh the benefits, as mentioned in the preceding question, especially in patients with uncontrolled hypertension, which, coupled with aspirin, can increase the risk of a hemorrhagic stroke.

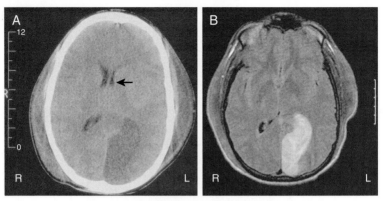

Figure 2-4. Stroke on computed tomography (CT) and magnetic resonance imaging (MRI) scans. **A,** The CT scan performed 3 days after a stroke shows a low-density area posteriorly on the left, with a mass effect and clear midline shift *(arrow)*. **B,** The MRI scan performed on the same day shows the infarcted area much more clearly. *(From Mettler FA Jr. Essentials of radiology. 2nd ed. Philadelphia: Saunders, 2004, Fig. 2-17.)*

11. **True or false: In the setting of an acute neurologic deficit, you should give aspirin before ordering brain imaging.**
    False. When a patient has an acute neurologic deficit, you do not know whether he or she is having a hemorrhagic stroke, ischemic stroke, or TIA. TIA is a retrospective diagnosis made once the symptoms clear and imaging has ruled out tissue injury. The first step should be to order a CT or MRI scan to rule out hemorrhagic stroke. If the CT or MRI scan is negative for blood, the patient should be given aspirin (160 to 325 mg) within 24 to 48 hours of TIA or stroke onset.

12. **What clues suggest carotid stenosis? How is it diagnosed?**
    The classic presentation of carotid stenosis is a TIA, especially with amaurosis fugax, which is the sudden onset of transient, unilateral blindness, sometimes described as a "shade pulled over one eye." Physical examination may reveal a carotid bruit. Ultrasound of the carotid arteries (duplex scan of the carotids) is used to diagnose and quantify the degree of stenosis.

13. **How is carotid stenosis managed?**
    In symptomatic patients, if the stenosis is **70% to 99%**, patients are usually advised to undergo CEA for the best long-term prognosis if their state of health allows them to tolerate the surgery. If the stenosis is 50% to 69%, the data are less clear and patient factors affect the decision. CEA is generally recommended for men, patients aged 75 years or older, patients with a recent stroke (not TIA), and patients with hemispheric symptoms other than transient monocular blindness (amaurosis fugax). Female patients, patients younger than 75 years, and those with mild symptoms generally do better with medical management if the stenosis is 50% to 69%. If the stenosis is less than 50%, medical management is indicated.
    Patients should not undergo CEA after a stroke that leaves them severely disabled, but small, nondisabling strokes are not contraindications to surgery. CEA should not be performed during a TIA or stroke in evolution. Surgery is always done electively, not on an emergency basis.
    In asymptomatic patients, if the stenosis is 60% to 99%, CEA is indicated. If the stenosis is less than 60%, medical management is indicated. Medical management includes antihypertensive agents, statins, and antiplatelet therapy.
    The role of carotid angioplasty and carotid stenting in carotid stenosis is not yet clearly defined. CEA remains the treatment of choice for suitable carotid stenosis.
    Because medical therapy has improved since the initial studies comparing CEA with medical management were performed, medical management of lower-grade carotid stenosis and asymptomatic carotid stenosis is gaining favor. This is an area that is still being clarified in the medical literature and likely will not be tested on the USMLE.

14. **In what setting does dural venous sinus thrombosis occur? How is it diagnosed and treated?**

    The risk factors are similar to those for deep venous thrombosis in other areas, including hypercoagulable state, trauma, dehydration, pregnancy, oral contraceptive use, infections (e.g., extension of sinusitis or mastoiditis intracranially), nephrotic syndrome, and local tumor invasion. The diagnostic test of choice is MRI. Although hemorrhagic infarcts are common with dural venous thrombosis, treatment with anticoagulation improves outcomes.

PERIPHERAL NERVE DISEASES

1. **What are the causes of lower motor neuron facial nerve paralysis?**
   - Bell palsy (discussed in more detail later in the chapter)
   - Herpes infection (Ramsay Hunt syndrome), which commonly involves the eighth nerve (look for vesicles on the pinna and inside the ear; encephalitis or meningitis may be present)
   - Lyme disease (one of the most common causes of bilateral facial nerve palsy)
   - Stroke
   - Middle ear or mastoid infections
   - Meningitis
   - Temporal bone fracture (look for the Battle sign and/or bleeding or CSF drainage from the ear)
   - Tumor, classically an acoustic schwannoma (i.e., neuroma) of the cerebellopontine angle
   Order a CT or MRI scan of the head if the cause is not apparent or if the history or physical examination raises suspicion, especially in the presence of additional neurologic signs.

2. **List the causative categories of peripheral neuropathy and give examples of each.**
   1. Metabolic/endocrine: diabetes mellitus (autonomic and sensory neuropathy), uremia, and hypothyroidism
   2. Nutritional: deficiencies of vitamin B_{12}, vitamin B_6 (look for history of isoniazid use), thiamine ("dry" beriberi), and vitamin E
   3. Toxins/medications: lead (the classic symptom is wrist or foot drop; look for coexisting CNS or abdominal symptoms) or other heavy metals, isoniazid, vincristine, ethambutol (optic neuritis), and aminoglycosides (especially CN VIII)
   4. Immunization and autoimmune disorders: Guillain-Barré syndrome, lupus erythematosus, polyarteritis nodosa, scleroderma, sarcoidosis, and amyloidosis
   5. Trauma: carpal tunnel syndrome (entrapment of the median nerve at the wrist; usually due to repetitive physical activity but may be a presentation of acromegaly or hypothyroidism; look for positive Tinel and Phalen signs), pressure paralysis (radial nerve palsy in alcoholics), and fractures (causing nerve compression)
   6. Infectious: Lyme disease, diphtheria, HIV, and leprosy

3. **What test can be used to prove the presence of a peripheral neuropathy, regardless of cause?**

   Nerve conduction velocity is slowed with a peripheral neuropathy.

4. **Cover the right-hand columns in the following table and specify the motor and sensory functions of the peripheral nerves listed. In what common clinical scenarios are the nerves often damaged?**

NERVE	MOTOR FUNCTION	SENSORY FUNCTION	CLINICAL SCENARIO
Radial	Wrist extension (watch for wrist drop)	Back of forearm, back of hand (first 3 digits)	Humeral fracture
Ulnar	Finger abduction (watch for "claw hand")	Front and back of last 2 digits	Elbow dislocation or fracture
Median	Pronation, thumb opposition	Palmar surface of hand (first 3 digits)	Carpal tunnel syndrome, humeral fracture

Continued

NERVE	MOTOR FUNCTION	SENSORY FUNCTION	CLINICAL SCENARIO
Axillary	Abduction, lateral rotation	Lateral shoulder	Upper humeral dislocation or fracture
Peroneal	Dorsiflexion, eversion (watch for foot drop)	Dorsal foot and lateral leg	Knee dislocation, fibula fracture

5. **What two diseases commonly cause isolated palsies of cranial nerves III, IV, and VI? How do you recognize them?**

Isolated palsies of cranial nerves III, IV, and VI are usually due to vascular complications of diabetes mellitus and hypertension. Symptoms generally resolve on their own within 2 months. In patients older than 40 years with a history of diabetes or hypertension and no other neurologic deficits or pain, observation is generally all that is required because hypertension and/or diabetes is the most likely cause. If resolution does not occur within 8 weeks, if the patient is younger than 40 years, if neither hypertension nor diabetes is present, or if the patient starts to develop pain or other neurologic deficits, order an MRI scan of the head to rule out tumor or aneurysm (i.e., benign cause less likely).

HEADACHE AND MOVEMENT DISORDERS

1. **Differentiate among tension, cluster, and migraine headaches. How is each treated?**

Tension headaches are the most common; look for a long history of headaches and stress, plus a feeling of tightness or stiffness, usually frontal or occipital and bilateral. Treat with stress reduction and acetaminophen or nonsteroidal antiinflammatory drugs (NSAIDs).

Cluster headaches are unilateral, severe, and tender; they occur in clusters (e.g., three in 1 week, then none for 2 months) and are usually accompanied by autonomic symptoms such as ptosis, lacrimation, rhinorrhea, and nasal congestion. Supplemental oxygen and subcutaneous sumatriptan are first-line therapy for acute attacks. In patients with cluster headaches, alcohol can precipitate attacks and should be avoided.

Migraine headaches are classically associated with an aura (a peculiar sensation, such as a noise or a flash of light, that lets the patient know that an attack is about to start). Signs and symptoms often include photophobia, nausea/vomiting, and a positive family history. Occasionally neurologic symptoms are seen during attacks. Migraines usually begin between the ages of 10 and 30 years. Medications used for acute treatment of migraines include NSAIDs, triptans, ergotamine, and antiemetics. Prophylaxis can be achieved with beta-blockers, tricyclic antidepressants, topiramate, valproic acid, and calcium channel blockers.

2. **How do you recognize a headache secondary to a brain tumor or intracranial mass?**

Such a headache is recognized by the presence of associated neurologic symptoms and signs of intracranial hypertension (papilledema; nausea/vomiting, which may be projectile; and mental status changes or ataxia). The classic headache occurs every day and is worse in the morning. Watch for a headache that wakes the patient from sleep. Headaches caused by an intracranial mass get worse with a Valsalva maneuver, exertion, or sex. There may be associated focal neurologic deficits. Perform a CT or MRI scan of the head.

3. **Define pseudotumor cerebri. How is it diagnosed and treated?**

Pseudotumor cerebri (now renamed **idiopathic intracranial hypertension** [IIH]) is a fairly benign condition that can mimic a tumor because both cause intracranial hypertension with papilledema and daily headaches that are classically worse in the morning and may be accompanied by nausea and vomiting. The difference, however, is that pseudotumor cerebri is usually found in young obese females who are unlikely to have a brain tumor. Negative

CT and MRI scans rule out a tumor or mass. The main worrisome sequela is vision loss. Large doses of vitamin A, tetracyclines, and withdrawal from corticosteroids are possible causes of pseudotumor cerebri. Weight loss may help; acetazolamide or topiramate may also help. Repeated lumbar punctures or a CSF shunt may be needed; when a lumbar puncture is performed, the opening pressure will be very high but studies will be otherwise negative.

4. **How do you recognize a headache caused by meningitis?**
   The adult patient has a fever, the **Brudzinski sign** or **Kernig sign,** and positive CSF findings (the classic findings in bacterial meningitis are significantly elevated white blood cells, decreased glucose, protein around 100 mg/dL, and increased opening pressure) if a lumbar puncture is performed. Photophobia is also common.

5. **What causes the "worst headache" of a patient's life?**
   This is a classic description for a subarachnoid hemorrhage. The most common causes are a ruptured congenital berry aneurysm or trauma. Look for blood around the brain or within sulci on a CT or MRI scan or grossly bloody CSF on lumbar puncture. Treatment is supportive. Aneurysms require surgical treatment to prevent rebleeding and death.

6. **What are the common extracranial causes of headache?**
   - Eye pain (optic neuritis, eyestrain from refractive errors, iritis, glaucoma)
   - Middle ear pain (otitis media, mastoiditis)
   - Sinus pain (sinusitis)
   - Oral cavity pain (toothache)
   - Herpes zoster infection with cranial nerve involvement
   - Nonspecific (e.g., malaise from any illness)

7. **What are the six general types of seizures that you should be able to recognize?**
   1. Simple partial
   2. Complex partial
   3. Absence (petit mal)
   4. Tonic-clonic
   5. Febrile
   6. Secondary

8. **Describe a simple partial seizure. How is it treated?**
   Simple partial (local or focal) seizures may be motor (e.g., jacksonian march), sensory (e.g., hallucinations), or psychic (cognitive or affective symptoms). The key point is that consciousness is *not* impaired. The first-line agents for treatment are carbamazepine, lamotrigine, oxcarbazepine, and levetiracetam.

9. **Describe complex partial seizures. How are they treated?**
   Complex partial (psychomotor) seizures are any simple partial seizure followed by impairment of consciousness. Patients perform purposeless movements and may become aggressive if restraint is attempted (however, individuals who get into fights or kill others are not having a seizure). The first-line agents for treatment are valproate, lamotrigine, and levetiracetam.

10. **Give the classic description of an absence seizure.**
    Absence (petit mal) seizures do not begin after the age of 20 years. They are brief (10 to 30 seconds in duration) generalized seizures in which the main manifestation is loss of consciousness, often with eye or muscle fluttering. The classic description is a child in a classroom who stares into space in the middle of a sentence, then 20 seconds later resumes the sentence where he left off. The child is *not* daydreaming; he or she is having a seizure. There is no postictal state (an important differential point). The first-line treatment agents are ethosuximide and valproate.

11. **How do you recognize a tonic-clonic seizure?**
    Tonic-clonic (grand mal) seizures are the classic seizures that we knew about before we went to medical school. They may be associated with an aura. Tonic muscle contraction is followed by clonic contractions, usually lasting for 2 to 5 minutes. Associated symptoms

may include incontinence and tongue lacerations. The postictal state is characterized by drowsiness, confusion, headache, and muscle soreness. The first-line agents for treatment are valproate, lamotrigine, and levetiracetam.

12. **Define febrile seizure.**

Children between the ages of 6 months and 5 years may have a seizure caused by fever. Always assume another cause outside this age range. The criteria for a simple febrile seizure are (1) febrile, (2) generalized seizure *at onset* with no focal features, (3) lasting less than 15 minutes, and (4) only occurring once within a 24-hour period. Febrile patients for whom criteria 2, 3, and 4 are not all met have a *complex* febrile seizure, which is more worrisome. No specific seizure treatment is required, but you should treat the underlying cause of the fever, if possible, and give acetaminophen to reduce the fever. Such children do *not* have epilepsy, and their chances of developing it are only barely higher than in the general population. Make sure that the child does not have meningitis, a tumor, or another serious cause of the seizure. The Step 3 question will give clues in the case description as to whether you should pursue a workup for a serious condition.

13. **What are the common causes of secondary seizures? How are they treated?**

- Mass effect (tumor, hemorrhage)
- Metabolic disorder (hypoglycemia, hypoxia, phenylketonuria, hyponatremia)
- Toxins (lead, cocaine, carbon monoxide poisoning)
- Drug withdrawal (alcohol, barbiturates, benzodiazepines, anticonvulsant withdrawal that is too rapid)
- Cerebral edema (severe or malignant hypertension; also watch for pheochromocytoma and eclampsia)
- CNS infections (meningitis, encephalitis, toxoplasmosis, cysticercosis)
- Trauma
- Stroke

Treat the underlying disorder and use acute benzodiazepine (lorazepam or diazepam) and/or phenytoin or fosphenytoin administration to control seizures. For all seizures (primary or secondary), secure the airway and, if possible, roll the patient onto his or her side to prevent aspiration.

14. **Define status epilepticus. How is it treated?**

Status epilepticus is a seizure that lasts for a sufficient length of time (previously defined as 30 minutes or longer, but newer guidelines favor 5 minutes or longer) or is repeated frequently enough that the individual does not return to neurologic baseline between seizures (e.g., still postictal when the second seizure begins). Status epilepticus may occur spontaneously or result from anticonvulsant withdrawal that is too rapid. Treat with intravenous lorazepam. Give fosphenytoin if the seizures persist. As with all seizures, remember the ABCs (airway, breathing, circulation). Protect the airway. Intubate if necessary and roll the patient on his or her side to prevent aspiration.

15. **True or false: Hypertension can cause seizures.**

True. Always remember hypertension as a cause of seizures, headache (although the association between hypertension and headache is tenuous at best unless the blood pressure is very high), confusion, stupor, and mental status changes.

16. **What do you need to remember when giving anticonvulsants to women?**

All anticonvulsants are teratogenic, and women of reproductive age need counseling about the risks of pregnancy. Perform a pregnancy test before starting anticonvulsant therapy and offer birth control. Valproic acid is a major contributor to the risk. Polypharmacy increases the risk. There is limited information on risks to the human fetus for the newer antiepileptic medications.

17. **What does cranial nerve V (CN V; trigeminal nerve) innervate? What classic peripheral nerve disorder affects its function?**

CN V innervates the muscles of mastication and facial sensation, including the afferent limb of the corneal reflex. Watch for **trigeminal neuralgia** (tic douloureux), which is classically described as unilateral shooting pains in the face in older adults and is often triggered by activity (e.g., brushing the teeth). This condition is best treated with antiepilepsy medications (e.g., carbamazepine). If the patient is younger and female or the symptoms are bilateral, consider multiple sclerosis and rule out other causes, such as tumor or stroke.

18. **What is the most common cause of lower motor neuron facial nerve paralysis? How does it present?**
    The most common cause is Bell palsy. Look for sudden unilateral onset, usually after an upper respiratory tract infection. The cause is thought to be reactivation of latent herpes simplex I infection in most cases. Patients may have *hyperacusis*, in which everything sounds loud because the stapedius muscle in the ear is paralyzed. In severe cases, patients may be unable to close the affected eye; if so, use drops to protect the eye. Most cases resolve spontaneously in about 1 month, although some have permanent sequelae. Oral prednisone and antiviral treatment for herpes (e.g., valacyclovir, acyclovir) may improve outcomes and lessen the duration of symptoms.

19. **What structures does CN VII innervate? What is the difference between an upper and lower motor neuron lesion of the facial nerve?**
    CN VII (facial nerve) innervates the muscles of facial expression, taste in the anterior two thirds of the tongue, the skin of the external ear, lacrimal and salivary glands (except the parotid gland), and the stapedius muscle. For an upper motor neuron lesion of CN VII the forehead is spared on the affected side and the cause is usually a stroke or tumor. For a lower motor neuron lesion the forehead is involved on the affected side and the cause is usually Bell palsy or a tumor.

20. **What brain lesions cause a resting tremor and an intention tremor? What about hemiballismus?**
    A resting tremor, if caused by a brain lesion, is generally a sign of basal ganglia disease, as is chorea. An intention tremor is usually due to cerebellar disease. Hemiballismus (random, violent, unilateral flailing of the limbs) is classically due to a lesion in the **subthalamic nucleus.**

21. **What conditions other than Parkinson disease cause a resting tremor?**
    A resting tremor may be due to hyperthyroidism, anxiety, drug withdrawal, drug intoxication, or benign (essential) hereditary tremor. Benign hereditary tremor is usually autosomal dominant; look for a positive family history and use beta-blockers to reduce the tremor. Also watch for Wilson disease (hepatolenticular degeneration), which can cause chorea-like movements; asterixis (slow, involuntary flapping of outstretched hands) may be seen in patients with liver failure.

22. **Describe Tourette syndrome. How is it treated?**
    Tourette syndrome is a motor tic disorder (eye blinking, grunting, throat clearing, grimacing, barking, or shoulder shrugging) that is exacerbated by stress and remits during activity or sleep. Although part of the classic description, coprolalia (swearing) affects only 10% to 30% of patients. Males are affected more often than females. Of interest, Tourette syndrome can be caused or unmasked by the use of stimulants (e.g., for presumed attention-deficit hyperactivity disorder). Antipsychotics (haloperidol) or dopamine receptor blockers (e.g., fluphenazine, pimozide) can be used if the symptoms are severe. Tourette syndrome tends to be a lifelong problem.

SLEEP DISORDERS

1. **Describe the hallmark findings of narcolepsy. How is it treated?**
   Narcolepsy is a sleep disorder characterized by daytime sleepiness in spite of a normal daily sleep regimen. Patients have decreased latency for rapid eye movement (REM) sleep (patients go into REM as soon as they fall asleep); cataplexy (random loss of muscle tone often triggered by strong emotions that causes patients to fall down); and hallucinations as they awaken (hypnopompic) or fall asleep (hypnagogic). Treat with **modafinil** (a nonamphetamine stimulant), methylphenidate, or amphetamines.

NEOPLASMS

1. **Describe the common presentations of brain tumors.**

   CNS tumors are the second most common tumors in children (second to leukemia); be suspicious in this age group. In adults, two thirds of primary tumors are supratentorial (i.e., above the tentorium cerebelli, a portion of the dura that separates the cerebellum from the cerebral hemispheres), whereas in children, two thirds are infratentorial (i.e., lower brainstem or cerebellum [posterior fossa]). In either group, look for new-onset seizures, neurologic deficits, or signs of intracranial hypertension (headache, blurred vision, papilledema, nausea, projectile vomiting). In children, also look for hydrocephalus (manifests as an inappropriate increase in head circumference), new clumsiness, ataxia, loss of developmental milestones, or a change in school performance or personality.

2. **What are the most common histologic types of primary CNS tumors in children and adults? How are primary brain tumors treated?**

   The most common primary type in **adults** is **glioma**. Most gliomas are astrocytomas, which are intraparenchymal and have little or no calcification. The second most common type in adults is **meningioma**, which is often calcified and is external to the brain substance. In **children** the most common types are **cerebellar astrocytoma** (benign pilocytic astrocytoma) and **medulloblastoma**, followed by ependymoma. Treat with surgical removal (if possible), followed by radiation and/or chemotherapy, depending on the tumor.

3. **Which cancers tend to metastasize to the brain?**

   Lung cancer, breast cancer, and melanoma are the most common and together account for 75% of brain metastases. Remember that a brain malignancy is more likely to be metastatic from another source than a primary brain malignancy.

4. **Metastatic cancer to the spine can cause spinal cord compression. How do you recognize and treat this medical emergency?**

   Spinal cord compression causes local spinal pain and neurologic symptoms (reflex changes, weakness, sensory loss, paralysis, incontinence, urinary retention). In rare cases it may be the first indication of a malignancy. The first step is to start high-dose corticosteroid therapy; then order an MRI scan. The next step is to treat with radiation. Surgical decompression is used if radiation fails or the tumor is known not to be radiosensitive. Prompt intervention is essential, and outcome is closely linked to pretreatment function.

5. **What diseases should come to mind for children with cerebellar findings?**
   - Brain tumor (cerebellar astrocytoma, medulloblastomas)
   - Hydrocephalus (enlarging head in an infant aged <6 months, Arnold-Chiari or Dandy-Walker malformations)
   - Friedreich ataxia (starts between ages 5 and 15 years; autosomal recessive; look for areflexia, loss of vibration/position sense, and cardiomyopathy)
   - Ataxia-telangiectasia (progressive cerebellar ataxia, oculocutaneous telangiectasias, and immune deficiency)

6. **What diseases should come to mind for adults with cerebellar findings?**

   Alcoholism, brain tumor, ischemia or hemorrhage, and multiple sclerosis.

7. **What tumor should you suspect in an adult with signs of CN VIII damage and increased intracranial pressure?**

   An acoustic neuroma (especially in the setting of neurofibromatosis). Coinvolvement of the facial nerve is not uncommon.

8. **What tumor should you suspect in children with intracranial calcifications on skull radiographs?**

   Craniopharyngioma (benign tumor that arises from remnants of the Rathke pouch and grows slowly from birth).

9. **What is the classic physical finding for a pituitary tumor? What is the most common type?**

   The classic physical finding is **bitemporal hemianopsia** caused by compression of the tumor on the optic chiasm. Order an MRI scan of the brain in any patient with this finding.

Patients may also have signs and symptoms of increased intracranial pressure. The most common type of pituitary tumor is a prolactinoma, which is associated with high prolactin levels, galactorrhea, and menstrual or sexual dysfunction. Other types of pituitary tumors may cause hyperthyroidism, Cushing disease, or acromegaly, or they may be nonfunctional (i.e., they do not secrete hormones).

INFECTIOUS DISEASES

1. **What is the classic age group for meningitis? Describe the physical findings.**
   Neonates are the classic age group for meningitis; 75% of all cases occur in children younger than 2 years. Deciding when to do a lumbar puncture is difficult, because patients often do not have classic physical findings (Kernig sign and Brudzinski sign). Look for lethargy, hyperthermia or hypothermia, poor muscle tone, a bulging fontanelle, vomiting, photophobia, altered consciousness, and signs of generalized sepsis (e.g., hypotension, jaundice, respiratory distress). Seizures also may be seen, but simple febrile seizures are common in the absence of meningitis if the patient is between 5 months and 6 years of age with a fever greater than 102° F (38.9° C). Remember that all neonates younger than 28 days with a fever should automatically get a full sepsis workup that includes a lumbar puncture to evaluate for meningitis.

2. **What should you do if you suspect bacterial meningitis?**
   In the absence of trauma, do a lumbar puncture immediately and begin (1) corticosteroids, (2) broad-spectrum antibiotics, and (3) IV fluids. Do *not* wait for culture or other results before starting antibiotic therapy.

3. **What is the most common neurologic sequela of meningitis?**
   Hearing loss. All pediatric and many adult patients need formal hearing evaluation after a bout of meningitis. Vision testing is also recommended. Other sequelae include mental retardation, motor deficits/paresis, epilepsy, and learning/behavioral disorders.

4. **What are the common viral (aseptic) causes of meningitis in children?**
   Mumps and measles meningitis may be seen in children who are not immunized. The best treatment is prevention via immunization. Watch for neonatal herpes encephalitis (HSV-2) if the mother has genital lesions of herpes simplex virus at the time of delivery. Other children and adults can develop HSV-1 herpes encephalitis, which classically affects the **temporal lobes** and can be seen on a head CT or MRI scan. Give intravenous acyclovir.

5. **Which types of bacterial meningitis require antibiotic prophylaxis in contacts?**
   Neisseria meningitidis and *Haemophilus influenzae*. If a case of meningitis is due to *Neisseria*, give all contacts rifampin, ciprofloxacin, ceftriaxone, or azithromycin as prophylaxis; rifampin is used as prophylaxis for *H. influenzae* meningitis.

TRAUMA AND TOXIC EFFECTS

1. **What are the two classic causes of a "floppy" (flaccid) baby? How do you differentiate the two?**
   Genetic disorders, the most common of which is Werdnig-Hoffmann disease (WHD), and infant botulism are the classic causes of this condition. History easily differentiates the two. WHD is an autosomal recessive degeneration of anterior horn cells in the spinal cord and brainstem (lower motor neuron disease). Most infants are hypotonic at birth, and all are affected by 6 months. Look for a positive family history and a long, slowly progressive disease course. Treatment is supportive only.
   Infant botulism is caused by a *Clostridium botulinum* toxin. Look for sudden onset and a history of ingestion of honey or other home-canned foods. Diagnosis is made by finding *C. botulinum* toxin or organisms in the feces. Treatment involves inpatient monitoring and support with close monitoring of respiratory status. The child may need intubation for respiratory muscle paralysis. Spontaneous recovery usually occurs within 1 week, and supportive care is all that is needed.

2. **After a history of head trauma, what does a dilated, unreactive pupil on one side mean until proven otherwise?**

In the setting of head trauma, a dilated, unreactive pupil on one side most likely represents impingement of the ipsilateral CN III and impending uncal herniation caused by increased intracranial pressure. Of the different intracranial hemorrhages, this scenario is seen most commonly with epidural hemorrhage. Do *not* perform a lumbar puncture in any patient with a "blown" pupil, because this procedure may precipitate uncal herniation and death. Instead, order a CT or MRI scan of the head. Emergency management includes hyperventilation, hyperosmolar therapy (mannitol or hypertonic saline), and emergency neurosurgery consultation for decompression.

3. **List the four classic signs of a basilar skull fracture.**
   1. Periorbital ecchymosis ("raccoon eyes")
   2. Postauricular ecchymosis (Battle sign)
   3. Hemotympanum (blood behind the eardrum)
   4. CSF otorrhea or rhinorrhea (leakage of CSF that is clear in appearance from the ears or nose)

4. **What is the imaging test of choice for skull fractures of the calvarium? How are they managed?**

Skull fractures of the calvarium (roof of the skull) are best seen on a CT scan (preferred over plain x-rays). Surgical indications include contamination (surgical cleaning and debridement), depression with impingement on the brain parenchyma, or open fracture with CSF leakage. Otherwise, such fractures can be observed and generally heal on their own.

5. **True or false: Severe, permanent neurologic deficits may occur after head trauma, even with a negative CT or MRI scan of the head.**

True. Head trauma can cause cerebral contusion or shear injury of the brain parenchyma, both of which may not show up on a CT or MRI scan but may cause temporary or permanent neurologic deficits.

6. **What finding suggests increased intracranial pressure?**

Increased intracranial pressure (intracranial hypertension) is highly suggested in the setting of bilaterally dilated and fixed pupils. Normal intracranial pressure is between 5 and 15 mm Hg. Less specific symptoms include headache, papilledema, nausea and vomiting, and mental status changes. Look also for the classic Cushing triad, which consists of increasing blood pressure, bradycardia, and respiratory irregularity.

7. **How should increased intracranial pressure be managed?**

The first step is to intubate the patient in the reverse Trendelenburg position (head up). Once intubated, the patient should be hyperventilated to rapidly lower the intracranial pressure via a decrease in intracranial blood volume (because of cerebral vasoconstriction). For longer-term treatment, **mannitol** diuresis can be tried to lessen cerebral edema. Furosemide is also used but is less effective. Ventriculostomy should be performed if hydrocephalus is identified. Barbiturate coma and decompressive craniotomy (burr holes) are last-ditch measures. Anticonvulsant therapy should be started if seizures are suspected; prophylactic anticonvulsant administration is controversial but may be warranted in some cases.

Remember that cerebral perfusion pressure equals blood pressure minus intracranial pressure. In other words, do *not* treat hypertension initially in a patient with increased intracranial pressure because hypertension is the body's way of trying to increase cerebral perfusion. Lowering the blood pressure in this setting may worsen symptoms or even cause a stroke.

8. **True or false: Lumbar puncture is the first test that should be performed in a patient with increased intracranial pressure.**

False. *Never* perform a lumbar puncture in any patient with signs of increased intracranial pressure until a CT scan is done first. If the CT scan is negative, you can proceed to a lumbar puncture, if needed. If you perform a lumbar puncture first, you may precipitate uncal herniation and death.

9. **What symptoms do patients with spinal cord trauma exhibit? How are they managed?**

Patients with spinal cord trauma often exhibit spinal shock (loss of reflexes and motor function) and neurogenic shock (hypotension caused by decreased catecholamine release if the lesion is higher in the cord). Order standard trauma radiographs (cervical spine, chest, pelvis) and additional spine radiographs or CT scans according to the physical examination. Moderate hypothermia is increasingly used in the management of patients with spinal cord trauma. Surgery is performed for incomplete neurologic injury (some residual function maintained) with external compression (e.g., subluxation, bone chip). An MRI scan can reveal cord injury noninvasively. For patients with neurogenic shock, early vasopressor use should be considered to replace the lack of endogenous catecholamines.

10. **What causes spinal cord compression? What symptoms do patients exhibit?**
Spinal cord compression is usually acute or subacute. Most cases of acute cord compression result from trauma. Look for the appropriate history. Subacute compression is often due to metastatic cancer but may also result from a primary neoplasm, subdural or epidural abscess (classically seen in diabetics and caused by *Staphylococcus aureus*), or hematoma (especially after a lumbar puncture or epidural/spinal anesthesia in a patient with a bleeding disorder or a patient on anticoagulation therapy).
   Patients present with local spinal pain (especially with bone metastases) and neurologic deficits below the lesion (e.g., hyperreflexia, positive Babinski sign, weakness, sensory loss).

11. **How should patients with subacute spinal cord compression be diagnosed and treated?**
The first step in the emergency department is to give high-dose corticosteroids and order an MRI scan (preferred over CT). If the cause is cancer or tumor, give local radiation if the metastases are from a known primary tumor that is radiosensitive. Surgical decompression can be used if the tumor is not radiosensitive. For a hematoma or subdural/epidural abscess, surgery is indicated for decompression and drainage. Prognosis is related most closely to pretreatment function; the longer you wait to treat, the worse the prognosis.

DISORDERS OF THE EYE

1. **What cause should be attributed for bitemporal hemianopsia until proven otherwise?**
A pituitary tumor (or other neoplasm) pressing on the optic chiasm.

2. **Use the visual field defect to localize the site of the brain lesion (Fig. 2-5).**

VISUAL FIELD DEFECT	LESION LOCATION
Right anopsia (monocular blindness)	Right optic nerve
Bitemporal hemianopsia	Optic chiasm
Left homonymous hemianopsia	Right optic tract
Left upper quadrant anopsia	Right optic radiations in the right temporal lobe
Left lower quadrant anopsia	Right optic radiations in the right parietal lobe
Left homonymous hemianopsia with macular sparing	Right occipital lobe (from posterior cerebral artery occlusion)

3. **How do you distinguish between benign and serious causes of a CN III deficit?**
For benign causes (e.g., hypertension and diabetes) of a CN III palsy, the pupil is normal in size and reactive; no treatment is needed. For serious causes (e.g., aneurysm, tumor, or uncal herniation), the pupil is dilated and nonreactive ("blown"). Urgent diagnosis and treatment are required. Additional neurologic symptoms also indicate a serious cause.
   The first step for serious cases is to obtain a CT or MRI scan of the head. Careful observation is preferred in benign cases, but if the patient does not improve within a few months or does not have hypertension or diabetes, you should order a CT or MRI scan of the head just in case.

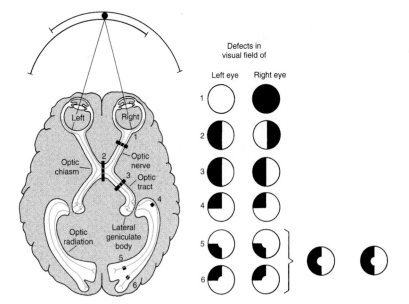

Figure 2-5. Visual field defects produced by lesions at various levels of the visual pathway. *1*, Right optic nerve; *2*, optic chiasm; *3*, optic tract; *4*, Meyer loop; *5*, cuneus; *6*, lingual gyrus; *bracket*, occipital lobe (with macular sparing). (*From Berne R et al. Physiology. 5th ed. Philadelphia: Mosby, 2003, Fig. 8-10.*)

4. **Describe the classic presentation of retinoblastoma.**
   Retinoblastoma classically presents in a child younger than 3 years with leukocoria (the pupillary red reflex changes to white) and/or unilateral exophthalmos. It may be bilateral in the inherited form.

5. **What is the hallmark of conjunctivitis?**
   Hyperemia of the conjunctival vessels.

6. **Distinguish among allergic, viral, and bacterial conjunctivitis in terms of the signs and symptoms and treatment.**

ETIOLOGY	SIGNS AND SYMPTOMS	TREATMENT
Allergic	Itching, bilateral, seasonal, long duration	Vasoconstrictors or topical antihistamines/mast cell destabilizers
Viral*	Preauricular adenopathy, highly contagious (look for affected contacts); clear, watery discharge	Supportive, hand washing to prevent spread
Bacterial	Purulent discharge; classic in neonates	Topical antibiotics with or without systemic antibiotics

*The leading viral cause is adenovirus.

7. **True or false: Conjunctivitis frequently causes loss of vision.**
   False. Other than transient blurriness (caused by tear film debris) that resolves with blinking, conjunctivitis should not affect vision. If vision is affected, think of other, more serious conditions.

8. **Define glaucoma. What are the risk factors for developing it? What are the two general types?**

    Glaucoma is best thought of as ocular hypertension (or elevated intraocular pressure, measured with a tonometer); its effects include visual field defects and blindness. The risk factors are age older than 40 years, black race, and positive family history. The two main types are open-angle and closed-angle glaucoma.

9. **Describe the physical findings for open-angle glaucoma. How common is it and how is it treated?**

    Open-angle glaucoma causes 90% of the cases of glaucoma; it is painless and does not involve acute attacks. The only signs are elevated intraocular pressure (usually 20 to 30 mm Hg), gradually progressive loss of visual field, and optic nerve changes (increased cup-to-disc ratio on funduscopic examination). Treatment may involve several different classes of medications, including beta-blockers, prostaglandins, alpha-adrenergic agonists, carbonic anhydrase inhibitors, and cholinergic agonists, as well as laser therapy and surgery. Although patients can have open-angle glaucoma with a normal intraocular pressure, for purposes of the USMLE, patients will always have elevated intraocular pressure.

10. **How does closed-angle glaucoma present? What should you do if you recognize it?**

    Closed-angle glaucoma presents with sudden ocular pain, seeing halos around lights, red eye, high intraocular pressure (>30 mm Hg), nausea and vomiting, sudden decreased vision, and a fixed, middilated pupil. It is an ophthalmologic emergency. Treat the patient immediately with **pilocarpine** and oral glycerin and/or acetazolamide to break the attack. Definitive surgery (peripheral iridectomy) is used to prevent further attacks. In rare cases, anticholinergic medications can trigger an attack of closed-angle glaucoma in a susceptible, previously untreated patient. Medications do not cause acute attacks in patients with open-angle glaucoma or in patients with surgically treated closed-angle glaucoma.

11. **How do steroids affect the eye?**

    Steroids, whether topical or systemic, can cause glaucoma and cataracts. Topical ocular steroids can worsen ocular herpes and fungal infections. For the Step 3 exam, do *not* give topical ocular steroids, especially if the patient has a dendritic corneal ulcer that is stained green by fluorescein. Such an ulcer represents herpes.

12. **Define ultraviolet keratitis. How is it treated?**

    Exposure to ultraviolet light can cause keratitis (corneal inflammation) with pain, foreign body sensation, red eye, tearing, and decreased vision. Patients have a history of welding, using a tanning bed or sunlamp, or snow skiing ("snow blindness"). Treat with an eye patch (for 24 hours) and a topical antibiotic. You can reduce pain with an anticholinergic eye drop that causes paralysis of the ciliary muscle (cycloplegia).

13. **What pediatric rheumatologic condition is commonly associated with uveitis?**

    Uveitis is common in juvenile rheumatoid arthritis (especially the pauciarticular form). Patients with juvenile rheumatoid arthritis need periodic ophthalmologic examination to check for uveitis.

14. **What is the most common cause of painless, slowly progressive loss of vision?**

    Cataracts, especially in the elderly. Treatment is surgical removal of the affected lens(es) and replacement with an artificial lens.

15. **What should cataracts in a neonate suggest?**

    Cataracts in a neonate may indicate a TORCH (toxoplasmosis, other [e.g., syphilis, HIV], rubella, cytomegalovirus, and herpes simplex virus) infection or an inherited metabolic disorder (the classic example is galactosemia).

16. **What changes in the retina and fundus are seen in diabetes and hypertension?**

    Diabetes is associated with dot-blot hemorrhages, microaneurysms, and neovascularization of the retina. **Hypertension** is associated with arteriolar narrowing, copper/silver wiring, and cotton-wool spots. Papilledema may be seen with severe hypertension and should alert you to the presence of a hypertensive emergency.

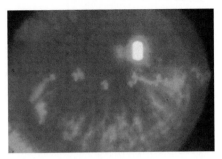

Figure 2-6. Varicella dendritic keratitis. Numerous dendrites are seen in this slit-lamp photograph with fluorescein staining of the dendritic lesions from active viral growth in the corneal epithelium. See Plate 2. (*From Krachmer JH et al. Cornea. 3rd ed. Philadelphia: Mosby, 2010, Figure 80.2.*)

17. **What is the most common cause of blindness in patients younger and older than 55 years and in black patients?**

    In the United States, diabetes is the leading cause of blindness in younger adults, and senile macular degeneration (look for macular drusen) is the most common cause of blindness in adults older than 55 years. Glaucoma is the leading cause of blindness in blacks of any age and is ranked third as the overall cause of blindness in the United States.

18. **Define proliferative diabetic retinopathy. How is it treated? How is nonproliferative diabetic retinopathy treated?**

    Proliferative diabetic retinopathy occurs after many years of established diabetes and is defined as the development of neovascularization (new, abnormal growth of vessels in the retina). Treatment involves application of a laser beam to the periphery of the entire retina (**panretinal photocoagulation**). Surgical or medical vitrectomy in used in some cases. Medical therapy for proliferative diabetic retinopathy is investigational but is used in some circumstances. The most promising therapeutics are vascular endothelial growth factor (VEGF) inhibitors (bevacizumab, ranibizumab, pegaptanib).

    Focal laser treatment is common for nonproliferative (background) retinopathy when macular edema is present; the laser is applied only to the affected area. In severe cases, panretinal photocoagulation may be used. Otherwise, nonproliferative retinopathy is treated supportively, primarily with tight control of blood glucose and follow-up eye examinations to watch for the development of macular edema or neovascularization.

19. **What is the key to managing chemical burns to the eye? Which is worse, acid or alkaline burns?**

    For chemical burns to the eye (acid or alkaline), the key to management is copious irrigation with the closest source of water. The longer you wait, the worse the prognosis. Do not wait to obtain additional history. Alkali burns have a worse prognosis because they tend to penetrate more deeply into the eye.

20. **Distinguish between a hordeolum (stye) and a chalazion. How are they treated?**

    A hordeolum is a painful red lump near the eyelid margin. A chalazion is a painless lump away from the eyelid margin. Treat both with warm compresses. For chalazions, use intralesional steroid injection or incision and drainage if warm compresses do not work.

21. **How do you recognize and treat herpes simplex keratitis?**

    Herpes simplex keratitis usually begins with conjunctivitis and vesicular lid eruption and then progresses to the classic dendritic keratitis (seen with fluorescein stain; Fig. 2-6). Treat with topical antivirals (e.g., idoxuridine, trifluridine). Corticosteroids are generally contraindicated in dendritic keratitis because they may make the condition worse.

22. **What findings suggest an ophthalmic herpes zoster infection?**

    Ophthalmic herpes zoster infection should be suspected in patients with involvement of the tip of the nose (Hutchinson sign) and/or medial eyelid, a typical zoster dermatomal skin rash, and eye complaints. Treat with oral acyclovir. Complications include uveitis, keratitis, and glaucoma.

23. **How do you recognize a central retinal artery occlusion? What causes it?**
Central retinal artery occlusion presents with sudden (within a few minutes) and painless unilateral loss of vision. The classic funduscopic appearance includes a pale, opaque fundus with a cherry red spot in the fovea (center) of the macula. No satisfactory treatment is available. The most common cause is emboli (from carotid plaque or heart), but watch for temporal arteritis as a cause on the Step 3 examination.

24. **Describe the symptoms of temporal arteritis. What should you do if you suspect it?**
Temporal arteritis is a vasculitis seen in older adults. Symptoms include jaw claudication, loss of vision (caused by central retinal artery occlusion), a tortuous temporal artery (as seen or palpated on examination), a markedly elevated erythrocyte sedimentation rate, and coexisting **polymyalgia rheumatica** (in 50%; causes proximal muscle pain and stiffness). If temporal arteritis is suspected in the setting of vision complaints, administer corticosteroids immediately before confirming the diagnosis with a temporal artery biopsy. Withholding of treatment until a formal diagnosis can be made may cause the patient to lose vision in the other eye.

25. **How do you recognize central retinal vein occlusion? Describe the cause and treatment.**
Central retinal vein occlusion also presents with sudden (within a few hours) and painless unilateral loss of vision. The classic funduscopic appearance includes distended, tortuous retinal veins; retinal hemorrhages; and a congested, edematous fundus. This is referred to as a "blood and thunder" appearance given the drastic funduscopic findings. No satisfactory treatment is available. The most common causes are hypertension, diabetes, glaucoma, and increased blood viscosity (e.g., leukemia). Complications are related to neovascularization, which commonly develops and leads to vision loss and glaucoma.

26. **Describe the classic history of a patient with retinal detachment.**
The classic history of a patient with retinal detachment includes sudden (instant) and painless unilateral loss of vision with "floaters" (small black spots that are seen no matter where the patient looks) and flashes of light. It is sometimes described as a "curtain or veil coming down in front of my eye." This history should prompt immediate referral to an ophthalmologist. Surgery may save the patient's vision by reattaching the retina.

27. **True or false: Cataracts and macular degeneration are common causes of bilateral painless loss of vision in older adults.**
True. Although one side may be worse than the other, bilateral complaints are not uncommon. The red reflex typically becomes black in the case of a significant cataract. Individuals with macular degeneration typically have focal yellow-white deposits called **drusen** in and around the macula on funduscopic examination. Treat cataracts with surgery; most cases (90%) of macular degeneration are the "dry" or nonexudative, subtype, which is treated supportively (e.g., magnification aids). "Wet" or exudative, macular degeneration is treated with intravenous VEGF inhibitors, thermal laser photocoagulation in selected patients, and photodynamic therapy.

28. **How do optic neuritis and papillitis present? What are the common causes?**
Optic neuritis and papillitis typically present with fairly quick (over hours to days) and painful unilateral or bilateral loss of vision. The optic disc margins may appear blurred on funduscopic examination, with papillitis, just as in papilledema.
    Multiple sclerosis (which can also cause internuclear ophthalmoplegia) is a very common cause of optic neuritis, especially in 20- to 40-year-old women. Lyme disease, malignancy, and syphilis are other causes.

29. **What is strabismus? Beyond what age is it abnormal in children?**
Strabismus is the medical term for a "lazy eye." The affected eye deviates, most commonly inward. Strabismus is normal only if intermittent and during the first 3 months of life. When strabismus is constant or persistent beyond 3 months, it requires ophthalmologic referral to prevent blindness (known as amblyopia) in the affected eye.

30. **Why does blindness develop in patients with strabismus?**
The visual system is still developing until the age of 7 or 8 years. For this reason, visual screening of both eyes is important in children. If one eye does not see well or is turned outward, the brain cannot fuse the two different images that it sees. Thus it suppresses the "bad" eye, which does not develop the proper neural connections. This eye will never see well and cannot be corrected with glasses because the problem is neural rather than refractive. This problem is treatable with special glasses or surgery if it is caught in time; the goal of treatment is to allow normal neural connections (and thus vision) to develop.

31. **What is presbyopia? When does it occur?**
Presbyopia occurs between the ages of 40 and 50 years, when the lens loses its ability to accommodate. Patients then need bifocal or reading glasses for near vision. Presbyopia is a normal part of aging.

DISORDERS OF THE EAR

1. **Describe how otitis externa typically presents. What causes it?**
Patients have erythematous, swollen skin in the auditory canal and pain on manipulation of the auricle. A foul-smelling discharge and conductive hearing loss may also be present. Swimming is a known risk factor for otitis externa (inflammation of the outer ear). It is most often due to infection with *Pseudomonas aeruginosa.* Treat with topical antibiotics (e.g., ofloxacin, neomycin, polymyxin B) and possibly topical steroids to reduce swelling.

2. **What causes otitis media? How do you recognize it?**
Otitis media (inflammation of the middle ear) is an extremely common pediatric infection, most often due to infection with *Streptococcus pneumoniae*, *H. influenzae*, or *Moraxella catarrhalis*. Patients have no pain on manipulation of the auricle; positive symptoms include earache, fever, erythematous and bulging tympanic membranes (the light reflex and landmarks are difficult to see on otoscopy), and nausea and vomiting.

3. **What are the complications of otitis media? How are they avoided?**
Complications include tympanic membrane perforation (bloody or purulent discharge), mastoiditis (fluctuance and inflammation over the mastoid process roughly 2 weeks after the onset of otitis media), labyrinthitis, palsies of CN VII and VIII, meningitis, cerebral abscess, dural sinus thrombosis, and chronic otitis media (because of permanent perforation of the tympanic membrane). Patients with chronic otitis media may develop cholesteatomas with marginal perforations that require surgical excision.
Otitis media is generally treated with antibiotics to avoid these complications (e.g., amoxicillin, second-generation cephalosporin such as cefuroxime, or a macrolide).

4. **What is the problem with recurrent otitis media? How is it treated?**
Recurrent otitis media is a common pediatric problem (along with prolonged secretory otitis, a result of incompletely resolved otitis media) and can cause hearing loss with resultant developmental problems (speech, cognitive functions). Treat with prophylactic antibiotics or tympanostomy tubes. Adenoidectomy is controversial but may help in some cases; it is thought to help prevent blockage of the eustachian tubes.

5. **What causes infectious myringitis? How do you recognize and treat it?**
Infectious myringitis, also known as *bullous myringitis*, is an inflammation of the tympanic membranes that can be diagnosed when otoscopy reveals vesicles on the tympanic membrane. Infectious myringitis is classically caused by *Mycoplasma* species, but *S. pneumoniae* or a virus may also be the culprit. Treat with erythromycin or clarithromycin to cover *Mycoplasma* species and *S. pneumoniae*.

6. **What are the common causes of hearing loss?**
The most common cause is **aging** (presbyacusis); prescribe a hearing aid if needed. The history may suggest other causes:
• Prolonged or intense exposure to loud noise (e.g., work related)
• Congenital TORCH infection

- Ménière disease (accompanied by severe vertigo, tinnitus, nausea and vomiting; treat acute episodes with benzodiazepines, anticholinergics [scopolamine], and antihistamines [meclizine or dimenhydrinate]; diuretics are often used for ongoing treatment; surgery may be used for refractory cases)
- Drugs (e.g., aminoglycosides, aspirin, quinine, loop diuretics, cisplatin)
- Tumor (classically, acoustic neuroma)
- Labyrinthitis (may be viral or follow or extend from meningitis or otitis media)
- Miscellaneous causes (diabetes, hypothyroidism, multiple sclerosis, sarcoidosis, pseudotumor cerebri)

7. In what situations should you worry about hearing loss?
- A bout of meningitis (hearing loss is the most common neurologic complication)
- Congenital TORCH infections
- Measles or mumps
- Chronic middle ear effusions or chronic or recurrent otitis media
- Use of ototoxic drugs (e.g., aminoglycosides)

8. Define otosclerosis. How is it treated?
In otosclerosis, the otic bones become fixed together and impede hearing. Otosclerosis is the most common cause of progressive conductive hearing loss in adults, whereas presbyacusis is the most common cause of sensorineural hearing loss in adults. Treat with a hearing aid or surgery.

9. What is the Weber test used to evaluate? How is it performed and interpreted?
The Weber test compares bone conduction in the two ears. A vibrating tuning fork is placed on the forehead and the patient is asked where the vibrating sound is heard best. The normal response is to hear the vibration in the middle (or equally in both ears). Patients with conductive hearing loss hear the sound best in the affected ear, whereas patients with sensorineural hearing loss hear the sound best in the unaffected ear.

10. What is the Rinne test used to evaluate? How is it performed and interpreted?
The Rinne test compares air conduction with bone conduction. A vibrating tuning fork is placed on the tip of the mastoid process. When the patient can no longer hear the sound, the tuning fork is removed from the mastoid and placed next to the auditory meatus of the external ear and the patient is asked if the sound can be heard.

Because air conduction is normally greater than bone conduction, patients can hear the tuning fork when it is placed next to the auditory meatus (air conduction) even after they can no longer hear it vibrating on the mastoid (bone conduction). In patients with conductive hearing loss, bone conduction is greater than air conduction; thus they cannot hear the tuning fork when it is placed next to the external auditory meatus. In patients with sensorineural hearing loss, both air and bone conduction are impaired, but the normal ratio (air conduction greater than bone conduction) is maintained. Thus patients still hear the tuning fork next to the ear after they can no longer hear it on the mastoid.

11. What is the usual cause of sudden deafness?
Sudden sensorineural hearing loss (SSNHL) involves acute unexplained hearing loss that is usually unilateral and occurs over hours (usually <72 hours). More than 90% of patients with SSNHL report tinnitus. Most cases are idiopathic but have been postulated to be attributable to viral causes, microvascular events, or autoimmune causes. Physical examination is unremarkable. MRI is indicated to rule out causes such as acoustic neuroma, multiple sclerosis, and vascular insufficiency. Glucocorticoids (administered orally or by intratympanic injection) are considered first-line therapy; antiviral agents are sometimes used, although there is not much evidence to support their use. Two thirds of patients will experience recovery, although the resolution is often not complete. Among those who recover, hearing usually returns within 2 weeks.

12. What is the most common cause of acquired hearing loss in children?
Bacterial meningitis. All children should undergo formal hearing testing after a bout of meningitis.

13. What are the common causes of vertigo?
Vertigo can result from the same CN VIII lesions that cause hearing loss (Ménière disease, tumor, infection, multiple sclerosis). Another common cause is benign positional

(paroxysmal) vertigo, which is induced by certain head positions, may be accompanied by nystagmus, and is not associated with hearing loss. This condition often resolves spontaneously; no treatment is required. The Epley maneuver, or modified Epley maneuvers, may help with resolution of symptoms. Ruling out central vertigo is an important distinction. For testing purposes, peripheral vertigo (more benign) has severe symptoms that last for a short time and are positional. For central vertigo (more serious, such as a cerebellar stroke), patients will have symptoms that are less severe, last for a longer duration, and are not particularly positional.

14. **Describe the function of CN VIII. What symptoms do lesions cause?**
    CN VIII (the vestibulocochlear nerve) is needed for hearing and balance. Lesions can cause deafness, tinnitus, and/or vertigo. In children, think of meningitis as a cause. In adults, symptoms may be due to a toxin or medication (e.g., aspirin, aminoglycosides, loop diuretics, cisplatin), infection (labyrinthitis), tumor, or stroke.

DISORDERS OF THE RESPIRATORY SYSTEM

CHAPTER 3

1. **What should you know about pulmonary function in the setting of surgery?**
   A baseline chest radiograph is not part of the standard preoperative evaluation but is often used for patients older than 60 years or patients with known pulmonary or cardiovascular disease. Preoperative pulmonary function testing is somewhat controversial, and the question will probably not appear in the Step 3 exam. Overall, the best indicator of possible postoperative pulmonary complications is preoperative pulmonary function. The best way to reduce pulmonary complications postoperatively is to advise patients to **stop smoking** preoperatively, especially if stopped at least 8 weeks before surgery. Aggressive pulmonary toilet, incentive spirometry, minimal narcotic administration, and early ambulation help to prevent or minimize postoperative pulmonary complications. Lastly, remember that the most common cause of a postoperative fever in the first 24 hours is atelectasis.

2. **Describe the effect of smoking on the lung.**
   Lung cancer and chronic obstructive pulmonary disease (COPD) are typically due to smoking. If the patient is very young or has no smoking history, you should consider **alpha$_1$-antitrypsin deficiency** as the cause of COPD. Although the changes of COPD are irreversible, the risk of death still decreases if the patient stops smoking.

3. **What about second-hand smoke?**
   It has been proven that second-hand smoke is a risk factor for lung cancer and other lung disease. The risk increases linearly with exposure. For parents who smoke, their children are at increased risk of asthma and upper respiratory tract infections, including otitis media, if exposed to second-hand smoke.

4. **What other bad effects does smoking have?**
   Smoking retards the healing of peptic ulcer disease, and cessation stops the development of **Buerger disease** (Raynaud symptoms in young male smokers). Smoking by a pregnant woman increases the risk of low birth weight, prematurity, spontaneous abortion, stillbirth, and infant mortality. Cessation of smoking preoperatively is the best way to decrease the risk of postoperative pulmonary complications, especially if smoking is stopped at least 8 weeks before surgery.

OBSTRUCTIVE AIRWAYS DISEASE

1. **What is the most common lethal genetic disease in whites? How do you recognize it?**
   Cystic fibrosis, which is an autosomal recessive disease. Always suspect cystic fibrosis in pediatric patients with rectal prolapse, meconium ileus, esophageal varices, recurrent pulmonary infections, or failure to thrive. The classic complaint reported by the mother is a "salty-tasting" baby. Patients also commonly have pancreatic insufficiency and infertility (98% of affected males and 50% of females); they also may develop cor pulmonale (right-sided heart failure).

2. **How is cystic fibrosis diagnosed and treated?**
   Diagnosis is made on the basis of an abnormal increase in electrolytes (sodium and chloride) in the patient's sweat and/or DNA testing. Treat with chest physical therapy, annual influenza vaccination, fat-soluble vitamin supplements, pancreatic enzyme replacement, bronchodilators, dornase alfa (DNA-cleaving enzyme that helps to clear pulmonary secretions), and aggressive treatment of infections with antibiotics that cover *Staphylococcus*, *Haemophilus influenzae*, and *Pseudomonas* spp.

3. **What is COPD? What are the risk factors for COPD?**

   Chronic obstructive pulmonary disease (COPD) is a lung disease characterized by persistent (not fully reversible) airflow limitation that is usually progressive and associated with an enhanced chronic inflammatory response in the airways and lungs to noxious particles and gases. Risk factors for COPD include cigarette smoking, second-hand smoke exposure, occupational dust and chemical exposure, advancing age, low socioeconomic status, and specific gene variants.

4. **What historical features should make you think of COPD? How do you diagnose COPD?**

   Look for the three cardinal symptoms of dyspnea, chronic cough, and sputum production in a middle-aged or older patient who has a smoking history. COPD is suspected clinically but is diagnosed by spirometry. Diagnosis requires a value of greater than 0.70 for the forced expiratory volume in 1 second (FEV_1) divided by the forced vital capacity (FVC). Classification of the severity of COPD (Gold stages 1 to 4) is based on airflow limitation as measured by FEV_1.

5. **What do you need to think of if you have a young patient with COPD?**

   If you have a patient younger than 45 years with minimal smoke exposure, think of alpha$_1$-antitrypsin deficiency.

6. **What are the treatment goals for chronic stable COPD? What are the treatment options?**

   The main treatment goals for stable COPD are symptom relief, improved exercise tolerance, prevention of disease progression, prevention of exacerbations, and reduced mortality. The general medication classes used to treat COPD are short-acting beta$_2$-agonists (e.g., albuterol), long-acting beta$_2$-agonists (e.g., salmeterol, formoterol), short-acting anticholinergics (e.g., ipratropium), long-acting anticholinergics (e.g., tiotropium), and inhaled corticosteroids (e.g., beclomethasone, fluticasone, budesonide). The selective phosphodiesterase-4 inhibitor roflumilast can be used in selected patients. Oxygen can be given to patients who are chronically hypoxemic. Do not forget to provide influenza and pneumococcal vaccinations for all patients with COPD.

7. **What is a COPD exacerbation? How is it treated?**

   A COPD exacerbation is an acute event characterized by worsening of respiratory symptoms beyond the normal day-to-day variations in a patient with COPD. It is most commonly caused by a viral infection of the upper respiratory tract. A chest x-ray is usually ordered to assess other contributing factors (e.g., pneumonia). The decision to hospitalize is based on the patient's overall status. Treatment includes a short-acting inhaled beta$_2$-agonist (albuterol) with a short-acting inhaled anticholinergic drug (ipratropium). Patients should also be given systemic steroids, typically prednisone 40 mg daily for 5 days. Antibiotics are indicated for patients with increased dyspnea, sputum volume, and sputum purulence, as well as those who have a need for mechanical ventilation. Oxygen is provided as needed.

8. **Describe the difference between obstructive and restrictive pulmonary disease on pulmonary function testing.**

   In COPD, FEV_1/FVC is less than the normal value (the normal value [0.75 to 0.80] should be given in the question). In restrictive lung disease, FEV_1/FVC is often normal. FEV_1 may be equal in both conditions, but the FEV_1/FVC ratio is always different.

9. **How do you recognize and treat asthma?**

   Watch for chronic wheezing in "allergic" children with a family history of asthma or allergies. In the acute setting, treat with a beta$_2$-agonist (albuterol). Use steroids if the attack is severe or does not respond to beta$_2$-agonists. Inhaled glucocorticoids (preferred agent), leukotriene modifiers (zafirlukast, montelukast, zileuton), long-acting beta-agonists, and cromolyn are prophylactic agents and are not used for acute attacks. Phosphodiesterase inhibitors (theophylline, aminophylline) are older agents that are now infrequently used. Do *not* prescribe beta-blockers for asthmatics or patients with COPD; they block the beta$_2$-receptors that are needed to open the airways.

10. **What is the concern regarding the use of long-acting beta-agonists (LABAs) in the treatment of asthma?**

    The U.S. Food Drug Administration (FDA) has recommended that LABAs should not be used as **solo** agents in the treatment of asthma in children or adults because of an increased risk of death. The advisory recommends that LABAs not be used alone as initial therapy for asthma of any severity, that they not be added when asthma control is actively deteriorating, that they only be used long term in patients whose asthma cannot be adequately controlled with other asthma controller medications, and that the LABA be discontinued, if possible, once asthma control is achieved. However, a LABA plus an inhaled corticosteroid does not carry this increased risk of death.

11. **What should you think if a patient with acute asthma stops hyperventilating or has a normal carbon dioxide (CO_2) level?**

Beware the asthmatic who is no longer hyperventilating or whose CO_2 is normal or rising. The patient should be hyperventilating, which causes low CO_2. If the patient seems calm or sleepy, do *not* assume that he or she is "okay." Such patients are probably crashing; they need an immediate arterial blood gas analysis and possible intubation. Fatigue alone is sufficient reason to intubate. Remember also that any patient with COPD may normally live with a higher CO_2 and lower oxygen (O_2) level. Treat the patient, not the laboratory value. If the patient is asymptomatic and talking to you, the laboratory value should not cause panic.

12. **When should you intubate?**

The four indications for intubation are (1) failure to ventilate, (2) failure to oxygenate, (3) expected clinical course, and (4) failure to protect airway. As a rough rule of thumb, think about intubation in any patient whose CO_2 is greater than 50 mm Hg or whose O_2 is less than 50 mm Hg, especially if the pH in either situation is less than 7.30 while the patient is breathing room air. Usually, unless the patient is crashing rapidly, a trial of oxygen via a nasal cannula or face mask is given first. If this does not work or if the patient becomes too tired (use of accessory muscles is a good clue to the work of breathing), intubate. Clinical correlation is always required; patients with chronic lung disease may be asymptomatic at laboratory value levels that seem to defy reason. Alternatively, laboratory values may look great, but if the patient is becoming tired from increased work of breathing, intubation may be needed because of the expected clinical course. Intubation is also indicated in obtunded or otherwise altered patients who are at risk of aspiration.

PNEUMOCONIOSIS/FIBROSING OR RESTRICTIVE PULMONARY DISORDERS

1. **What is sarcoidosis? What symptoms do patients exhibit?**

Sarcoidosis is a multisystem granulomatous disorder of unknown cause. Affected individuals exhibit bilateral hilar lymphadenopathy, pulmonary reticular opacities, and skin, joint, and/or eye lesions. Sarcoidosis is three to four times more common in black populations and typically affects young adults. In approximately half of cases it is detected in asymptomatic patients because of incidental radiographic abnormalities. In symptomatic patients, look for fever, cough, malaise, dyspnea, chest pain, weight loss, and arthritis. The features of sarcoidosis can be remembered by the mnemonic GRUELING: **g**ranulomas, **r**heumatoid arthritis, **u**veitis, **e**rythema nodosum, **l**ymphadenitis, **i**nterstitial fibrosis, **n**egative purified protein derivative (PPD), **g**ammaglobulinemia. Look for bilateral hilar lymphadenopathy and/or infiltrates on chest x-ray. Hypercalcemia is common. Pulmonary function tests reveal a restrictive or mixed restrictive-obstructive pattern.

2. **How is the diagnosis made?**

Sarcoidosis is a diagnosis of exclusion. Evaluate for other causes such as lymphoma, tuberculosis, HIV, fungal infection, and idiopathic pulmonary fibrosis. Do a complete physical examination and order a chest x-ray, pulmonary function tests (PFTs), complete blood count (CBC), serum chemistries including calcium, serum angiotensin-converting enzyme (ACE) level (classically elevated), urinalysis, electrocardiogram (ECG), PPD, and ophthalmologic evaluation. PFTs typically show a restrictive pattern. Diagnosis is made on the basis of a tissue biopsy revealing noncaseating granulomas without organisms.

3. **How is sarcoidosis treated?**

Most cases of sarcoidosis do not require treatment because patients are often asymptomatic and nonprogressive and some experience spontaneous remission. Treat symptomatic patients with prednisone.

4. **What is pneumoconiosis?**

A pneumoconiosis is an interstitial lung disease that results from dust inhalation and is almost always occupational. The main types of pneumoconiosis are coal worker's pneumoconiosis, asbestosis, and silicosis. Look for a patient with chronic shortness of breath, the right occupational exposure, a restrictive pattern on PFTs, and a chest x-ray revealing patchy, subpleural, bibasilar interstitial infiltrates or honeycombing.

5. **What is asbestosis? What are the symptoms? With what malignancy is asbestos exposure associated?**

Asbestosis is pneumoconiosis caused by inhalation of asbestos fibers that results in a slowly progressive pulmonary fibrosis. There is usually a latency period of 20 to 30 years between exposure and the development of symptoms, most commonly dyspnea with exertion. There is usually no cough, wheezing, or sputum production. Asbestos exposure is associated with an increased risk of mesothelioma, which is discussed in more detail later in this chapter.

6. **How is asbestosis diagnosed? What is the treatment?**

Asbestosis is a clinical diagnosis based on a history of exposure, certain findings on high-resolution chest computed tomography (CT), the presence of interstitial fibrosis, and the absence of other causes of parenchymal lung disease. There is no specific treatment, but supportive measures should be instituted. These include avoidance of further exposure to asbestos, smoking cessation, pneumococcal and influenza vaccines, and oxygen supplementation if needed.

7. **What symptoms do patients with pulmonary fibrosis exhibit?**

Interstitial lung diseases (ILDs) are a heterogeneous group of disorders that result in pulmonary fibrosis. Look for progressive dyspnea with exertion, a persistent nonproductive cough, a history of appropriate occupational exposure (e.g., dust, chemicals), a history of connective tissue disease, an abnormal chest x-ray, and/or lung function abnormalities on spirometry. On examination, look for pulmonary crackles and clubbing of the digits.

8. **How do you evaluate suspected pulmonary fibrosis?**

The workup is quite involved because of all of the possible causes of pulmonary fibrosis. Most patients should have a CBC, a chemistry panel, liver function tests, creatine kinase, urinalysis, chest x-ray and high-resolution CT of the chest, PFTs, and bronchoalveolar lavage. Other typical laboratory tests include rheumatoid factor, antibodies against cyclic citrullinated peptide, antinuclear antibody, antisynthetase antibody, aldolase, scleroderma antibodies, and Sjögren antibodies.

RESPIRATORY FAILURE AND PULMONARY VASCULAR DISEASE

1. **How do you recognize pulmonary hypertension? How is pulmonary hypertension diagnosed?**

Look for exertional dyspnea, lethargy, and fatigue. Peripheral edema, exertional chest pain, and exertional syncope may be present in more advanced cases in which right ventricular hypertrophy and failure are present. Many cases of pulmonary hypertension can be diagnosed by echocardiography. If the diagnosis is in doubt, proceed to right-sided heart catheterization and look for a mean pulmonary artery pressure greater than or equal to 25 mm Hg at rest.

2. **What are the causes of pulmonary hypertension? How is each treated?**

There are five main causes of pulmonary hypertension, and treatment with diuretics, oxygen, anticoagulation, digoxin, and exercise can be considered for all five groups. The five causes are:

1. **Idiopathic.** Primary therapy is typically ineffective, and advanced therapies are usually required.
2. **Secondary to left-sided heart disease.** Treat the underlying heart disease.
3. **Secondary to hypoxemia** from causes such as COPD, ILD, and sleep-disordered breathing. Treat the underlying cause.
4. **Thromboembolic disease.** Treat with anticoagulation.
5. **Multifactorial mechanisms** such as hematologic disorders (e.g., myeloproliferative disorders) and systemic disorders (e.g., sarcoidosis).

3. **How do you recognize and treat adult respiratory distress syndrome (ARDS)?**
   ARDS results from acute lung injury and causes noncardiogenic pulmonary edema, respiratory distress, and hypoxemia. Common causes are sepsis, major trauma, pancreatitis, shock, near-drowning, and drug overdose. Look for ARDS to develop within 24 to 48 hours of the initial insult. The classic patient has mottled/cyanotic skin, intercostal retractions, rales or rhonchi, and no improvement in hypoxia on oxygen administration. Radiographs show pulmonary edema with a normal cardiac silhouette (no cardiomegaly). Treat with intubation, mechanical ventilation with low tidal volumes (6 to 8 mL/kg), and high positive end-expiratory pressure (PEEP) while addressing the underlying cause (if possible).

4. **What is the most common cause of fever in the first 24 hours after surgery?**
   Atelectasis. Prevent and treat atelectasis with early ambulation, chest physiotherapy/percussion, incentive spirometry, and proper pain control. Too much pain or excessive narcotic administration (both can decrease respiratory effort) increase the risk of atelectasis.

5. **In what clinical settings does pulmonary embolus (PE) occur? Describe the symptoms and signs.**
   PE commonly follows deep vein thrombosis, delivery (amniotic fluid embolus), or long bone fractures (fat emboli). The classic patient has had recent surgery or immobilization (long car/plane ride) or has an active malignancy. Symptoms include tachypnea, dyspnea, chest pain, hemoptysis (if a lung infarct has occurred), hypotension, syncope, or death in severe cases. In rare instances, the chest radiograph shows a wedge-shaped defect due to a pulmonary infarct.

6. **How is PE diagnosed?**
   Use a CT pulmonary angiogram or ventilation/perfusion (V/Q) scan if CT is not available to evaluate for PE. If the test is positive, PE is diagnosed and treatment is started. If the test is indeterminate, a conventional pulmonary angiogram can be used to confirm the diagnosis. Conventional pulmonary angiography is the gold standard, but it is invasive and carries substantial risks. If a CT angiogram or V/Q scan is negative, it is highly unlikely that the patient has a significant PE so no treatment is needed. In the setting of a low-probability V/Q scan and high clinical suspicion, a CT angiogram or conventional pulmonary angiogram is needed.

7. **How is PE treated?**
   PE is treated initially with low–molecular-weight heparin or intravenous unfractionated heparin to prevent further clots and emboli. Then the patient is switched gradually to oral warfarin, which must be taken for at least 3 to 6 months. Direct thrombin inhibitors (dabigatran) and factor Xa inhibitors (rivaroxaban) are emerging treatment modalities but are less likely to be tested on the USMLE. In patients with recurrent clots on anticoagulation or contraindications to anticoagulation, an inferior vena cava filter (e.g., Greenfield filter) should be used. In patients with massive PE, embolectomy (surgical or catheter embolectomy) or pharmacologic thrombolysis (e.g., giving tissue plasminogen activator) may be attempted.

UPPER RESPIRATORY TRACT CONDITIONS

1. **What are the three common causes of rhinitis?**
   Viral, allergic, and bacterial infection.

2. **How do you recognize and treat viral rhinitis?**
   Viral rhinitis (the common cold) may be due to rhinovirus (the most common cause), influenza, parainfluenza, Coxsackie virus, adenovirus, respiratory syncytial virus (RSV), coronavirus, or echovirus. Treatment involves relief of symptoms. Vasoconstrictors such as phenylephrine can be used for short-term symptomatic relief, but they may cause rebound congestion when discontinued.

3. **How do you recognize and treat allergic rhinitis?**
   Allergic rhinitis (hay fever) is associated with seasonal flare-ups, boggy and bluish turbinates, onset before 20 years of age, nasal polyps, sneezing, pruritus, conjunctivitis, wheezing or

asthma, eczema, positive family history, eosinophils in nasal mucous, and elevated serum immunoglobulin E. Skin tests may identify an allergen. Treat with avoidance of known antigens (e.g., pollen). Antihistamines, nasal steroids, and/or cromolyn may be used for more severe symptoms. Desensitization is also an option.

4. **What are the common bacterial causes of sinusitis? How is this condition recognized clinically?**
   Sinusitis is often due to *Streptococcus pneumoniae*, *H. influenzae*, or other streptococcal or staphylococcal species. Look for tenderness over the affected sinuses, headache, and a purulent nasal discharge (yellow or green). Associated symptoms are headache and/or toothache (maxillary sinusitis). Radiograph or CT used to confirm the diagnosis and show opacification of the sinus, classically with an air-fluid level in acute sinusitis; CT scans are preferred to evaluate chronic sinusitis or suspected extension of infection outside the sinus (watch for high fever and chills). Treat with antibiotics (amoxicillin, trimethoprim-sulfamethoxazole, a second- or third-generation cephalosporin, a macrolide, or amoxicillin clavulanate for 10 to 14 days or for up to 6 weeks in chronic cases). Culture is usually not necessary unless the patient fails to respond to antibiotics. Operative intervention (drainage procedure, sinus obliteration) may be required for resistant cases.

5. **When do the sinuses develop in children?**
   The maxillary and ethmoid sinuses are present at birth and continue to grow through adolescence. The frontal sinus begins to develop around the age of 7 years and continues through adolescence. The sphenoid sinus does not begin to develop until adolescence.

6. **How is a deviated nasal septum treated in patients with recurrent bacterial sinusitis?**
   Surgical correction.

7. **What causes nosebleeds?**
   The most common cause of nosebleed is trauma; for example, nose picking is a common cause in children. Also watch out for the following causes:
   - Local tumor (nasopharyngeal angiofibroma; seen in adolescent boys with no history of trauma or blood dyscrasia; signs include recurrent nosebleeds and/or obstruction)
   - Leukemia (from pancytopenia; typically in children with associated fever and anemia)
   - Other causes of thrombocytopenia (e.g., idiopathic thrombocytopenic purpura, hemolytic uremic syndrome)

8. **How do you recognize a nasal fracture? What complication may result?**
   A nasal fracture can be seen on radiographs or CT scans. Watch for a septal hematoma, which must be removed surgically to prevent pressure-induced septal necrosis.

9. **What are the symptoms of streptococcal pharyngitis? How do you diagnose and treat it?**
   Look for a sore throat with fever, tonsillar exudate, enlarged tender cervical nodes, and leukocytosis. A positive streptococcal throat culture confirms the diagnosis. Elevated titers of antistreptolysin O (ASO) and anti-DNase antibody can be used for a retrospective diagnosis in patients with rheumatic fever or poststreptococcal glomerulonephritis. Treat streptococcal pharyngitis with penicillin, amoxicillin, cephalosporin, macrolide, or clindamycin to avoid rheumatic fever and scarlet fever.

10. **What are the symptoms of peritonsillar abscess?**
    A peritonsillar abscess (PTA) typically has symptoms of severe sore throat, fever, and a muffled voice. Drooling may be present and patients often have trismus. On examination, look for a swollen and fluctuant tonsil with deviation of the uvula to the opposite side.

11. **How is PTA evaluated and treated?**
    PTA is a clinical diagnosis by history and physical examination. No specific testing may be required. Bedside ultrasound can confirm the presence of a PTA, and definitive treatment is needle aspiration or incision and drainage. PTAs are usually polymicrobial, so clindamycin is usually the preferred agent. In otherwise healthy patients, once a PTA is drained, the patient can be discharged on oral antibiotics.

In cases that are not as straightforward, CT of the neck with IV contrast may be required to confirm the diagnosis and/or establish the presence of other diagnoses (e.g., retropharyngeal abscess). Throat swabs for rapid group A streptococcal (GAS) antigen or a throat culture can confirm the presence of GAS, but will not rule in or out PTA.

NEOPLASMS

1. **How should you manage a patient with a solitary pulmonary nodule on a chest radiograph?**
   The first step is comparison with previous chest radiographs (if available). If the nodule has remained the same size for more than 2 years, it is very unlikely to be cancer. CT scans are used to evaluate and follow a solitary pulmonary nodule. A nodule that has a low probability of being malignant can be followed with serial CT scans.
   A nodule that has increased in size on serial imaging should be biopsied or excised. If no old films are available and the patient is older than 35 years or has more than a 5-year history of smoking, obtain a CT scan (and possibly a positron emission tomography [PET] scan). PET scans are generally used to evaluate nodules of intermediate probability. If the nodule is not definitely benign, get a biopsy of the nodule (via bronchoscopy or transthoracic needle biopsy, if possible) for tissue diagnosis.
   If the patient is younger than 35 years or has no smoking history, the cause is most likely infection (tuberculosis or fungi), hamartoma, or collagen vascular disease. The patient should undergo a CT scan and careful observation, with follow-up imaging in 3 to 6 months. Investigate for infection if the history is suspicious.

2. **What classic clues in the Step 3 exam point to the cause of a solitary pulmonary nodule?**
   - Immigrant: think of tuberculosis; do a skin test.
   - Southwest United States exposure: think of *Coccidioides immitis*.
   - Cave explorer, exposure to bird droppings or Ohio/Mississippi River valleys (Midwest): think of histoplasmosis.
   - Smoker older than 50 years: think of lung cancer; order bronchoscopy and biopsy.
   - Person younger than 40 years with none of the previous indications: think of hamartoma.

3. **What clinical vignette should make you suspect lung cancer?**
   The classic clue is a change in the chronic cough of a smoker. The more pack years of tobacco use, the more suspicious you should be. Patients may also exhibit hemoptysis, pneumonia, or weight loss. The chest radiograph may show a mass or pleural effusion. Put a needle in the fluid and examine for malignant cells.

4. **How do you diagnose and treat lung cancer?**
   As with all cancers, you need a tissue biopsy (e.g., via bronchoscopy, CT-guided biopsy, open-lung biopsy) to confirm malignancy and to define the histologic type. Non–small-cell lung cancer may be treated with surgery if the cancer remains within the lung parenchyma (i.e., without involvement of the opposite lung, pleura, chest wall, spine, or mediastinal structures). Early metastases of small-cell lung cancer make surgery inappropriate. Small-cell lung cancer and extensive non–small-cell lung cancer are treated with chemotherapy with or without radiation. A platinum-containing chemotherapy regimen (e.g., cisplatin) is typically used.

5. **What consequences can result from an apical (Pancoast) lung cancer?**
   Horner syndrome: from invasion of the cervical sympathetic chain. Look for unilateral ptosis, miosis, and anhidrosis (no sweating).
   Superior vena cava syndrome: caused by compression of the superior vena cava with impaired venous drainage. Look for edema and plethora (redness) of the neck and face and central nervous system symptoms (headache, visual symptoms, and altered mental status).
   Unilateral diaphragm paralysis: from phrenic nerve involvement (apical tumor not required); will result in an elevated hemidiaphragm on chest x-ray.
   Hoarseness: from recurrent laryngeal nerve involvement (apical tumor not required).

6. What is a paraneoplastic syndrome? What are the commonly tested paraneoplastic syndromes of lung cancer?

A paraneoplastic syndrome is a condition caused by a malignancy but not directly by destruction or invasion by tumor. Classic examples in lung cancer are as follows:

Cushing syndrome: from production of adrenocorticotropic hormone (histologic type: small-
cell carcinoma).

Syndrome of inappropriate antidiuretic hormone secretion (SIADH): from production of
antidiuretic hormone (histologic type: small-cell carcinoma).

Hypercalcemia: from production of parathyroid-like hormone (histologic type: squamous-
cell carcinoma).

Eaton-Lambert syndrome: myasthenia-gravis–like disease from lung cancer that spares the
ocular muscles. The muscles become stronger with repetitive stimulation, which is the
opposite of myasthenia gravis (histologic type: small-cell carcinoma).

7. What are the symptoms of mesothelioma? What is the typical x-ray finding? How
is mesothelioma diagnosed?

Look for gradual-onset chest pain, dyspnea, cough, fatigue, and weight loss, particularly in a
patient with a history of asbestos exposure. A chest x-ray typically reveals a unilateral pleural
abnormality with a large unilateral pleural effusion. Perform thoracentesis and send the fluid
for cytology. Pleural biopsy is usually indicated to establish a tissue diagnosis.

8. What two points do you need to know about nasopharyngeal cancer?

This condition usually is seen in Asians and is associated with **Epstein-Barr virus.**

9. What cancers are more likely in smokers?

Smoking increases the risk of cancers of the lung (smoking causes 85% to 90% of cases);
oral cavity (90% of cases); esophagus (70% to 80% of cases); larynx, pharynx, bladder
(30% to 50% of cases); kidney (20% to 30%); pancreas (20% to 25%); cervix, stomach,
colon, and rectum.

LUNG INFECTIONS

1. Cover up the right-hand column in the following table and describe the preferred
treatment for tuberculosis on the basis of the clinical scenario.

CLINICAL SETTING/FINDINGS	TREATMENT
Exposed adult with negative PPD skin test	None
Exposed child <5 yr of age with negative PPD	Isoniazid (INH) for 3 mo, then repeat PPD
Prophylaxis for PPD conversion (negative to positive), no active disease	INH for 9 mo
Active pulmonary disease/positive culture	INH/rifampin/pyrazinamide/ethambutol for 2 mo, then INH/rifampin for 4 mo in most patients

PPD, Purified protein derivative.

2. Name some other important tuberculosis treatment issues.

- Multidrug-resistant strains are an increasing problem and require four-drug therapy (pyrazinamide, isoniazid, ethambutol, and rifampin) in most circumstances.
- If the patient is noncompliant, directly observed therapy (someone watches the patient
take medications every day) is recommended.
- Consider supplementation with vitamin B_6 (pyridoxine) for patients on isoniazid (INH) or
watch for signs of deficiency such as neuropathy, confusion, angular cheilitis, and a seborrheic dermatitis-like rash.
- Watch for liver dysfunction in patients on therapy. Patients should be advised to abstain
from alcohol while on treatment and should have their transaminase levels monitored.

3. **How is pneumonia diagnosed?**
   The diagnosis of pneumonia is usually based on clinical findings (fever and rales or rhonchi) plus an elevated white blood cell count and an abnormal chest radiograph consistent with pneumonia. For patients being admitted to the hospital, sputum and blood cultures are usually obtained before empiric antibiotic therapy is begun.

4. **What is the difference between typical and atypical pneumonia?**
   Typical pneumonia is usually caused by bacteria such S. *pneumoniae* (most common), *H. influenzae*, and *Moraxella catarrhalis*. Atypical pneumonia may be caused by influenza virus, *Mycoplasma*, *Chlamydia* spp., *Legionella*, or adenovirus. Pneumonia is also divided into treatment categories on the basis of where it was acquired: community-acquired pneumonia, health-care–associated pneumonia (for outpatients with extensive health-care contact), hospital-acquired pneumonia (develops after 48 hours as an inpatient), and ventilator-associated pneumonia (develops after 48 hours on a ventilator).

	TYPICAL PNEUMONIA	**ATYPICAL PNEUMONIA**
Prodrome	Short (<2 days)	Long (>3 days) (headache, malaise, body aches)
Fever	High (>102° F [38.9° C])	Low (<102° F [38.9° C])
Age	>40 yr	<40 yr
Chest radiograph	One distinct lobe involved	Diffuse or multilobe involvement
Bug	*Streptococcus pneumonia*	Many (*Haemophilus, Mycoplasma, Chlamydia* spp.)
Antibiotic*	Ceftriaxone, broad spectrum	Macrolides (e.g., azithromycin), doxycycline, or certain fluoro-quinolones (e.g., levofloxacin, moxifloxacin)

*Avoid the temptation to pull out the "bigger gun" antibiotics (very wide spectrum, potent) unless the patient is crashing or unstable.

5. **What are the classic clinical clues in the Step 3 exam for the different causative organisms in pneumonia?**
   College student: think of *Mycoplasma* spp. (look for cold agglutinins) or *Chlamydia* spp.
   Alcoholic: think of *Klebsiella* spp. ("currant jelly" sputum), *Staphylococcus aureus*, and other enteric organisms (aspiration).
   Cystic fibrosis: think of *Pseudomonas* spp. or *S. aureus*.
   Immigrant: think of tuberculosis.
   COPD: think of *H. influenzae* or *Moraxella* spp.
   Known tuberculosis with pulmonary cavitation: think of *Aspergillus* spp.
   Silicosis: (metal, granite, pottery workers) think of tuberculosis.
   Exposure to air conditioner or aerosolized water: think of *Legionella* spp.
   HIV/AIDS: think of *Pneumocystis jirovecii* or cytomegalovirus (if you are shown koilocytosis).
   Exposure to bird droppings: think of *Chlamydia psittaci* or histoplasmosis.
   Child younger than 1 year: think of RSV.
   Child 2 to 5 years of age: think of parainfluenza (croup).

6. **What should you suspect if a child has recurrent pneumonias?**
   If the pneumonia always occurs in the same spot (especially the right middle and/or right lower lobe), it is probably due to foreign body aspiration. Remember that a foreign body is most likely to go down the right mainstem bronchus. This diagnosis should be considered especially if the child has no other signs of immunodeficiency (e.g., other types of infection, symptoms of cystic fibrosis) before or during the episodes. If immunodeficiency is the cause of recurrent pneumonia, the child should have a history of chronic bilateral lung problems and other types of infection.

7. **What is "round" pneumonia?**

Pneumonia may appear round, typically in children, which causes it to simulate a mass. In such cases involving children, assume pneumonia and treat appropriately. A follow-up x-ray can be obtained to confirm resolution, which is not usually required in children, who almost never develop lung malignancies. In an adult, a round pneumonia should be viewed with suspicion (more likely to be a malignancy) and further workup with a CT scan is typically employed.

8. **Why should you order a follow-up chest x-ray for all people older than 40 years who develop pneumonia?**

A follow-up chest x-ray is routine in those older than 40 years who develop pneumonia to make sure the condition clears after appropriate antibiotic treatment. If pneumonia does not clear by 4 to 6 weeks, suspect something other than bacterial pneumonia. The classic culprit is malignancy, specifically **bronchoalveolar carcinoma**, which is a subtype of adenocarcinoma. In addition, recurrent pneumonia in the same location in an adult may be due to an endobronchial mass, whether benign or malignant.

9. **What is the most common cause of pneumonia? What are the classic symptoms?**

Streptococcus pneumoniae is the most common cause. Look for rapid onset of shaking chills after 1 to 2 days of symptoms of an upper respiratory tract infection (sore throat, runny nose, dry cough), followed by fever, pleurisy, and productive cough (yellowish-green or rust-colored from blood), especially in older adults. Chest radiographs show lobar consolidation (Fig. 3-1) and the white blood cell count is high with a large percentage of neutrophils. Treat with a macrolide (e.g., azithromycin, clarithromycin), doxycycline, third-generation cephalosporin, or a fluoroquinolone that provides atypical coverage (e.g., levofloxacin, moxifloxacin).

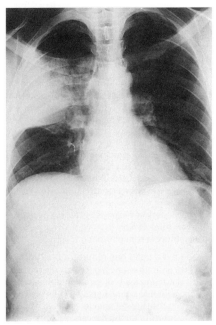

Figure 3-1. Pneumococcal pneumonia with lobar consolidation. (*From Mason RJ, Broaddus VC, Martin TR et al. Murray and Nadel's textbook of respiratory medicine. 5th ed. Philadelphia: Saunders, 2010, Fig. 32-1.*)

10. **What is the best prevention against *S. pneumoniae*?**

Vaccination is the best prevention. Give pneumococcal vaccine to all children, as well as adult patients older than 65 years, splenectomized patients, patients with sickle cell disease (who have autosplenectomy) or splenic dysfunction, immunocompromised patients (HIV, malignancy, organ transplant), and all patients with chronic disease (e.g., diabetes, cardiac disease, asthma and other pulmonary disease, renal disease, liver disease, or tobacco use).

11. **How do you recognize and treat *H. influenzae* pneumonia?**

H. influenzae is now uncommon in children because of vaccination but is still an important cause of pneumonia in the elderly and in those with underlying lung disease such as COPD. It often resembles pneumococcal pneumonia clinically, but look for gram-negative coccobacilli on a sputum Gram stain. Treat with amoxicillin or a second- or third-generation cephalosporin.

12. **Describe the hallmarks of *S. aureus* pneumonia.**

S. aureus tends to cause hospital-acquired (nosocomial) pneumonia and pneumonia in patients with cystic fibrosis (along with *Pseudomonas* spp.), intravenous drug abusers, and patients with chronic granulomatous disease (look for recurrent lung abscesses). Empyema and lung abscesses are relatively common with *S. aureus* pneumonia.

13. **In what clinical situations do you tend to see gram-negative pneumonias?**

Pseudomonas infection is classically associated with cystic fibrosis, *Klebsiella* infection with alcoholics and those who are homeless (watch for the classic description of "currant jelly" sputum), and infection by enteric gram-negative organisms (e.g., *Escherichia coli*) with aspiration, neutropenia, and hospital-acquired pneumonia. These pneumonias often have a high mortality rate because of the type of patient affected and the severity of the pneumonia (abscesses are common). Treat empirically with an antipseudomonal penicillin (e.g., ticarcillin, piperacillin) with or without a beta-lactamase inhibitor (e.g., clavulanate, tazobactam). Alternatives include ceftazidime and ciprofloxacin.

14. **How do you recognize *Mycoplasma* pneumonia?**

Mycoplasma infection is most common in adolescents and young adults (the classic patient is a college student or soldier who lives in a dormitory/barracks and has sick contacts). It is one of the atypical pneumonias because the symptoms differ from those for a typical pneumonia caused by *S. pneumoniae*. For example, *Mycoplasma* pneumonia has a long prodrome with gradual worsening of malaise, headaches, a dry nonproductive cough, and sore throat; the fever tends to be low grade. Chest radiographs show a patchy, diffuse bronchopneumonia that classically looks terrible, although the patient often does not feel that bad. Look for positive titers for **cold-agglutinin antibodies**, which may cause hemolysis or anemia. Atypical pneumonia is treated empirically with a macrolide antibiotic (azithromycin), doxycycline, or a broad-spectrum fluoroquinolone (e.g., levofloxacin or moxifloxacin).

15. **What about chlamydial pneumonia?**

Chlamydia is second only to *Mycoplasma* as the cause of atypical pneumonia in adolescents and young adults. It has similar symptoms but has negative cold-agglutinin antibody titers. Treat with erythromycin in children younger than 8 years of age and either azithromycin or doxycycline in children older 8 years of age, adolescents, and adults.

16. **What kind of pneumonia should you suspect in a homeless alcoholic patient?**

Aspiration pneumonia. Look for enteric organisms (anaerobes, *E. coli*, streptococci, staphylococci) as the cause. Think of *Klebsiella* spp. if the sputum resembles currant jelly or thick mucoid capsules are mentioned in culture reports.

17. **How do you recognize *P. jirovecii* pneumonia (PCP)?**

For the Step 3 exam, think of PCP first in any patient with HIV and pneumonia, even though community-acquired pneumonia is more common, even in patients with AIDS. Look for severe hypoxia with normal radiographs or diffuse, bilateral interstitial infiltrates (Fig. 3-2). Patients usually have a dry, nonproductive cough. PCP may be detected with silver stains (Wright-Giemsa, Giemsa, or methenamine silver) applied to induced sputum; if not, you can use bronchoscopy with bronchoalveolar lavage and brush biopsy to make the diagnosis. High levels of lactate dehydrogenase are suspicious in the appropriate setting. PCP is now usually treated presumptively (typically with trimethoprim-sulfamethoxazole),

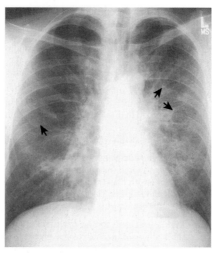

Figure 3-2. Posteroanterior chest radiograph of a HIV-seropositive patient with *Pneumocystis* pneumonia showing bilateral, predominantly perihilar, granular opacities and three pneumatoceles (*arrows*). Pneumatoceles may predispose patients to pneumothorax. (*Reproduced with permission from L. Huang.*)

with diagnostic testing reserved for those in whom the diagnosis is unclear or initial treatment fails. Corticosteroids are added in the treatment of suspected PCP in patients with (1) hypoxemia on pulse oximetry, (2) PaO_2 less than or equal to 70 mm Hg on room air, or (3) an alveolar-arterial gradient greater than or equal to 35 mm Hg for arterial blood gas (ABG).

18. **In what setting do you see PCP and cytomegalovirus (CMV) pneumonia?**
   In HIV-positive patients with CD4 counts less than 200/mm³ (AIDS) and other severely immunosuppressed patients (e.g., organ transplant recipients taking powerful immuno-suppressants or patients on cancer chemotherapy). In AIDS, PCP is the most common opportunistic pneumonia and may require bronchoalveolar lavage for diagnosis. PCP can be seen with silver stains and typically causes bilateral interstitial lung infiltrates. Treat with trimethoprim-sulfamethoxazole with or without corticosteroids. CMV pneumonia is characterized by intracellular inclusion bodies. Treat with valganciclovir.

19. **What is the best time to treat PCP?**
   Before it happens! PCP is acquired when the CD4 count is less than 200/mm³. At that point you should institute PCP prophylaxis with trimethoprim-sulfamethoxazole in HIV-positive patients. Alternatives include dapsone and atovaquone.

20. **What is a common cause of wheezing in children younger than 2 years of age?**
   RSV infection, which classically occurs in the winter and causes a fever. Asthma may also be the cause but is usually associated with a chronic history.

21. **What are the "big three" respiratory infections in patients younger than 5 years?**
   Croup, epiglottitis, and RSV infection (bronchiolitis). These three diseases are of high yield on the USMLE.

22. **How do you recognize croup (acute laryngotracheobronchitis)? Describe the cause and treatment.**
   Look for a child of 1 to 2 years of age. Croup usually occurs in the fall or winter. Some 50% to 75% of cases are due to infection with parainfluenza virus; the other common causative agent is influenza virus. The disease begins with symptoms of viral upper respiratory tract infection (e.g., rhinorrhea, cough, fever). Roughly 1 to 2 days later, patients develop a "barking" cough, hoarseness, and inspiratory stridor. The **steeple sign** (describes subglottic narrowing of the trachea; Fig. 3-3) is classic on a frontal radiograph of the chest or neck. Treat with dexamethasone, racemic epinephrine, and humidified oxygen.

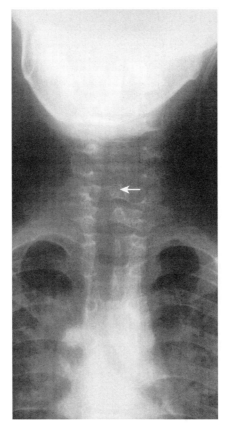

Figure 3-3. Anteroposterior radiograph of the neck region of child with croup. Note the steeple sign *(white arrow)*. *(From Wetmore RF. Pediatric otolaryngology: the requisites in pediatrics. 1st ed. Philadelphia: Mosby, 2007, Fig. 11-1.)*

23. **How do you recognize epiglottitis? Describe the cause and treatment.**
    Epiglottitis usually occurs in children aged 2 to 5 years. The main cause is *Haemophilus influenzae* type b; widespread vaccination has significantly reduced the incidence of this condition. *S. aureus, Streptococcus pyogenes,* and *S. pneumoniae* are other potential causes. Look for little or no prodrome, with rapid progression to high fever, toxic appearance, drooling, and respiratory distress with no coughing. The **thumb sign** (describes a swollen, enlarged epiglottis; Fig. 3-4) is classic on lateral radiographs of the neck. Do not examine the throat or irritate the child in any way. You may precipitate airway obstruction. When a case of epiglottitis is diagnosed, the first step is to be prepared to establish an airway (intubation and, if needed, tracheostomy). Treat with a combination of oxacillin or cefazolin or clindamycin or vancomycin plus cefotaxime or ceftriaxone.

24. **Describe the classic clinical vignette for bronchiolitis. What is the cause? How is it treated?**
    Bronchiolitis generally affects children aged 0 to 18 months and usually occurs in the fall or winter. More than 75% of cases are caused by RSV; other causes are parainfluenza and influenza viruses. Patients first develop symptoms of viral upper respiratory tract infection, followed 1 to 2 days later by rapid respirations, intercostal retractions, and expiratory wheezing. The child may have crackles on auscultation of the chest. Diffuse hyperinflation of the lungs is classic on chest radiographs; look for a flattened diaphragm.

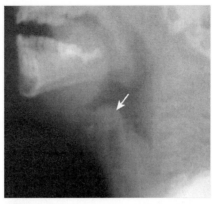

Figure 3-4. Lateral neck radiograph demonstrating epiglottis with the thumb sign. (*From Zaoutis LB, Chiang VW. Comprehensive pediatric hospital medicine. 1st ed. Philadelphia: Mosby, 2007, Fig. 66-3.*)

Treat supportively (e.g., oxygen, bronchodilators, intravenous fluids). Use ribavirin only in patients with severe symptoms or at high risk (e.g., patients with cyanosis or other chronic health problems).

25. **What "old school" pediatric infection causes pseudomembranes and myocarditis? What about whooping cough?**
    Diphtheria (*Corynebacterium diphtheriae*) and pertussis (*Bordetella pertussis*). Diphtheria is quite uncommon in the United States because of mandatory vaccination. Pertussis was uncommon, but the incidence has been increasing significantly over the last 20 years. If a child is not immunized (e.g., child of immigrants), do not forget these two entities. Diphtheria causes grayish pseudomembranes (necrotic epithelium and inflammatory exudate) on the pharynx, tonsils, and uvula, as well as myocarditis. Pertussis is associated with severe paroxysmal coughing and a high-pitched whooping inspiratory noise (traditionally called whooping cough), particularly in children and especially those younger than 1 year. Treat diphtheria with antitoxin and either penicillin or erythromycin. Treat pertussis with azithromycin or erythromycin.

TRAUMA AND TOXIC EFFECTS

1. **How are patients managed after a nonfatal drowning episode?**
   Some (not all) physicians believe that fresh water is worse than salt water in drownings, because aspirated fresh water can cause hypervolemia, electrolyte disturbances, and hemolysis. Intubate patients after a near-drowning episode if they are unconscious, and monitor arterial blood gases if they are conscious. Patients who drown in cold water often do better than those who drown in warm water because of decreased metabolic needs. Death is usually due to hypoxia and/or cardiac arrest.

2. **What six thoracic injuries can be rapidly fatal?**
   1. Airway obstruction
   2. Open pneumothorax (also known as a *sucking chest wound*)
   3. Tension pneumothorax
   4. Cardiac tamponade
   5. Massive hemothorax
   6. Flail chest
   You may be asked to recognize and/or treat any of these six conditions on the USMLE.

3. **How do you recognize and treat airway obstruction?**
   Patients with airway obstruction have no audible breath sounds, cannot answer questions even if awake, and may be gurgling. Treat with intubation. If intubation fails, perform a cricothyroidotomy (or a tracheostomy in the operating room if time allows).

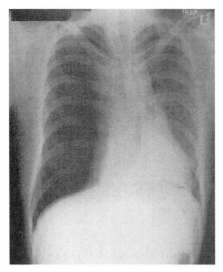

Figure 3-5. Radiograph of tension pneumothorax. The right hemithorax is dark (lucent) because the mediastinum has shifted to the left. (*From Marx JA. Rosen's emergency medicine. 7th ed. Philadelphia: Mosby, 2009, Fig. 75-3*).

4. **How do you recognize and treat an open pneumothorax?**
   An open pneumothorax (sucking chest wound) is an open defect in the chest wall with decreased or absent breath sounds on the affected side. This condition causes poor ventilation and oxygenation. Treat with closure of the defect in the chest wall by applying an occlusive dressing and taping it on three sides only. This creates a one-way valve that allows excessive pressure to escape so that you do not convert an open pneumothorax into a tension pneumothorax.

5. **How do you recognize and treat a tension pneumothorax?**
   A tension pneumothorax may occur after blunt or penetrating trauma to the chest. Air forced into the pleural space cannot escape and collapses the affected lung, and then shifts the mediastinum and trachea to the opposite side of the chest (Fig. 3-5). Findings include absent breath sounds on the affected side and a hypertympanic percussion sound. Hypotension and/or distended neck veins may result from impaired cardiac filling. Treat with needle thoracostomy followed by insertion of a chest tube.

6. **Define massive hemothorax. How is it diagnosed and treated?**
   Massive hemothorax is defined as a loss of more than 1.5 L of blood into the thoracic cavity. Patients have decreased (not absent) breath sounds in the affected area, a dull note on percussion, hypotension, collapsed neck veins (from blood leaving the vascular tree), and tachycardia. Placement of a chest tube allows the blood to come out. Give intravenous fluids and/or blood before you place the chest tube if the diagnosis is known in advance. If the bleeding stops after the initial outflow, order a chest radiograph or CT scan to check for remaining blood or pathology. Treat supportively. In cases of massive hemothorax or if the bleeding does not stop, emergent thoracotomy is required.

7. **How do you recognize and treat flail chest?**
   Flail chest occurs when several adjacent ribs are broken in multiple places, causing the affected part of the chest wall to move paradoxically during respiration (inward during inspiration, outward during expiration). Almost all patients have an associated pulmonary contusion, which, combined with pain, may make respiration inadequate. When you are in doubt or the patient is not doing well, intubate and give positive-pressure ventilation.

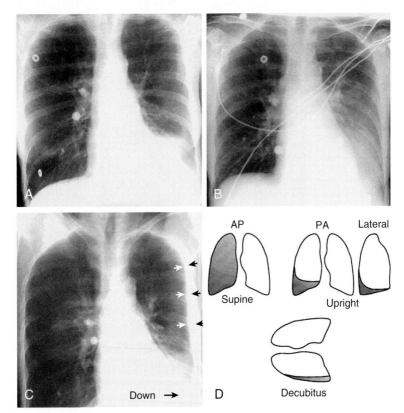

Figure 3-6. The appearance of pleural effusions depends on patient position. **A,** On an upright posteroanterior chest x-ray, a large left-sided pleural effusion obscures the left hemidiaphragm, the left costophrenic angle, and the left cardiac border. **B,** On a supine anteroposterior view, the fluid runs posteriorly, causing a diffuse opacity over the lower two thirds of the left lung while the left hemidiaphragm remains obscured. This can easily mimic an infiltrate or atelectasis of the left lower lobe. **C,** With a left lateral decubitus view, the left side of the patient is dependent and the pleural effusion is seen as freely moving and layering (*arrows*) along the lateral chest wall. **D,** These findings are also shown diagrammatically for a right-sided pleural effusion. (*From Mettler FA Jr. Essentials of radiology. 2nd ed. Philadelphia: Saunders, 2004, Fig. 3-80.*)

8. **What clues suggest a diagnosis of diaphragmatic rupture? How is it treated?**
   Diaphragm rupture usually occurs after blunt trauma and on the left side (because the liver protects the right side of the diaphragm). You may hear bowel sounds when listening to the chest or see bowel that has herniated into the chest on a chest radiograph. Treatment is surgical repair of the diaphragm.

9. **How should a choking victim be managed?**
   Always leave choking patients alone if they are speaking, coughing, or breathing. If they stop doing all of these, perform the Heimlich maneuver.

10. **What should you do if a patient has a pleural effusion?**
    If you do not know the cause of the effusion (Fig. 3-6), consider thoracocentesis to examine the fluid in an attempt to determine its cause. Common tests ordered for pleural fluid include a Gram stain, culture and sensitivity testing (including tuberculosis culture), a cell count with differential, glucose (low with infection), protein (high with infection), cytology (to look for malignancy), amylase (if pancreatitis is a suspected cause of effusion), triglycerides (if a chylous effusion is suspected), albumin, and lactate dehydrogenase (the last two tests help to determine whether the fluid is an exudate or transudate).

CHAPTER 4

CARDIOVASCULAR DISORDERS

1. **What is the most common cause of syncope? What other conditions should you consider that mimic syncope?**

   Vasovagal syncope is the most common cause and is classically seen after stress or fear. Arrhythmias and orthostatic hypotension are also common. Always remember to consider hypoglycemia as a cause. The other main categories to worry about are as follows:

   1. Cardiac problems (arrhythmias, hypertrophic cardiomyopathy, valvular disease, tamponade) Always check an electrocardiogram (ECG). Further testing with echocardiography or treadmill stress testing can be performed according to the ECG findings and degree of suspicion.
   2. Neurologic disorders (e.g., seizures, migraine headache, brain tumor). Consider an electroencephalogram or a computed tomography (CT) or magnetic resonance imaging (MRI) scan if the history suggests seizures or an intracranial lesion.
   3. Vascular disease (consider transient ischemic attacks or carotid stenosis, which can be ruled out with carotid artery ultrasound/duplex scanning, although this is not a common cause of syncope).
   4. Medication effects (e.g., anticholinergic agents, beta-blockers, narcotics, vasodilators, alpha-agonists, antipsychotics).

   As many as half of patients have syncope of unknown cause according to a standard diagnostic evaluation.

HYPOTENSION

1. **What class of antihypertensive agents is best known for severe, first-dose orthostatic hypotension?**

   Alpha$_1$-antagonists such as terazosin.

2. **Define shock.**

   Shock is a state in which blood flow to and perfusion of peripheral tissues are inadequate for sustaining life. Although they are not included in a rigid definition of shock, hypotension, lactic acidosis (inadequate perfusion leading to anaerobic metabolism), and oliguria or anuria (inadequate renal perfusion) are associated findings for board purposes. Tachycardia is also usually present as a compensatory response.

3. **List the four primary categories of shock.**

   Hypovolemic shock (e.g., dehydration, hemorrhage), cardiogenic shock, distributive shock (e.g., septic shock, anaphylactic shock, neurogenic shock in which vasodilation causes poor distribution of blood flow), and obstructive shock (e.g., tension pneumothorax causing impeded venous return, cardiac tamponade with poor cardiac filling due to pressure from fluid in the pericardial space).

4. **What should you do if a patient is in shock?**

   Keep the patient alive according to the ABC protocol (airway, breathing, and circulation) while you try to determine the cause of the shock. Give oxygen and fluids while you are thinking unless the patient is in congestive heart failure (CHF). If CHF is present, avoid fluids.

5. **How should fluids be given if a patient is in shock?**

   Many patients in shock need fluid. The standard intravenous bolus is 10 to 20 mL/kg of normal saline or lactated Ringer solution; infuse 1 to 2 L as fast as it will go. Then reassess the patient to determine whether the bolus helped; positive signs include increases in blood pressure and urine output. Do *not* be afraid to give a second bolus if the first bolus leads to no improvement. You should watch for fluid overload, which may cause CHF. Make sure that no bilateral crackles can be heard on lung examination. Place a Foley catheter to ensure accurate monitoring of urine output. In the case of hemorrhagic shock, blood products are preferred over crystalloid solutions. For septic and anaphylactic shock, resuscitation with a large amount of fluid is generally required; the most recent sepsis guidelines recommend 30 mL/kg at a minimum. Neurogenic shock is due to decreased sympathetic tone, so fluids are usually not as effective as vasopressors but can be given initially.

6. **What should you do if fluid challenges fail to raise a patient's blood pressure?**
   Consider the use of vasoactive agents to increase tissue perfusion. Norepinephrine (Levophed) is the first-line treatment for septic and cardiogenic shock. Epinephrine is the first line of treatment for anaphylactic shock. Blood transfusions and source control are the mainstays of treatment for hemorrhagic shock. The use of invasive hemodynamic monitoring (e.g., central venous catheter or Swan-Ganz catheter) can help to determine the cause of the shock and guide therapeutic decisions.

7. **What are the classic parameters for each type of shock?**

TYPE OF SHOCK	CO	PCWP	SVR	SVO$_2$
Septic (early)	High	Low	Low	High
Hypovolemic	Low	Low	High	Low
Cardiogenic	Low	High	High	Low
Neurogenic	Low	Low	Low	Low
Anaphylactic	High (but can be variable)	Low	Low	Low

CO, Cardiac output; PCWP, pulmonary capillary wedge pressure; SVO$_2$, systemic venous oxygen saturation; SVR, systemic vascular resistance.

For **anaphylactic shock,** the cause is usually obvious because of a temporal relation to a common culprit.

8. **Specify the usual findings in patients with neurogenic shock.**
   Patients usually have a history of severe central nervous system trauma or hemorrhage and flushed skin. The heart rate may be normal. These patients require early vasopressors as a substitute for their endogenous sympathetic tone, which they have lost.

9. **How do you recognize septic shock?**
   Look for fever, leukocytosis (unless the patient is on chemotherapy or has an immunosuppressive condition such as AIDS), skin that is flushed and warm to the touch, and extremes of age. Start broad-spectrum antibiotics after "pan culturing" (blood, sputum, and urine cultures plus others as dictated by the history). Sepsis and septic shock are discussed in further detail in Chapter 13.

10. **What clues suggest cardiogenic shock?**
    Look for a history of myocardial infarction (MI), CHF, or chest pain. Assess patients for risk factors for coronary artery disease. Most patients have cold, clammy skin and look pale. Distended neck veins and pulmonary congestion (as demonstrated by a physical exam and/or chest radiograph) are usually present.

11. **How do you recognize hypovolemic shock?**
    Look for a history of fluid loss (hemorrhage, diarrhea, vomiting, sweating, use of diuretics, inability to drink water). Patients have cold, clammy skin and look pale. Fluid loss may be internal, as in the case of a ruptured abdominal or thoracic aortic aneurysm and obstruction or infarction of the spleen, pancreas, or bowel. The postoperative state may also lead to hypovolemic shock. Patients usually have orthostatic hypotension, tachycardia, sunken eyes, tenting of the skin, and a sunken fontanelle (young children).

12. **What clues suggest anaphylactic shock?**

    Look for a history of recent exposure to the common culprits: bee stings, peanuts, shellfish, penicillins, sulfa drugs, or any new medication. Treat with **epinephrine** and fluids. Administer oxygen, and intubate if necessary. A tracheostomy or cricothyroidotomy should be performed if laryngeal edema prevents intubation. Antihistamines are helpful primarily when the reaction is mild, but will only treat the cutaneous symptoms. Use corticosteroids, but understand that they take several hours to take effect. Monitor all patients for at least 6 hours after the initial reaction.

13. **What clues suggest pulmonary embolus as a cause of shock?**

    Look for deep venous thrombosis (DVT; positive **Homan sign** with a painful, swollen leg) or risk factors for DVT. Remember the **Virchow triad:** endothelial damage, stasis, and hypercoagulable state. Watch for postoperative status (especially after orthopedic or pelvic surgery) or a history of recent delivery (amniotic fluid embolus) or bone fractures (fat emboli). Patients classically have chest pain, tachypnea, shortness of breath, hypoxia, right-axis shift on ECG, and a positive CT pulmonary angiography or ventilation/perfusion scan. Heparin or its low–molecular-weight form should be administered to prevent further clotting and emboli. Thrombolysis with tissue plasminogen activator (t-PA) is indicated in hemodynamically unstable patients.

14. **How do you recognize pericardial tamponade as a cause of shock?**

    Look for the Beck triad: hypotension, distended neck veins, and muffled heart sounds. Look for a compatible history such as penetrating chest trauma or aortic dissection. Also consider risk factors for pericardial effusion: malignancy, pericarditis, autoimmune disease, and uremia. Perform emergent pericardiocentesis in the setting of tamponade and arrange for definitive surgical management.

15. **Explain toxic shock syndrome.**

    Toxic shock syndrome classically occurs in a woman of reproductive age who leaves her tampon in too long. Look for skin desquamation. The syndrome is caused by a *Staphylococcus aureus* toxin.

16. **What clues suggest Addison disease as a cause of shock?**

    Patients usually have a history of steroid use, hyperkalemia, and hyponatremia. Treat with steroids and large volumes of normal saline.

17. **What is the most important point to remember if a patient is in shock?**

    The ABCs. Patients in shock often need heroic measures to survive and are among the exceptions to the "wait and see" and "be conservative" rules that are usually favored by USMLE examiners. Intubate at the drop of a hat, do not feed the patient, and avoid narcotics if possible. Mental status changes are often an important clue to impending doom. Also monitor the ECG, vital signs, Swan-Ganz parameters (although these are no longer being used as much), urine output, arterial blood gas, and hemoglobin/hematocrit.

18. **Discuss the use of norepinephrine, dobutamine, dopamine, and isoproterenol to support blood pressure in the setting of shock.**

    Norepinephrine is used for its $alpha_1$-agonist effects, but it also has $beta_1$-agonist effects. It is given primarily to patients with hypotension to increase peripheral resistance so that perfusion to vital organs can be maintained. It is the first line of therapy for septic and cardiogenic shock.

    Dobutamine is a $beta_1$-agonist used to increase cardiac output by increasing contractility; it is the intensive care equivalent of digoxin.

    Dopamine affects dopamine receptors at low doses and results in selective vasodilation (the traditional use for renal perfusion has been disproven). At higher doses, its $beta_1$-agonist effects increase contractility. At the highest doses, dopamine has $alpha_1$-agonist effects and causes vasoconstriction. Note that this differential effect is debated but could still be tested. The $beta_1$-agonist activity of dopamine makes it a first-line agent for many cases of symptomatic bradycardia.

    Isoproterenol is used for its $beta_1$-agonist and $beta_2$-agonist effects in hypovolemic, septic, and cardiogenic shock.

19. What about the use of phenylephrine, epinephrine, and milrinone in the setting of shock?

Phenylephrine is used for its pure alpha$_1$-agonist effects; it is similar to norepinephrine but has no beta effects.

Epinephrine is used in patients with cardiac arrest and anaphylaxis for its alpha and beta effects.

Milrinone and **amrinone** are phosphodiesterase inhibitors. They are used in patients with refractory heart failure (they are not first-line agents) because they have a positive inotropic effect via potentiation of cyclic adenosine monophosphate (cAMP), but they cannot be used in hypotensive patients.

ISCHEMIC HEART DISEASE AND ATHEROSCLEROSIS

1. How often should you screen for hypertension?

Although there is no absolutely correct answer, all individuals should be screened roughly every 2 years, starting at the age of 3 years.

2. Define hypertension

Persistent blood pressure greater than 140/90 mm Hg. Individuals with a systolic blood pressure of 120 to 139 mm Hg or a diastolic pressure of 80 to 89 mm Hg should be considered as prehypertensive. Remember that 145/60 mm Hg is hypertension, as is 115/95 mm Hg (isolated systolic and diastolic hypertension, respectively). In grading the severity of hypertension, use the worst number, whether it is diastolic or systolic. Table 4-1 lists the 2003 Joint National Committee (JNC-7) classification. Please note that this classification system was not addressed in the updated 2013 JNC-8 classification.

3. What is the "two measurement" rule in the diagnosis of hypertension?

Blood pressure should be measured two times on each of two separate office visits before the diagnosis and pharmacologic treatment of hypertension. However, if asked, institute conservative measures and address associated comorbidities (e.g., obesity, diabetes) after the first abnormal measurement. There are a few important exceptions to the "start conservative and remeasure" strategy, however, and more aggressive approaches are gaining favor. Patients with marked blood pressure elevation (generally >200/120 mm Hg) and acute end-organ damage (e.g., encephalopathy, MI, unstable angina, pulmonary edema, stroke) require hospitalization and parenteral drug therapy. Patients with markedly elevated blood pressure but without end- organ damage usually do not require hospitalization but should be given immediate combination oral antihypertensive therapy. In pregnant or recent postpartum women, preeclampsia may be the cause of hypertension. Waiting to treat in this setting can have devastating consequences for the mother and fetus.

Table 4-1. 2003 Joint National Committee (JNC-7) Hypertension Classification

SYSTOLIC BP* (mm Hg)	DIASTOLIC BP* (mm Hg)	CLASSIFICATION
<120	<80	Normal
120-139	80-89	Prehypertension
140-159	90-99	Stage I hypertension
≥160	≥100	Stage II hypertension

BP, Blood pressure.

*Classification is based on the worst number (e.g., 168/60 mm Hg is considered stage II hypertension even though the diastolic pressure is normal). Adapted from the National Heart, Lung, and Blood Institute. The Seventh Report of the Joint National Committee on Prevention, Detection, Evaluation, and Treatment of High Blood Pressure (JNC-7). Available from: https://www.nhlbi.nih.gov/guidelines/hypertension/jnc7full. htm. Accessed March 10, 2014.

4. **When should you initiate therapy for hypertension for various groups according to JNC-8? What are the blood pressure targets in these groups?**

GROUP	INITIATE THERAPY	GOAL BLOOD PRESSURE
General population aged ≥60 yr	≥150/90 mm Hg	<150/90 mm Hg
General population aged <60 yr	≥140/90 mm Hg	<140/90 mm Hg
Individuals aged ≥18 yr with CKD or DM	≥140/90 mm Hg	<140/90 mm Hg

Data from James PA, Oparil S, Carter BL, et al. 2014 evidence-based guideline for the management of high blood pressure in adults: report from the panel members appointed to the Eighth Joint National Committee (JNC 8). JAMA 2014;311:507-520.
CKD, Chronic kidney disease; DM, diabetes mellitus.

5. **What does lowering of blood pressure accomplish?**
Hypertension is the leading modifiable risk factor for strokes. Lowering of blood pressure decreases the incidence of heart disease, MI, atherosclerosis, stroke, renal failure, and aortic aneurysms.

6. **What are the conservative (i.e., nonpharmacologic) treatments for hypertension?**
Dietary changes (i.e., low salt, low fat, low calorie), reduced smoking and alcohol intake, weight loss, and exercise may each have a positive effect on blood pressure and, in some cases, return the patient to the normotensive range.

7. **List the first-line medications for treatment of hypertension.**
JNC-8 recommends treatment with an angiotensin-converting enzyme inhibitor (ACEI), angiotensin receptor blocker (ARB), and calcium channel blocker (CCB) or diuretic. There are a few groups for whom treatment is more specific. In the general black population, including those with diabetes, initial antihypertensive treatment should include a thiazide-type diuretic or CCB. In the population aged 18 years or older with chronic kidney disease (CKD) and hypertension, initial (or add-on) antihypertensive treatment should include an ACEI or ARB to improve kidney outcomes. This applies to all CKD patients with hypertension regardless of race or diabetes status. In some cases, medications from multiple classes may be needed to reach blood pressure goals. Beta-blockers and alpha-blockers are not recommended for initial management.

DRUG CLASS	USE IN PATIENTS WITH	AVOID IN PATIENTS WITH
Thiazides	Heart failure, diabetes, high risk for CAD or stroke, osteoporosis	Gout, electrolyte disturbances (e.g., hyponatremia), pregnancy
ACE inhibitors	Heart failure, diabetes, acute coronary syndrome/unstable angina, acute or prior MI, high risk for CAD or stroke, chronic kidney disease	Pregnancy (and generally women of childbearing age), angioedema, renovascular hypertension (may cause renal failure)
ARBs	Heart failure, diabetes, chronic kidney disease	Pregnancy (and generally women of childbearing age), renovascular hypertension (may cause renal failure)
Calcium channel blockers	Raynaud syndrome, atrial tachyarrhythmias	Heart block, sick sinus syndrome, congestive heart failure (all related to central-acting agents), pregnancy

Continued

DRUG CLASS	USE IN PATIENTS WITH	AVOID IN PATIENTS WITH
Beta-blockers*	Stable angina, acute coronary syndrome/unstable angina, acute or prior MI, high risk for CAD, atrial tachycardia/fibrillation, thyrotoxicosis (short term), essential tremor, migraines	Asthma, chronic obstructive pulmonary disease, heart block, sick sinus syndrome

ACE, Angiotensin-converting enzyme; ARBs, angiotensin receptor blockers; CAD, coronary artery disease; MI, myocardial infarction.
*Not recommended for initial management of hypertension in the general population.

Note: In diabetes, ACEIs reduce progression to nephropathy and neuropathy. All patients with stable CHF or diabetes should take an ACEI (if they can tolerate it) even in the absence of hypertension.

8. **What about women of reproductive age and pregnant women with hypertension?**
   Labetalol, hydralazine, and alpha-methyldopa are safe. If preeclampsia is present, remember that magnesium sulfate lowers blood pressure and is the first-line agent of choice.

9. **Define hypertensive urgency. How is it different from hypertensive emergency?**
   Hypertensive **urgency** is defined as blood pressure greater than 200/120 mm Hg without symptoms. Hypertensive **emergency** is defined as blood pressure greater than 200/120 mm Hg with symptoms or evidence of end-organ damage. Examples include acute left ventricular failure, chest pain or angina, MI, encephalopathy (watch for headaches, confusion, retinal hemorrhages, papilledema, mental status changes, vomiting, blurry vision, dizziness, and/or seizures), or acute renal failure (from necrotizing arteriolitis). Hypertensive emergency requires immediate treatment with intravenous antihypertensives such as nitroprusside, labetalol, and nicardipine. Patients with hypertensive urgency should be started on oral antihypertensives as an outpatient.

10. **What causes hypertension?**
    Roughly 90% to 95% of cases are idiopathic, multifactorial, or essential hypertension. About 5% to 10% of cases are due to secondary (known) causes.

11. **What are the common causes of secondary hypertension in younger men and women?**
    In younger men, a common cause of secondary hypertension is excessive alcohol intake (get the patient to quit!). In younger women, common and classic causes are birth control pills (stop them!) and renal artery stenosis (RAS) from fibromuscular dysplasia (which may cause a bruit and should be treated with balloon angioplasty).

12. **List less common causes of secondary hypertension.**
    Pheochromocytoma. Look for wild swings in blood pressure with diaphoresis and confusion. As a screening test, order 24-hour urine collection to assess catecholamine products (metanephrines, vanillylmandelic acid, homovanillic acid).
    RAS. Unlike young patients with fibromuscular dysplasia, elderly patients typically have RAS caused by atherosclerosis. A renal artery bruit is classically present (although not sensitive); an MRI scan or conventional angiography aids in making a definitive diagnosis. Giving ACEIs to patients with RAS may precipitate acute renal failure (sometimes the first diagnostic clue to its presence).
    Polycystic kidney disease. Look for a flank mass, a positive family history (autosomal-dominant pattern of inheritance), and elevations in creatinine and blood urea nitrogen.
    Cushing syndrome. Look for stigmata of Cushing syndrome on examination. Order a 24-urine collection to assess free cortisol or a dexamethasone suppression test.
    Conn syndrome (primary hyperaldosteronism). The cause is an aldosterone-secreting adrenal neoplasm. Look for high aldosterone levels, low renin levels, hypernatremia, hypokalemia, metabolic alkalosis, and/or an adrenal mass on a CT scan. The screening test of choice is the ratio of plasma aldosterone to plasma rennin activity; a ratio of greater than 30 is indicative of primary hyperaldosteronism.

Coarctation of the aorta. Look for hypertension in the upper extremities only, with unequal pulses, radiofemoral delay, and rib notching on a chest radiograph; this condition is associated with Turner syndrome. MRI or angiography can aid in making a definitive diagnosis.

Renal failure from any cause. In children, watch for poststreptococcal glomerulonephritis or hemolytic uremic syndrome.

13. **What tests should be ordered for every patient with a diagnosis of hypertension? Why?**
    1. **ECG:** to determine whether the heart has been affected (e.g., left ventricular hypertrophy).
    2. **Chemistry 7 panel** (i.e., basic metabolic panel): clues to possible secondary cause of hypertension (e.g., electrolyte disturbances in Conn syndrome) and evaluation for diabetes and renal dysfunction.
    3. **Urinalysis:** clues to possible secondary cause of hypertension (e.g., red blood cell casts in poststreptococcal glomerulonephritis) and for kidney damage (proteinuria).
    4. **Hemoglobin and hematocrit:** to evaluate for anemia or polycythemia.
    5. **Lipid panel:** to evaluate for dyslipidemia as an additional risk factor for coronary artery disease.

14. **When is cholesterol screening performed?**
    Although no protocol is universally accepted, measurement of total cholesterol and high-density lipoprotein (HDL) cholesterol every 5 years once a person turns 20 years of age is considered reasonable by most authorities. Start sooner and screen more frequently for obese patients and patients with a family history of hypercholesterolemia.

15. **Why is cholesterol so important?**
    Cholesterol is one of the main known modifiable risk factors for atherosclerosis. Atherosclerosis is involved in about half of all deaths in the United States and one third of deaths between the ages of 35 and 65 years. Atherosclerosis is the most important cause of permanent disability and accounts for more hospital days than any other illness.

16. **What physical findings will the Step 3 test use as clues to hypercholesterolemia?**
    Xanthelasma, tendon xanthomas (cholesterol deposits in the skin, classically over tendons in the lower extremities), corneal arcus in younger patients, milky-appearing serum, and obesity are possible markers for familial hypercholesterolemia. Family members should be tested if a case of familial hypercholesterolemia is found. Pancreatitis in the absence of obvious risk factors may be a marker for familial hypertriglyceridemia.

17. **What are the current recommendations for management of cholesterol levels?**
    The following information is from the 2013 American College of Cardiology/American Heart Association (ACC/AHA) Guidelines on the Treatment of Blood Cholesterol to Reduce Atheroscleroitc Cardiovascular Risk in Adults. This new guideline differs from the previous recommendations in that it moves away from specific low-density lipoprotein (LDL) targets. Instead, overall LDL reduction is recommended.

GROUP	LDL REDUCTION GOAL	RECOMMENDED THERAPY
Anyone with LDL ≥190 mg/dL	Reduce by >50%	High-intensity statin
Diabetics aged 40-75 yr with LDL >70 mg/dL	Reduce by 30-50%	Moderate-intensity statin
Anyone with current or past CVD (angina, MI, PAD) and LDL >70 mg/dL	Reduce by >50%	High-intensity statin
Anyone with ≥7.5% chance of developing atherosclerotic CVD in the next 10 yr, using a specific calculator*	Reduce by 30-50%	Moderate-intensity statin

CVD, Cardiovascular disease; LDL, low-density lipoprotein; MI, myocardial infarction; PAD, peripheral arterial disease.

*The Pooled Cohort Equations. Available at http://my.americanheart.org/professional/Statements Guidelines/Prevention-Guidelines_UCM_457698_SubHomePage.jsp.

18. **What is meant by high-intensity and moderate-intensity statins?**

High-dose statin means a statin at a sufficient dose to reduce LDL by at least 50%. This includes atorvastatin 40 to 80 mg and rosuvastatin 20 to 40 mg. Moderate-dose statin means a statin at a sufficient dose to reduce LDL by 30% to 50%. This includes atorvastatin 10 to 20 mg, simvastatin 20 to 40 mg, rosuvastatin 5 to 10 mg, pravastatin 40 to 80 mg, and lovastatin 40 mg.

19. **What about nonstatin cholesterol-lowering drugs such as ezetimibe and the fibrates?**

These medications are not included in the current ACC/AHA guidelines because there is insufficient evidence that they reduce atherosclerotic coronary vascular disease (ASCVD) events.

20. **List the major risk factors for coronary heart disease (CHD).**

Although elevated levels of LDL and total cholesterol are risk factors for CHD, do not count them as risk factors when deciding whether or not to treat high cholesterol. The following factors should be counted:

- **Age** (men aged ≥45 years; women aged ≥55 years or with premature menopause and no estrogen replacement therapy)
- **Family history of premature heart attack** (defined as definite MI or sudden death in a first-degree male relative aged <55 years or a first-degree female relative aged <65 years)
- **Cigarette smoking**
- **Hypertension** (≥140/90 mm Hg or prescription for antihypertensive medications)
- **Diabetes mellitus**
- **Low HDL** (<40 mg/dL)

Note: A HDL level greater than or equal to 60 mg/dL is considered protective and negates one risk factor.

21. **Discuss other possible risk factors for heart disease that may affect a decision to prescribe a statin.**

The 2013 ACC/AHA cholesterol guidelines address other factors that may indicate an elevated risk for ASCVD. In selected individuals who are in one of the four statin benefit groups and for whom a decision to initiate statin therapy is otherwise unclear, additional factors may be considered to inform treatment decision making. These factors include:

- Primary LDL greater than or equal to 160 mg/dL
- Family history of premature ASCVD with onset younger than 55 years in a first-degree male relative or younger than 65 years in a first-degree female relative
- High-sensitivity C-reactive protein greater than or equal to 2 mg/L
- Coronary artery calcium (CAC) score greater than or equal to 300 Agatston units or greater than or equal to the 75th percentile for age, sex, and ethnicity
- Ankle-brachial index greater than 0.9
- Elevated lifetime risk of ASCVD (yes, this is vague)

22. **How is HDL affected by alcohol? Estrogens? Exercise? Smoking? Progesterone?**

High HDL is protective against atherosclerosis and is increased by moderate alcohol consumption (1 to 2 drinks/day; but not by high alcohol intake), exercise, and estrogens. HDL is decreased by smoking, androgens, progesterone, and hypertriglyceridemia.

23. **What causes hypercholesterolemia?**

Genetic factors certainly play a role (e.g., familial hyperlipidemia), but most cases are thought to be multifactorial. A Western diet and an inactive lifestyle certainly contribute. Secondary causes of increased cholesterol include uncontrolled diabetes, hypothyroidism, uremia, nephrotic syndrome, obstructive liver disease, excessive alcohol intake (which increases triglycerides), and medications (e.g., birth control pills, glucocorticoids, thiazides, beta-blockers).

24. **In a patient with chest pain, what elements of the history and physical examination steer you away from a diagnosis of MI?**

Wrong age: in the absence of known heart disease, strong family history, or multiple risk factors for coronary artery disease, a patient younger than 40 years is extremely unlikely to have an MI.

Lack of risk factors: a 60-year-old marathon runner who eats well and has a high HDL level and no cardiac risk factors (other than age) is unlikely to have a heart attack.

Physical characteristics of pain: if the pain is reproducible by palpation, it is from the chest wall, not the heart. The pain associated with an MI is usually not sharp or well localized. The pain should not be related to certain foods or eating.

Having said all of this, many physicians still want to make sure that a heart attack has not occurred with at least an ECG and possibly one or more sets of cardiac enzyme levels. For the Step 3 exam, however, these clues should steer you toward an alternative diagnosis.

25. **What clues suggest the common noncardiac causes of chest pain?**

Gastroesophageal reflux/peptic ulcer disease: look for a relation to certain foods (spicy foods, chocolate), smoking, caffeine, or lying down. Pain is relieved by antacids or acid-reducing medications. Patients with peptic ulcer disease often test positive for *Helicobacter pylori*.

Chest wall pain (costochondritis, bruised or broken ribs): pain is well localized and reproducible on chest wall palpation.

Esophageal problems (achalasia, nutcracker esophagus, or esophageal spasm): this is often a difficult differential diagnosis. The question will probably give negative results for a workup for MI or mention the lack of atherosclerosis risk factors. Look for abnormalities on a barium swallow (achalasia) or esophageal manometry. Treat achalasia with pneumatic dilation or botulism toxin administration, and treat nutcracker esophagus or esophageal spasm with CCBs. If medical treatments are ineffective, surgical myotomy may be needed.

Pericarditis: look for a viral infection prodrome for the upper respiratory tract. The ECG shows diffuse ST-segment elevation, the erythrocyte sedimentation rate is elevated, and a low-grade fever is present. Classically, the pain is relieved by sitting forward. The most common cause is infection with Coxsackie virus. Other causes include tuberculosis, uremia, malignancy, and lupus erythematosus or other autoimmune diseases (Fig. 4-1).

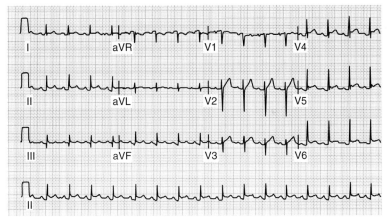

Figure 4-1. Acute pericarditis in a 30-year-old man with pleuritic chest pain. The electrocardiogram demonstrates ST-segment elevation most clearly seen in leads I, II, aV$_F$, and V$_3$ to V$_6$, diffuse PR-segment depression, and PR-segment elevation in lead aV$_R$. (*From Demangone D. ECG manifestations: noncoronary heart disease. Emerg Med Clin North Am 24:113-131.*)

Pneumonia: chest pain is due to pleuritis. Patients also have a cough, fever, and/or sputum production. Ask about possible sick contacts.

Aortic dissection: associated with a severe tearing or ripping pain that may radiate to the back. Look for hypertension or evidence of Marfan syndrome (tall, thin patient with hyperextensible joints). Blunt chest trauma can cause aortic laceration and pseudoaneurysm, which are different conditions that are often managed similarly.

26. **What historical points should steer you toward a diagnosis of MI?**

Patients often have a history of angina or previous chest pain, murmurs, arrhythmias, risk factors for coronary artery disease, hypertension, or diabetes. They also may be taking digoxin, furosemide, cholesterol medications, antihypertensive agents, or other cardiac medications.

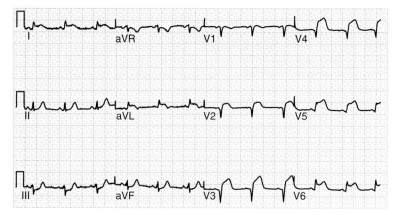

Figure 4-2. An anterolateral acute myocardial infarction caused by a lesion in the proximal left anterior descending artery. ST-segment elevation is seen in leads I, aV_L, and V_2 through V_6. (*From Marx J, Hockberger R, Walls R. Rosen's emergency medicine: concepts and clinical practice. 6th ed. Philadelphia: Mosby, 2006, Fig. 77-6.*)

27. **What findings on ECG should make you suspect an MI?**
    After a heart attack you should see flipped or flattened T waves, ST-segment elevation (depression means ischemia; elevation means injury), and/or Q waves in a segmental distribution (e.g., leads II, III, and aV_F for an inferior MI) (Fig. 4-2).

28. **Describe the classic pattern of chest pain in an MI.**
    The pain is classically described as a crushing or pressure sensation; it is a poorly localized substernal pain that may radiate to the shoulder, arm, or jaw. The pain is usually not reproducible on palpation, and in patients with a heart attack often does not resolve with nitroglycerin (as it often does in angina). The pain usually lasts for at least half an hour.

29. **Describe the classic physical examination findings in patients with MI.**
    Patients are often diaphoretic, anxious, tachycardic, tachypneic, and pale; they may have nausea and vomiting. For large heart attacks that cause heart failure, look for bilateral pulmonary rales in the absence of other pneumonia-like symptoms, distended neck veins, S_3 or S_4 heart sounds, new murmurs, hypotension, and/or shock.

30. **What tests are used to diagnose an MI?**
    Other than an ECG, a patient with a possible MI should have serial determinations of troponin (usually three times at 8-hour intervals before a heart attack is ruled out, but shorter intervals between troponin tests are becoming more well accepted). Troponin levels remain elevated for up to a week. Radiographs may show cardiomegaly and/or pulmonary congestion; echocardiography may show abnormalities in ventricular wall motion.

31. **Describe the treatment for an ST-elevation MI (STEMI).**
    Treatment involves admission to the intensive or cardiac care unit. Several basic principles should be kept in mind:
    1. Early reperfusion is crucial. Percutaneous coronary intervention (PCI) is the preferred method (i.e., balloon angioplasty/stent). Bringing the patient to the catheterization laboratory should be the priority for all patients with STEMI. Fibrinolytic therapy with t-PA is only indicated in patients who cannot receive PCI within 2 hours of medical contact. Fibrinolytics can only be given within 12 hours of symptom onset. There is a long list of contraindications to t-PA given its risk for severe hemorrhage.
    2. Administer **aspirin.**
    3. ECG monitoring is essential. If ventricular tachycardia occurs, use amiodarone (or cardioversion if the patient is hemodynamically unstable).
    4. Give oxygen to maintain an oxygen saturation of greater than 90%.

5. Administer **nitroglycerin** for symptomatic relief if the patient's blood pressure can tolerate this vasodilatory medication; avoid nitroglycerin for inferior MIs because a decrease in the patient's preload can lead to hypotension in the case of a right ventricular infarction.
6. Control pain with **morphine**, which may improve pulmonary edema, if present.
7. Administer **unfractionated or low–molecular-weight heparin.**
8. Administer **clopidogrel.**
9. **Beta-blockers**, which patients without contraindications should take for life, reduce the MI mortality rate and the incidence of a second heart attack.
10. An **ACEI** or **ARB** should be started within 24 hours.
11. Administer an **HMG-CoA reductase inhibitor** (statin).

32. **When is heparin indicated in the setting of chest pain and MI?**

Heparin should be started if acute coronary syndrome is diagnosed (unstable angina, non-STEMI [NSTEMI], or STEMI), if the patient has a cardiac thrombus, or if severe CHF is seen on echocardiography. The Step 3 exam will not ask about other indications, which are not as clear cut. Do not give heparin to patients with contraindications to its use (e.g., active bleeding).

33. **How can you recognize stable angina?**

The chest pain of stable angina begins with exertion or stress and remits with rest or on calming down. The key to a diagnosis of stable angina is that it is stable, not increasing in duration of pain, not occurring with less exertion, and not becoming more frequent. The pain is described as a pressure or squeezing pain in the substernal area and may radiate to the shoulders, neck, and/or jaw. It often is accompanied by shortness of breath, diaphoresis, and/or nausea. The pain is usually relieved by nitroglycerin. An ECG performed during an acute attack often shows ST-segment depression, but in the absence of pain, the ECG is often normal. The pain should last for less than 20 minutes or be relieved after sublingual nitroglycerin administration; otherwise, there may be progression to unstable angina or MI.

34. **Define unstable angina. How is it diagnosed and treated?**

In strict terms, unstable angina is defined as a change from previously stable angina. If a patient used to experience angina once a week and now experiences it once a day, the patient technically has unstable angina. Patients with unstable angina usually exhibit normal or only minimally elevated cardiac enzymes, ECG changes (ST depression), and prolonged chest pain that does not respond to nitroglycerin initially (like a heart attack). The pain often begins at rest. Treatment is similar to that for MI. The patient is admitted to the coronary or intensive care unit. Initial treatment begins with oxygen, aspirin, and nitroglycerin administration. The patient should be given a beta-blocker, clopidogrel, and heparin (unfractionated or the low–molecular-weight form). A glycoprotein IIb/IIIa receptor inhibitor should be administered to patients with continuing ischemia or with other high-risk features. An ACEI or ARB should be given as well. Consider emergent percutaneous tranluminal coronary angiography (PTCA) if the pain does not resolve. Almost all patients have a history of stable angina and coronary artery disease risk factors.

35. **Describe variant (Prinzmetal) angina.**

This rare type of angina is characterized by pain at rest (unrelated to exertion) and ST-segment elevation; cardiac enzymes are normal. The cause is coronary artery spasm. Prinzmetal angina usually responds to nitroglycerin and is treated over the long term with CCBs, which reduce arterial spasms.

36. **Define silent MI. How common is it?**

Patients with a silent MI do not develop chest pain. Their symptoms include CHF, shock, or confusion and delirium (especially elderly patients). MIs are silent in up to 25% of cases (especially in diabetics with neuropathy).

37. **Injury to what organ (other than the heart) causes elevated levels of creatine kinase (CK)?**

Muscle. Watch for trauma, rhabdomyolysis, HMG-CoA reductase inhibitors (which can cause muscle damage), and burns. CK-MB is a subtype of CK that is more specific to the myocardium.

38. **What is the relationship between aspirin and MI?**

It has been proved that low-dose aspirin is of benefit in reducing the risk of MI in patients who have had a previous MI and patients with stable or unstable angina who have not had an MI. The 2012 American College of Chest Physicians (ACCP) clinical practice guidelines on antithrombotic and thrombolytic therapy recommend that all patients with chronic stable angina or other clinical or laboratory evidence of coronary artery disease receive aspirin indefinitely. There is strong medical literature support for the net benefit of aspirin for primary prevention of a first MI in individuals at moderate to high risk. Aspirin is recommended in all diabetic patients with cardiovascular disease and for primary prevention in diabetic patients with one or more risk factors (e.g., age >40 years, cigarette smoking, hypertension, hyperlipidemia, obesity, albuminuria, or family history of cardiovascular disease). The risks of aspirin prophylaxis may outweigh the benefits in patients with a history of liver disease, kidney disease, peptic ulcer disease or gastrointestinal bleeding, poorly controlled hypertension, or a bleeding disorder.

39. **True or false: Patients should be given aspirin as soon as possible in the emergency department for a suspected MI or unstable angina.**

True, but beware the patient with chest pain who ends up having an aortic dissection (aspirin should be avoided in such patients).

40. **How is smoking related to heart disease?**

Smoking is the best risk factor to eliminate for prevention of deaths related to heart disease; it is responsible for 30% to 45% of such deaths in the United States. This risk is decreased by 50% within 1 year of quitting, and by 15 years after quitting, the risk is the same as for someone who has never smoked.

41. **What is the most common cause of death during vascular surgery?**

MI, regardless of the procedure performed. Peripheral vascular and aortic diseases are generalized markers for atherosclerosis, and almost all patients have significant coronary artery disease. Always evaluate patients for modifiable and treatable atherosclerosis risk factors (i.e., hyperlipidemia, hypertension, smoking, diabetes).

42. **Describe the classic symptoms of chronic mesenteric ischemia.**

The classic patient has a long history of postprandial abdominal pain (also known as intestinal angina; eating exercises the intestines), which causes fear of food and extensive weight loss. This diagnosis is difficult because, like all atherosclerotic disease, it occurs in patients older than 40 years who have other conditions that may cause the same problem (e.g., peptic ulcer disease, pancreatic cancer, stomach cancer). Look for a history of extensive atherosclerosis (known coronary artery disease, peripheral vascular disease, stroke, or multiple risk factors), abdominal bruit, Hemoccult-positive stool, and lack of jaundice (jaundice suggests pancreatic cancer). Most patients undergo a CT scan of the abdomen; negative results raise the suspicion of ischemia. The diagnosis can be made on the basis of selective angiography of the superior mesenteric artery. MRI angiography and CT angiography are emerging tools, but angiography is still the preferred modality. Patients are treated with surgical revascularization because of the risks of bowel infarction and malnutrition.

43. **What are the symptoms of an acute bowel infarction?**

Classically, a patient with a history of atrial fibrillation, atherosclerosis, or multiple atherosclerosis risk factors has symptoms of abdominal pain and bloody diarrhea. Patients classically have pain out of proportion to the examination, but may have peritoneal signs (e.g., rebound tenderness, guarding). Watch for the thumbprinting sign (thickened bowel walls that resemble thumbprints) on abdominal radiographs. Patients may also have tachycardia, hypotension, and/or shock.

CONGESTIVE HEART FAILURE

1. **What are the general symptoms and signs of CHF?**
   - Fatigue
   - Ventricular hypertrophy on ECG

- Dyspnea
- S_3 or S_4 sound on cardiac examination
- Cardiomegaly on chest radiography
- Specific left-sided and right-sided findings (see the next question)

2. **What symptoms and signs help to determine whether CHF is due to left or right ventricular failure?**
   Left ventricular failure: orthopnea (shortness of breath when lying down; the patient sleeps on more than one pillow or even sitting up); paroxysmal nocturnal dyspnea; pulmonary congestion (rales); Kerley B lines on chest radiography; pulmonary vascular congestion and edema; bilateral pleural effusions.
   Right ventricular failure: peripheral edema, jugular venous distention, hepatomegaly, ascites, underlying lung disease (cor pulmonale; see later discussion).
   Note: Both ventricles are commonly affected, so a mixed pattern is often seen.

3. **How is chronic CHF treated?**
   Chronic CHF is treated on an outpatient basis with sodium restriction, ACEIs (first-line agents that reduce mortality), beta-blockers (somewhat counterintuitive but proven to work), diuretics (furosemide, spironolactone, metolazone), digoxin (not used in diastolic dysfunction; usually reserved for moderate to severe CHF with a low ejection fraction or systolic dysfunction), and vasodilators (arterial and venous).

4. **How is acute CHF treated?**
   Acute CHF exacerbations are often treated on an inpatient basis by addressing (1) oxygenation, (2) preload reduction, and (3) contractility.
   1. Arrange for upright positioning of the patient. Titrate O_2 to greater than 92% with supplemental oxygen and noninvasive positive-pressure ventilation continuous positive airway pressure/biphasis positive airway pressure (CPAP/BiPAP) as needed. Severe exacerbations may require intubation.
   2. Preload reduction is accomplished through the use of diuretics (furosemide). In cases of respiratory distress, nitroglycerin can rapidly reduce preload by causing vasodilation.
   3. In cases of cardiogenic shock, norepinephrine is used to maintain tissue perfusion. Digoxin may be used if the patient is stable. Intravenous sympathomimetics (dobutamine, dopamine, amrinone) may also be required for severe CHF.

5. **What factors precipitate exacerbations in previously stable patients with CHF?**
   The most common factor is noncompliance with dietary recommendations or medication regimens, but watch for **MI**, severe hypertension, arrhythmias, infections and fever, pulmonary embolus, anemia, thyrotoxicosis, and myocarditis.

6. **Define cor pulmonale. With what clinical scenarios is it associated?**
   Cor pulmonale is right ventricular enlargement, hypertrophy, and heart failure caused by primary lung disease. Common causes are chronic obstructive pulmonary disease and pulmonary embolus. In a young woman (20 to 40 years of age) with no other medical history or risk factors, think of idiopathic pulmonary arterial hypertension. Treat with prostacyclins (parenteral epoprostenol), antiendothelins (bosentant), phosphodiesterase 5 inhibitors, and CCBs while awaiting heart-lung transplantation. Sleep apnea can also cause cor pulmonale; look for an obese snorer who is sleepy during the day. Patients with cor pulmonale may have tachypnea, cyanosis, clubbing, parasternal heave, and loud P_2 and right-sided S_4 sounds, in addition to the signs and symptoms of pulmonary disease.

DYSRHYTHMIAS

1. **What ECG abnormalities do you need to know about for the Step 3 exam? How are they treated?**
   Figures 4-3 through 4-15 demonstrate the arrhythmias noted in the following table. Always check for electrolyte disturbances as a cause of any arrhythmia.

ARRHYTHMIA	TREATMENT AND WARNINGS
Atrial fibrillation	In symptomatic patients, first slow the ventricular rate with a beta-blocker, CCB, or digoxin: • If acute (onset <48 hr), cardiovert with amiodarone, procainamide, or DC-synchronized cardioversion • If chronic, first anticoagulate, evaluate for thrombus with transesophageal echocardiogram, then cardiovert; if this approach fails or atrial fibrillation recurs, leave the patient on rate-control medications (beta-blocker, CCB, or digoxin) and warfarin
Atrial flutter	Treat as for atrial fibrillation
Heart Block	
First degree	No treatment, but avoid beta-blockers and CCBs, which slow conduction
Second degree	For Mobitz type I, use a pacemaker or atropine only in symptomatic patients; use a pacemaker in all patients with Mobitz type II
Third degree	Use a pacemaker
WPW with AVRT or atrial fibrillation	Use procainamide or quinidine; avoid digoxin and verapamil
Ventricular tachycardia	If pulseless, treat with standard ACLS and defibrillation followed by an antiarrhythmic to prevent recurrence (e.g., procainamide); if a pulse is present and the patient is stable, treat with procainamide, amiodarone, or synchronized cardioversion; if a pulse is present and the patient is unstable, treat with synchronized cardioversion
Ventricular fibrillation	Immediate defibrillation followed by epinephrine, vasopressin, amiodarone, or lidocaine
PVCs	Usually not treated; if severe and symptomatic, consider beta-blockers or amiodarone
Sinus bradycardia	Usually not treated; use atropine, dopamine, or pacing if severe and symptomatic (e.g., after heart attack); avoid beta-blockers, CCBs, and other conduction-slowing medications
Sinus tachycardia	Usually none; correct the underlying cause; use a beta-blocker or CCB if symptomatic

ACLS, Advanced cardiovascular life support; AVRT, atrioventricular reentrant tachycardia; CCB, Calcium channel blocker; DC, direct current; PVCs, premature ventricular complexes; WPW, Wolff-Parkinson-White.

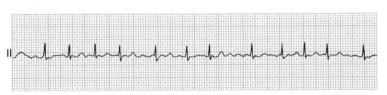

Figure 4-3. Atrial fibrillation. There are no true P waves and the ventricular rate is irregular. (*From Goldberger AL. Clinical electrocardiography: a simplified approach. 7th ed. Philadelphia: Mosby, 2006, Fig. 15-4.*).

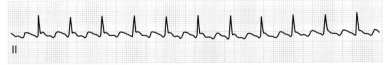

Figure 4-4. An example of atrial flutter. In contrast to atrial fibrillation, atrial flutter is regular. The baseline has a sawtooth shape. (*From Walsh D. Palliative medicine. 1st ed. Philadelphia: Saunders, 2008, Fig. 80-2.*)

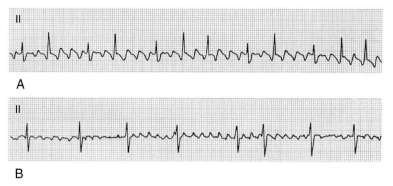

Figure 4-5. Atrial flutter with variable block (**A**) and coarse atrial fibrillation (**B**) may be easily confused. Notice that for atrial fibrillation the ventricular rate is erratic and the atrial waves are not identical from segment to segment, whereas these atrial waves are identical for atrial flutter. (*From Goldberger A. Clinical electrocardiography: a simplified approach. 7th ed. Philadelphia: Mosby, 2006, Fig. 23-3.*)

First-degree AV block

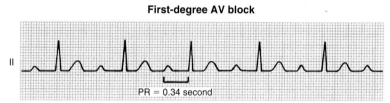

Figure 4-6. First-degree atrioventricular block with a PR interval that is prolonged to more than 0.20 seconds with each electrical cycle (0.12 to 0.20 seconds is normal). (*From Goldberger A, Goldberger ZD, Shvilkin A. Goldberger's clinical electrocardiography: a simplified approach. 8th ed. Philadelphia: Saunders, 2012, Fig. 17-2.*)

Mobitz type I (Wenckebach) second-degree AV block

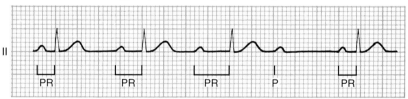

Figure 4-7. Mobitz type I second-degree atrioventricular (AV) block (Wenckebach; a second-degree AV block in which the PR interval progressively lengthens from cycle to cycle until the AV node no longer conducts a stimulus from above). Notice the progression of the PR interval before the impulse is completely blocked. (*From Goldberger A, Goldberger ZD, Shvilkin A. Goldberger's clinical electrocardiography: a simplified approach. 8th ed. Philadelphia: Saunders, 2012, Fig. 17-3.*)

Mobitz II AV block with sinus rhythm

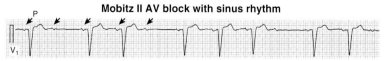

Figure 4-8. Mobitz type II second-degree atrioventricular block (an intermittent dropped QRS). Note the abrupt appearance of sinus P waves that are not followed by QRS complexes (nonconducted or dropped beats). (*From Goldberger A, Goldberger ZD, Shvilkin A. Goldberger's clinical electrocardiography: a simplified approach. 8th ed. Philadelphia: Saunders, 2012, Fig. 17-5.*)

Third-degree (complete) AV block

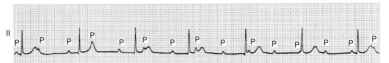

Figure 4-9. A third-degree atrioventricular block (none of the atrial depolarizations conduct to the ventricles) is characterized by independent atrial (P) and ventricular (QRS complex) activity. The atrial rate is always faster than the ventricular rate. (*From Goldberger A, Goldberger ZD, Shvilkin A. Goldberger's clinical electrocardiography: a simplified approach. 8th ed. Philadelphia: Saunders, 2012, Fig. 17-7.*)

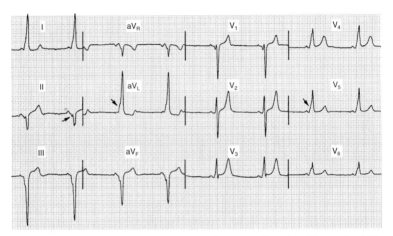

Figure 4-10. Wolff-Parkinson-White syndrome. Triad of a wide QRS complex, a short PR interval, and delta waves (*arrows*). (*From Goldberger AL. Clinical electrocardiography: a simplified approach. 7th ed. Philadelphia: Mosby, 2006, Fig. 12-3.*)

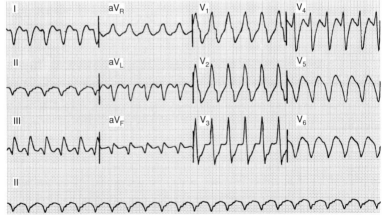

Figure 4-11. Ventricular tachycardia. Tachycardia with a wide QRS complex. (*From Goldberger AL. Clinical electrocardiography: a simplified approach. 7th ed. Philadelphia: Mosby, 2006, Part 4, Case 3.*)

Ventricular fibrillation

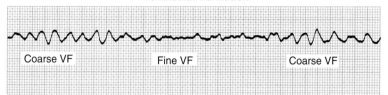

Figure 4-12. Ventricular fibrillation. Fibrillatory waves in an irregular pattern. (*From Goldberger AL. Clinical electrocardiography: a simplified approach. 7th ed. Philadelphia: Mosby, 2006, Fig. 16-13.*)

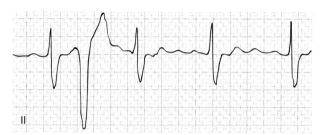

Figure 4-13. A single premature ventricular complex. (*From Marx J, Hockberger R, Walls R. Rosen's emergency medicine. 7th ed. Philadelphia: Mosby, 2009, Fig. 77-22.*)

Sinus bradycardia

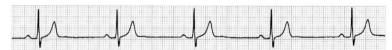

Figure 4-14. Sinus bradycardia at a rate of about 40 beats/min. (*From Goldberger A, Goldberger ZD, Shvilkin A. Goldberger's clinical electrocardiography: a simplified approach. 8th ed. Philadelphia: Saunders, 2013, Fig. 20-1.*)

Sinus tachycardia

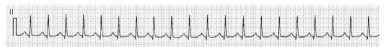

Figure 4-15. Sinus tachycardia at a rate of about 150 beats/min. (*From Goldberger A, Goldberger ZD, Shvilkin A. Goldberger's clinical electrocardiography: a simplified approach. 8th ed. Philadelphia: Saunders, 2013, Fig. 13-2.*)

2. What endocrine disease is suggested when a patient has sinus tachycardia or atrial fibrillation?
   Hyperthyroidism. Check the level of thyroid-stimulating hormone (TSH) as a screening test.

3. Which patients with atrial fibrillation should receive anticoagulation?
   The $CHADS_2$ score is used to estimate the risk of stroke in patients with nonrheumatic atrial fibrillation. The score is used to determine whether the patient should be treated with an anticoagulant (warfarin or dabigatran) or aspirin.

The points in the following table are added to determine the CHADS$_2$ score.
A score of 0 indicates low risk of stroke, so aspirin can be used.
A score of 1 indicates moderate risk, so aspirin or warfarin can be used.
A score of 2 or greater indicates moderate or high risk, so warfarin should be used unless contraindicated (e.g., significant fall risk).

	CONDITION	POINTS
C	Congestive heart failure	1
H	Hypertension: blood pressure consistently >140/90 mm Hg (or taking antihypertension medication)	1
A	Age >75 yr	1
D	Diabetes mellitus	1
S$_2$	Prior stroke or transient ischemic attack	2

4. **What are the classic symptoms of Wolff-Parkinson-White syndrome?**
A child becomes dizzy or dyspneic or passes out after playing and then recovers and has no other symptoms. The cause is a transient arrhythmia via the accessory pathway. ECG shows the infamous delta wave and shortened PR interval. The treatment of choice for such patients is radiofrequency catheter ablation of the pathway.

DISORDERS OF THE GREAT VESSELS

1. **What is the most common cause of immediate death after an automobile accident or a fall from a great height?**
Aortic rupture. Look for a widened mediastinum on a chest radiograph and an appropriate history of trauma. Order a CT scan or angiogram if a contained aortic rupture is suspected (of those who survive to be admitted to the hospital, 50% will die in the first 24 hours). Aortic laceration, traumatic aortic injury, and traumatic pseudoaneurysm all describe the phenomenon seen in initial survivors: an aortic rupture contained by a hematoma or an inadequate amount of surrounding tissue (e.g., adventitia only). Treat with immediate surgical repair.

2. **What are the classic findings in a patient with an abdominal aortic aneurysm? How is this condition evaluated?**
Abdominal aortic aneurysm classically involves a pulsatile abdominal mass that may cause abdominal pain. If pain is present, rupture or leakage of the aneurysm should be suspected, although an unruptured aneurysm may cause some degree of pain. Ultrasound or a CT scan is used for initial evaluation and diagnostic confirmation in stable patients, as well as for serial monitoring.

3. **How is an abdominal aortic aneurysm managed? What clues indicate that the aneurysm has ruptured?**
If the aneurysm is smaller than 5 cm, you can follow it with serial ultrasound examinations to ensure that it is not enlarging. These small aneurysms should be managed with risk factor reduction (smoking cessation and treatment of hypertension and dyslipidemia). If the aneurysm is larger than 5 cm, symptomatic, or rapidly enlarging, surgical correction should be advised if the patient can tolerate the surgery. Before surgery, the patient's condition can be medically optimized by administration of a beta-blocker (esmolol) to a target heart rate of 60 beats/min and with nitroprusside or nicardipine to a target systolic blood pressure of 100 to 120 mm Hg.

A **pulsatile abdominal mass plus hypotension** requires emergent laparotomy for a presumed ruptured aneurysm, which carries a mortality rate of roughly 90%. Management of an abdominal aortic aneurysm dissection depends on the location of the dissection. Patients who survive the initial tear typically have a severe sharp or tearing sensation in the back or chest. Acute dissections involving the ascending aorta are considered surgical emergencies.

Dissections confined to the descending aorta are treated medically unless the dissection progresses or continues to bleed.

VALVULAR HEART DISEASE

1. Describe the cause and classic history of the various heart valve abnormalities.

VALVE PROBLEM	CAUSE	HISTORY
Mitral stenosis	RF is the most common cause	Dyspnea, orthopnea, and PND
Mitral regurgitation	Typically results from RF or chordae tendinae rupture after MI	Fatigue, dyspnea, orthopnea
Aortic stenosis	Typically seen in the elderly; bicuspid or unicuspid valves may lead to symptoms in childhood	Usually asymptomatic for years and begins with DOE; progresses to angina, syncope, and heart failure, with the mortality rate increasing through this progression
Aortic regurgitation	**CREAM** mnemonic: **c**ongenital, **r**heumatic damage, **e**ndocarditis, **a**ortic dissection/**a**ortic root dilation, **M**arfan syndrome	Symptoms in acute cases include severe dyspnea, acute pulmonary congestion, and cardiogenic shock; symptoms in chronic cases include DOE, orthopnea, and PND

DOE, Dyspnea on exertion; *MI,* myocardial infarction; *PND,* paroxysmal nocturnal dyspnea; *RF,* rheumatic fever.

2. What physical examination findings are associated with various heart valve abnormalities?

VALVE PROBLEM	PHYSICAL CHARACTERISTICS	OTHER FINDINGS
Mitral stenosis	Late diastolic blowing murmur (best heard at the apex)	Opening snap, loud S_1, AF, LAE, PH
Mitral regurgitation	Holosystolic murmur (radiates to the axilla)	Soft S_1, LAE, PH, LVH
Aortic stenosis	Harsh systolic ejection murmurs (best heard in the aortic area; radiates to the carotid arteries)	Slow pulse upstroke, S_3/S_4, ejection click, LVH, cardiomegaly; syncope, angina, heart failure
Aortic regurgitation	Early diastolic decrescendo murmur (best heard at apex)	Widened pulse pressure, LVH, LV dilation, S_3
Mitral prolapse	Midsystolic click, late systolic murmur	Panic disorder

AF, Atrial fibrillation; *LAE,* left atrial enlargement; *LV,* left ventricle; *LVH,* left ventricular hypertrophy; *PH,* pulmonary hypertension.

3. Describe the treatment of each of the aforementioned valvular disorders.
Mitral stenosis is a mechanical problem and requires balloon valvotomy or surgery if it becomes severe. Medical management (diuretics, digoxin, beta-blockers) is only adjunctive

to either percutaneous or surgical intervention. **Mitral regurgitation** is treated with corrective surgery if certain indications are present (flail leaflet, severe regurgitation). Vasodilators (nitroprusside, hydralazine) may be used in symptomatic patients. Atrial fibrillation is common because of left atrial enlargement and is treated with either cardioversion or rate control and anticoagulation. as appropriate, if it is present. Aortic valve replacement should be performed in essentially all patients with symptomatic **aortic stenosis.** Aortic valve replacement or repair is indicated in symptomatic patients with chronic **aortic regurgitation.** Aortic valve replacement or repair may be indicated for asymptomatic patients under certain circumstances, such as progressive left ventricular enlargement (along with specific echocardiographic findings that are beyond the scope of the USMLE). Vasodilators may be used to reduce the hemodynamic burden and possibly delay the need for surgery in asymptomatic patients.

4. True or false: An understanding of the pathophysiology behind the various changes associated with longstanding valvular heart disease is of high yield for the Step 3 exam.
   True. For example, it is advisable to understand why right ventricular failure may occur with longstanding mitral stenosis. This is not memorization but rather an ability to determine rationally which changes are associated with each type of valvular dysfunction.

5. What are the recommendations for endocarditis prophylaxis?
   The 2008 American Heart Association recommendations conclude that only an extremely small number of cases of infective endocarditis might be prevented by antibiotic prophylaxis for dental procedures. Cardiac conditions for which prophylaxis for dental procedures is recommended include a prosthetic cardiac valve, previous infectious endocarditis, congenital heart disease, and a cardiac transplant in recipients who develop valvulopathy. Antibiotic prophylaxis is no longer recommended for genitourinary or gastrointestinal procedures.

   If a prophylactic antibiotic is indicated, it should be administered in a single dose before the procedure. Amoxicillin is the preferred choice for oral therapy. Cephalexin, clindamycin, azithromycin, or clarithromycin may be used in patients with penicillin allergy. Ampicillin, cefazolin, ceftriaxone, or clindamycin may be used for patients unable to take oral medication.

6. Describe the two clinical types of endocarditis. What are the causative organisms?
   1. **Acute (fulminant) endocarditis** typically affects normal heart valves and is most commonly caused by S. aureus.
   2. **Subacute endocarditis** has an insidious onset and typically affects previously damaged or prosthetic valves. The most common cause is Streptococcus viridans, but other streptococcal and staphylococcal species may also cause endocarditis (e.g., Staphylococcus epidermis, Streptococcus bovis, and enterococci). Suspect colon cancer if S. bovis is detected in a blood culture.

7. What elements of a medical history point to endocarditis?
   Look for patients who are more likely to be affected by endocarditis:
   • Intravenous drug abusers, who usually have right-sided lesions, although left-sided lesions are much more common in the general population
   • Patients with abnormal heart valves (e.g., prosthetic valves, rheumatic valvular disease, and congenital heart defects such as tetralogy of Fallot)
   • Postoperative patients (especially after dental surgery)

8. How is endocarditis diagnosed and treated?
   The diagnosis is generally made on the basis of blood cultures. Empiric treatment is started until the culture and sensitivity results are known. An antistaphylococcal penicillin (such as oxacillin or nafcillin, or vancomycin if methicillin-resistant S. aureus is suspected) plus an aminoglycoside is a good choice for native valve endocarditis. A third-generation penicillin or cephalosporin plus an aminoglycoside is a reasonable choice. Empiric treatment

for prosthetic valve endocarditis is vancomycin plus gentamicin plus either cefepime or a carbapenem.

9. **What are the classic signs and symptoms of endocarditis?**
   Look for general signs of infection (e.g., fever, tachycardia, malaise) plus a new-onset heart murmur, embolic phenomena (stroke and other infarcts), **Osler nodes** (painful nodules on the tips of the fingers), **Janeway lesions** (*nontender* erythematous lesions on the palms and soles), **Roth spots** (round retinal hemorrhages with white centers), and septic shock (more likely for acute than subacute disease).

10. **What are the major and minor Jones criteria for rheumatic fever? Why is rheumatic fever less common today?**
    The five major Jones criteria include migratory polyarthritis, carditis, chorea, erythema marginatum, and subcutaneous nodules. The minor Jones criteria include elevations in the erythrocyte sedimentation rate, C-reactive protein, white blood cell count, and antistreptolysin O titer; prolonged PR interval on ECG; and arthralgia. The diagnosis of rheumatic fever requires a history of streptococcal infection and the presence of two of the major criteria, or one major criterion plus two minor criteria. Treatment of streptococcal pharyngitis with antibiotics markedly reduces the incidence of rheumatic fever; thus the condition is less common today. Give all patients affected by rheumatic fever endocarditis prophylaxis before surgical procedures. A way to remember the major Jones criteria is with the mnemonic JONES: joints, obvious (the heart!), nodules, erythema marginatum, Syndenham chorea.

PERIPHERAL ARTERIAL VASCULAR DISEASES

1. **What are the symptoms of thoracic outlet syndrome? How is it treated?**
   Thoracic outlet obstruction involves symptoms caused by obstruction of the nerves or blood vessels that serve the arm as the neurovascular bundle passes from the thoracocervical region to the axilla. Affected patients have upper extremity paresthesias (nerve impingement), weakness, cold temperature (arterial compromise), edema, and/or venous distention (venous compromise). The absence of central nervous system symptoms helps to differentiate this condition from subclavian steal syndrome. Causes include cervical ribs (ribs arising from a cervical vertebrae that are usually asymptomatic but may compromise subclavian blood flow) or muscular hypertrophy (classic in young male weightlifters). Treat with surgical intervention (e.g., cervical rib resection).

2. **Define Leriche syndrome. For what is it a marker?**
   Leriche syndrome is the combination of claudication in the buttocks, buttock atrophy, and impotence in men, and is due to aortoiliac occlusive disease. Most patients need an aortoiliac bypass graft.

3. **Define claudication. What are the associated physical findings?**
   Claudication is pain, usually in the lower extremity, brought on by exercise and relieved by rest. It occurs with severe atherosclerotic disease and is the equivalent of angina for the extremities. Associated physical findings include cyanosis (with dependent rubor), atrophic changes (thickened nails, loss of hair, shiny skin), decreased temperature, and decreased (or absent) distal pulses.

4. **How are patients with claudication managed?**
   The best treatment is conservative: cessation of smoking, exercise, and good control of cholesterol, diabetes, and hypertension. Antiplatelet agents are warranted in patients with claudication. Aspirin is preferred, but clopidogrel may be used for patients who cannot tolerate aspirin. Cilostazol may be used for the treatment of intermittent claudication. Beta-blockers may worsen claudication (as a result of $beta_2$-receptor blockade) but the benefits may outweigh the risks in some patients (e.g., prior MI). If claudication progresses to pain at rest (forefoot pain, generally at night, that is classically relieved by hanging the foot over the edge of the bed) or interferes with lifestyle or work obligations, perform arterial duplex ultrasonography for diagnosis and use angioplasty or surgical revascularization for treatment.

Because claudication and peripheral vascular disease are general markers for atherosclerosis, check for other atherosclerosis risk factors.

5. **What is the probable cause of sudden onset of SEVERE foot pain in patients with no previous history of foot pain, trauma, or associated chronic physical findings?**
This scenario may indicate an embolus (look for atrial fibrillation; the pulse may be absent in the affected area) or compartment syndrome (common after revascularization procedures).

DISEASES OF VEINS

1. **True or false: The lupus anticoagulant causes a clotting tendency.**
True. Although the lupus anticoagulant may cause a prolonged partial thromboplastin time (PTT), the patient has a tendency toward thrombosis. Look for associated lupus symptoms, positive results on the Venereal Disease Research Laboratory (VDRL) or rapid plasma reagin (RPR) tests for syphilis, or a history of miscarriages to help you recognize this condition.

2. **What genetic and acquired causes of an increased tendency toward clot formation may appear on the Step 3 exam?**
The list keeps growing. Watch for factor V Leiden mutation (or activated protein C resistance), prothrombin G20210A mutation, hyperhomocysteinemia, elevated factor VIII level, and deficiencies in protein C, protein S, or antithrombin III as genetic causes of an increased tendency toward thrombosis. Acquired causes include antiphospholipid syndrome (lupus anticoagulant and anticardiolipin antibody), hyperhomocysteinemia, pregnancy, cancer, and estrogen-containing medications. Note that hyperhomocysteinemia can be genetic or acquired. All are treated with anticoagulant therapy to prevent DVT and pulmonary embolus. Suspect these conditions if a patient develops recurrent clots or develops a clot in the absence of risk factors for clot development.

3. **What is the Virchow triad?**
The Virchow triad consists of three findings associated with DVT: endothelial damage, venous stasis, and hypercoagulable state. These three broad categories should help you remember when to think about the possibility of DVT.

4. **List the common clinical scenarios for the development of DVT.**
   • Surgery (especially orthopedic, pelvic, abdominal, or neurosurgery)
   • Malignancy
   • Trauma
   • Immobilization
   • Pregnancy
   • Use of birth control pills
   • Disseminated intravascular coagulation
   • Hypercoagulable states such as factor V (Leiden), antithrombin III deficiency, protein C deficiency, protein S deficiency, prothrombin G20210A gene mutation, hyperhomocysteinemia, and antiphospholipid antibodies

5. **Describe the physical signs and symptoms of DVT. How is it diagnosed?**
Signs and symptoms include unilateral leg swelling, pain or tenderness, and/or the **Homan sign** (present in 30% of cases). Superficial palpable cords imply superficial thrombophlebitis rather than DVT (see later discussion). DVT is best diagnosed by Doppler compression ultrasonography of the veins of the extremity. The gold standard is venography, but this invasive test is reserved for situations in which the diagnosis is not clear.

6. **How is DVT treated? For how long?**
Systemic anticoagulation is necessary. Use intravenous heparin or subcutaneous low–molecular-weight heparin initially, followed by crossover to oral warfarin. Patients should be maintained on warfarin for at least 3 to 6 months, and possibly for life if more than one episode of clotting occurs.

7. **What is the best way to prevent DVT in patients undergoing surgery?**
Prophylactic measures for patients undergoing surgery depend on the risk of developing DVT or pulmonary embolism. Early ambulation is recommended for low-risk patients.

Low–molecular-weight heparin, low-dose unfractionated heparin, or fondaparinux is recommended for patients at moderate risk. High-risk patients should be given low–molecular-weight heparin, fondaparinux, or an oral vitamin K antagonist. Pneumatic compression stockings should be used instead if the patient is at moderate or higher risk and at high risk of bleeding.

8. **True or false: DVT can lead to a stroke.**
False, with one rare exception. Embolization of left-sided heart clots (caused by atrial fibrillation, ventricular wall aneurysm, severe CHF, or endocarditis) leads to arterial infarcts (stroke and renal, gastrointestinal, or extremity infarcts), **not** pulmonary emboli. Deep venous thrombi (or right-sided heart clots) that embolize cause pulmonary emboli, **not** arterial emboli. The exception is a patient with a right-to-left shunt, such as a patent foramen ovale, atrial or ventricular septal defect, or pulmonary arteriovenous fistula. In such patients, a venous clot may embolize and cross over to the left side of the circulation, causing an arterial infarct. This event is quite rare.

9. **True or false: A superficial palpable cord is a fairly specific sign of DVT.**
False. A superficial palpable cord usually represents superficial thrombophlebitis.

10. **Describe the usual history of a patient with superficial thrombophlebitis. How is the condition treated?**
Patients often have a history of varicose veins and exhibit localized leg pain with superficial cordlike induration, reddish discoloration, and mild fever. Superficial thrombophlebitis is not a significant risk factor for pulmonary embolus and patients do not need anticoagulation. Treatment is usually conservative and includes nonsteroidal antiinflammatory drugs (NSAIDs) and warm compresses. The condition generally subsides on its own within a few days. A thrombectomy under local anesthesia can be performed for severe or nonresolving symptoms.

11. **True or false: Superficial thrombophlebitis is a risk factor for pulmonary embolus.**
False. Superficial thrombophlebitis (erythema, tenderness, edema, and a palpable clot in a superficial vein) affects superficial veins and does not cause pulmonary emboli. It is considered a benign condition, although recurrent superficial thrombophlebitis can be a marker for underlying malignancy (e.g., Trousseau syndrome, or migratory thrombophlebitis, is a classic marker for pancreatic cancer). Treat affected patients with NSAIDs and warm compresses.

12. **What are the signs and symptoms of venous insufficiency? How is it treated?**
Venous insufficiency generally occurs in the lower extremities. Patients may have a history of DVT, varicose veins, and/or swelling in the extremity with pain, fatigability, or heaviness. Symptoms are relieved by elevating the extremity. Patients may also have increased skin pigmentation around the ankles with possible skin breakdown and ulceration.
   Treatment is at first conservative, including elastic compression stockings, elevation with minimal standing, and treatment of ulcers with cleaning and wet-to-dry dressings, and antibiotics if cellulitis occurs.

CONGENITAL DISEASE

1. **What do you need to know about the common congenital heart defects?**

DEFECT	SYMPTOMS, TREATMENT*, OTHER INFORMATION
Patent ductus arteriosus	Constant, machine-like murmur at the upper left sternal border; dyspnea and possible CHF. Close with indomethacin or surgery (if indomethacin fails). Keep open with prostaglandin E_1. Associated with congenital rubella and high altitudes.
Ventricular septal defect (VSD)	*Most common congenital heart defect.* Characterized by holosystolic murmur next to the sternum. Most cases resolve on their own. Watch for fetal alcohol, TORCH, or Down syndrome.

DEFECT	SYMPTOMS, TREATMENT*, OTHER INFORMATION
Atrial septal defect	Often asymptomatic until adulthood. Characterized by fixed split S_2 and palpitations. Most defects do not require correction (unless very large).
Tetralogy of Fallot	*Most common cyanotic congenital heart defect.* Characterized by four anomalies: VSD, RVH, pulmonary stenosis, and overriding aorta. Look for "tet" spells (squatting after exertion).
Coarctation of aorta	Upper-extremity hypertension only; radiofemoral delay; systolic murmur heard over mid-upper back; rib notching on radiographs; associated with Turner syndrome.

CHF, Congestive heart failure; RVH, right ventricular hypertrophy; TORCH, *Toxoplasma*, other, rubella, cytomegalovirus, and herpes infections.

*Endocarditis prophylaxis is required for all of these cardiac defects except an asymptomatic secundum-type atrial septal defect.

2. Name the noncyanotic congenital heart defects.
   Noncyanotic heart diseases result in left-to-right shunts in which oxygenated blood from the lungs is shunted back into the pulmonary circulation, resulting in a "pink baby." These noncyanotic heart conditions can be remembered by the three Ds: ventricular septal defect (VSD), atrial septal defect (ASD), and patent ductus arteriosus (PDA).

3. Name the cyanotic congenital heart defects.
   Cyanotic heart disease results in a right-to-left shunt in which deoxygenated blood is shunted into the systemic circulation, resulting in a "blue baby." These cyanotic heart conditions can be remembered by the five Ts and the mnemonic 12345:
   1. **T**runcus arteriosus; there is just **one** common vessel leaving the ventricles.
   2. **T**ransposition of the great vessels; the **two** great vessels (aorta and pulmonary artery) are transposed.
   3. **T**ricuspid atresia; **three** for **tri**cuspid.
   4. **T**etralogy of Fallot; **four** for **tetra**logy.
   5. **T**otal anomalous pulmonary venous return; there are **five** words in TAPVR.

DISEASES OF THE MYOCARDIUM

1. What causes restrictive cardiomyopathy? How is it different from constrictive pericarditis?
   Restrictive cardiomyopathy involves a problem with the ventricles and is usually due to amyloidosis, sarcoidosis, hemochromatosis, or myocardial fibroelastosis. A ventricular biopsy is abnormal in all of these conditions. **Constrictive pericarditis** can be fixed simply by removing an abnormal pericardium; look for a pericardial knock on examination, calcification of the pericardium, and a normal ventricular biopsy. Watch for an S_4 sound (which indicates stiff ventricles) and signs of right-sided heart failure (jugular venous distention and peripheral edema) in both conditions. These two disorders are mentioned together because both can cause a restrictive-type cardiac physiology, but the treatments are quite different.

2. What is the most common kind of cardiomyopathy? What causes it?
   Dilated cardiomyopathy, which is most commonly caused by chronic coronary artery disease or ischemia, although by strict definition this is not a true cardiomyopathy. For the USMLE, watch for alcohol, myocarditis, or doxorubicin as the cause of dilated cardiomyopathy.

3. Which cardiomyopathy is likely in a young person who passes out or dies while exercising or playing sports and has a family history of sudden death?
   Hypertrophic cardiomyopathy, which may be autosomal dominant. This idiopathic condition causes asymmetric ventricular hypertrophy that reduces cardiac output (an example of diastolic dysfunction). Look for a systolic ejection murmur along the left sternal border

(similar to aortic stenosis) that increases with standing or with a Valsalva maneuver (these maneuvers decrease the volume of blood in the left ventricle). Treat with beta-blockers or disopyramide (to allow the ventricle more time to fill). Competitive sports should be avoided. Positive inotropes (e.g., digoxin), diuretics, and vasodilators are contraindicated because they worsen the condition.

DISEASES OF THE PERICARDIUM

1. **Describe the usual symptoms of cardiac tamponade. How is it diagnosed and treated?**
   Cardiac tamponade is classically associated with penetrating trauma to the left chest. Patients classically have the Beck triad: hypotension (caused by impaired cardiac filling), distended neck veins, and muffled heart sounds. Patients will have normal breath sounds, which can distinguish tamponade from tension pneumothorax. **Pulsus paradoxus** is an exaggerated fall in blood pressure on inspiration that occurs in tamponade. If the patient is unstable, treat with pericardiocentesis; put a catheter through the skin and into the pericardial sac and aspirate blood and fluid. If the patient is stable, you can first perform echocardiography to confirm the diagnosis.

TRAUMA AND TOXIC EFFECTS

1. **What are the side effects of diuretics?**
   Thiazide diuretics cause calcium retention, hyperglycemia, hyperuricemia, hyperlipidemia, hyponatremia, hypokalemic metabolic alkalosis, and hypovolemia.
   Loop diuretics cause hypokalemic metabolic alkalosis, hypovolemia (more potent than thiazides), ototoxicity, and calcium excretion. All are sulfa drugs, with the exception of ethacrynic acid.
   Carbonic anhydrase inhibitors cause metabolic acidosis.
   Potassium-sparing diuretics (e.g., spironolactone) may cause hyperkalemia.

2. **What are the side effects of beta-blockers?**
   Like many antihypertensive agents, beta-blockers can cause sedation, depression, and sexual dysfunction. They also cause bradycardia and heart block in susceptible patients and should be avoided in patients with these conditions, as should central-acting CCBs (e.g., verapamil and diltiazem). Beta-blockers can also precipitate asthmatic attacks and mask the symptoms of hypoglycemia, so they should be avoided or used with caution in asthmatic patients and those with chronic obstructive pulmonary disease. A $beta_1$-selective beta-blocker (atenolol, metoprolol) or a combined beta-blocker and alpha-blocker (carvedilol) is preferred if a beta-blocker is needed to treat another condition such as heart disease. Use in diabetic patients requires an analysis of the risks and benefits; if other equivalent medications are available, use them instead.

3. **What antihypertensive agent is best known for causing depression?**
   Methyldopa. Beta-blockers may also cause depression.

CHAPTER 5

NUTRITIONAL AND DIGESTIVE SYSTEM DISORDERS

MOUTH, SALIVARY GLANDS, AND ESOPHAGUS

1. **What causes parotid gland swelling?**

   The classic cause is mumps. The best treatment for mumps and the complication of infertility is prevention through immunization. Parotid gland swelling may also be due to a neoplasm, of which pleomorphic adenoma is the most common type; Sjögren syndrome; sialolithiasis (a stone in the parotid duct); sarcoidosis; or bulimia. Alcoholism can cause parotid gland hypertrophy as well. Remember too that the parotid gland contains lymph nodes within its parenchyma (unique in this regard), which can become enlarged in a number of conditions, as with lymph nodes elsewhere.

2. **Define stomatitis. What does it suggest?**

   Stomatitis is an inflammation of the mucous membranes of the mouth. The classic finding is fissuring of the corners of the mouth (angular stomatitis). Watch for deficiencies of B-complex vitamins (riboflavin, niacin, pyridoxine) or vitamin C.

3. **What factors increase the risk of oral cancers? Describe the typical appearance.**

   Smoking or chewing tobacco and alcohol consumption are the main risk factors for oral cancer; their effects are synergistic. Also look for poor oral hygiene. Lesions often begin as leukoplakia (white patch) or malakoplakia (red patch). Oral hairy leukoplakia can resemble leukoplakia somewhat but is an unrelated condition affecting HIV-positive patients and is associated with the Epstein-Barr virus. The clinical setting should help you distinguish the two.

4. **What are the common causes of a neck mass?**

   In **children**, watch for thyroglossal duct cysts, which have a *midline* location and elevate with tongue protrusion; branchial cleft cysts, which are *lateral* in location and often become infected; cystic hygroma, a benign tumor also known as lymphangioma that is associated with Turner syndrome and treated with surgical resection; and cervical lymphadenitis. Cervical lymphadenitis is usually due to streptococcal pharyngitis, Epstein-Barr virus (common in the second and third decades), cat-scratch disease, or mycobacterial infection (scrofula). In terms of malignancy in children, cervical lymphadenopathy may be present in cases of leukemia or lymphoma.

   In **adults**, suspect malignancy, either lymphadenopathy from a primary tumor (lymphoma) or a metastatic neoplasm (usually squamous cell carcinoma). The mass may also represent the tumor itself (especially with thyroid cancer).

5. **Describe the workup for an unknown cancer in the neck.**

   The workup includes random biopsy of the nasopharynx, palatine tonsils, and base of the tongue, as well as laryngoscopy, bronchoscopy, and esophagoscopy (with biopsies of any suspicious lesions). This approach is known as triple endoscopy with triple biopsy.

6. **How are bleeding esophageal varices treated?**

   First, think of the ABCs (**a**irway, **b**reathing, and **c**irculation). Stabilize the patient with intravenous fluids and blood if needed. If indicated, correct any clotting factor deficiencies with fresh frozen plasma, fresh blood, and vitamin K. Give octreotide to cause splanchnic vasoconstriction and decrease bleeding. Give prophylactic antibiotics (oral norfloxacin, IV ciprofloxacin, or IV ceftriaxone) before endoscopy. Endoscopy of the upper gastrointestinal (GI) tract is performed to determine the cause of the upper GI tract bleed (there are many possibilities in an alcoholic). Once varices are identified on endoscopy, sclerotherapy of the veins is attempted with cauterization, banding, or vasopressin administration. The mortality rate is high and rebleeding is common. If you must choose, try a transjugular intrahepatic portasystemic shunt (TIPS) over an open surgical portacaval shunt for more definitive management, if needed. The most physiologic shunt type among the surgical options is a splenorenal shunt. However, open surgical shunt procedures are now rarely performed.

7. **How are varices with no history of bleeding treated?**
With nonselective beta-blockers (propranolol, nadolol, timolol) to relieve portal hypertension, provided that there is no contraindication to their use.

8. **Define gastroesophageal reflux disease (GERD). What causes it?**
GERD involves reflux of stomach acid into the esophagus. It is due to inappropriate intermittent relaxation of the lower esophageal sphincter. The incidence is much higher in patients with a hiatal hernia (see Question 11).

9. **Describe the classic symptoms of GERD. How is it treated?**
The main complaint is usually heartburn, often related to eating and lying supine. GERD may also cause abdominal or chest pain. Initial treatment is to elevate the head of the bed and to avoid coffee, alcohol, tobacco, spicy and fatty foods, chocolate, and medications with anticholinergic properties. If this approach fails, antacids, histamine-2 blockers, and proton-pump inhibitors may be tried. Many patients have already tried over-the-counter remedies before presentation, and many physicians begin empiric treatment at the first visit, because lifestyle modifications usually fail. Surgery (Nissen fundoplication) is reserved for severe or resistant cases.

10. **What are the sequelae of GERD?**
Sequelae of GERD include esophagitis, esophageal stricture (which may mimic esophageal cancer), esophageal ulcer, hemorrhage, Barrett esophagus, and esophageal adenocarcinoma. Dysphagia, odynophagia, early satiety, and weight loss are all red flag symptoms that warrant endoscopic evaluation.

11. **What is a hiatal hernia?**
A hiatal hernia is a sliding hernia, whereby the whole gastroesophageal junction moves above the diaphragm, pulling the stomach with it. This common and benign finding may predispose individuals to GERD. In a paraesophageal hernia (a type of hiatal hernia), the gastroesophageal junction stays below the diaphragm, but the stomach herniates through the diaphragm into the thorax. This type of hernia is uncommon but serious; it may become strangulated and should be repaired surgically.

12. **What are the classic symptoms of esophageal disease?**
Dysphagia (difficulty in swallowing) and/or odynophagia (painful swallowing). Patients may also have atypical chest pain.

13. **Define achalasia. How is it diagnosed and treated?**
Achalasia is caused by incomplete relaxation of a hypertensive lower-esophageal sphincter and loss or derangement of peristalsis. It is usually idiopathic but may be secondary to **Chagas disease** (South America). Patients have intermittent dysphagia for solids and liquids but no heartburn because the lower esophageal sphincter stays tightly closed and does not allow acid reflux. A barium swallow reveals a dilated esophagus with distal "bird-beak" narrowing. The diagnosis is often confirmed by esophageal manometry. Treat with calcium channel blockers, pneumatic balloon dilation, or botulism toxin injection. Surgery (myotomy) is a last resort. Patients with achalasia have a higher risk of esophageal carcinoma.

14. **What are the symptoms and signs of esophageal spasm? How is it treated?**
Both diffuse esophageal spasm and nutcracker esophagus (best thought of as a special variant of esophageal spasm) are characterized by irregular, forceful, and painful esophageal contractions that cause intermittent chest pain. Diagnose with esophageal manometry. Treat with calcium channel blockers and, if needed, surgery (myotomy).

15. **What clues suggest scleroderma as the cause of esophageal complaints?**
Scleroderma may cause aperistalsis because of esophageal fibrosis and atrophy of smooth muscle. The lower esophageal sphincter often becomes incompetent, and many patients

have heartburn (opposite of achalasia). Look for antinuclear antibody positivity and mask-like facies, as well as other autoimmune symptoms. Remember also the **CREST** syndrome, which is now known as limited scleroderma, consisting of **c**alcinosis, **R**aynaud phenomenon, **e**sophageal dysmotility, **s**clerodactyly, and **t**elangiectasias. (An alternative mnemonic is C-CREST, which includes the point that limited scleroderma has positive anticentromere antibodies).

16. **What do you need to know about the epidemiology of esophageal cancer?**
First, the epidemiology has recently changed, because adenocarcinoma is now more common than squamous cell carcinoma. Adenocarcinoma is due to the longstanding effects of gastric acid reflux and thus occurs in the distal esophagus. Squamous cell carcinoma is usually caused by alcohol and tobacco (synergistic effects) and is classically seen in black men over the age of 40 years who smoke and drink alcohol. Patients complain of weight loss and food "sticking" in the chest (solids more than liquids). Squamous cell carcinoma usually occurs in the proximal esophagus.

17. **What is the relationship between Barrett esophagus and esophageal cancer?**
Barrett esophagus, which is usually caused by longstanding GERD, predisposes individuals to esophageal adenocarcinoma. Barrett esophagus describes a columnar metaplasia of the normally squamous cell epithelium of the esophageal mucosa. Once Barrett esophagus is seen on endoscopy and confirmed by endoscopic biopsy, periodic biopsies must be done to monitor for the development of esophageal cancer.

18. **Distinguish between Mallory-Weiss and Boerhaave tears in the esophagus. How are they diagnosed?**
Mallory-Weiss tears are superficial erosions in the esophageal mucosa, whereas Boerhaave tears are full-thickness esophageal ruptures. Both may cause a GI bleed and are usually seen with vomiting and retching (alcoholics and bulimic patients) if they are not iatrogenic (caused by endoscopy). Diagnosis is usually made endoscopically (bleeding vessels should be sclerosed) and/or from contrast radiographs. Mallory-Weiss tears usually stop bleeding on their own or with endoscopic treatment, but Boerhaave tears require immediate surgical repair and drainage.

19. **What is the rule about bowel contrast when a GI perforation is suspected?**
For all GI studies, barium is preferred because it provides higher-quality images. However, do not use barium for suspected GI perforation because it can cause chemical peritonitis or mediastinitis when a perforation or leak is present. Instead, use water-soluble contrast (e.g., Gastrografin). The decision is tricky in patients with a significant risk of aspiration, because the lungs tolerate barium well but develop chemical pneumonitis from water-soluble contrast. When in doubt, give water-soluble contrast first, followed by barium once perforation has been excluded.

20. **Describe the classic presentation of esophageal cancer. What is the most common cell type?**
The presentation depends on the histologic type. The classic patient with squamous cell carcinoma is a chronic smoker and alcohol drinker between the ages of 40 and 60 years (blacks more than whites) with weight loss, anemia, and the complaint that food is sticking, which progresses to dysphagia for liquids. The other cell type is adenocarcinoma, which is typically due to malignant degeneration of Barrett esophagus (columnar metaplasia of the esophageal squamous epithelium caused by acid reflux); thus patients have a long history of acid reflux and heartburn. The prognosis is usually quite poor for either type because of late presentation. Squamous cell carcinomas used to predominate, but squamous cell carcinoma and adenocarcinoma now occur with almost equal frequency.

STOMACH

1. **What are the risk factors for stomach cancer? What are the symptoms?**
Risk factors include Asian race, increasing age, smoking history, ingestion of smoked meat, and *Helicobacter pylori* infection. Symptoms and signs include anemia, weight loss, early satiety, abdominal pain, and a nonhealing gastric ulcer. All gastric ulcers must be biopsied

to exclude malignancy. Consider follow-up endoscopy to document resolution of an ulcer, although this is somewhat controversial. Be especially suspicious if the question describes a nonhealing ulcer in a patient with weight loss.

2. **What is a Virchow node?**
A Virchow node is left supraclavicular node enlargement caused by spread of visceral cancer (classically stomach cancer). The reason for this is that this node is located close to the thoracic duct, which is responsible for lymphatic drainage from the entire abdomen.

3. **What are the symptoms of peptic ulcer disease (PUD)?**
PUD classically involves chronic, intermittent epigastric pain (burning, gnawing, or aching) that is localized and often relieved by antacids or milk. Look for epigastric tenderness. Other signs and symptoms include occult blood in the stool and nausea or vomiting. PUD is more common in men. The two types of PUD are gastric and duodenal ulcers.

4. **Explain the classic differences between duodenal and gastric ulcers.**

	DUODENAL	GASTRIC
Cases (%)	75	25
Acid secretion	Normal to high	Normal to low
Main cause	*Helicobacter pylori*	Use of nonsteroidal antiinflammatory drugs, including aspirin
Peak age	Forties	Fifties
Blood type	O	A
Eating food	Pain gets better, then worse 2-3 hr later	Pain not relieved or made worse

5. **What is the diagnostic study of choice for PUD?**
The gold standard is endoscopy (most sensitive test), but a barium study of the upper GI tract is cheaper and less invasive. Empiric treatment with medications may be tried in the absence of diagnostic studies if the symptoms are typical. If endoscopy is performed, a biopsy of any gastric ulcer is mandatory to exclude malignancy. Duodenal ulcers do not have to be biopsied initially, because malignancy is rare.

6. **What is the most feared complication of PUD? What should you suspect if an ulcer does not respond to treatment?**
The most feared complication of PUD is **perforation.** Look for peritoneal signs, a history of PUD, and free air on an abdominal radiograph. Treat with antibiotics (such as ceftriaxone and metronidazole) and laparotomy with repair of the perforation. If ulcers are severe, recurrent, atypical (e.g., located in the jejunum), or nonhealing, think about stomach cancer or Zollinger-Ellison syndrome (gastrinoma; check gastrin levels). PUD is also a cause of GI bleeding, which can be severe in some cases.

7. **How is PUD treated initially?**
First, remember that dietary changes are not thought to help heal ulcers, although reduced alcohol and tobacco use may speed healing. Stop all nonsteroidal antiinflammatory drug use. Start treatment with proton-pump inhibitors, test for *H. pylori* infection, and treat any such infection with antibiotics. Many regimens exist, but the most commonly used is triple therapy with a proton pump inhibitor, clarithromycin, and amoxicillin.

8. **List the surgical options for ulcer treatment. What complications may occur?**
Surgical options are generally only considered if medical treatment has failed or if complications are present (perforation, bleeding). Surgical procedures for PUD include antrectomy, vagotomy, and Billroth I or II procedures. After surgery (especially Billroth procedures) watch for dumping syndrome (weakness, dizziness, sweating, and nausea or vomiting after eating). Patients also develop hypoglycemia 2 to 3 hours after a meal, which causes recurrence of the same symptoms, as well as afferent loop syndrome (bilious vomiting after a meal relieves abdominal pain), bacterial overgrowth, and vitamin deficiencies (vitamin B_{12} and/or iron, causing anemia).

9. **Describe the usual history of a perforated ulcer. How is it treated?**
   Patients often have no history of alcohol abuse or gallstones (pancreatitis risk factors). Abdominal radiographs classically show free air under the diaphragm, and a history of PUD is often included in the patient description. Remember that a perforated bowel can cause increases in amylase and lipase levels. Treat with surgery.

10. **Define Zollinger-Ellison syndrome. What clues point to the diagnosis?**
    Zollinger-Ellison syndrome is a gastrinoma that causes acid hypersecretion (gastrin stimulates acid secretion) and PUD. Peptic ulcers are often multiple and resistant to therapy and may be found in unusual locations (distal duodenum or jejunum). More than half of these pancreatic islet-cell tumors are malignant. Diagnosis is made on the basis of an elevated fasting serum gastrin level or a secretin stimulation test. Remember that a patient on a proton-pump inhibitor will also have elevated gastrin levels because of its feedback mechanism.

11. **Define achlorhydria. What causes it?**
    Achlorhydria is an absence of hydrochloric acid secretion. It is most commonly due to **pernicious anemia**, in which antiparietal cell antibodies destroy acid-secreting parietal cells and thus cause achlorhydria and vitamin B_{12} deficiency. It is often associated with other endocrine autoimmune disorders (e.g., hypothyroidism, vitiligo, diabetes, hypoadrenalism). Achlorhydria may also be caused by surgical gastric resection.

12. **What are the classic differences between upper and lower GI tract bleeds?**

	UPPER GI TRACT BLEED	LOWER GI TRACT BLEED
Location	Proximal to ligament of Treitz	Distal to ligament of Treitz
Common causes	Gastritis, ulcers, varices, esophagitis	Vascular ectasia, diverticulosis, colon cancer, colitis, inflammatory bowel disease, hemorrhoids
Stool	Tarry, black stool (melena)	Bright red blood seen in stool (hematochezia)
NGT aspirate	Positive for blood	Negative for blood

NGT, Nasogastric tube.

13. **How is a GI bleed treated?**
    The first step is to *make sure that the patient is stable* (ABCs [airway, breathing, circulation]; intravenous fluids and blood, if needed) before you try to reach a diagnosis. Next, place a nasogastric tube and test the aspirate for blood to help determine whether the patient has an upper or lower GI tract bleed. Patients with upper GI tract bleeds are started on intravenous proton-pump inhibitors. Octreotide and antibiotics are started if variceal bleeding is suspected. **Endoscopy** is usually the first test performed (upper or lower tract, depending on symptoms and nasogastric tube aspirate). Endoscopically treatable lesions include ulcers, polyps, vascular ectasias, and varices.

14. **What radiologic imaging studies can be done to localize a GI bleed? Does surgery have a role?**
    Radionuclide (i.e., nuclear medicine) scans can detect slow or intermittent bleeds if a source cannot be found by endoscopy. Angiography can detect more rapid bleeds, and embolization of bleeding vessels can be performed during the procedure. Surgery is reserved for severe or resistant bleeds and typically involves resection of the affected bowel (usually colon).

15. **Define acute abdomen. What physical examination signs suggest its presence?**
    Acute abdomen generally refers to an inflamed peritoneum (peritonitis), which is often due to a surgically correctable problem. Patients with an acute abdomen often receive a laparotomy and/or laparoscopy because it signifies a potentially life-threatening condition. The best physical examination confirmations of peritonitis are **rebound tenderness** and **involuntary guarding.** Rebound tenderness is elicited by letting go quickly after deep palpation of the abdomen; acute pain occurs in the area of palpation (with generalized peritonitis) or at the location of localized

inflammation (e.g., Rovsing sign in appendicitis). Involuntary guarding describes a muscle spasm of the abdominal wall that cannot be controlled. Voluntary guarding (person reflexively or willfully tenses his or her abdomen during attempted palpation) and tenderness to palpations are softer signs often present in benign diseases.

16. **What should you do if you are not sure whether a stable patient has acute abdomen?**
When you are in doubt and the patient is stable, use minimal pain medications as needed (to avoid masking symptoms before you have a diagnosis), perform serial abdominal examinations, and consider a computed tomography (CT) scan. If the patient becomes unstable, proceed to laparoscopy and/or laparotomy.

17. **Name a few causes of peritonitis that do not require laparotomy or laparoscopy.**
Pancreatitis, many cases of diverticulitis, and spontaneous bacterial peritonitis.

18. **Specify which conditions are associated with pain and peritonitis in the abdominal areas listed.**

AREA	ORGAN (CONDITIONS)
Upper right quadrant	Gallbladder/biliary (cholecystitis, cholangitis) or liver (abscess)
Upper left quadrant	Spleen (rupture with blunt trauma)
Lower right quadrant	Appendix (appendicitis), pelvic inflammatory disease (PID)
Left lower quadrant	Sigmoid colon (diverticulitis), PID
Epigastric area	Stomach (peptic ulcer) or pancreas (pancreatitis)

SMALL INTESTINE/COLON AND RECTUM

1. **Specify the classic differences between Crohn disease and ulcerative colitis.**

	CROHN DISEASE	ULCERATIVE COLITIS
Place of origin	Distal ileum, proximal colon	Rectum
Thickness of pathology	Transmural	Mucosa/submucosa only
Progression	Irregular (skip lesions)	Proximal, continuous from rectum; no skipped areas
Location	From mouth to anus	Involves only colon, rarely extends to ileum
Bowel habit changes	Obstruction, abdominal pain	Bloody diarrhea
Classic lesions	Fistulas/abscesses, cobblestoning, string sign on barium x-ray	Pseudopolyps, lead-pipe colon on barium x-ray, toxic megacolon
Colon cancer risk	Slightly increased	Markedly increased
Surgery	No (may make worse)	Yes (proctocolectomy with ileoanal anastomosis)

2. **Describe the extraintestinal manifestations of inflammatory bowel disease.**
Both forms of inflammatory bowel disease can cause uveitis, arthritis, ankylosing spondylitis, erythema nodosum, erythema multiforme, primary sclerosing cholangitis, failure to thrive or grow in children, toxic megacolon, anemia of chronic disease, and fever. Toxic megacolon is more common in ulcerative colitis; look for a markedly distended colon on an abdominal radiograph.

3. **How is inflammatory bowel disease treated?**
Patients are treated with 5-aminosalicylic acid, with or without a sulfa drug (e.g., sulfasalazine), when stable. Steroids and other immune modulators (e.g., azathioprine) are used during severe disease flare-ups.

4. **What causes toxic megacolon? How is it treated?**

   Toxic megacolon is classically seen with inflammatory bowel disease (especially ulcerative colitis) and infectious (especially *Clostridium difficile*) colitis. It may be precipitated by the use of antidiarrheal medications, which for this reason are usually not given for infectious diarrhea. Most patients have a high fever, leukocytosis, abdominal pain, rebound tenderness, and a dilated segment of colon on abdominal radiography. Toxic megacolon is an emergency! Start treatment by discontinuing all antidiarrheal medications. Do not allow the patient to eat, place a nasogastric tube, start intravenous fluids, and give antibiotics to cover bowel flora (such as ceftriaxone and metronidazole), as well as steroids if the cause is inflammatory bowel disease. Surgery is required if perforation occurs (free air is seen on an abdominal radiograph).

5. **True or false: Children may develop inflammatory bowel disease and irritable bowel syndrome.**

   True. Abdominal pain may be the result of inflammatory bowel disease or irritable bowel syndrome. Diarrhea, fever, bloody stools, anemia, joint pains, and poor growth are more concerning for inflammatory bowel disease. GI complaints may be due to anxiety or psychiatric problems. Watch for separation anxiety, children who do not want to go to school, depression, and child abuse.

6. **Define diverticulosis. What are its complications?**

   Diverticulosis is characterized by sac-like mucosal projections through the muscular layer of the colon and/or rectum. It is extremely common and the incidence increases with age. It is thought to be caused in part by a low-fiber, high-fat diet. Complications include GI bleeding (common cause of painless lower GI bleeds) and diverticulitis (inflammation of a diverticulum), which can lead to abscess, fistula formation, sepsis, or large bowel obstruction.

7. **What is the cause of left lower quadrant pain and fever in a patient older than 50 years until proved otherwise? How is it treated?**

   Diverticulitis. Treat medically with broad-spectrum antibiotics (e.g., ciprofloxacin plus metronidazole), avoidance of eating, and a nasogastric tube if nausea and vomiting are present. For disease that recurs or is refractory to medical therapy, consider sigmoid colon resection.

8. **How do you diagnose and treat diverticulitis? What test should a patient have after a treated episode of diverticulitis?**

   Signs and symptoms of diverticulitis include left lower quadrant pain or tenderness, fever, diarrhea or constipation, and increased white blood cell count. The pathophysiology is thought to be similar to that for appendicitis. Stool or other debris impacts within the diverticulum and causes obstruction, leading to bacterial overgrowth and inflammation. The diagnosis can be confirmed by a CT scan, if needed, which can also help to rule out complications such as perforation or abscess. In the absence of complications, the treatment is antibiotics that cover bowel flora (e.g., a fluoroquinolone plus metronidazole) and bowel rest (i.e., no oral intake). Surgery is needed for perforation or abscess.

   After a treated episode of diverticulitis, all patients need colon cancer screening with colonoscopy (colon carcinoma with perforation can mimic diverticulitis clinically and on CT scans). These studies should be avoided during active diverticulitis, however, because of an increased risk of perforation.

9. **Define irritable bowel syndrome. How do you recognize it?**

   Irritable bowel syndrome is a common cause of GI complaints. Patients may be anxious or neurotic and have a history of diarrhea aggravated by stress; bloating; abdominal pain relieved by defecation; and/or mucus in the stool. Look for psychosocial stressors in the history and normal physical findings and test results. Irritable bowel syndrome is a diagnosis of exclusion; you must perform at least basic laboratory tests, a rectal examination, a stool examination, and sigmoidoscopy. Because it is so common, however, irritable bowel syndrome is the most likely diagnosis if the question gives no positive findings, especially in young adults (female-to-male ratio of 3:1).

10. **How is diarrhea categorized according to its causes?**
    - Systemic: any illness can cause diarrhea as a systemic symptom, especially in children (e.g., infection)
    - Osmotic

- Secretory
- Malabsorptive
- Infectious
- Exudative
- Altered intestinal transit

11. **Define osmotic diarrhea. How can an easy diagnosis be made?**
Osmotic diarrhea is caused by nonabsorbable solutes that remain in the bowel, where they retain water (e.g., lactose or other sugar intolerance). When the patient stops ingesting the offending substance (e.g., avoidance of milk or a trial of not eating), the diarrhea stops—an easy diagnosis. Artificial sweeteners such as sorbitol are an often-tested cause of osmotic diarrhea.

12. **What causes secretory diarrhea?**
Secretory diarrhea results when the bowel secretes too much fluid. It is often due to bacterial toxins (cholera, some species of *Escherichia coli*), VIPoma (pancreatic islet cell tumor that secretes vasoactive intestinal peptide [VIP]), or bile acids (after ileal resection). Secretory diarrhea continues when the patient stops eating.

13. **What are the common causes of malabsorptive diarrhea?**
Celiac disease (look for dermatitis herpetiformis, and avoid gluten in the diet), Crohn disease, and postgastroenteritis (caused by depletion of brush-border enzymes). Malabsorptive diarrhea improves when the patient stops eating.

14. **What are the common clues to infectious diarrhea? What are the common causes?**
In patients with infectious diarrhea, look for fever and white blood cells in the stool (only with invasive bacteria such as *Shigella*, *Salmonella*, *Yersinia*, and *Campylobacter* spp.; not found with toxigenic bacteria). Travel history (traveler's diarrhea caused by enterotoxigenic *E. coli*) is also a tip-off. Enterotoxigenic *E. coli* is treated with ciprofloxacin. Hikers and stream-drinkers may have *Giardia* infection, which presents with steatorrhea (fatty, greasy, malodorous stools that float) caused by small bowel involvement and unique protozoal cysts in the stool. Treat *Giardia* infections with metronidazole. Also watch for *C. difficile* diarrhea in patients with a history of antibiotic use. Test the stool for *C. difficile* toxin; if the result is positive, treat with oral metronidazole (oral vancomycin is a second-line agent if metronidazole is not an option).

15. **What causes exudative diarrhea?**
Exudative diarrhea results from inflammation in the bowel mucosa that causes seepage of fluid. Mucosal inflammation is usually due to inflammatory bowel disease (Crohn disease or ulcerative colitis) or cancer. Patients commonly have fever and white blood cells in the stool, as in infectious diarrhea, but a lack of pathogenic organisms, chronicity, and nonbowel symptoms are clues.

16. **What are the common causes of diarrhea that is due to altered intestinal transit?**
This type of diarrhea is seen after bowel resections, in patients taking medications that interfere with bowel function, and in patients with hyperthyroidism or neuropathy (e.g., diabetic diarrhea). Watch for factitious diarrhea, which is caused by secret laxative abuse and is classically found to have melanosis coli, a darkening of the colonic mucosa.

17. **What should you do if a patient has diarrhea?**
In all patients with diarrhea, watch for and treat dehydration and electrolyte disturbances, especially metabolic acidosis and hypokalemia. Diarrhea is a common and preventable cause of death in underdeveloped countries. Perform a rectal examination, look for occult blood in the stool, and examine the stool for bacteria (Gram stain and culture), ova and parasites, fat content (steatorrhea), and white blood cells.

18. **What should you watch for in children after a bout of bacterial diarrhea?**
After bacterial (especially *E. coli* or *Shigella* spp.) diarrhea in children, watch for **hemolytic uremic syndrome**, which is characterized by thrombocytopenia, hemolytic anemia (schistocytes, helmet cells, and fragmented red blood cells on a peripheral blood smear), and acute renal failure. Treatment is supportive. Patients may need dialysis and/or transfusions.

19. What is the most common cause of diarrhea in children?

As a primary cause, viral gastroenteritis is probable (e.g., Norwalk virus, rotavirus). Remember, however, that diarrhea is often a nonspecific sign of any systemic illness (e.g., otitis media, pneumonia, urinary tract infection).

20. Describe the classic presentation of appendicitis. How is it treated?

Appendicitis classically occurs in 10- to 30-year-old individuals with a history of crampy, poorly localized periumbilical pain followed by nausea and vomiting. Then the pain localizes to the right lower quadrant, and peritoneal signs develop with worsening of nausea and vomiting. It is said that a patient who is hungry and asking for food does not have appendicitis (called the hamburger sign), but up to a quarter of patients with appendicitis will not have anorexia. A classic clue to the diagnosis is the **Rovsing sign:** when you palpate a different quadrant and then quickly release your hand, the patient feels pain at the McBurney point (two thirds of the way from the umbilicus to the anterior superior iliac spine). The McBurney point is the area of maximal tenderness in the right lower quadrant and the site where an open appendectomy incision is made. CT scanning is increasingly used to confirm the diagnosis before surgery in stable patients.

21. What are the hallmarks of small bowel obstruction? How is it treated?

Small bowel obstruction commonly causes bilious vomiting (early symptom), abdominal distention, constipation, hyperactive bowel sounds (high-pitched, rushing sounds), and usually poorly localized abdominal pain. Radiographs show multiple air-fluid levels. Patients often have a history of previous surgery (most common overall) or have a hernia (most common cause in patients without a history of surgery).

Start treatment by withholding food, placing a nasogastric tube set to low intermittent wall suction, and giving intravenous fluids. If the obstruction does not resolve or if peritoneal signs develop, laparotomy is usually needed. CT scanning can confirm an uncertain diagnosis in stable patients and may reveal the underlying cause of the obstruction and localize the exact area of the obstruction if surgery is planned.

22. What are the common causes of a small bowel obstruction?

In adults, the most common cause is **adhesions,** which usually develop from prior surgery. Incarcerated hernias and Crohn disease are other common causes. Other causes include Meckel diverticulum and intussusception (both typically seen in children).

23. Describe the signs and symptoms of large bowel obstruction. What causes it? How is it treated?

The presentation for large bowel obstruction usually involves gradually increasing abdominal pain, abdominal distention, constipation, and feculent vomiting (late symptom). In older adults, the most common causes are diverticulitis, colon cancer, and volvulus. In children, watch for Hirschsprung disease. Treat early by withholding food and placing a nasogastric tube for nausea and vomiting. Sigmoid volvulus can often be decompressed with an endoscope, whereas cecal volvulus often requires surgery. Other causes or refractory cases require surgery to relieve the obstruction.

24. List the primary risk factors for colon cancer.

Age (incidence begins to increase after the age of 40 years; peak incidence between 60 and 75 years)

Family history (especially with familial polyposis or Gardner, Turcot, Peutz-Jeghers, or Lynch syndromes)

Inflammatory bowel disease (ulcerative colitis more than Crohn disease, but both are associated with increased risk)

Low-fiber, high-fat diet

25. What symptoms do patients with colon cancer tend to have?

Patients may have asymptomatic blood in the stool (visible streaks of blood on the stool or a positive occult blood test). Anemia is classic with right-sided colon cancer. A change in stool caliber ("pencil stool") or frequency (alternating constipation and frequency) is a classic symptom of left-sided colon cancer. Colon cancer is also a common cause of large bowel obstruction in adults. As with any cancer, look for weight loss.

26. **What is the rule about occult blood in the stool of a patient over age 40 years?**
Occult blood in the stool of a person older than 40 years should be considered colon cancer until proven otherwise. To rule out colon cancer, perform a colonoscopy.

27. **How is colon cancer treated?**
Treatment is primarily surgical, with resection of involved bowel. Adjuvant chemotherapy is sometimes given (e.g., 5-fluorouracil with leucovorin, irinotecan, oxaliplatin, cetuximab and panitumumab, or bevacizumab) for lymph node involvement. Distant metastases frequently go to the liver first (as with all GI tumors). Surgical resection of a solitary liver metastasis is often attempted. For metastases elsewhere, chemotherapy is the only option and prognosis is poor.

28. **What is the classic tumor marker for colon cancer? How is it used clinically?**
Carcinoembryonic antigen (CEA) may be elevated in colon cancer. If a patient is found to have colon cancer, the CEA level is usually measured before surgery. If it is elevated preoperatively (not always), the CEA level should return to normal after surgical removal of the tumor. Periodic monitoring of CEA after surgery may then help to detect recurrence before it is clinically apparent. CEA is *not* used as a screening tool for colon cancer; it is used only to follow known cancer because it is neither sensitive nor specific (can be elevated with other visceral tumors).

29. **What are the symptoms of carcinoid tumors? Where are they most commonly found?**
Carcinoid tumors secrete serotonin-like products that can cause symptoms, but the liver breaks down serotonin and other vasoactive secretions, so the tumor is initially asymptomatic. Once a carcinoid tumor metastasizes to the liver and vasoactive products reach the systemic circulation, symptoms begin (carcinoid syndrome), including episodic cutaneous flushing, abdominal cramps, diarrhea, and right-sided heart valve damage. The most common location is in the small bowel, but carcinoid tumors are also the most common appendiceal tumor (sometimes found at the time of appendectomy in patients with appendicitis).

30. **What laboratory test detects carcinoid tumors?**
Urinary levels of 5-hydroxyindoleacetic acid (5-HIAA, a serotonin breakdown product) are increased, but not all carcinoid tumors cause elevated 5-HIAA levels. If the diagnosis is still suspected, octreotide scintigraphy can reliably identify all types and locations of carcinoid tumors.

GALLBLADDER AND BILE DUCT

1. **What are the classic symptoms and signs of gallstone disease?**
Classic gallstone disease symptoms include postprandial colicky pain in the right upper quadrant with bloating and/or nausea and vomiting. The pain usually begins 15 to 60 minutes after a meal (especially a fatty meal). Look for the **Murphy sign** (palpation of the right upper quadrant under the rib cage causes arrest of inspiration because of pain) as the main physical examination finding for cholecystitis.

2. **What are the six Fs of cholecystitis? How do the demographics of patients with pigment stones differ from those of patients with cholesterol stones?**
The first five Fs summarize the demographics of individuals with cholesterol gallstones: fat, forty, fertile, female, and flatulent; the sixth F is febrile, which indicates that such patients have now developed acute cholecystitis. Patients with pigment (i.e., calcium bilirubinate) stones are classically young patients with hemolytic anemia (e.g., sickle cell disease, hereditary spherocytosis).

3. **How is a clinical suspicion of cholecystitis confirmed and treated?**
Ultrasound is the best first imaging study for suspected gallbladder disease. It may show gallstones, a thin layer of fluid around the gallbladder (termed pericholecystic fluid), and/or a thickened gallbladder wall. A more specific ultrasonographic Murphy sign using direct visualization of the gallbladder can be obtained (variant anatomy and significant obesity can

create uncertainty). A nuclear hepatobiliary scintigraphic study (e.g., hepatoiminodiacetic acid [HIDA] scan) confirms the diagnosis for a nonvisualized gallbladder. The treatment comprises pain control and cholecystectomy (antibiotics may be indicated if infection is suspected); a laparoscopic approach is generally preferred over an open procedure.

4. **Define cholangitis. How does it differ from cholecystitis? How is it treated?**
Cholangitis is inflammation of the bile ducts, whereas cholecystitis is inflammation of the gallbladder. Cholangitis is classically due to biliary obstruction with subsequent bile stasis and infection. Choledocholithiasis (a gallstone in the common bile duct) and malignancy are common causes of obstruction. Autoimmune cholangitis (e.g., sclerosing cholangitis) and primary infection (e.g., *Clonorchis sinensis* and other parasite infections common in some parts of Asia) are other causes. Cholangitis classically involves the **Charcot triad:** (1) right upper quadrant pain, (2) fever or shaking chills, and (3) jaundice. As patients worsen and develop sepsis from their cholangitis, they can develop the **Reynold pentad**, which also includes (4) hypotension and (5) altered mental status. Patients may have a history of gallstones. Start broad-spectrum antibiotics to cover bowel flora (e.g., piperacillin with tazobactam), then manage more definitively depending on the circumstances (treatment of cholangitis caused by gallstones is endoscopic retrograde cholangiopancreatography [ERCP] to remove stones in the common bile duct, with subsequent cholecystectomy to remove the gallbladder; biliary stent placement is the most common treatment for unresectable obstruction caused by malignancy).

5. **What usually precipitates cholangitis? What is the tip-off to its presence? How is it treated?**
Cholangitis is usually precipitated by a gallstone that blocks the common bile duct, with subsequent infection of the bile duct system. The tip-off is the presence of the **Charcot triad:** fever, right upper quadrant pain, and jaundice. Treatment is as described in the previous question.

6. **Who typically gets primary sclerosing cholangitis?**
Primary sclerosing cholangitis usually occurs in young adults with inflammatory bowel disease (usually ulcerative colitis). The symptoms are similar to bacterial cholangitis. Fever, chills, pruritis, and abdominal pain in the right upper quadrant are common.

7. **What signs and symptoms suggest biliary tract obstruction as a cause of jaundice?**
- Elevated conjugated bilirubin (conjugated bilirubin is more elevated than unconjugated bilirubin because the liver still functions and can conjugate bilirubin, but conjugated bilirubin cannot be excreted because of biliary tract disease)
- Markedly elevated alkaline phosphatase
- Pruritus
- Clay-colored stools
- Dark urine that is strongly positive for conjugated bilirubin (unconjugated bilirubin is not excreted in the urine because it is tightly bound to albumin)

8. **What are the types of biliary tract obstruction commonly tested in the USMLE?**
Bile duct obstruction, cholestasis, cholangitis, primary biliary cirrhosis, and primary sclerosing cholangitis.

9. **What are the two major causes of common bile duct obstruction? How are they distinguished?**
The most common cause is obstruction by a gallstone (choledocholithiasis). Look for a history of gallstones or the four Fs (female, forty, fertile, and fat). Ultrasound often images the stone; if not, use magnetic resonance cholangiopancreatography (MRCP) or ERCP. Treatment involves endoscopic removal of the stone. The second major cause of common bile duct obstruction is cancer. Look for weight loss. Pancreatic cancer is the most common type; look for the **Courvoisier sign** (jaundice with a palpably enlarged gallbladder). Sometimes cholangiocarcinoma or bowel cancer blocks the common bile duct.

10. **What are the two common causes of cholestasis?**
Medications (e.g., birth control pills, trimethoprim-sulfamethoxazole, phenothiazines, androgens) and pregnancy.

11. **What clues suggest a diagnosis of primary biliary cirrhosis?**
    This condition is usually seen in middle-aged women with no risk factors for liver or biliary disease. It causes marked pruritus, jaundice, and positive **antimitochondrial antibodies.** The rest of the workup is negative. Cholestyramine helps with symptoms, but the only treatment is liver transplantation.

12. **Which diseases can cause elevated levels of alkaline phosphatase? What laboratory test is used to distinguish among these diseases?**
    Alkaline phosphatase can be elevated in biliary disease, bone disease, and pregnancy (the placenta produces alkaline phosphatase). If the elevation is due to biliary disease, gamma-glutamyltranspeptidase (GGT) and/or 5′-nucleotidase (5′-NT) should also be elevated; however, both values are normal in bone disease and pregnancy.

LIVER

1. **List the common findings for acute liver disease.**
   - Elevated liver function tests (aspartate aminotransferase [AST], alanine aminotransferase [ALT], bilirubin, alkaline phosphatase, and/or prothrombin time (PT) and international normalized ratio [INR])
   - Jaundice
   - Nausea and vomiting
   - Right upper quadrant pain or tenderness
   - Hepatomegaly

2. **List the common causes of acute liver disease.**
   - Alcohol
   - Medications
   - Infection (usually hepatitis)
   - Reye syndrome
   - Biliary tract disease
   - Autoimmune disease

3. **What are the classic causes of drug-induced hepatitis?**
   Acetaminophen, isoniazid and other tuberculosis drugs (e.g., rifampin and pyrazinamide), halothane, HMG-CoA reductase inhibitors, and carbon tetrachloride. The first step in treatment is to stop the drug.

4. **When should you suspect idiopathic autoimmune hepatitis? What is the serologic marker?**
   Idiopathic autoimmune hepatitis is classically seen in 20- to 40-year-old women with antibodies against smooth muscle or antinuclear antibodies and no risk factors or laboratory markers for other causes of hepatitis. Treat with steroids.

5. **What are the usual causes of chronic liver disease?**
   Alcohol, hepatitis, and metabolic diseases. Watch for the stigmata of chronic liver disease: gynecomastia, testicular atrophy, palmar erythema, spider angiomas on the skin, and ascites.

6. **What is the most common cause of cirrhosis and esophageal varices?**
   Alcohol.

7. **Define hemochromatosis. How do you recognize it?**
   Hemochromatosis, in its primary form, is usually autosomal recessive; look for a family history. Nearly 1 in 250 people in the United States are homozygous for this condition, although penetrance and clinical expression are variable. The pathophysiology is incompletely understood but includes excessive iron absorption by the intestine. Excessive iron is deposited in the liver (potentially causing cirrhosis and/or hepatocellular carcinoma), pancreas (potentially causing diabetes), heart (resulting in dilated cardiomyopathy), skin (causing pigmentation classically known as **bronze diabetes**), and joints (arthritis). Men are symptomatic earlier and more often because women lose iron during menstruation. Treat with phlebotomy. Secondary iron overload can cause secondary hemochromatosis,

which is classically due to an anemia that results in ineffective erythropoiesis (e.g., thalassemia) and excessive iron intake.

8. **Define Wilson disease. How do you recognize it? How is it treated?**
   Wilson disease is an autosomal-recessive disease caused by excessive serum copper. Serum **ceruloplasmin** (a copper transport protein) is usually low or absent, but serum copper may be normal. Biopsy shows excessive copper in the liver. Patients classically have liver disease with central nervous system and psychiatric manifestations (caused by copper deposits in the basal ganglia; another name for this disease is hepatolenticular degeneration) and **Kayser-Fleischer** rings in the eye. Treat with penicillamine (copper chelator).

9. **What are the clues to a diagnosis of alpha₁-antitrypsin (AAT) deficiency?**
   The classic case is a young adult who develops cirrhosis and/or emphysema without risk factors for either. AAT deficiency has an autosomal-recessive inheritance pattern; look for a positive family history. Diagnosis requires serum AAT of less than 11 μmol/L and a severe deficiency genotype.

10. **What metabolic derangements accompany liver failure?**
    Coagulopathy: prolonged PT. In severe cases the partial thromboplastin time (PTT) may also be prolonged. The liver is responsible for synthesizing vitamin-K–dependent clotting factors II, VII, IX, and X; protein C; and protein S. However, administration of vitamin K does not solve the problem because it cannot be utilized by the damaged liver. Symptomatic patients must be treated with fresh frozen plasma.
    Jaundice/hyperbilirubinemia: elevated conjugated and unconjugated bilirubin with hepatic damage (vs. biliary tract disease; see later discussion).
    Hypoalbuminemia: the liver synthesizes albumin.
    Ascites: caused by portal hypertension and/or hypoalbuminemia. Ascites can be detected on physical examination as a shifting dullness or a positive fluid wave. A possible complication is **spontaneous bacterial peritonitis** (SBP) caused by infected ascitic fluid that can lead to sepsis. Look for fever and/or a change in mental status in a patient with known ascites. Perform paracentesis, examine the ascitic fluid for elevated white blood cell count (especially neutrophils; a neutrophil count of >250/mm³ is diagnostic for SBP), and perform a Gram stain, culture and sensitivity tests, and glucose (low with infection) and protein (high with infection) measurements. The usual causes are *E. coli*, *Streptococcus pneumoniae*, and other enteric organisms. Treat with broad-spectrum antibiotics (cefotaxime is a common choice).
    Portal hypertension: seen with cirrhosis (chronic liver disease); causes hemorrhoids, varices, and caput medusae (engorged veins on the abdominal wall).
    Hyperammonemia: the liver clears ammonia. Treat with decreased protein intake (source of ammonia) and lactulose administration (prevents absorption of ammonia). The last choice is neomycin (which is no longer used as much as it once was), which kills bowel flora species that produce ammonia.
    Hepatic encephalopathy: mostly caused by hyperammonemia; often precipitated by protein intake, a GI bleed, or infection. Look for asterixis and/or mental status changes.
    Hepatorenal syndrome: liver failure may cause kidney failure (believed to be due to splanchnic vasodilation, increased renin-angiotensia-aldosterone (RAA) activity, and renal vasoconstriction).
    Hypoglycemia: the liver stores glycogen.
    Disseminated intravascular coagulation: activated clotting factors are cleared by the liver.

11. **What are the classic physical stigmata of liver disease in alcoholics?**
    - Abdominal wall varices (caput medusae)
    - Testicular atrophy
    - Esophageal varices
    - Encephalopathy
    - Hemorrhoids (internal)
    - Asterixis
    - Jaundice

- Scleral icterus
- Ascites
- Edema
- Palmar erythema
- Spider angiomas
- Gynecomastia
- Terry nails (white nails with a ground glass appearance and no lunula)
- Fetor hepaticus (so-called breath of the dead, which is a sweet, fecal smell)
- Dupuytren contractures (contracture of the palmar fascia)

12. **What are the classic laboratory findings for liver disease in alcoholics?**
    - Anemia (classically macrocytic)
    - Prolonged PT
    - Hyperbilirubinemia
    - Hypoalbuminemia
    - Thrombocytopenia

13. **Describe the classic derangement of AST and ALT in alcoholic hepatitis.**
    The ratio of AST (also known as serum glutamate oxaloacetate transaminase [SGOT]) to ALT (also known as serum glutamate pyruvate transaminase [SGPT]) is at least 2:1, although levels of both may be elevated. Other causes of hepatitis are usually associated with the opposite ratio or equal elevation of both AST and ALT.

14. **What increases the risk of hepatocellular cancer of the liver? What is the classic tumor marker for liver cancer?**
    The same factors that increase the risk of cirrhosis. The three leading causes are alcohol, chronic hepatitis (hepatitis C is now a more likely culprit than hepatitis B in countries that routinely vaccinate against hepatitis B), and hemochromatosis. Hepatocellular carcinoma may develop in patients with hepatitis B before the onset of cirrhosis. **Alpha-fetoprotein** is often elevated and can be measured postoperatively to detect recurrences. It is also used for screening in high-risk populations (e.g., those with cirrhosis) in addition to serial ultrasound scans. The most common cause of a new liver mass in any patient with cirrhosis is hepatocellular carcinoma.

15. **What symptoms do patients with liver cancer exhibit? How is liver cancer treated?**
    Patients often have a history of alcoholism, hepatitis, and/or hemochromatosis or other causes of cirrhosis. They exhibit weight loss, right upper quadrant pain, and an enlarged liver. The prognosis is poor. Treatment options for hepatocellular carcinoma include surgical resection, radiofrequency ablation, and transcatheter arterial chemoembolization (TACE) in selected candidates.

16. **What other tumors of the liver may appear in the USMLE? What clues suggest their presence?**
    Hemangioma: most common primary tumor of the liver; benign and generally left alone. Surgery is performed only if symptoms (pain, bleeding) are present.
    Hepatic adenoma: benign tumor in women of reproductive age who take **birth control pills.** Stop the birth control pills; the tumor may regress. If not, surgery is usually preferred to prevent hemorrhage and rare malignant transformation.
    Cholangiocarcinoma: malignant. Fifty percent of patients have inflammatory bowel disease (especially ulcerative colitis); liver flukes (*Clonorchis* spp.) increase the risk in some immigrant populations (China, Japan, Taiwan, Vietnam, Korea, far eastern Russia).
    Angiosarcoma: malignant. Look for industrial exposure to vinyl chloride.
    Hepatoblastoma: malignant; the most common primary liver malignancy in children.
    Metastases: Look for the presence of multiple liver masses.

17. **Name three medications that cause hepatic enzyme induction and three that cause hepatic enzyme inhibition.**
    Barbiturates, antiepileptics, and rifampin are classic enzyme inducers; cimetidine, erythromycin, and ketoconazole are classic enzyme inhibitors. The end result may be ineffectiveness or

toxicity of other administered drugs (e.g., warfarin, oral contraceptives, and antiepileptics). Other classically tested substances include an enzyme inhibitor, grapefruit juice, and an enzyme inducer, St. John's wort.

18. **What happens after an overdose of acetaminophen?**

High doses of acetaminophen cause liver toxicity caused by depletion of glutathione and resultant cellular damage from the metabolite N-acetyl-p-benzoquinone imine (NAPQI). Treat with **acetylcysteine** to decrease liver injury.

PANCREAS

1. **Describe the classic symptoms of pancreatic cancer. How is it treated? What is the cell of origin?**

The classic patient is a smoker in the 40- to 80-year-old range who has lost weight and has jaundice. Other signs and symptoms include depression, epigastric pain, migratory thrombophlebitis (**Trousseau syndrome,** which may also be seen with other visceral cancers), and a palpable, nontender gallbladder (**Courvoisier sign**). Pancreatic cancer is more common in men than in women, in diabetic than in nondiabetic patients, and in blacks than in whites. Surgery (Whipple procedure) is rarely curative and the prognosis is generally dismal. Chemotherapy is minimally successful at prolonging survival. The cells of origin in pancreatic cancer are ductal epithelial cells.

2. **What is the most common islet cell tumor of the pancreas? How is it diagnosed?**

Insulinomas (beta-cell tumors) are the most common islet cell tumors. Look for two parts of the **Whipple triad**: hypoglycemia (glucose <50 mg/dL) and resultant symptoms of the central nervous system (confusion, stupor, loss of consciousness). As a good doctor, you provide the third part of the Whipple triad: administration of glucose to relieve symptoms. Ninety percent of insulinomas are benign; they should be cured with resection, if possible. In your workup, take a history and check the C-peptide level first to make sure that the patient is not diabetic and taking too much insulin or a patient with a factitious disorder. C-peptide levels are high with insulinoma and sulfonylurea overdose and low with factitious insulin administration (commercial preparations of insulin do not have C-peptide).

3. **Name the other two islet cell tumors. What should islet cell tumors make you think about?**

   1. **Glucagonomas** (alpha cell tumors) cause hyperglycemia with high glucagon levels and migratory necrotizing skin erythema.
   2. **VIPomas** (tumors that secrete VIP) cause watery diarrhea, hypokalemia, and achlorhydria.

   Watch for multiple endocrine neoplasia (MEN) syndrome in patients with islet cell tumors.

4. **Describe the typical history and the physical examination and laboratory findings for pancreatitis. How is it treated?**

Look for epigastric pain that radiates to the back in an alcohol abuser or a patient with a history of (or risk factors for) gallstones. Serum amylase and/or lipase levels should be elevated. If these values are not given, order the tests! Other common signs include decreased bowel sounds, localized ileus (sentinel loop of bowel on abdominal radiography) nausea, vomiting, and/or anorexia.

Treat pancreatitis supportively. Narcotics are often needed for pain control; hydromorphone and fentanyl are now common choices; meperidine, which has a risk of seizures, has traditionally been favored over morphine because of concern about sphincter of Oddi spasms, although clinical evidence of this is lacking. Do not feed the patient initially; place a nasogastric tube as needed for nausea and vomiting, and give intravenous fluids and any other supportive care needed. Watch for the complications of pseudocyst and pancreatic abscess, both of which can be diagnosed by CT scanning and may require surgical intervention. Increasing evidence of the benefit of early nutrition in patients with pancreatitis is emerging.

5. **What causes acute pancreatitis?**
More than 80% of cases are due to alcohol or gallstones. Other causes include hypertriglyceridemia, viral infections (mumps, Coxsackie virus), trauma, hypercalcemia, PUD, medications (e.g., isoniazid, furosemide, simvastatin, steroids, azathioprine), and scorpion bites.

6. **Other than pancreatic disease, what else can cause elevated levels of amylase?**
Damage to the salivary glands or bowel, renal failure, and ruptured tubal pregnancy may cause elevated amylase levels. Lipase is more specific for pancreatic pathology, and elevation of both amylase and lipase levels in the same patient is usually due to pancreatitis. The boards may try to trick you with isolated elevation of the amylase level.

7. **What are the complications of acute pancreatitis?**
Complications include pseudocyst formation (drain surgically if symptomatic and persistent for several weeks), abscess or infection (treat with antibiotics and drainage if needed), and chronic pancreatitis.

8. **What causes chronic pancreatitis? How is it treated?**
Chronic pancreatitis in the United States is almost always due to alcoholism and usually results from repeated bouts of acute pancreatitis. Gallstones do not cause chronic pancreatitis. Chronic pancreatitis may lead to diabetes, steatorrhea (excessive fat in the stool due to lack of pancreatic enzymes), calcification of the pancreas (which may be seen on a plain abdominal radiograph), and fat-soluble vitamin deficiencies (caused by malabsorption). The incidence of pancreatic cancer is slightly higher in patients with pancreatitis, although smoking is a greater risk factor than alcohol for pancreatic cancer.
Treat chronic pancreatitis with alcohol abstinence, oral pancreatic enzyme replacement, and fat-soluble vitamin supplements.

NUTRITIONAL DISORDERS

1. **What may happen if you give glucose to an alcoholic without giving thiamine first?**
You may precipitate Wernicke encephalopathy. **Always give thiamine before glucose** to avoid this complication.

2. **What is the difference between Wernicke and Korsakoff syndromes? What causes each?**
Wernicke syndrome is an acute encephalopathy characterized by ophthalmoplegia, nystagmus, ataxia, and/or confusion. It can be fatal but can often be reversed by thiamine administration.
Korsakoff syndrome is a chronic psychosis characterized by anterograde amnesia (inability to form new memories) and confabulation (lying) to cover up the amnesia. Korsakoff syndrome is generally irreversible, and it is thought that it is due to damage to the mamillary bodies and thalamic nuclei. Both conditions result from thiamine deficiency.

3. **Which vitamin deficiencies may lead to neurologic signs or symptoms?**
Vitamin B_{12}: dementia, peripheral neuropathy, loss of vibration sense in the lower extremities, loss of position sense, ataxia, spasticity, hyperactive reflexes, and positive Babinski sign.
Thiamine: peripheral neuropathy, confusion, ophthalmoplegia, nystagmus, ataxia, confusion, delirium, and dementia.
Vitamin E: loss of proprioception/vibratory sensation, areflexia, ataxia, and gaze palsy.
Vitamin A: vision loss.
Vitamin B_6: peripheral sensory neuropathy (watch for isoniazid as a cause, and give prophylactic B_6 to patients taking isoniazid, if given the choice).

4. Specify the signs and symptoms of the various vitamin deficiencies and toxicities.

VITAMIN	DEFICIENCY	TOXICITY
A	Night blindness, scaly rash, xerophthalmia (dry eyes), Bitot spots (debris on conjunctiva); increased infections	Pseudotumor cerebri, bone thickening, teratogenic
C	Scurvy (hemorrhages/skin petechiae, bone, gums; loose teeth; gingivitis), poor wound healing, hyperkeratotic hair follicles, bone pain (from periosteal hemorrhages)	
D	Rickets, osteomalacia, hypocalcemia	Hypercalcemia, nausea, renal toxicity
E	Anemia, peripheral neuropathy, ataxia	Necrotizing enterocolitis (infants)
K	Hemorrhage, prolonged prothrombin time	Hemolysis (kernicterus)
B1 (thiamine)	Wet beriberi (high-output cardiac failure), dry beriberi, (peripheral neuropathy), Wernicke and Korsakoff syndromes	
B$_2$ (riboflavin)	Angular stomatitis, dermatitis	
B$_3$ (niacin)	Pellagra (dementia, dermatitis, diarrhea), stomatitis	
B$_6$ (pyridoxine)	Peripheral neuropathy, stomatitis, convulsions in infants, microcytic anemia, seborrheic dermatitis	Peripheral neuropathy (only B vitamin with toxicity)
B$_{12}$ (cobalamin)	Megaloblastic anemia *plus* neurologic symptoms	
Folic acid	Megaloblastic anemia *without* neurologic symptoms	

5. Specify the signs and symptoms of the various mineral deficiencies and toxicities.

MINERAL	DEFICIENCY	TOXICITY
Iron	Microcytic anemia, koilonychia (spoon-shaped fingernails)	Hemochromatosis
Iodine	Goiter, cretinism, hypothyroidism	Myxedema
Fluoride	Dental caries (cavities)	Fluorosis with mottling of teeth and bone exostoses
Zinc	Hypogeusia (decreased taste), rash, slow wound healing	
Copper	Menkes syndrome (X-linked; kinky hair, mental retardation)	Wilson disease
Selenium	Cardiomyopathy and muscle pain	Loss of hair and nails
Manganese	"Manganese madness" in miners of ore (behavioral changes/psychosis)	
Chromium	Impaired glucose tolerance	

6. What are the fat-soluble vitamins? In what general category of patients are they deficient?

Vitamins A, D, E, and K are fat soluble. Deficiency of any of these vitamins may be due to malabsorption (e.g., cystic fibrosis, cirrhosis, celiac disease, duodenal bypass, bile duct obstruction, pancreatic insufficiency, chronic giardiasis). In such patients, parenteral supplements are required if high-dose oral supplements fail.

7. **What vitamin, mineral, and electrolyte deficiencies are classically seen in alcoholics?**
Any can be seen, but watch especially for folate, thiamine, phosphorus, and magnesium deficiencies.

8. **What is the most common cause of vitamin B_{12} deficiency? How is it diagnosed?**
Pernicious anemia, in which antiparietal cell antibodies destroy the ability to secrete intrinsic factor. Conditions associated with pernicious anemia include other autoimmune conditions such as hypothyroidism, type I diabetes, and vitiligo. Diagnosis of B_{12} deficiency is confirmed by a low serum B_{12} level. The presence of antibodies against intrinsic factor is highly confirmatory for pernicious anemia. The Schilling test is of historic interest but is no longer commonly used in the diagnosis of B_{12} deficiency.

9. **What else may cause vitamin B_{12} deficiency?**
Gastrectomy, terminal ileum resection or disease (e.g., Crohn disease), a strict vegan diet, chronic pancreatitis, and the infamous *Diphyllobothrium latum* (fish tapeworm) infection. A peripheral smear looks the same as in folate deficiency (macrocytes, hypersegmented neutrophils), but patients have **neurologic deficiencies** (e.g., loss of sensation and position sense, paresthesias, ataxia, spasticity, hyperreflexia, positive Babinski sign, dementia).

10. **How is vitamin B_{12} deficiency treated?**
Vitamin B_{12} supplements are given. The usual replacement is via parenteral (intramuscular) injection or high-dose oral replacement. Because of the potential for erratic absorption, oral replacement may be best utilized after levels have been normalized via the parenteral route. Supplementation may be required for life.

11. **What is the classic iatrogenic cause of vitamin B_6 deficiency?**
Prolonged therapy with isoniazid (especially in young people). Pyridoxine supplementation is recommended for patients on isoniazid therapy for tuberculosis.

12. **What causes folate deficiency? In what patient populations is it commonly seen?**
Folate deficiency is commonly seen in alcoholics (poor intake) and pregnant women (increased need). All women of reproductive age should take folate supplements (ideally before pregnancy occurs) to prevent neural tube defects in their offspring. Rare causes of folate deficiency include a poor diet (e.g., tea and toast), methotrexate, prolonged therapy with trimethoprim-sulfamethoxazole, anticonvulsant therapy (especially phenytoin), and malabsorption. Look for macrocytes and **hypersegmented neutrophils** (either one should make you think of folate or B_{12} deficiency) with no neurologic symptoms or signs (unlike B_{12} deficiency) and low folate levels in serum or red blood cells. Treat with oral folate once the level of vitamin B_{12} is known to be normal; treating folate deficiency when there is concomitant B_{12} deficiency can cause worsening of the B_{12} deficiency and irreversible neurologic damage.

13. **Which medications may cause folate deficiency?**
Anticonvulsants (especially phenytoin), methotrexate, and trimethoprim.

14. **What are the physical findings for rickets (vitamin D deficiency in children)?**
   • Craniotabes (poorly mineralized skull; bones feel like a ping-pong ball)
   • Rachitic rosary sign (costochondral beading; small round masses on the anterior rib cage)
   • Delayed fontanelle closure
   • Bossing of the skull
   • Kyphoscoliosis
   • Bow legs and knock knees
Bone changes appear first at the lower end of the radius and ulna.

15. **Describe the relationship between vitamin K and broad-spectrum antibiotics.**
Prolonged therapy with broad-spectrum antibiotics is a potential cause of vitamin K deficiency. These medications can eliminate the normal gut bacteria that synthesize much of the vitamin K required daily.

16. **What is the classic Step 3 description of a patient with vitamin C deficiency?**
An elderly person with a diet of "hot dogs and soda" or "tea and toast" who presents with bleeding gums and bone pain.

INFECTIONS

1. **What clues suggest hepatitis A virus (HAV) infection? Describe the diagnostic serology.**
   Look for outbreaks from a foodborne source. There are no long-term sequelae of infection, although acute liver failure is a remote possibility. Immunoglubulin M (IgM) antibodies to HAV are positive during jaundice or shortly thereafter. The incubation period for HAV is about 4 weeks, although IgM may be detected by the time symptoms begin.

2. **How is hepatitis B virus (HBV) acquired? What is the best treatment?**
   HBV is acquired through sharing of needles, sex, or perinatal transmission. Transfused blood is now screened for HBV, but this risk of transmission is still about 1 in 200,000 according to the American Red Cross. A history of transfusion years ago is still a risk factor (screening by blood banks began in 1972 in the United States). Prevention is the best treatment (vaccination). Interferon alfa-2b, peginterferon alfa-2a, adefovir, dipivoxil, entecavir, telbivudine, or tenofovir can be tried in patients with chronic hepatitis and elevated liver enzyme levels.

3. **Describe the serology of HBV infection, including the surface, core, and "e" markers.**
   An HBV surface antigen (HBsAg) test is positive in any unresolved infection (acute or chronic). The HBV "e" antigen (HBeAg) is a marker for infectivity; patients positive for the HBV "e" antibody (HBeAb) have a low likelihood of spreading disease. The first antibody to appear is the IgM HBV core antibody (HBcAb), which appears during the window phase, when both HBsAg and HBV surface antibody (HBsAb) are negative. Positive HBsAb means that the patient is immune (as a result of either recovery from infection or vaccination); HBsAb never appears if the patient has chronic hepatitis.
   Make sure you know and understand Table 5-1. It is of high yield.

4. **What are the possible sequelae of chronic HBV or hepatitis C virus (HCV) infection?**
   Cirrhosis and hepatocellular cancer (only with chronic, not acute, infection).

5. **What should be given to individuals acutely exposed to HBV?**
   It has been demonstrated that HBV immunoglobulin and HBV vaccination or HBV vaccination alone is effective in preventing transmission after exposure to HBV.

6. **Which type of viral hepatitis is the new "king" of chronic hepatitis?**
   Hepatitis C. HCV is the most likely cause of hepatitis after a blood transfusion. Although blood is now screened for HBV and HCV, the HCV test was developed later (screening in the United States began in 1972 for HBV and in 1992 for HCV). HCV infection is also more likely than HBV infection to progress to chronic hepatitis, cirrhosis, and cancer. Because of the relatively high prevalence in the "baby boomer" generation and the lack of symptoms, the Centers for Disease Control has recommended that all Americans born between 1945 and 1965 have a one-time screening test for HCV.

Table 5-1. Serologic Markers at Different Stages of Disease

	HBsAg	HBeAg	HBeAb	HBsAb	HBcAb
Incubation	+	+	–	–	–
Acute stage	+	+	–	–	+
Persistent carrier	+	+/–	–/+	–	+
Recovery (immune)	–	–	+	+	+
Immunization	–	–	–	+	–

The presence of HBeAg and HBeAb depends on the degree of infectivity.
(Adapted from Cohen J, Powderly WG, Berkley SF, et al. Infectious diseases. 2nd ed. Edinburgh: Mosby, 2004, p 2015, with permission.)

7. Describe the serology and treatment for HCV infection.
   Positivity for HCV antibodies means that the patient has had an infection in the past but does not mean the infection has been cleared. Many patients become chronic carriers of the virus. A test for HCV RNA is available to detect and quantify the virus. Treatment is with pegylated interferon alfa and ribavirin (plus a protease inhibitor for those with genotype 1). Success rates depend on the type of infection. Genotype 1 is the most common in the United States, but treatment success rates are higher for genotypes 2 and 3.

8. When is hepatitis D virus (HDV) infection seen? Describe the serology.
   HDV is seen only in patients with HBV infection. It may become chronic (with HBV coinfection) and is acquired in the same ways as HBV. IgM antibodies to the HDV antigen demonstrate resolution of recent infection. The presence of the HDV antigen, HDV RNA, and high levels of IgM antibodies to HDV indicates chronicity.

9. How is hepatitis E virus (HEV) transmitted? What is special about the infection in pregnant women?
   HEV is transmitted like HAV (via food and water; no chronic state). It is often fatal in pregnant women (for unknown reasons).

10. Which hepatitis viruses can lead to chronic liver disease?
    HBV, HCV, and HDV. HDV can cause infection only in the setting of coexisting HBV.

TRAUMA AND TOXIC EFFECTS

1. Which GI malformations are common in children? How can they be distinguished?

NAME	PRESENTING AGE	VOMIT DESCRIPTION	FINDINGS/KEY WORDS
Pyloric stenosis	3-6 wk	Nonbilious, projectile	Males >> females; palpable olive-shaped mass in the epigastrium; low Cl/low K metabolic alkalosis
Intestinal atresia	0-1 wk	Bilious	Double-bubble sign, Down syndrome
Trans-esophageal fistula*	0-2 wk	Food regurgitation	Respiratory compromise with feeding, aspiration pneumonia, inability to pass a nasogastric tube into the stomach, gastric distention (from air)
Hirschsprung disease	0-1 yr	Feculent	Abdominal distention, obstipation, no nerve ganglia seen on rectal biopsy; males >> females
Anal atresia	0-1 wk	Late, feculent	Detected on initial examination in the nursery; males > females
Choanal atresia	0-1 wk	—	Cyanosis with feeding, relieved by crying; inability to pass a nasogastric tube through the nose

*The most common variant (85% of cases) includes esophageal atresia with a fistula from the bronchus to the distal esophagus. The result is gastric distention, because each breath transmits air to the GI tract. Be able to recognize a sketch of this most common variant (Fig. 5-1).

Treat each of the conditions listed with **surgical repair.**

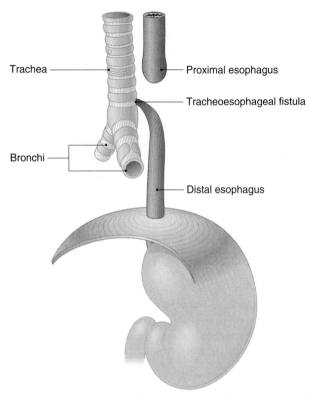

Figure 5-1. Tracheoesophageal fistula. Diagram of the most common type of esophageal atresia and tracheoesophageal fistula. (*From Gilbert-Barness E. Potter's pathology of the fetus, infant and child. 2nd ed. Philadelphia: Mosby, 2007, Fig. 25.6*).

2. What other pediatric GI conditions are commonly found on the Step 3 board exams? How are they distinguished?

NAME	PRESENTING AGE	VOMIT DESCRIPTION	FINDINGS/KEY WORDS
Intussusception	3 mo to 2 yr	Bilious	Currant-jelly stools (blood and mucus), palpable sausage-shaped mass; treat with pneumatic or hydrostatic enema guided by fluoroscopy or ultrasound (diagnostic and therapeutic)
Necrotizing enterocolitis	0-2 mo	Bilious	Premature baby, fever, rectal bleeding, air in bowel wall; treat with nil by mouth, orogastric tube, IV fluids, and antibiotics
Meconium ileus	0-1 wk	Feculent, late	Manifestation of cystic fibrosis (as is rectal prolapse)
Midgut volvulus	0-2 yr	Bilious	Sudden onset of pain, distention, rectal bleeding, peritonitis, bird beak sign on abdominal radiography; treat with surgery

Continued

NAME	PRESENTING AGE	VOMIT DESCRIPTION	FINDINGS/KEY WORDS
Meckel diverticulum	0-2 yr	Varies	Rule of 2s*; GI ulceration or bleeding; use a Meckel scan to detect; treat with surgery
Strangulated hernia	Any age	Bilious	Physical examination reveals bowel loops in the inguinal canal

*Rule of 2s for Meckel diverticulum: 2% of the population affected (most common GI tract abnormality), 2 inches long, within 2 feet of the ileocolic junction, appears in the first 2 years of life. Meckel diverticulum can cause intussusception, obstruction, or volvulus.

3. How are omphalocele and gastroschisis differentiated?

An **omphalocele** is in the midline, the sac contains multiple abdominal organs, the umbilical ring is absent, and other anomalies are common. **Gastroschisis** is to the right of the midline, only small bowel is exposed (no true hernia sac), the umbilical ring is present, and other anomalies are rare.

4. List and differentiate the three common types of groin hernias.

1. **Indirect hernias** are the most common type in both sexes and all age groups. The hernia sac travels through the inner and outer inguinal rings (protrusion begins lateral to the inferior epigastric vessels) and into the scrotum or labia because of a patent processus vaginalis (congenital defect).
2. **Direct hernias** (no sac) protrude medial to the inferior epigastric vessels because of weakness in the abdominal musculature of the Hesselbach triangle.
3. **Femoral hernias** are more common in women. The hernia (no sac) goes through the femoral ring onto the anterior thigh (located below the inguinal ring).

Of the three types, femoral hernias are the most susceptible to incarceration and strangulation. All three types are treated with elective surgical repair to prevent this.

5. Define incarcerated and strangulated hernias.

Incarceration occurs when a herniated organ is trapped and becomes swollen and edematous. Incarcerated hernias are the most common cause of small bowel obstruction in patients who have had no previous abdominal surgery and are the second most common cause in patients who have had previous abdominal surgery. The treatment is prompt surgery.

Strangulation occurs after incarceration when the entrapment becomes so severe that the blood supply is cut off. Strangulation can lead to necrosis and is a surgical emergency. Patients may have symptoms of small bowel obstruction and shock.

6. How do you manage a patient with blunt abdominal trauma?

In patients with blunt abdominal trauma, the initial findings determine the appropriate course of action. If the patient is awake and stable and your examination is benign, observe the patient and repeat the abdominal examination later. You can also perform a FAST (focused assessment by sonography in trauma) scan to check for free fluid in the abdomen and pelvis in a hypotensive patient. A positive FAST examination in an unstable patient mandates that the patient be brought to the operating room before a CT scan. Stable patients for whom there is significant concern for intraabdominal injury can undergo a CT scan with IV contrast.

If the patient is hemodynamically unstable (hypotension and/or shock that does not respond to fluid challenge) and has a positive FAST examination (i.e., free fluid in the abdomen), proceed directly to laparotomy. For patients who are hemodynamically unstable with a negative FAST examination, other sources of fluid loss should be considered (e.g., massive hemothorax, pelvic fracture with retroperitoneal bleeding, obstructive shock from a tension pneumothorax).

If the patient has an altered mental status or has an unreliable abdominal examination and is hemodynamically stable, order a CT scan of the abdomen and pelvis with IV contrast (also get a CT scan of the head and cervical spine in the case of altered mental status). Diagnostic peritoneal lavage is no longer used because it has been replaced by the noninvasive and more rapid FAST examination.

7. How is penetrating abdominal trauma managed?

In patients with penetrating abdominal trauma (e.g., gunshot, stab wound), the type of injury and the initial findings determine the course of action. For any gunshot wound that may have violated the peritoneal cavity, proceed directly to laparotomy. For a wound from a sharp instrument, management is more controversial. Either proceed directly to laparotomy (your best choice if the patient is unstable) or perform a CT scan if the patient is stable. For nonoperative management, perform serial abdominal examinations. No imaging or operative management is required for superficial penetrating abdominal trauma that does not violate the peritoneum; these are simple lacerations and can be treated as such if peritoneal violation has been ruled out.

8. What should you always remember when a question mentions that a child was given aspirin?

Reye syndrome, which causes encephalopathy and/or liver failure. This usually occurs after aspirin is given for influenza or varicella infection. Use acetaminophen in children to avoid this rare (but often tested) condition.

CHAPTER 6

BEHAVIORAL AND EMOTIONAL DISORDERS

1. **What is the difference between objective and subjective psychological tests?**
   Objective tests are generally multiple-choice tests that are scored by a computer; the classic example is the IQ test. **Subjective tests** have no right answers and are scored by the test-giver (the classic example is the Rorschach test).

2. **Characterize each of the following psychological tests as objective or subjective and briefly describe its use.**

TEST NAME	DESCRIPTION
Stanford-Binet	Objective IQ test for adults
Wechsler Intelligence Scale for Children	Objective IQ test for children (4-17 yr)
Rorschach Test	Subjective test in which patients describe what they see in an inkblot
Thematic Apperception Test	Subjective test in which the patient describes what is going on in a cartoon drawing of people
Beck Depression Inventory	Objective tests to look for depression
Minnesota Multiphasic Personality Inventory	Objective tests to measure personality type
Halstead-Reitan Battery	Objective tests used to determine the location and effects of specific brain lesions
Luria-Nebraska Neuropsychological Battery	Objective tests that assess many cognitive functions, as well as cerebral dominance (left or right)

Note that psychological tests can be used to aid in a difficult diagnosis; they are not used or needed for a straightforward case.

PSYCHOTIC DISORDERS

1. **What are the five main diagnostic criteria for schizophrenia?**
   1. Delusions
   2. Hallucinations
   3. Disorganized speech
   4. Grossly disorganized or catatonic behavior
   5. Negative symptoms (i.e., flat affect, avolition)

2. **Why is the duration of symptoms important in psychosis?**
   The time frame is important because given the exact same symptoms, a patient is given one of three diagnoses based only on symptom duration:
   • Less than 1 month: acute psychotic disorder
   • 1 to 6 months: schizophreniform disorder
   • More than 6 months: schizophrenia

3. **List the positive symptoms of schizophrenia.**
   - Delusions
   - Bizarre behavior
   - Hallucinations
   - Thought disorder (e.g., tangentiality, "clanging")

   These symptoms respond well to all currently used antipsychotics. Positive symptoms are symptoms that occur *in addition* to normal behavior; normal individuals do not exhibit these symptoms.

4. **List the negative symptoms of schizophrenia.**
   - Flat affect
   - Anhedonia
   - Alogia (no speech)
   - Poor attention
   - Avolition (apathy)

   These symptoms respond poorly to traditional antipsychotics (e.g., haloperidol) but may respond to atypical agents such as risperidone, olanzapine, aripiprazole, paliperidone, quetiapine, and ziprasidone. Negative symptoms are symptoms for which patients have *lost* some form of normal behavior; they have lost behaviors that normal individuals typically have.

5. **What features of schizophrenia suggest a poor prognosis?**
   - Poor premorbid functioning (most important)
   - Family history of schizophrenia
   - Early onset
   - Negative symptoms
   - No precipitating factors
   - Poor support system
   - Single, divorced, or widowed status

6. **What features suggest a good prognosis?**
   - Good premorbid functioning (most important)
   - Family history of mood disorders
   - Late onset
   - Positive symptoms
   - Obvious precipitating factors
   - Good support system
   - Married status

7. **What is the difference in age of onset for schizophrenia in males and females?**
   The typical age of onset is 15 to 25 years for males (look for someone going to college and deteriorating) and 25 to 35 years for females.

8. **True or false: Roughly 1% of the population has schizophrenia in almost every country in the world.**
   True.

9. **True or false: In the United States, most schizophrenic people are born in the summer months.**
   False. Most schizophrenic patients in the United States are born in the winter (reason unknown).

10. **Roughly what percentage of patients with schizophrenia commit suicide?**
    In the United States, roughly 10% of patients with schizophrenia eventually commit suicide (a past attempt is the best predictor of eventual success).

11. **True or false: Psychosocial treatment improves outcomes in schizophrenia.**
    True. Antipsychotic medications are the mainstay of therapy, but it has been shown that psychosocial treatment improves outcome. Medications are needed first, but the best treatment (as in most psychiatric illnesses) is medications plus therapy.

12. Differentiate among the classes of antipsychotic drugs.

	HIGH POTENCY	LOW POTENCY	ATYPICAL AGENTS*
Prototype drug	Haloperidol	Chlorpromazine	Risperidone, olanzapine, aripiprazole, paliperidone, quetiapine, ziprasidone
EPS side effects	High incidence	Low incidence	Low incidence
ANS side effects†	Low incidence	High incidence	Medium incidence
Positive symptoms	Works well	Works well	Works well
Negative symptoms	Works poorly	Works poorly	Works fairly well

ANS, Autonomic nervous system; EPS, extrapyramidal system.

*Atypical, newer antipsychotic agents are generally first-line treatment and maintenance therapy because of their reduced EPS side effects and efficacy for negative symptoms. Choose them over older agents.

†ANS side effects include anticholinergic effects (dry mouth, urinary retention, blurry vision, mydriasis), alpha1 blockade (orthostatic hypotension), and antihistamine effects (sedation).

13. What are the four commonly tested extrapyramidal side effects of antipsychotics?

Acute dystonias, akathisia, parkinsonism, and tardive dyskinesia.

14. Define acute dystonia. How is it treated?

Acute dystonia is an extrapyramidal movement disorder that occurs in the first few hours or days of treatment. Patients develop muscle spasms or stiffness (e.g., torticollis, trismus), tongue protrusions and twisting, opisthotonos, and/or oculogyric crisis (forced sustained deviation of the head and eyes). Acute dystonia is most common in young men. Treat with antihistamines (e.g., diphenhydramine) or anticholinergic drugs (e.g., benztropine, trihexyphenidyl).

15. Define akathisia.

Akathisia occurs in the first few days of treatment. The patient has a subjective feeling of restlessness and may pace constantly, alternate between sitting and standing, and be unable to sit still. Beta-blockers can be tried for treatment.

ANXIETY DISORDERS

1. How do you recognize and treat panic disorder?

Panic disorder classically affects 20- to 40-year-old patients who often think that they are dying or having a heart attack, although in fact they are healthy and have a negative workup for organic disease. Patients often hyperventilate and are extremely anxious. They may experience tingling of the extremities. Remember the association between panic disorder and agoraphobia (fear of leaving the house). Treat with selective serotonin reuptake inhibitors (SSRIs; e.g., fluoxetine), which are favored over benzodiazepines.

2. What is generalized anxiety disorder? How is it treated?

Patients with generalized anxiety disorder worry about everything (e.g., career, family, future, relationships, and money) at the same time. Symptoms are not as dramatic as in panic disorder; the patient is simply a severe worrier. Treat with cognitive behavioral therapy and medications: buspirone (partial agonist of 5-hydroxytryptamine 1A serotonin receptor; non-addictive, nonsedating, but slow onset of action), SSRIs (especially if depressive symptoms coexist), or benzodiazepines (addictive, sedating).

3. Give the classic examples of simple phobias. How are they treated?

Classic examples of simple phobias include fear of needles, blood products, animals, and heights. Treat with behavioral therapy, including flooding (sudden, intense exposure to the feared object without chance for escape), systematic desensitization (gradual increase in intensity and type of exposure until the person is comfortable with intense exposure to the feared object), and biofeedback (learning to control autonomic variables such as heart rate during anxiety-inducing maneuvers).

4. **What is social anxiety disorder?**

Social anxiety disorder, also known as social phobia, is a specific type of simple phobia (fear of social situations) best treated with behavioral therapy. To reduce symptoms, beta-blockers may be used before a public appearance that cannot be avoided, and SSRIs are increasingly being used as a primary treatment. Serotonin-norepinephrine reuptake inhibitors (SNRIs) and benzodiazepines also may be used.

5. **Describe obsessive-compulsive disorder. How is it treated?**

Obsessive-compulsive disorder (OCD) is marked by recurrent thoughts or impulses (obsessions) or recurrent behaviors (compulsions) that cause dysfunction in the occupational or interpersonal life of affected individuals. Look for washing rituals (e.g., washing the hands 30 times per day) and checking rituals (e.g., checking to see if the door is locked 40 times per day). Onset is usually in adolescence or early adulthood. Treat with SSRIs (especially fluvoxamine) or clomipramine (serotonin-specific tricyclic antidepressant). Therapies such as cognitive behavioral therapy and flooding may be effective.

6. **How do you recognize and treat posttraumatic stress disorder?**

Look for someone who has been through a life-threatening event (e.g., war, severe accident, rape), repeatedly reexperiences the event (nightmares, flashbacks), and tries to avoid thinking about it. As a result, patients have depression or poor concentration. Treat with peer group therapy; if you have to choose a medication, use an antidepressant, usually an SSRI. Note that posttraumatic stress disorder must have symptoms for longer than 1 month (symptoms for < 1 month indicate acute stress disorder).

MOOD DISORDERS

1. **Define depression.**

Depression, or *major depressive disorder* as it is technically called, is defined by the Diagnostic and Statistical Manual of Mental Disorders, 5th edition (DSM-V) as a depressed mood or a loss of interest or pleasure in daily activities for longer than 2 weeks. There is impaired function in social, occupational, or educations roles. At least five of the following nine symptoms are present nearly every day: depressed mood or irritability, decreased interest or pleasure in most activities, significant weight change or change in appetite, change in sleep, change in activity, fatigue or loss of energy, guilt or feelings of worthlessness, diminished ability to think or concentrate, and suicidality.

2. **True or false: Patients with depression often do not complain about it directly.**

True. Patients often do not come out and say, "I'm depressed." You must watch for the clues: a change in sleep habits (classically insomnia), vague somatic complaints, anxiety, low energy or fatigue, a change in appetite (classically decreased appetite), poor concentration, psychomotor retardation, and/or anhedonia (loss of pleasure). The history may or may not reveal obvious precipitating factors, such as loss of a loved one, divorce, separation, unemployment, retirement, chronic disease, or debilitating disease.

3. **How do you treat depression?**

As with most psychiatric illnesses, the treatment of choice includes both medications (antidepressants) and psychotherapy. The combination is more effective than medications alone. SSRIs are usually the preferred first-line agents. Other options include SNRIs and tricyclic antidepressants. Bupropion and mirtazapine have unique modes of action.

4. **Is depression more common in males or females?**

Depression is more common in females.

5. **What is an adjustment disorder with depressed mood?**

A diagnosis that you must be able to distinguish from major depression. In adjustment disorder, a patient goes through a normal life experience (e.g., relationship break-up, grade failure, job loss) but does not handle it well. There is marked distress that exceeds what would be expected for exposure to the stressor or that causes significant impairment in social or occupational functioning. Although patients may have a depressed mood, they do not meet the criteria for full-blown major depression. An example is a woman who divorces her husband, seems to cry a lot for the next few weeks, and leaves work early on most days. Another example is a high-school boy who doesn't make the basketball team and mopes around the house, crying and not wanting to go to school or out with his friends for a few weeks.

6. **True or false: Antidepressants can trigger mania or hypomania.**
   True, especially in bipolar patients. Remember to ask about any history of manic episodes when considering treatment for depression.

7. **How do SSRIs work? Why are they preferred over tricyclic antidepressants?**
   SSRIs (e.g., fluoxetine, citalopram, paroxetine, sertraline, fluvoxamine, escitalopram) prevent reuptake of serotonin only. They have less serious side effects (insomnia, anorexia, jitteriness, headache, sexual dysfunction) and are not dangerous in overdose. Tricyclic antidepressants used to be the leading cause of prescription drug overdose in the United States.

8. **How do SNRIs work?**
   SNRIs (e.g., venlafaxine, duloxetine, desvenlafaxine) prevent reuptake of serotonin and norepinephrine. The side effects of SNRIs are similar to those of SSRIs but also include noradrenergic symptoms such as sweating and dizziness.

9. **What are monoamine oxidase (MAO) inhibitors? Describe their side effects.**
   MAO inhibitors (e.g., phenelzine, tranylcypromine) are older medications that are not used as first-line agents for treatment of depression. They may be good for atypical depression (look for hypersomnia and hyperphagia—the opposite of classic depression) that fails to respond to other agents. When patients taking MAO inhibitors eat tyramine-containing foods (especially wine and cheese), they may experience a hypertensive crisis. Do *not* give MAO inhibitors at the same time as SSRIs or meperidine; severe reactions can occur, possibly even death.

10. **What is the most notorious side effect of trazodone?**
    Priapism (persistent, painful erection in the absence of sexual desire that may lead to permanent impotence if not treated).

11. **True or false: Children with depression frequently exhibit an irritable rather than a depressed mood.**
    True.

12. **Define bipolar disorder. What are the classic symptoms?**
    Mania is the only criterion required for a diagnosis of bipolar disorder, but a history of depression is classically present. Classic symptoms of mania include a decreased need for sleep, pressured speech, sexual promiscuity, shopping sprees, and exaggerated self-importance or delusions of grandeur. Look for initial onset between the ages of 16 and 30 years.

13. **How is bipolar disorder treated?**
    Both lithium and valproic acid are mood stabilizers and first-line agents. Typical antipsychotics (haloperidol), atypical antipsychotics (risperidone, quetiapine, clozapine, ziprasidone, and aripiprazole), carbamazepine, and gabapentin are second-line agents. Antipsychotics or antidepressants may be needed if the patient becomes psychotic or depressed; use at the same time as the mood stabilizer.

14. **Define bipolar II disorder and cyclothymia.**
    Bipolar II disorder is hypomania (mild mania without psychosis that does not cause occupational dysfunction) plus major depression. Cyclothymia involves at least 2 years of hypomania alternating with depressed mood, but there are no full-blown episodes of mania or major depression.

15. **List the major risk factors for suicide.**
    - Age greater than 45 years
    - Prior psychiatric history
    - Alcohol or substance abuse
    - Depression
    - History of rage or violence
    - Recent loss or separation
    - Prior suicide attempts
    - Loss of health

- Male gender (men commit suicide three times more often than women, but women attempt it four times more often than men)
- Unemployed or retired status
- Single, widowed, or divorced status

16. **What is the best predictor of future suicide?**
A past suicide attempt.

17. **True or false: Some psychiatric patients can be hospitalized against their will.**
True. Patients can be hospitalized against their will if they are a danger to themselves (suicidal or unable to take care of themselves) or others (homicidal).

18. **True or false: Be careful in asking about suicide, because you may plant the idea in the patient's head.**
False. Always ask a patient about suicidal thoughts; it does not make them more likely to commit suicide. If necessary, you should temporarily hospitalize an acutely suicidal patient against his or her will.

19. **True or false: When patients are just emerging from a deep depression, they are at an increased risk of suicide.**
True. When the antidepressant begins to work, the patient gets a little more energy—possibly just enough to carry out a suicide plan.

20. **True or false: The highest suicide rates are in individuals aged 15 to 24 years.**
False. Suicide rates are rising most rapidly in 15- to 24-year-olds, but the greatest absolute risk is in individuals older than 65 years.

21. **What are the symptoms of postpartum depression? When can the symptoms occur?**
Symptoms of postpartum depression include sadness, hopelessness, fatigue, crying episodes, feeling overwhelmed, feelings of inadequacy in taking care of the baby, emptiness, guilt, irritability, anxiety, anhedonia, changes in sleeping patterns, changes in appetite, social withdrawal, and reduced libido.
   Symptoms of postpartum depression can occur any time in the first year after delivery, but postpartum depression is defined as depression with onset during pregnancy or within 4 weeks after childbirth.

22. **How common is postpartum depression?**
Prevalence rates are unclear, but reported rates are 5% to 25%.

23. **What are the risk factors for postpartum depression?**
There are numerous risk factors for postpartum depression including previous history of postpartum depression (the biggest risk factor), previous history of depression, poor social support, high life stress, physical limitations after childbirth, bipolar disorder, and a family history of depression or bipolar disorder.

24. **What is postpartum psychosis?**
A disturbance in a patient's perception of reality, often including delusions, hallucinations, and thought disorganization. Postpartum psychosis classically occurs within the first weeks after childbirth, but may present several months later.

SOMATOFORM DISORDERS

1. **Explain the concept of somatic symptom disorders (previously called somatoform disorders).**
A patient with somatoform disorder experiences psychiatric stress and expresses it through physical symptoms. Patients do not do so on purpose.

2. **Describe the four major somatic symptom disorders.**
Somatization disorder: the patient has multiple complaints in multiple organ systems over many years and has had extensive negative workups in the past. Mnemonic: patients with **soma**tization disorder have **so ma**ny physical complaints.

Conversion disorder: the patient has an obvious precipitating factor (e.g., fight with boy-friend) and then develops unexplainable neurologic symptoms (e.g., blindness, stocking-glove numbness). This is thought to be a physical manifestation of emotional distress. The patient is not malingering and truly believes the symptom is real.

Hypochondriasis: the patient continues to believe that he or she has a disease despite extensive negative workup. These patients tend to be excessively worried about a minor symptom and are not reassured by multiple negative workups.

Body dysmorphic disorder: the patient is preoccupied with an imagined physical defect; for example, a teenager who thinks that his or her nose is too big when it is normal in size.

3. **How are somatic symptom disorders treated?**
    Treat all somatic symptom disorders with frequent return visits to the clinic and/or psycho-therapy. Screen for and treat any coexisting depression.

4. **Distinguish among somatic symptom disorders, factitious disorders, and malingering.**
    In **somatic symptom disorders,** the patient does not intentionally create symptoms (unconscious process). In **factitious disorders,** patients intentionally create an illness or symptoms (e.g., they inject insulin to create hypoglycemia) and subject themselves to pro-cedures to assume the role of a patient (no financial or other secondary gain). In **malinger-ing,** patients intentionally create their illness for secondary gain (e.g., money, release from work or jail).

5. **How do you recognize dissociative fugue (also called psychogenic fugue or fugue state)?**
    Dissociative fugue is reversible amnesia for personal identity including the memories, per-sonality, and other identifying characteristics of individuality. It usually involves unplanned travel or wandering. There is complete amnesia for the fugue episode. The classic patient develops amnesia, travels, and assumes a new identity but does not remember the event upon returning.

EATING DISORDERS AND OTHER IMPULSE-CONTROL DISORDERS

1. **How do you recognize anorexia?**
    The classic patient is a female adolescent who is a good athlete or student with a perfection-ist personality. The criteria for the diagnosis are body weight at least 15% below normal and an intense fear of gaining weight or feeling fat despite emaciation. Roughly 10% to 15% of patients die from complications of starvation or coexisting bulimia (electrolyte imbalances, cardiac arrhythmias, infections). Although more positive therapies are preferred, patients sometimes need to be hospitalized against their will for intravenous nutrition. Patients with anorexia may be of a restrictive type (severely restricted caloric intake) or a binge-purge type (self-induced vomiting or laxative abuse).

2. **Define bulimia. What are the classic findings for the mouth and fingers?**
    Bulimic patients have binge-eating episodes, during which they feel a lack of control and then engage in purging behavior (vomiting, taking laxatives, exercising, fasting). Those affected are typically normal-weight or overweight adolescent females. If these patients ever meet criteria for anorexia, they are diagnosed with the binge-purge type of anorexia (i.e., the anorexia diagnosis trumps the bulimia diagnosis). Patients may require hospital-ization for electrolyte disturbances. Classic findings include eroded tooth enamel caused by frequent vomiting and eroded skin over the knuckles from putting the fingers into the throat.

3. **Name some of the recognized impulse-control disorders.**
    Pathologic gambling, pyromania, intermittent explosive disorder, kleptomania, and impulse-control disorders not otherwise specified, which include sexual compulsion, internet addic-tion, and compulsive shopping.

4. **What are the five behavioral stages that characterize impulsivity? How are impulse-control disorders treated?**
The five behavioral stages are the (1) impulse, (2) growing tension, (3) pleasure on acting, (4) relief from the urge, and (5) guilt. SSRIs (specifically fluvoxamine) and clomipramine are effective treatment options. Cognitive behavioral therapies can also be helpful, albeit to varying degrees, depending on the disorder.

DISORDERS ORIGINATING IN INFANCY, CHILDHOOD, OR ADOLESCENCE

1. **Define conduct disorder. With what adult disorder is it associated?**
Conduct disorder is the pediatric form of **antisocial personality disorder.** Look for fire setting, cruelty to animals, lying, stealing, and/or fighting. As adults, patients often have antisocial disorder. **Note:** Evidence of conduct disorder as a child is required for a diagnosis of antisocial personality disorder in adults.

2. **Describe the behavior of a child who has oppositional defiant disorder.**
The child displays negative, hostile, and defiant behavior toward authority figures (e.g., parents, teachers). He or she exhibits such behavior around adults but behaves normally around peers and is *not* a cruel, lying criminal (unlike patients with conduct disorder).

3. **Give the classic description of children with separation anxiety disorder.**
Affected children refuse to go to school because they think that something will happen to them or their parents if they separate. They will do anything to avoid separation (e.g., feign stomach ache, headache, temper tantrum).

4. **Define attention-deficit hyperactivity disorder (ADHD).**
As the name implies, patients are hyperactive and have short attention spans. ADHD is more common in males than females. Look for a fidgety child who is impulsive and cannot pay attention but is not cruel. These symptoms must be present in two different settings (e.g., at home and school). Treat with a stimulant (paradoxic calming effect) such as methylphenidate (Ritalin), an amphetamine, or atomoxetine. Stimulants and amphetamines may cause insomnia, abdominal pain, anorexia, weight loss, and growth suppression. Atomoxetine is an SNRI and an alternative to stimulant therapy, but it has serious potential side effects including cardiovascular events and suicidal thinking.

5. **What is a learning disorder?**
Learning disorders describe isolated impairment in math, reading, writing, speech, language, or coordination. All other skills are normal; no mental retardation is present (e.g., "Johnny just can't do math.").

6. **How do you recognize autism spectrum disorder?**
Autism symptoms start at a very young age, beginning as early as 6 months and becoming well established by the age of 2 or 3 years. Look for impaired social interaction (isolative, unaware of surroundings), impaired verbal and nonverbal communication (strange words, babbling, repetition), and restricted activities and interests (head banging, strange movements). Autism is a spectrum of disorders in which patients may range from very highly functioning (previously called Asperger syndrome) to severely intellectually disabled. Most individuals with autism exhibit some degree of intellectual disability that is typically moderate in severity.
   No single cause has been identified for the development of autism. Genetic origins are suspected on the basis of twin studies and a higher incidence among siblings. Possible contributing factors include fetal alcohol exposure, infections (congenital rubella infection), other perinatal factors, and immunologic causes.

PERSONALITY DISORDERS

1. **Define personality disorders.**
Personality disorders are lifelong disorders that affect the way in which a person interacts with the world. Look for a history dating back to childhood or the teenage years. No real treatment is available, although psychotherapy can be tried.

2. Give a one- or two-sentence description of each of the following ten personality disorders.

Cluster A (odd disorders)

- **Paranoid:** Patients are paranoid and think that everyone is out to get them; they often initiate lawsuits.
- **Schizoid:** Patients are classic loners who have no friends and no interest in having friends.
- **Schizotypal:** Patients have bizarre beliefs (cults, superstitions) and a bizarre manner of speaking but no psychosis.

Cluster B (dramatic, emotional, or erratic disorders)

- **Histrionic:** Patients are overly dramatic, attention seeking, and inappropriately seductive; they must be the center of attention.
- **Narcissistic:** Patients are egocentric, lack empathy, and use others for their own gain; they have a sense of entitlement.
- **Antisocial:** The most frequently tested personality disorder. Patients have long criminal records (e.g., con artists) and tortured animals or set fires as children. A history of pediatric conduct disorder is required for this diagnosis. Patients are aggressive and do not pay their bills or support their children. They are liars and have no remorse or conscience. Antisocial personality disorder has a strong association with alcoholism, drug abuse, and somatization disorder. Most patients are male.
- **Borderline:** Patients have unstable moods, behaviors, relationships (many are bisexual), and self-image. Look for splitting; that is, these patients identify other individuals as all good or all bad and may frequently change categories. Other clues include suicidal gestures, micropsychotic episodes (2 minutes of psychosis), impulsiveness, and constant crisis.

Cluster C (anxious or fearful disorders)

- **Avoidant:** Patients have no friends but want them; they avoid others out of fear of criticism and rejection (inferiority complex). This is distinguished from schizoid personality disorder, in which the patient is isolated but has no desire for social contact.
- **Dependent:** Patients cannot be or do anything alone. A wife may stay with her abusive husband despite continued abuse.
- **Obsessive-compulsive:** Patients are obsessed with rules, perfection, and organization. They may seem anal retentive and stubborn. Rules are more important than objectives, and affect is restricted. Money is a frequent concern and is often hoarded.

PSYCHOSOCIAL PROBLEMS

1. Distinguish between normal grief and pathologic grief (i.e., depression).

Initial grief after a loss (e.g., death of a loved one) may include a state of shock, a feeling of numbness or bewilderment, distress, crying, sleep disturbances, decreased appetite, difficulty in concentrating, weight loss, and guilt (survivor guilt) for up to 1 year—in other words, the same symptoms as depression. It is normal to have an illusion or hallucination about the deceased, but a normal grieving person knows that it is an illusion, whereas a depressed person believes that it is real. Intense yearning (even years after the death) and even searching for the deceased are normal. Feelings of worthlessness, psychomotor retardation, and suicidal ideation are not signs of normal grief; they are signs of depression.

SUBSTANCE ABUSE DISORDERS

1. Discuss the epidemiology of alcohol abuse.

Roughly 10% to 15% of the population abuses alcohol. Alcohol abuse is more common in men. The genetic component is passed most easily from father to son.

2. What diseases and conditions may be caused by chronic alcohol intake?

- Gastritis
- Fatty changes in the liver
- Mallory-Weiss tears

- Hepatitis
- Pancreatitis (acute or chronic)
- Cirrhosis
- Peripheral neuropathy (via thiamine deficiency and a direct effect)
- Wernicke or Korsakoff syndromes
- Cerebellar degeneration (ataxia, past pointing)
- Dilated cardiomyopathy
- Rhabdomyolysis (acute or chronic)

3. **With which cancers is alcohol intake associated?**
Cancers of the oral cavity, larynx, pharynx, esophagus, liver, and lung. It may also be associated with gastric, colon, pancreatic, and breast cancer.

4. **Describe the relationship between alcohol and accidental or intentional death (i.e., suicide and murder).**
Alcohol is involved in roughly 50% of fatal car accidents, 67% of drownings, 67% of homicides, 35% of suicides, and 70% to 80% of deaths caused by fire.

5. **True or false: Alcohol withdrawal can be fatal.**
True. Alcohol withdrawal needs to be treated on an inpatient basis because it can result in death (mortality rate of 1% to 5% with delirium tremens).

6. **How is alcohol withdrawal treated?**
With benzodiazepines (or, in rare cases, barbiturates). The dose is tapered off gradually over several days until symptoms have resolved.

7. **What are the stages of alcohol withdrawal?**
Acute withdrawal syndrome (12 to 48 hours after the last drink): tremors, sweating, hyperreflexia, and seizures (so-called rum fits).
Alcoholic hallucinosis (24 to 72 hours after the last drink): auditory and visual hallucinations and illusions without autonomic signs.
Delirium tremens (2 to 7 days after the last drink, possibly longer): hallucinations and illusions, confusion, poor sleep, and autonomic lability (sweating, increased pulse and temperature). Death is usually associated with this stage.
These stages may overlap. Delirium tremens may occur several days after the last drink. The classic example is a patient who develops delirium on postoperative day 2 but was fine before the surgery. He or she could be a closet alcoholic, assuming that other causes for delirium have been ruled out.

8. **What is the best treatment for alcoholism?**
Alcoholics Anonymous and other peer-based support groups have had the best success rates. Disulfiram (an aldehyde dehydrogenase enzyme inhibitor that makes individuals sick when they drink) can be used in some patients. Be sure to warn patients that metronidazole and certain cephalosporins have a similar effect on those who drink alcohol.

9. **What is the most commonly abused illicit drug? Describe its effects on users.**
Marijuana. Watch for a teenager who is withdrawn and shows a decline in school performance. Other symptoms include amotivational syndrome (chronic use results in laziness and lack of motivation), time distortion, and the so-called munchies (eating binges during intoxication). No physical symptoms have been reported for withdrawal, but psychological cravings may be present. Marijuana is not dangerous in overdose (although patients may experience temporary dysphoria) and is a controversial teratogen (evidence is weak).

10. **What is the basic rule of thumb about the difference in symptoms between intoxication and withdrawal for the same drug?**
The symptoms are usually the opposite of each other. For example, stimulants (e.g., cocaine, amphetamines) cause insomnia with intoxication and hypersomnolence in withdrawal, whereas depressants (e.g., alcohol, benzodiazepines, barbiturates) cause sedation with intoxication and insomnia in withdrawal.

11. **Describe the effects of opioids. What symptoms are seen in withdrawal?**

Heroin and other opioids cause euphoria, analgesia, drowsiness, miosis, constipation, and central nervous system (CNS) depression. Overdoses can be fatal because of respiratory depression, which should be treated with **naloxone.** Because the drug is often taken intravenously, associated morbidity and mortality include endocarditis, HIV infection, hepatitis, cellulitis, and talc damage. Withdrawal is not life threatening, but patients act as though they are going to die. Symptoms of withdrawal include gooseflesh, diarrhea, insomnia, abdominal cramping, and pain. Methadone or buprenorphine can be used to reduce acute withdrawal symptoms.

12. **True or false: Benzodiazepines and barbiturates can be fatal in overdose but not in withdrawal.**

False. Both can be fatal in overdose and withdrawal.

13. **Describe the symptoms and signs of benzodiazepine or barbiturate intoxication.**

Benzodiazepines and barbiturates cause sedation and drowsiness, as well as disinhibition and reduced anxiety. They can be fatal in overdose as a result of respiratory depression; treat acute overdoses of a benzodiazepine with **flumazenil** (although this may precipitate seizures). In withdrawal, death may result from seizures and/or cardiovascular collapse. Treat withdrawal on an inpatient basis with a long-acting benzodiazepine, and gradually taper off the dose over several days. Benzodiazepines and barbiturates are especially dangerous when mixed with alcohol because all three are CNS depressants.

14. **What symptoms are associated with cocaine intoxication and withdrawal?**

Cocaine causes sympathetic stimulation (insomnia, tachycardia, mydriasis, hypertension, sweating) with hyperalertness, and possible paranoia, aggressiveness, delirium, psychosis, or formication (so-called cocaine bugs; patients think that insects are crawling on them). Overdose can be fatal as a result of arrhythmia, myocardial infarction, seizure, or stroke. During withdrawal, the patient is sleepy, hungry (vs. anorexic with intoxication), and irritable, with possible severe depression. Cocaine withdrawal is not dangerous, but psychological cravings are usually severe. Cocaine is teratogenic, causing vascular disruptions in the fetus.

15. **Describe the symptoms of amphetamine intoxication.**

Amphetamines are longer acting and associated more commonly with psychotic symptoms (patients may appear to be full-blown schizophrenics), but basically their effects are similar to those of cocaine.

16. **How do you recognize intoxication with lysergic acid diethylamide (LSD) or hallucinogenic mushrooms?**

Symptoms of intoxication with LSD or mushrooms include hallucinations (usually visual vs. auditory in schizophrenia), mydriasis, tachycardia, diaphoresis, and perception and mood disturbances. Neither is dangerous in overdose, unless the patient thinks that he or she can fly and jumps out a window. No withdrawal symptoms or teratogenic effects have been reported. Users may experience flashbacks (brief feelings of being on the drug again even though none was taken) months to years later or a bad trip (acute panic reaction or dysphoria), which should be treated with reassurance or a benzodiazepine or antipsychotic, if needed.

17. **What about phencyclidine (PCP) intoxication?**

PCP intoxication causes LSD/mushroom symptoms plus confusion, agitation, and aggressive behavior. Also look for vertical and/or horizontal nystagmus and possible schizophrenic-like symptoms (e.g., paranoia, auditory hallucinations, disorganized behavior and speech). Overdose can be fatal because of convulsions, coma, and respiratory arrest. Treat with supportive care and urine acidification to hasten elimination. No withdrawal symptoms have been reported.

18. **Describe the symptoms and signs of inhalant intoxication. Who is likely to abuse inhalants?**

Inhalant intoxication (e.g., gasoline, glue, varnish remover) causes euphoria, dizziness, slurred speech, a feeling of floating, ataxia, and a sense of heightened power. It is usually seen in younger teenagers (11 to 15 years of age) because these substances are cheap, legal to buy, and readily available. Inhalants can be fatal in overdose as a result of respiratory depression, cardiac arrhythmias, or asphyxiation and may cause severe permanent sequelae (CNS, liver, or kidney toxicity; peripheral neuropathy). There is no known withdrawal syndrome.

19. What are the symptoms of caffeine withdrawal?
Headaches and fatigue.

TOXIC EFFECTS

1. Describe the relationship between antipsychotics and parkinsonism.
Parkinsonism usually occurs in patients taking antipsychotics within the first few months of treatment. It is thought that parkinsonism develops because of dopamine depletion but that psychosis develops because of too much dopamine in the brain (a gross oversimplification). Thus antipsychotics create an iatrogenic decrease in effective dopamine in the brain by blocking dopamine receptors. The patient develops stiffness, cogwheel rigidity, a shuffling gait, mask like facies, and drooling. Parkinsonism is most common in older women. Treat with antihistamines (e.g., diphenhydramine) or anticholinergic agents (e.g., benztropine, trihexyphenidyl).

2. Define tardive dyskinesia. When does it occur?
Tardive dyskinesia appears after years of treatment with antipsychotics. Most commonly, the patient develops perioral movements (darting, protruding movements of the tongue; chewing; grimacing; and puckering). The patient may also have involuntary choreoathetoid movements of the head, limbs, and trunk. There is no known treatment for tardive dyskinesia. If you are asked to make a choice when a patient develops tardive dyskinesia, discontinue the current antipsychotic and consider switching to a second-generation agent (e.g., clozapine, risperidone).

3. What is neuroleptic malignant syndrome? How do you recognize and treat it?
Neuroleptic malignant syndrome is a life-threatening condition that can occur at any time during antipsychotic treatment. Patients classically develop rigidity, mutism, obtundation, agitation, high fever (up to 107° F [41.7° C]), very **high levels of creatine phosphokinase** (>10 times the normal upper limit), sweating, and myoglobinuria. Treat by discontinuing the antipsychotic; then give supportive care for fever and potential renal failure caused by myoglobinuria (primarily IV fluids). Lastly, consider dantrolene (just as in malignant hyperthermia, which is thought to be a similar condition).

4. Describe the relationship between antipsychotic agents and prolactin levels.
Dopamine blockade causes increases in prolactin levels because dopamine is a prolactin-inhibiting factor in the tuberoinfundibular tract of the brain. The end result may be high serum prolactin levels, resulting in **galactorrhea** and impotence, menstrual dysfunction, and/or decreased libido.

5. What are the classic side effects of thioridazine, chlorpromazine, and clozapine?
   - Thioridazine: retinal pigment deposits
   - Clozapine: agranulocytosis (white blood cell counts must be monitored)
   - Chlorpromazine: jaundice and photosensitivity

6. What are the side effects of the atypical antipsychotic agents?
   - Olanzapine: weight gain, sedation, hypotension, dry mouth
   - Quetiapine: sedation, orthostatic hypotension, akathisia, weight gain, dry mouth
   - Ziprasidone: nausea, weakness, mild QT prolongation
   - Aripiprazole: headache, nausea, akathisia, tremor, constipation
   - Paliperidone: parkinsonism, dystonia, dyskinesia, akathisia, QT prolongation
   - Clozapine: orthostatic hypotension, weight gain, metabolic syndrome, sedation, constipation

7. What are the side effects of lithium, valproic acid, and carbamazepine?
   - Lithium: renal dysfunction (diabetes insipidus), thyroid dysfunction, tremor, and CNS effects at toxic levels
   - Valproic acid: liver dysfunction
   - Carbamazepine: bone marrow suppression

8. How do tricyclic antidepressants work? What are their side effects?

Tricyclic antidepressants (e.g., nortriptyline, amitriptyline) prevent reuptake of norepinephrine and serotonin. They also block alpha-adrenergic receptors (watch for orthostatic hypotension, dizziness, or falls) and muscarinic receptors (watch for anticholinergic effects such as dry mouth, blurred vision, constipation, and urinary retention), cause sedation (antihistamine effect), and lower the seizure threshold (especially bupropion, which is technically not tricyclic). Tricyclic antidepressants are dangerous in overdose primarily because of **cardiac arrhythmias,** which may respond to bicarbonate. Remember the three Cs of tricyclic antidepressant overdose: coma, convulsions, and cardiotoxicity.

CHAPTER 7

DISORDERS OF THE MUSCULOSKELETAL SYSTEM

DEGENERATIVE/METABOLIC DISORDERS

1. **What is the most common form of arthritis?**
   Osteoarthritis (at least 75% of cases), which is also called degenerative joint disease.

2. **If the cause of arthritis is in doubt, what should you do?**
   When in doubt, or if you suspect something other than osteoarthritis, perform an x-ray of and aspirate fluid from the affected joint. Examine the fluid for cell count and differential, glucose, bacteria (Gram stain and culture), and crystals.

3. **How do you distinguish among the common causes of arthritis?**

	OA	RA	GOUT	PSEUDOGOUT	SEPTIC
Usual age/sex	Older adults	Women 20-45 yr	Older men	Older adults	Any age
Classic joints	DIP, PIP, hip, knee	PIP, MCP, wrist	Big toe	Knees, elbows	Knee
Joint fluid WBCs (cells/mL)	<2000	>2000	>2000	>2000	>50,000
Neutrophils (%)	<25	>50	>50	>50	>75

DIP, Distal interphalangeal joint; MCP, metacarpophalangeal joint; OA, osteoarthritis; PIP, proximal interphalangeal joint; RA, rheumatoid arthritis; WBCs, white blood cells.

4. **What other clues point to a diagnosis of osteoarthritis?**
   Osteoarthritis typically occurs in those older than 40 years of age and has few signs of inflammation on examination; thus the joints are not hot, red, or tender as in the other four types of arthritis listed in Question 3. Look for Heberden nodes (visible and palpable distal interphalangeal joint osteophytes) and Bouchard nodes (proximal interphalangeal joint osteophytes), worsening of symptoms after use and in the evening, bony spurs, and increasing incidence with age. Treat with weight reduction and nonsteroidal antiinflammatory drugs (NSAIDs) or acetaminophen as needed.

5. **What clues point to a diagnosis of gout?**
   Gout classically begins with podagra (gout in the big toe). Also look for high uric acid levels (not always present), tophi (subcutaneous uric acid deposits that look like punched-out lesions on bone radiographs), **needle-shaped crystals with negative birefringence** in the joint fluid, and male gender (more commonly affected than female gender). Alcohol and protein-rich foods may precipitate an attack. Colchicine or NSAIDs (but *not* aspirin, which causes decreased excretion of uric acid by the kidney) are used for acute attacks. For maintenance therapy, a high fluid intake, alkalinization of the urine, and/or allopurinol or probenecid (neither drug is used for acute attacks) may be used.

6. **What causes pseudogout? How is it diagnosed?**
   Pseudogout is caused by deposition of calcium pyrophosphate crystals in joints. Look for **rhomboid crystals** with **weakly positive birefringence** (vs. negative birefringence for gout crystals in the joint fluid).

7. **Name some other causes of arthritis.**
   - Prior trauma
   - Lupus and other collagen vascular diseases (e.g., scleroderma)

- Psoriasis
- Inflammatory bowel disease
- Lyme disease
- Ankylosing spondylitis
- Reactive arthritis
- Lyme disease
- Hemophilia
- Paget disease
- Hemochromatosis, Wilson disease
- Neuropathy (i.e., Charcot joint)

8. **Why do patients with hemophilia get arthritis?**
Recurrent hemarthroses (bleeding into the joints), which can cause a debilitating arthritis. Treatment is with acetaminophen. Avoid aspirin and other NSAIDs because of the risk of bleeding.

9. **Why do patients with sickle cell disease often have arthritis?**
Patients frequently experience arthralgias (pain) from ischemic sickle crises, but the classic cause of arthritis is avascular necrosis (e.g., hip arthritis from avascular necrosis of the femoral head).

10. **How do hemochromatosis and Wilson disease cause arthritis?**
Via deposition of excessive iron (hemochromatosis) or copper (Wilson disease) in the joints.

11. **True or false: One of the major Jones criteria for the diagnosis of rheumatic fever is arthritis.**
True. Migratory polyarthritis is one of the major Jones criteria. Look for a history of streptococcal throat infection. The other major criteria are carditis, chorea, erythema marginatum, and subcutaneous nodules. Remember the mnemonic JONES for the major Jones criteria (joints, obvious [the heart!], nodules [subcutaneous], erythema marginatum, and Sydenham chorea).

12. **What are the risk factors for avascular necrosis? What is the best test for making the diagnosis?**
Avascular necrosis describes local intravascular coagulation with subsequent bone ischemia and necrosis of cancellous bone and marrow. The presenting symptom is pain in the affected area. There are many potential causes and associations, including:
- Trauma (usually in the setting of a fracture)
- Corticosteroid excess (endogenous or iatrogenic)
- Sickle cell disease or other hemoglobinopathy
- Alcohol abuse
- Lupus and other connective tissue disorders
- Decompression sickness
- Slipped capital femoral epiphysis
- Pancreatitis
The best test for making the diagnosis is a magnetic resonance imaging (MRI) scan, which can detect avascular necrosis earlier than regular x-rays.

13. **What are the most common locations of intervertebral disc herniations? What symptoms do they cause?**
Lumbar disc herniation is a common, often correctable cause of low back pain. The most common location is the L5-S1 disc, which affects the S1 nerve root. Look for decreased ankle jerk, weakness of plantar flexors in the foot, pain from the midgluteal area to the posterior calf, and a positive straight leg-raise test. The second most common location for herniation is the L4-L5 disc, which affects the L5 nerve root. Look for a decreased biceps femoris reflex, weakness of the foot extensors, and pain in the hip or groin.

   After the lumbar area, the second most common location is the cervical spine. The classic symptom of cervical disc disease is neck pain. Herniation is most common at the C6-C7 disc, which affects the C7 nerve root. Look for decreased triceps reflex/strength and weakness of forearm extension.

14. How is intervertebral disc herniation diagnosed and treated?

Diagnosis is made on the basis of an MRI scan (preferred) or a computed tomography (CT) scan or myelography. Conservative treatment with analgesics is usually tried first because roughly 90% of cases resolve with conservative management. Epidural steroid injection may help. Surgery (discectomy) may be required if conservative treatment fails or a significant neurologic deficit is present (to prevent permanent nerve damage).

INFLAMMATORY OR IMMUNOLOGIC DISORDERS

1. What generalized systemic signs of inflammation may suggest an autoimmune disorder?

Systemic signs and symptoms of inflammation include elevations in the erythrocyte sedimentation rate (ESR) and C-reactive protein (CRP), fever, anemia of chronic disease, fatigue, and weight loss. If these symptoms are present (especially in a woman of reproductive age), you should consider the possibility of an autoimmune disease.

2. Describe the hallmarks of ankylosing spondylitis.

Ankylosing spondylitis is associated with human leukocyte antigen B27 (**HLA-B27**). Most often a 20- to 40-year-old man with a positive family history has symptoms of back pain and morning stiffness. Patients may assume a bent-over posture. The sacroiliac joints are primarily affected, and radiographs may reveal a so-called **bamboo spine**. Patients have other autoimmune-type symptoms, such as fever, elevation of ESR and CRP, and anemia. Some develop uveitis. Treat with NSAIDs, methotrexate, sulfasalazine, or tumor necrosis factor (TNF) antagonists (etanercept, infliximab, adalimumab).

3. What clues point to a diagnosis of rheumatoid arthritis?

Rheumatoid arthritis often causes systemic symptoms (fever, malaise, subcutaneous nodules, pericarditis, pleural effusion, uveitis), prolonged morning stiffness, and swan neck and boutonnière deformities. The diagnosis is often made on the basis of elevated ESR or CRP and a positive rheumatoid factor (RF), which is present in most adults but often negative in children. Antibodies to cyclic citrullinated peptide have similar sensitivity to RF but are more specific. Radiographs and MRI scans can also support the diagnosis. General treatment strategies reflect the fact that destruction of affected joints because of inflammation occurs early in the course of rheumatoid arthritis. The patient should be offered treatment with disease-modifying antirheumatic drugs (DMARDs) as soon as possible after disease onset. Escalate the intensity of the treatment until synovitis and inflammation have improved.

There are five general medication classes used to treat rheumatoid arthritis, with DMARDs forming the backbone of treatment. Treatment options include the following: analgesics (from acetaminophen to narcotics), NSAIDs, glucocorticoids, nonbiologic DMARDs (methotrexate, sulfasalazine, leflunomide, hydroxychloroquine, and minocycline), and biologic DMARDs. Biologic DMARDs include TNF inhibitors (etanercept, infliximab, and adalimumab), an interleukin-1 receptor antagonist (anakinra), a monoclonal antibody (rituximab), and biologic response modifiers (abatacept).

4. If a pediatric patient has uveitis and an inflammatory arthritis, but RF is negative, what disease should you suspect?

Juvenile idiopathic arthritis (previously called juvenile rheumatoid arthritis). RF is often negative in the pauciarticular variant. Affected patients commonly develop uveitis.

5. True or false: Psoriasis can cause an arthritis that resembles osteoarthritis.

False. The arthritis resembles rheumatoid arthritis. In the Step 3 exam, look for psoriatic skin lesions to make an easy diagnosis (Fig. 7-1). The arthritis usually affects the hands and feet, and although it resembles rheumatoid arthritis, RF is negative. NSAIDs are first-line therapy. Other treatments include nonbiologic DMARDS (methotrexate, Psoralens plus ultraviolet A [PUVA], retinoic acid derivatives, and cyclosporine) and biologic DMARDS, including TNF inhibitors (etanercept, infliximab, adalimumab, and golimumab).

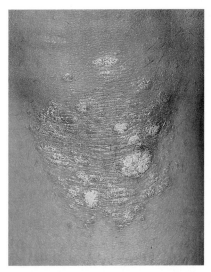

Figure 7-1. Psoriasis. Typical oval plaque with well-defined borders and silvery scale. *(From Habif TP. Clinical dermatology. 5th ed. St. Louis: Mosby, 2009).*

6. **What about lupus erythematosus and other autoimmune disorders as a cause of arthritis?**

   For lupus erythematosus, inflammatory bowel disease, and other autoimmune diseases, symptoms of the primary disease help in making these diagnoses in the USMLE.

7. **What is tenosynovitis? How does it occur? What are the presenting symptoms?**

   Tenosynovitis is inflammation of a tendon and its synovial sheath; the cause is usually an infection. Infections can result from trauma with direct inoculation (e.g., puncture wound or bite), direct spread from adjacent soft tissues, or hematogenous spread. Many organisms can cause tenosynovitis, but skin flora such as *Staphylococcus* and streptococcal species are most common. Look for tenderness along the course of a tendon and enlargement and slight flexion of the affected digit. Ultrasound or an MRI scan may be helpful in confirming the diagnosis. Treat with surgery and antibiotic therapy.

8. **Describe the presentation of the various inflammatory myopathies.**

   There are multiple subtypes of inflammatory myopathies, including dermatomyositis, polymyositis, inclusion body myositis, and overlap syndromes that occur with another rheumatic disease. All subtypes feature immune-mediated muscle injury. For dermatomyositis and polymyositis, look for elevated muscle enzymes (creatine kinase, lactate dehydrogenase, aldolase, alanine aminotransferase, and aspartate aminotransferase), positive autoantibodies such as antinuclear antibodies, and elevated serum and urine myoglobin. Electromyography abnormalities are common, but muscle biopsy is most useful in making a diagnosis and distinguishing the subtypes.

   Dermatomyositis typically involves symmetric proximal muscle weakness that gradually worsens, as well as characteristic skin findings such as heliotrope eruption (an erythematous to violaceous eruption on the upper eyelids, sometimes with eyelid edema) and Gottron papules (erythematous to violaceous papules over the dorsal aspects of the metacarpophalangeal and interphalangeal joints). There are other less common skin eruptions that are unlikely to be tested on the Step 3 USMLE. There is an increased risk of malignancy with dermatomyositis.

   The presentation for polymyositis is similar but without the characteristic skin eruptions, which is a key distinguishing factor. Interstitial lung disease may occur with both polymyositis and dermatomyositis.

   Inclusion body myositis and overlap syndromes (which occur with diseases such as systemic lupus erythematosus and systemic sclerosis) are unlikely to appear on the Step 3 USMLE.

HEREDITARY DEVELOPMENTAL DISORDERS

1. Describe genu valgum and genu varum. What is the appropriate management for each?

   Genu valgum is knock-knees, whereas genu varum is bowlegs. Distinguishing normal from abnormal development is important in determining when orthopedic evaluation is indicated. At birth, the normal alignment of the legs is varus. The amount of varus often increases as the child begins to walk. Alignment should be neutral at 18 to 24 months of age. Alignment progresses to valgus from the age of 2 to 4 years, and then the valgus alignment decreases to the normal adult alignment (slight valgus to neutral) by the age of 7 years.

   Pathologic causes of genu valgum include trauma, neoplasms, rickets, and skeletal dysplasia. Clues to pathologic causes include severe valgus deformity, asymmetric valgus deformity, progressive deformity after the age of 4 years, and short stature. X-rays and orthopedic consultation are indicated for suspected pathologic valgus deformity.

   Clues to pathologic causes of genu varum include severe bowing, progressive or persistent bowing after 3 years of age, asymmetric bowing, and short stature. Management is the same as for genu valgum.

2. Specify the age at presentation, epidemiology, symptoms and signs, and treatment for the three classically tested pediatric hip disorders.

NAME	AGE	EPIDEMIOLOGY	SYMPTOMS/SIGNS	TREATMENT
CHD	At birth	Female, first born, breech delivery	Barlow and Ortolani signs	Observation, abduction splint, or open or closed reduction
LCPD	4-10 yr	Short male with delayed bone age	Knee, thigh, or groin pain; limp	Orthoses
SCFE	9-13 yr	Overweight male adolescent	Knee, thigh, or groin pain; limp	Surgical pinning

CHD, Congenital hip dysplasia; LCPD, Legg-Calvé-Perthes disease; SCFE, slipped capital femoral epiphysis.

Note: All of these conditions may occur in an adult as arthritis of the hip.

3. If you forget everything else about differentiating the three pediatric hip disorders, what historical point will help you the most on the USMLE?

   Age at onset of symptoms.

4. How do you check for scoliosis? Who is usually affected? What is the treatment?

   Check for scoliosis by having patients touch their toes while you look at the spine. If scoliosis is present, you will see an abnormal lateral curvature of the spine. Scoliosis usually affects prepubertal girls and is idiopathic. Treat with a brace for anything other than very minor (<15 degrees) curvature. If the deformity is severe (e.g., with respiratory compromise, rapid progression), surgery should be considered.

5. What is the most common type of muscular dystrophy? How is it inherited? What are the classic findings?

   The most common type is Duchenne muscular dystrophy, an X-linked recessive disorder of dystrophin that is usually identified in boys between the ages of 3 and 7 years. Look for muscle weakness, markedly elevated levels of creatine phosphokinase, pseudohypertrophy of the calves (caused by fatty and fibrous infiltration of the degenerating muscle), and often a lower-than-normal IQ. The Gower sign is also classic: the patient "walks" his hands and feet toward each other to rise from a prone position. Muscle biopsy establishes the diagnosis. Treatment is supportive. Most patients die by age 20.

6. List the five less common types of muscular dystrophy.

   1. Becker muscular dystrophy: also an X-linked recessive dystrophin disorder but milder than the Duchenne type.

2. Fascioscapulohumeral dystrophy: an autosomal-dominant disorder that affects the areas in the name (face, shoulder girdle, upper arms). Symptoms begin between the ages of 7 and 20 years. Life expectancy is normal.
3. Limb-girdle dystrophy: affects pelvic and shoulder muscles; begins in adulthood.
4. Mitochondrial myopathies: of interest because they are inherited mitochondrial defects (passed only from mother to offspring; cannot be transmitted by men). The key phrase is *ragged red fibers* on a biopsy specimen. Ophthalmoplegia is usually present.
5. Myotonic dystrophy: an autosomal-dominant disorder that presents between the ages of 20 and 30 years. Myotonia (inability to relax muscles) classically manifests as an **inability to relax the grip or release a handshake.** Look for coexisting mental retardation, baldness, and testicular or ovarian atrophy. Treatment is supportive and includes genetic counseling. The diagnosis is clinical.

7. **What class of inherited metabolic disorders affects muscle and may resemble muscular dystrophy?**
The rare glycogen storage diseases (autosomal-recessive inheritance) can cause muscular weakness, especially **McArdle disease,** a deficiency in glycogen phosphorylase that is relatively mild and involves weakness and cramping after exercise because of lactic acid build up.

NEOPLASMS

1. **What is the most common type of bone tumor?**
Metastatic (especially from breast, lung, or prostate cancer).

2. **What is a pathologic fracture? What is the most common cause of a pathologic fracture?**
A pathologic fracture is one that occurs in bone previously weakened by another disease. Osteoporosis (especially in elderly, thin women) is the most common cause, but you should always think about the possibility of malignancy.

3. **What is a unicameral bone cyst? Who gets it? Describe the classic presentation.**
A unicameral bone cyst is an expansile, lytic, well-demarcated benign lesion in the proximal portion of the humerus in children and adolescents (Fig. 7-2). Although benign, it may weaken the bone enough to cause a pathologic fracture of the humerus (the classic presentation).

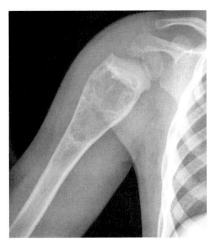

Figure 7-2. Plain film of unicameral bone cyst manifesting as a large, expansile, completely cystic intramedullary lesion that has well-defined focally sclerotic borders. (*From Gilbert-Barness E. Potter's pathology of the fetus, infant and child. 2nd ed. Philadelphia: Mosby, 2007.*)

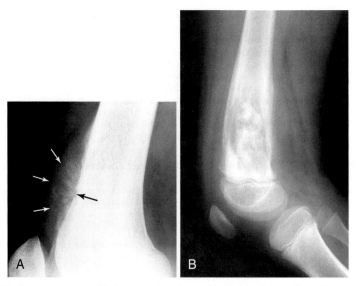

Figure 7-3. Osteogenic sarcoma of the knee. **A,** A lateral view of the knee in a 19-year-old man shows a sunburst-type periosteal reaction (*arrows*). Knowing that the distal femur is the most common site of osteogenic sarcoma, that periosteal reaction is a feature, and that this patient is a teenager should make osteogenic sarcoma very high on your differential diagnostic list. **B,** A destructive central lesion is seen here in the distal femur of an 8-year-old girl. (*From Mettler F. Essentials of radiology. 2nd ed. Philadelphia: Saunders, 2004.*)

4. **Give the basic facts for Paget disease. How is it linked to cancer?**

In Paget disease, bone is broken down and regenerated, often simultaneously. The disease is usually seen in individuals older than 40 years and is more common in men. It is often discovered in an asymptomatic patient through a radiograph. Classic cases involve the pelvis and skull; watch for a person who has had to buy larger-sized hats. Patients may complain of bone pain, arthritis, or hearing loss. **Alkaline phosphatase** is markedly elevated in the presence of normal calcium and phosphorus levels. The risk of osteosarcoma is increased in affected bones. The main treatment is antiresorptive agents (e.g., zoledronic acid, alendronate, risedronate, pamidronate).

5. **What do you need to know about osteosarcomas for the Step 3 exam?**

Osteosarcomas are most commonly seen around the knee in 10- to 30-year-old patients. The classic x-ray finding is a sunburst periosteal reaction (Fig. 7-3) in the distal femur or proximal tibia in association with a mass. In older adults, the risk is increased in bones with long-standing Paget disease or osteomyelitis.

INFECTIONS

1. **Which bacteria are the most common cause of septic arthritis? In what scenario should you think of another cause?**

Septic arthritis is most commonly due to *Staphylococcus aureus*, but in sexually active adults (especially those who are young and/or promiscuous), suspect *Neisseria gonorrhoeae*. Aspirate the joint and order a Gram stain, culture, and cell count with differential if infection is suspected. Obtain blood cultures because the organism usually reaches the joint via hematogenous spread. Also perform urethral swabs and cultures in appropriate patients. In patients with sickle cell disease, although *S. aureus* is most common, there is also an increased risk of *Salmonella* septic arthritis, which is commonly tested.

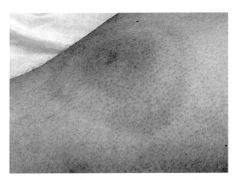

Figure 7-4. Erythema migrans rash of Lyme disease. Bull's-eye lesion on lateral thigh. *(From Firestein GS, Budd RC, Gabriel SE, et al. Kelley's textbook of rheumatology. 9th ed. Philadelphia: Saunders, 2012. Courtesy Juan Salazar, MD, University of Connecticut Health Center.)*

2. **What clues point to Lyme disease as the cause of arthritis?**
   Look for a history of a tick bite or hiking in the woods, **erythema chronicum migrans** rash (Fig. 7-4), and migratory arthritis (later). Treat *Borrelia burgdorferi*, the causative bacterium of Lyme disease, with doxycycline, amoxicillin, or cefuroxime. Avoid doxycycline in children younger than 8 years and in pregnant or lactating women.

3. **How do you recognize reactive arthritis as the cause of arthritis?**
   Reactive arthritis is also associated with HLA-B27. The classic triad of symptoms consists of **urethritis** (caused by chlamydial infection), **conjunctivitis,** and **arthritis** (*"can't pee, can't see, can't climb a tree"*). Reactive arthritis may also follow enteric bacterial infections. Superficial oral and penile ulcers are common. Diagnose and treat the sexually transmitted disease, and use NSAIDs for arthritis. Also treat the patient's sexual partners.

4. **What is the most common bacterial cause of osteomyelitis? In what clinical scenarios should you think of other causes?**
   Osteomyelitis is most commonly caused by *S. aureus*. Think of gram-negative bacteria in immunocompromised patients or intravenous drug abusers. A *Salmonella* species is the most likely cause in patients with sickle cell disease. Think *Pseudomonas aeruginosa* if there is a puncture wound through a tennis shoe. Diabetic patients who develop a so-called diabetic foot with subsequent osteomyelitis usually have a polymicrobial infection. Aspirate and biopsy the affected joint or bone, and order a Gram stain, culture, and cell count of the fluid or tissue if osteomyelitis is suspected. Check the serum ESR or CRP level.

TRAUMATIC INJURIES

1. **What are the common findings for ligament injuries of the knee? How do you distinguish injuries of the anterior cruciate, posterior cruciate, medial collateral, and lateral collateral ligaments on physical examination?**
   Ligament injuries in the knee commonly cause pain, joint effusions, instability of the joint, and a history of the joint *popping, buckling,* or *locking up.*
   - **Anterior cruciate ligament (ACL)** tears are the most common. Watch for the *anterior drawer test*. The knee is placed in 90 degrees of flexion and pulled forward (like opening a drawer). If the tibia pulls forward more than normal (e.g., more than the unaffected side), the test is positive and the patient has an ACL tear.
   - **Posterior cruciate ligament (PCL)** tears can be diagnosed with the *posterior drawer test*. Push the tibia back with the knee in 90 degrees of flexion. If the tibia pushes back more than normal, the test is positive, and a PCL tear is present.
   - **Medial collateral ligament (MCL)** tears are suggested during the *abduction* or *valgus* stress test. With the knee in 30 degrees of flexion, abduct the ankle while holding the knee. If

the knee joint abducts to an abnormal degree, the test is positive and a medial compartment injury is present.

- **Lateral collateral ligament (LCL)** tears are suggested during the *adduction* or *varus* stress test. Adduct the ankle while holding the knee. If the knee joint adducts to an abnormal degree, the test is positive and a lateral compartment injury is present.

An MRI scan and/or arthroscopy can be used to confirm suspected tears and look for other injuries.

2. **What type of radiographs should you order if you suspect a fracture?**

For any suspected fracture, order at least two views (usually anteroposterior and lateral) of the site, and consider radiographs of the joints above and below the fracture site.

3. **How should you treat a patient with severe pain after trauma and negative x-rays?**

Treat the patient conservatively. Assume that there is a fracture and have the patient rest the injured area. Splinting may be appropriate for distal extremity injuries. Obtain follow-up radiographs 7 to 14 days after the injury if symptoms persist; many occult fractures will become visible at this time. The exception to waiting is a suspected hip fracture in an elderly person—proceed to a CT or MRI scan of the hip to allow earlier diagnosis and treatment, which decrease operative morbidity and length of hospital stay compared with delayed diagnosis and treatment. In children, pain over the growth plates can indicate a fracture (called a Salter Harris I fracture), even in the absence of any radiographic changes, and this mandates immobilization.

4. **What fracture is usually diagnosed in trauma patients with pain in the anatomic "snuff box"?**

Scaphoid bone fracture (Fig. 7-5), classically after a fall onto an outstretched hand. X-rays may not show a fracture initially, so if a patient has had a fall onto an outstretched hand and has pain in the anatomic snuff box, treat such an injury as a fracture. Repeat x-rays can be performed 1 to 2 weeks later. An MRI scan is the most sensitive test, but it is not routinely ordered.

5. **What orthopedic fractures are associated with the highest mortality rate?**

Pelvic fractures, because patients can bleed to death. If the patient is unstable, consider heroic measures such as military antishock trousers (MAST trousers) and an external fixator. For traumatic pelvic bleeding in the setting of a pelvic fracture in an unstable patient, angioembolization is the preferred treatment.

6. **Why should areas distal to the fracture site be assessed by physical examination?**

Areas distal to the fracture site should be assessed for neurologic and vascular compromise, either of which may be an emergency.

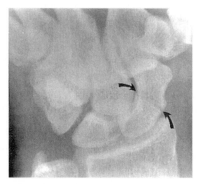

Figure 7-5. A film of a patient with snuff-box tenderness shows a fracture line at the midwaist of the scaphoid (*curved arrows*). (*From Katz DS, Math KR, Groskin SA, eds. Radiology secrets. Philadelphia: Hanley & Belfus, 1998, p. 436.*)

7. **Distinguish between an open and a closed fracture.**

   In an open (compound) fracture, the skin is broken over the fracture site. In closed fractures, the skin is intact over the fracture site.

8. **Explain the difference in the management of open and closed fractures.**

   For closed fractures, closed reduction and casting can generally be carried out. For open fractures, you should give antibiotics with coverage for gram-positive and gram-negative organisms (cefuroxime is appropriate; fluoroquinolones are an alternative). If the patient is at risk of methicillin-resistant *Staphylococcus aureus* (MRSA) infection, add vancomycin. Carry out surgical debridement, give a tetanus vaccine booster, lavage fresh wounds (if <8 hours old), and perform **open reduction**. The main risk for open fractures is infection, which is usually not a problem for closed fractures because the skin is intact.

9. **What are the indications for open reduction other than an open fracture?**
   - Intraarticular fractures or articular surface malalignment
   - Nonunion or failed closed reduction
   - Compromise of blood supply
   - Multiple trauma (to allow mobilization at the earliest possible point)
   - A need for perfect reduction to optimize extremity function (e.g., professional athletes)

10. **Define compartment syndrome. What is the cause?**

    Compartment syndrome is a problem of muscle compartments that are limited by the fascia in which they are contained. It is seen in the extremities (most commonly in the calf) when edema or hemorrhage causes swelling inside a muscle compartment. Rising pressure inside the fascial compartment can result in permanent nerve damage and muscle necrosis.

    The three common clinical scenarios in which compartment syndrome is seen are fractures (classically midshaft tibial fractures or supracondylar fractures of the humerus in children), burns (especially electrical and circumferential burns), and vascular compromise (or after vascular surgery procedures).

11. **What are the symptoms and signs of compartment syndrome? How is it treated?**
    - Pain (especially pain on passive movement out of proportion to the injury)
    - Paresthesias, hypesthesia, and numbness (decreased sensation and two-point discrimination)
    - Cyanosis or pallor
    - Firm-feeling muscle compartment
    - Paralysis (late, ominous sign)
    - Elevated compartment pressure (>30 mm Hg)

    In the USMLE, diagnosis of compartment syndrome often has to be made clinically without a pressure reading. Although pulses may be slightly decreased, they are usually palpable (or detectable with Doppler ultrasound) in compartment syndrome. Lack of palpable pulses is an ominous, late sign. Compartment syndrome is an emergency, and quick action can save an otherwise doomed limb. Treatment is immediate fasciotomy; incising the fascial compartment relieves the pressure.

12. **Define Charcot joint. What causes it? How is it managed?**

    Charcot joints (neuropathic joints) are seen in patients with diabetes mellitus or other conditions causing peripheral neuropathy (e.g., tertiary syphilis). A lack of sensation and proprioception causes the patient to overuse or misuse joints, resulting in arthropathy and joint deformity. The best treatment is prevention. To rule out a fracture, radiographs are warranted for patients with neuropathy in the feet after even seemingly minor trauma.

13. **What is reflex sympathetic dystrophy (RSD)? What symptoms do patients have?**

    RSD is a poorly understood disorder that generally occurs in an extremity and is characterized by pain, swelling, and signs of autonomic dysfunction (vasomotor instability with alternating warmth and coolness and/or sweating and dryness of the area). In most (but not all) cases it is posttraumatic in origin. The associated trauma is classically mild, and symptoms may begin days or several weeks after the injury. Patients classically have severe, intermittent pain, often described as burning, with associated temperature changes and sweating during episodes. A minor stimulus (e.g., a light touch) may trigger severe pain. The diagnosis can be confirmed with radiographs or a nuclear medicine scan. A presumptive diagnosis is often made in the appropriate setting if a sympathetic nerve block (i.e., injection of local anesthetic into the involved nerve) relieves symptoms. This procedure can be repeated as part of therapy if it is initially successful.

14. **True or false: There is a high incidence of vascular injury with posterior knee dislocations.**
    True. Order an angiogram if pulses are asymmetric (i.e., weaker or absent on the affected side) to check for injury to the popliteal artery.

15. **To what site is pain from hip inflammation or dislocation/fracture classically referred?**
    The knee (especially in children).

16. **Define Osgood-Schlatter disease. How is it recognized and treated?**
    Osgood-Schlatter disease is osteochondritis of the tibial tubercle. It is often bilateral and usually occurs in boys between 10 and 15 years of age. Symptoms and signs include pain, swelling, and tenderness in the knee (remember that the pediatric hip problems previously described have referred pain in the knee but no knee swelling or tenderness on palpation of the knee). Treat with rest, activity restriction, and NSAIDs. Most cases resolve on their own.

CHAPTER 8

DISORDERS OF THE SKIN AND SUBCUTANEOUS TISSUE

1. Cover the two right-hand columns in the following table and define the common terms used in dermatology to describe skin findings.

TERM	DEFINITION	EXAMPLES
Macule	Flat spot <1 cm (nonpalpable, just visible)	Freckles, tattoos
Patch	Same as macule but >1 cm	Port-wine birthmarks
Papule	Solid, elevated lesion <1 cm (palpable)	Wart, acne, lichen planus
Plaque	Same as papule but >1 cm and flat topped	Psoriasis
Nodule	Palpable, solid lesion >1 cm and not flat topped	Small lipoma, erythema nodosum
Vesicle	Elevated, circumscribed lesion <5 mm containing clear fluid (small blister)	Chickenpox, genital herpes
Bulla	Same as vesicle but >5 mm (large blister)	Contact dermatitis, pemphigus
Wheal	Itchy, transiently edematous area	Allergic reaction

SKIN ERUPTIONS

1. **Define vitiligo. With what diseases is it associated?**
   Vitiligo is characterized by skin depigmentation because of destruction of melanocytes. The exact cause is unknown, but it is associated with autoimmune conditions such as pernicious anemia, hypothyroidism, Addison disease, and type I diabetes. Patients often have antibodies to melanin, parietal cells, thyroid hormones, or other factors.

2. **Name several conditions to think about in the Step 3 exam for patients with pruritus.**
   Think of serious conditions first, such as obstructive biliary disease, uremia, and polycythemia rubra vera (classically seen after a warm shower or bath). Pruritus may also be caused by contact or atopic dermatitis, scabies, and lichen planus.

3. **Define contact dermatitis. How do you recognize it? What are the classic culprits?**
   Contact dermatitis is usually due to a type IV hypersensitivity reaction, although it may also be due to an irritating or toxic substance. Look for new exposure to a classic offending agent, such as poison ivy, nickel earrings, or deodorant. The rash is well circumscribed and occurs only in the area of exposure. The skin is red and itchy and often has vesicles or bullae (Fig. 8-1). Avoidance of the agent is required. Patch testing can be done, if needed, to determine the antigen.

4. **Define atopic dermatitis. What history points to this diagnosis?**
   Atopic dermatitis is a chronic allergic-type condition that begins in the first year of life, with red, itchy, weeping skin on the head, upper extremities, and sometimes around the diaper area. The clue to diagnosis is a family and/or personal history of allergies (e.g., hay fever) and asthma. The biggest problem is scratching of affected skin, which leads to skin breaks and possible bacterial infection. Treatment involves avoidance of drying soaps and use of antihistamines, moisturizing creams, topical steroids, and immunomodulating agents (topical pimecrolimus or tacrolimus).

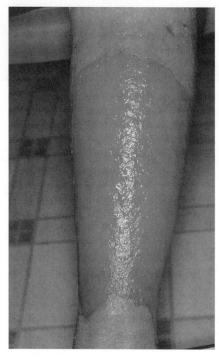

Figure 8-1. Allergic contact dermatitis of the leg caused by an elastic wrap. Notice the well-marginated distribution that differentiates it from cellulitis. See Plate 3. *(From Auerbach PS. Wilderness medicine, 6th ed. Philadelphia: Mosby, 2011, Fig. 82-46.)*

5. **What is diaper dermatitis? Name the main causes.**

   Diaper dermatitis is the term used for any inflammatory skin eruption that occurs in the diaper-covered region. Diaper-associated causes include irritant dermatitis, *Candida* dermatitis, and allergic dermatitis. Non–diaper-associated causes include seborrhea, atopic dermatitis, bacterial causes (impetigo and group A streptococcal infection), herpes simplex virus, psoriasis, scabies, and congenital syphilis. Child abuse must always be considered.

6. **How are the most common causes of diaper dermatitis treated?**

   Irritant dermatitis can be treated by avoiding skin contact with the diaper, such as allowing some time without the diaper on. Topical barriers such as petrolatum and zinc oxide can also be helpful. Candidal dermatitis can be treated with topical nystatin, clotrimazole, or miconazole. Classically, irritant dermatitis is present on the convex surfaces of the skin, with the intertriginous (skin fold) areas spared because the irritant does not get into the folds. This is in contrast to candidal dermatitis, which prefers the moist areas in skin folds.

7. **Define rosacea. In what age group is it seen? How do you treat it?**

   Rosacea often looks like acne but begins in middle age. There are numerous triggers for rosacea including sun exposure, emotional stress, alcohol consumption, spicy foods, and hot weather. Look for **rhinophyma** (bulbous red nose) and coexisting blepharitis. Treat with topical metronidazole or oral tetracycline. The pathogenesis is incompletely understood, but rosacea is not related to diet.

8. **Describe the classic psoriatic lesion.**

   Psoriatic lesions classically are described as dry, well-circumscribed, silvery, scaling papules and plaques that are *not* pruritic. Peeling of the scale will reveal pinpoint bleeding (Auspitz sign). Classic lesions are found on the scalp and extensor surfaces of the elbows and knees.

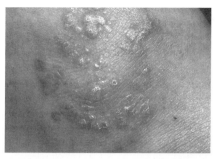

Figure 8-2. Lichen planus. Flat-topped, purple polygonal papules of lichen planus. See Plate 4. *(From Kliegman RM. Nelson textbook of pediatrics, 19th ed. Philadelphia: Saunders, 2011, Fig. 649-10.)*

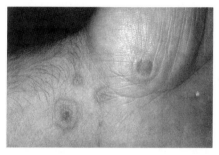

Figure 8-3. Erythema multiforme. Bull's-eye annular lesions with central vesicles and bullae. See Plate 5. *(From Goldman L, Schafer AI. Goldman's Cecil medicine, 24th ed. Philadelphia: Saunders, 2011, Fig. 447-10)*

9. **What other historical points and physical findings may be seen with psoriasis? How is it diagnosed and treated?**
   A family history of psoriasis is often present, and the disease occurs mostly in whites, with onset in early adulthood. Lesions may develop at sites of previous trauma (Koebner phenomenon). Affected patients may have pitting of the nails and an arthritis that resembles rheumatoid arthritis but is rheumatoid factor–negative. A diagnosis of psoriasis can often be made on the basis of appearance alone, but a biopsy can be used in doubtful cases. Treatment is complex and involves exposure to ultraviolet light, lubricants, topical corticosteroids, and keratolytics (e.g., coal tar, salicylic acid, anthralin). Oral therapies may include immunosuppressive and immunomodulating drugs such as methotrexate, cyclosporine, and biologic agents.

10. **What are the four *P*'s that clinch a diagnosis of lichen planus?**
    Pruritic, **p**urple, **p**olygonal **p**apules, classically on the wrists or lower legs, usually of adults (Fig. 8-2). Oral mucosal lesions (whitish with a lacelike pattern) may also be present. These oral lesions must be monitored because they may increase the risk of oral cancer.

11. **Describe the classic lesion of erythema multiforme. What virus is classically associated with it?**
    Look for the classic target (iris) lesions (Fig. 8-3). The classic cause is herpes infection, although Epstein-Barr virus and hepatitis C virus are also implicated. Some cases are idiopathic. Erythema multiforme used to be considered on the same spectrum as **Stevens-Johnson syndrome**; however, it is now generally considered to be an independent entity. Stevens-Johnson syndrome is usually a drug reaction. It may be fatal because of severe, widespread skin involvement. Patients with Stevens-Johnson syndrome are treated supportively with therapy similar to what a burn victim would receive (wound care, fluid and electrolyte management, pain control, nutritional support, and monitoring for and treatment of superinfections).

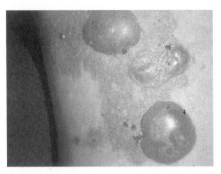

Figure 8-4. Bullous pemphigoid. Tense subepidermal bullae on an erythematous base. See Plate 6. (*From Goldman L, Schafer AI. Goldman's Cecil medicine, 24th ed. Philadelphia: Saunders, 2011, Fig. 447-6.*)

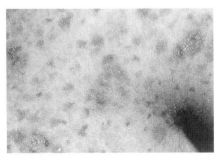

Figure 8-5. Dermatitis herpetiformis is characterized by pruritis, urticarial papules, and small vesicles. See Plate 7. (*From Feldman M, Friedman LS, Brandt LJ. Sleisenger and Fordtran's gastrointestinal and liver disease, 9th ed. Philadelphia: Saunders, 2010, Fig. 22-26. Courtesy Dr. Timothy Berger, San Francisco, CA.*)

12. **Define and describe pemphigus vulgaris. How is it different from bullous pemphigoid?**

    Pemphigus vulgaris is a potentially life-threatening autoimmune disease of middle-aged and elderly patients. The presenting symptoms are multiple bullae, starting in the oral mucosa and spreading to the skin of the rest of the body. Biopsy tissue can be stained for an immunoglobulin G (IgG) antibody to desmoglein 3 (which is associated with desmosomes) and shows a lacelike or fishnet immunofluorescence pattern. Treat with oral corticosteroids. Pemphigus vulgaris is associated with the Nikolsky sign, in which skin sloughs off on light pushing. A way to remember this is Nikolsky mouth is vulgar (pemphigus **vulgar**is, Nikolsky sign, oral lesions).

    Bullous pemphigoid is a similar but milder condition that results in a linear immunofluorescence pattern (different antibody) and is treated similarly (Fig. 8-4). It does not have oral involvement and does not have the Nikolsky sign, unlike pemphigus vulgaris.

13. **What skin disease is associated with celiac disease (gluten intolerance or sensitivity)? How is it treated?**

    Dermatitis herpetiformis is associated with celiac disease. Patients have intensely pruritic vesicles, papules, and wheals on the extensor aspects of the elbows and knees and possibly on the face or neck (Fig. 8-5). Look for diarrhea and weight loss (caused by gluten sensitivity). On biopsy, the skin has IgA deposits, even in unaffected areas. Test for celiac disease and treat both conditions with a gluten-free diet.

14. **What are decubitus ulcers? What is the best method of prevention?**
    Decubitus ulcers (bedsores or pressure sores) are skin ulcers caused by prolonged pressure
    against the skin. The best treatment is prophylaxis. Periodic turning of paralyzed, bedridden, or
    debilitated patients (the populations in which they are most common) and the use of special
    air mattresses prevent bedsores. Cleanliness and dryness also help to prevent decubitus ulcers.
    Periodic skin inspection can ensure that the problem is recognized early. When missed, the
    lesions can ulcerate down to the bone and become infected, possibly leading to sepsis and
    death. Treat major skin breaks with aggressive surgical debridement; if signs of infection are
    present, administer antibiotics.

15. **How are decubitus ulcers staged?**
    Stage 1 is intact skin with nonblanchable redness of a localized area. Stage 2 is partial-thick-
    ness loss of the dermis presenting as a shallow open ulcer. This stage may also present as an
    intact or ruptured blister. Stage 3 is full-thickness tissue loss. Subcutaneous fat may be visible,
    but bone, tendon, and muscle are not exposed. Stage 4 is full-thickness skin loss with exposed
    bone, tendon, or muscle. An unstageable ulcer has full-thickness loss in which the base of
    the ulcer is covered with slough or eschar. The true depth of the ulcer cannot be determined
    until the slough or eschar is removed.

DISORDERS OF NAILS/HAIR/SWEAT GLANDS

1. **How is acne described in medical terms? What bacteria may be involved in its
   pathogenesis?**
   The description of acne includes comedones (whiteheads and blackheads), papules, pustules,
   inflamed nodules, superficial pus-filled cysts, and/or possible inflammatory skin changes,
   including scar formation. *Propionibacterium acnes* is thought to be involved in the pathogenesis, as is blockage of pilosebaceous glands.

2. **What are the treatment options for acne?**
   Treatment options are multiple. Start with topical benzoyl peroxide; then try topical
   clindamycin or retinoid, either with or without an oral antibiotic (typically a tetracycline or
   erythromycin for *P. acnes* eradication). Oral isotretinoin is the *last resort*. Although highly
   effective, isotretinoin is teratogenic; pregnancy testing in women before and during therapy,
   as well as contraceptive use, is mandatory. In addition, isotretinoin may cause dry skin and
   mucosae, muscle and joint pain, and liver function abnormalities.

3. **Define seborrheic dermatitis. What part of the body does it involve? How is it
   treated?**
   Seborrheic dermatitis causes the common conditions known as cradle cap and dandruff, as
   well as blepharitis (eyelid inflammation). Look for scaling skin, with or without erythema,
   on the hairy areas of the head (scalp, eyebrows, eyelashes, mustache, beard), as well as on
   the forehead, nasolabial folds, external ear canals, and postauricular creases. Treat with dandruff shampoo (e.g., selenium or tar shampoo), topical corticosteroids, and/or ketoconazole
   cream.

4. **What should you think about if hirsutism is described in the Step 3 exam?**
   Hirsutism is most commonly idiopathic, but other signs of virilization (e.g., deepening voice,
   clitoromegaly, frontal balding) suggest an androgen-secreting ovarian tumor. In the absence
   of virilization, consider Cushing syndrome, polycystic ovary syndrome, and drugs (minoxidil,
   corticosteroids, and phenytoin).

5. **What are the common pathologic causes of baldness?**
   Watch out for trichotillomania (a psychiatric disorder in which patients pull out their
   hair; baldness is patchy and irregular) and alopecia areata (idiopathic but associated with
   antimicrosomal and other autoantibodies). Baldness may also be seen in patients with lupus
   erythematosus or syphilis and after cancer chemotherapy.

6. **What causes ordinary male-pattern baldness?**
   Although the exact pathophysiology is still not clear, male-pattern baldness is considered a
   genetic disorder that requires androgens for expression.

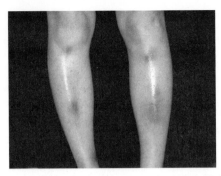

Figure 8-6. Erythema nodosum on the legs of a young woman. See Plate 8. (*From Hochberg MA, Silman AJ, Smolen JS, Weinblatt ME. Rheumatology, 5th ed. Philadelphia: Mosby, 2010, Fig. 159-13.*)

7. **What is hyperhidrosis? What causes it? How is it treated?**

Hyperhidrosis is sweating in amounts greater than what is required for thermoregulation. It typically occurs both awake and while sleeping, is bilateral, and affects the face, palms, soles, or axillae. Hyperhidrosis can have significant social and emotional consequences. Most cases are chronic and idiopathic, but consider medical conditions (e.g., hyperthyroidism, tuberculosis, human immunodeficiency virus (HIV), malignancy, endocarditis) and medications (e.g., hypoglycemic agents, antidepressants, hormonal agents, sympathomimetics) as possible causes. Treatment typically starts with 20% aluminum chloride in ethanol (Drysol) topically. Beta-blockers or benzodiazepines can be considered for cases of hyperhidrosis attributed to stress. Anticholinergic agents and clonidine may help but are limited by side effects. Axillary hyperhidrosis can be treated with botulinum toxin. Palmar hyperhidrosis that is refractory to topical and systemic therapies can be treated with endoscopic thoracic sympathectomy.

LUMPS/TUMORS OF THE SKIN

1. **Describe the classic lesion of erythema nodosum. With what diseases is it commonly associated?**

Erythema nodosum (Fig. 8-6) is an inflammation of the subcutaneous tissue and skin, classically over the shins (pretibial). Look for tender, red nodules. Sarcoidosis, coccidioidomycosis, or ulcerative colitis classically accompanies this condition on the USMLE, although multiple other infections (e.g., streptococci, tuberculosis) and drugs (e.g., sulfonamides) can also result in this finding.

2. **What are the ABCDEs of moles?**

ABCDE characteristics of a mole that should make you suspicious of malignant transformation (Fig. 8-7): **a**symmetry, **b**orders (irregular), **c**olor (change in color or multiple colors), **d**iameter (the bigger the lesion, the more likely it is malignant), and **e**volving over time. Excise any mole (or perform a biopsy if the lesion is very large) if it enlarges suddenly, develops irregular borders, darkens or becomes inflamed, changes color (even if only one small area of the mole changes color), begins to bleed, begins to itch, or becomes painful.

3. **Define dysplastic nevi syndrome. How is it managed?**

Dysplastic nevus syndrome is a genetic condition with multiple dysplastic-appearing nevi (usually more than 100 moles). Also look for a family history of melanoma. Treat with careful follow-up, excision or biopsy of any suspicious lesions, avoidance of sun and ultraviolet light exposure, and sunscreen use.

4. **Why is keratoacanthoma of note?**

Keratoacanthoma can mimic skin cancer (especially squamous cell cancer). Look for a flesh-colored lesion with a central crater that contains keratinous material, classically on the face (Fig. 8-8). Keratoacanthoma has a very rapid onset and grows to its full size in 1 to 2 months

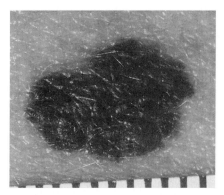

Figure 8-7. Melanoma (superficial spreading type). See Plate 9. *(From Goldman L, Schafer AI. Goldman's Cecil medicine, 24th ed. Philadelphia: Saunders, 2011, Fig. 210-3.)*

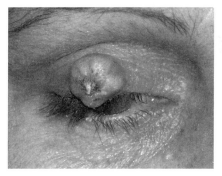

Figure 8-8. Keratoacanthoma on the right upper lid. Lesions are solitary, smooth, dome-shaped red papules or nodules with a central keratin plug. See Plate 10. *(From Albert DM, Miller JW. Albert and Jakobiec's principles and practice of opthalmology, 3rd ed. Philadelphia: Saunders, 2008, Fig. 250-3.)*

(which almost never happens with squamous cell cancer). The lesion involutes spontaneously in a few months and requires no treatment. If unsure, the best step is a biopsy, but choose observation as the answer for patients with a classic history of keratoacanthoma.

5. **Describe the classic lesion of basal cell cancer. What should you do if you suspect it?**
   Basal cell cancer classically begins as a shiny papule on a skin-exposed area (the head is classic) and slowly enlarges and develops an umbilicated center (which later may ulcerate) with peripheral telangiectasias (Fig. 8-9). Like all skin cancers, sunlight exposure increases the risk. It is more common in elderly, light-skinned people. Treat with excision. Biopsy any suspicious skin lesions in the elderly.

6. **True or false: Basal cell skin cancer almost never develops metastases.**
   True. However, it may be locally invasive and destructive.

7. **From what lesion does squamous cell cancer classically develop? What is Bowen disease?**
   Squamous cell cancer (Fig. 8-10) often develops in areas with preexisting actinic keratoses (hard, sharp, red, often scaly lesions in sun-exposed areas; Fig. 8-11) or burn scars. The lesions become nodular, warty, or ulcerated; perform a biopsy if such transformation occurs. Squamous cell cancer in situ is known as Bowen disease. Although metastases are rare in squamous cell cancer, they occur more frequently than in basal cell cancer.

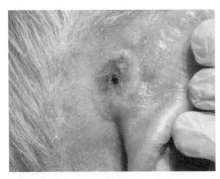

Figure 8-9. An ulcerated basal cell carcinoma with rolled borders on the posterior ear. See Plate 11. (*From Abeloff MD, Armitage JO, Niederhuber JE, Kastan MB, McKenna WG. Abeloff's clinical oncology, 4th ed. Philadelphia: Churchill Livingstone, 2008, Fig. 74-2.*)

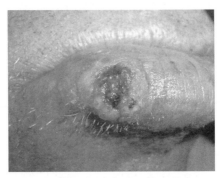

Figure 8-10. Squamous cell carcinoma on the lower lip. See Plate 12. (*From Rakel D, Rakel RE. Textbook of family medicine, 8th ed. Philadelphia: Saunders, 2011, Fig. 33-85. Copyright Richard P. Usatine.*)

8. **To what parameter is the prognosis of a malignant melanoma most closely related?**

   The thickness of the tumor. The 10-year survival rate decreases with increasing tumor thickness. Tumors less than 1.0 mm thick have the best prognosis.

9. **What type of melanoma do black patients tend to develop? How do you recognize it?**

   Although uncommon in blacks, melanoma in this population tends to be of the acrolentiginous type. Look for black dots on the palms or soles or under the fingernail (Fig. 8-12) that start to change in appearance or cause symptoms.

10. **Describe Paget disease of the nipple. What is its significance?**

    The presentation for Paget disease of the nipple is a unilateral, red, oozing or crusting nipple in an adult woman that fails to respond to typical dermatology treatments (Fig. 8-13). Although rare (roughly 1% to 2% of breast cancers), it signifies an underlying breast cancer (usually invasive ductal carcinoma or ductal carcinoma in situ) with extension to the skin.

11. **What is the classic clinical manifestation of Kaposi sarcoma?**

    A rash that does not respond to multiple treatments in a HIV-positive patient. Kaposi sarcoma is a vascular skin tumor that commonly begins as a papule or plaque on the upper body or in the oral cavity (Fig. 8-14). It is highly associated with herpesvirus (human herpesvirus 8 [HHV-8]) infection.

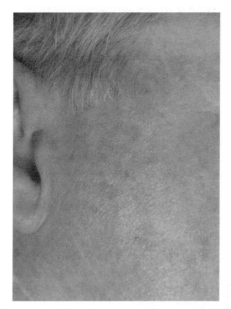

Figure 8-11. Multiple actinic keratoses visible as thin, red, scaly lesions. See Plate 13. (*From Goldberg D. Procedures in cosmetic dermatology: lasers and lights. Vol. 1, 2nd ed. Philadelphia: Saunders, 2008, Fig. 5-2.*)

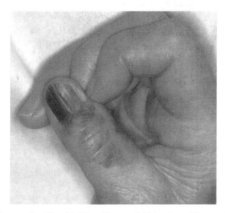

Figure 8-12. Nailbed melanoma. See Plate 14. (*From Dartmouth University and Dermnet Weekly Clinic, July 30, 2001.*)

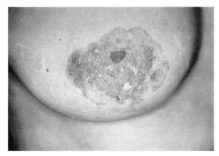

Figure 8-13. Paget disease of the nipple. Note the erythematous plaques around the nipple. See Plate 15. (*From Bolognia JL, Jorizzo JL, Rapini RP. Dermatology, 1st ed. Edinburgh: Mosby, 2003, Fig. 53-8.*)

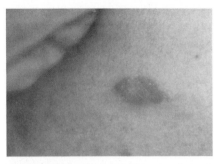

Figure 8-14. Kaposi sarcoma. See Plate 16. (*From Hoffman R.* Hematology: basic principles and practice, *5th ed. Philadelphia: Churchill Livingstone, 2008, Fig. 121-35.*)

12. **What is the main risk factor for skin cancer?**
    Ultraviolet light exposure.

13. **What are the two major cytologic clues for histiocytosis?**
    CD1-positive cells and Birbeck granules (cytoplasmic inclusion bodies that look like tennis rackets).

14. **Describe the clinical findings in tuberous sclerosis.**
    The findings for this autosomal-dominant disorder are hypopigmented skin macules (ash leaf spots), seizures, mental retardation, and central nervous system hamartomas (tubers). There is an increased risk of cardiac rhabdomyomas and renal tumors known as angiomyolipomas (because they comprise vascular, muscle, and fatty tissue). Look for a positive family history, although most cases are new mutations.

15. **How are capillary hemangiomas treated?**
    Capillary hemangiomas (also known as strawberry hemangiomas) are benign vascular tumors that are often first noticed a few days after birth. They tend to increase in size after birth (sometimes becoming quite large) and gradually resolve within the first 2 years of life (Fig. 8-15). The best treatment is to do nothing but observe and follow. Laser therapy can be considered in cases in which a capillary hemangioma is causing impairment (such as covering an eye or the mouth).

16. **Describe the skin lesions of neurofibromatosis type 1 (NF1). What else do you need to know about NF1?**
    Café-au-lait macules (Fig. 8-16) and cutaneous neurofibromas (Fig. 8-17) are the hallmark lesions of NF1. There is increased risk of mental retardation with NF1. There is also an increased lifetime risk of malignancy in patients with NF1 (5% to 10% of patients will develop peripheral nerve-sheath tumors; also look for malignancies such as pheochromocytoma and leukemia). Most patients with NF1 have macrocephaly, and many have short stature. Scoliosis is common. Hypertension may result from renovascular disease, coarctation of the aorta, or tumors that secrete vasoactive substances. Gastrointestinal neurofibromas can cause obstruction or anemia from bleeding. Seizures may result from intracranial tumors.

INFECTIONS

1. **Name the various dermatologic fungal infections.**
   Known as dermatophytosis, tinea, and *ringworm*, fungal infections include the following:
   Tinea corporis (body/trunk): look for red, ring-shaped lesions with raised borders that tend to clear centrally as they expand peripherally (Fig. 8-18).
   Tinea pedis (athlete's foot): look for macerated, scaling web spaces between the toes that often itch and may be associated with thickened, distorted toenails (onychomycosis). Good foot hygiene is part of treatment.
   Tinea unguium (onychomycosis): thickened, distorted nails with debris under the nail edges.

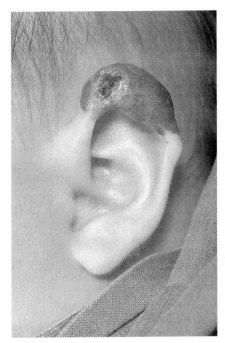

Figure 8-15. Infantile hemangioma. These lesions grow rapidly during the first few months of life once they appear (20% at birth), but they are asymptomatic unless they bleed, become infected, or obstruct a vital structure. Complete resolution is typical before the age of 7 years, and no treatment is usually required. See Plate 17. (*From du Vivier A.* Atlas of clinical dermatology, *3rd ed. New York: Churchill Livingstone, 2002, Fig. 8-28.*)

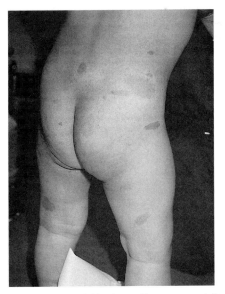

Figure 8-16. Multiple café-au-lait macules on a child with neurofibromatosis type 1. See Plate 18. (*From Eichenfield LF Frieden IJ, Esterly NB.* Neonatal dermatology, *2nd ed. Philadelphia: Saunders, 2007, Fig. 22-2.*)

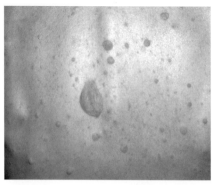

Figure 8-17. Discrete neurofibromas in a patient with neurofibromatosis type 1. (*From Ferri FF. Ferri's clinical advisor 2014, 1st ed. Philadelphia: Mosby, 2013, Fig. E1-586.*)

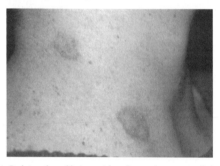

Figure 8-18. Tinea corporis. Red ring-shaped lesions with scaling and some central clearing. See Plate 19. (*From Kliegman RM. Nelson textbook of pediatrics, 19th ed. Philadelphia: Saunders, 2011, Fig. 658-8.*)

Tinea capitis (scalp): mainly affects children (highly contagious), who have scaly patches of hair loss and may have an inflamed, boggy granuloma of the scalp (known as a kerion) that usually resolves on its own.

Tinea cruris (jock itch): more common in obese males; usually found in the crural folds of the upper, inner thighs.

2. **What organisms cause fungal infections?**

Most fungal infections are due to *Trichophyton* species. In tinea capitis, if the hair fluoresces under a Wood lamp, a *Microsporum* species is the cause; if not, *Trichophyton* is probably the cause.

3. **How are fungal infections diagnosed and treated?**

Formal diagnosis of any fungal infection can be made by scraping the lesion and examining a potassium hydroxide (KOH) preparation to visualize the fungus via a microscope or by culturing the sample. Because they are so common clinically, empiric treatment without a formal diagnosis is common, but for the USMLE, get a formal diagnosis before treating. Oral antifungals must be used to treat tinea capitis and onychomycosis; other infections can be treated with topical antifungals (imidazoles such as miconazole, clotrimazole, and ketoconazole) or griseofulvin, which is better for severe or persistent infections.

4. **True or false: Candidiasis is often a normal finding in some women and children.**

True. Oral thrush (creamy white patches on the tongue or buccal mucosa that can be scraped off) is seen in normal children, and *Candida* vulvovaginitis is seen in normal women, especially during pregnancy or after taking antibiotics. However, at other times and in different patients, candidal infections may be a sign of diabetes or immunodeficiency; for example, thrush in a man should make you think about the possibility of AIDS, and recurrent vulvovaginal candidiasis should prompt screening for diabetes.

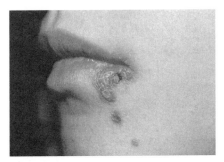

Figure 8-19. Impetigo. Multiple crusted and oozing lesions. See Plate 20. (*From Kliegman RM. Nelson textbook of pediatrics, 19th ed. Philadelphia: Saunders, 2011, Fig. 657-1.*)

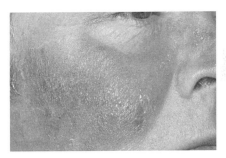

Figure 8-20. Sharply defined erythema and edema characteristic of erysipelas. See Plate 21. (*From Zaoutis LB, Chiang VW. Comprehensive pediatric hospital medicine, 1st ed. Philadelphia: Mosby, 2007, Fig. 156-2.*)

5. **How is candidiasis treated?**
   Treat with local/topical nystatin or imidazoles (e.g., miconazole, clotrimazole). Oral therapy (nystatin or ketoconazole) is used for extensive or resistant disease.

6. **How do you recognize and treat the rash of impetigo? What causes it?**
   In patients with impetigo, which is caused by *Streptococcus* and *Staphylococcus* species, look for a history of a break in the skin (e.g., previous chickenpox, insect bite, scabies, cut). The rash starts as thin-walled vesicles that rupture and form yellowish crusts (Fig. 8-19). The skin is classically described as "weeping". Typical lesions appear on the face and tend to be localized. The rash is infectious; look for a history of sick contacts. Treat with dicloxacillin, cephalexin, or clindamycin to cover both *Streptococcus* and *Staphylococcus* species. Topical mupirocin may also be used.

7. **Distinguish between impetigo and erysipelas.**
   Both are superficial skin infections caused by streptococci or *Staphylococcus aureus* and often occur after a break in the skin (e.g., trauma, scabies, insect bite). **Impetigo** classically changes, first from maculopapules to vesicopustules and bullae and then to honey-colored, crusted lesions. Staphylococci are a more frequent cause than streptococci. Definitely think of staphylococci if a furuncle or carbuncle is present; think of streptococci if glomerulonephritis develops. Impetigo is contagious; watch for sick contacts. If there are a limited number of lesions without bullae, topical mupirocin may be used. If there are bullous or many lesions, treat with dicloxacillin, cephalexin, or clindamycin. **Erysipelas** (Fig. 8-20) is a superficial cellulitis that appears red, shiny, and swollen; it is tender and may be associated with vesicles and bullae, fever, and lymphadenopathy. Treat with penicillin or amoxicillin, although erysipelas may require parenteral therapy with a cephalosporin (ceftriaxone or cefazolin) if systemic symptoms such as fever and chills are present.

8. **What organisms typically cause cellulitis? What special circumstances should make you think of atypical causes?**

   Streptococci and staphylococci cause most cases. Think of *Pseudomonas* species for burns or severe trauma; of *Pasteurella multocida* after a dog or cat bite (treat with ampicillin); and of *Vibrio vulnificus* in fishermen or other patients exposed to salt water (treat with tetracycline). Diabetic patients with foot ulcers tend to have polymicrobial infections and need powerful, broad-spectrum antibiotic coverage.

9. **Describe the physical findings for cellulitis.**

   In patients with cellulitis, the involved overlying skin is red, hot, and frequently tender. It looks like erysipelas but involves deeper subcutaneous tissues. Antibiotic selection depends on whether the cellulitis is purulent or nonpurulent. These are newer terms and are designations within the 2011 Infectious Diseases Society of America clinical practice guidelines for methicillin-resistant *S. aureus* (MRSA). The idea is that a purulent infection may be caused by *S. aureus*. Oral treatment options for purulent cellulitis are trimethoprim-sulfamethoxazole, doxycycline, clindamycin, and linezolid, which all cover *S. aureus*. Oral treatment options for nonpurulent cellulitis are dicloxacillin, cephalexin, and clindamycin, which all cover *Streptococcus pyogenes*, the most common cause of non-purulent cellulitis.

10. **Define necrotizing fasciitis. How is it treated?**

    Necrotizing fasciitis is defined as progression of cellulitis to necrosis and gangrene. Watch for crepitus and signs of systemic toxicity (e.g., tachycardia, fever, and hypotension). Multiple organisms are often involved (aerobes and anaerobes), but if one organism is involved, it is usually a group A *Streptococcus*. Treat with intravenous fluids, incision and drainage (I and D) or surgical debridement, and broad-spectrum antibiotics. This includes a carbapenem (imipenem or meropenem) plus clindamycin. Clindamycin is added because it shuts off protein synthesis and therefore stops the bacteria from producing further toxins.

11. **What is folliculitis? What is a carbuncle? What is a furuncle?**

    Folliculitis is a superficial bacterial infection of the hair follicles with purulent material in the epidermis but not the deeper soft tissue. A carbuncle is a coalescence of several inflamed follicles into one mass with purulent drainage from multiple follicles. A furuncle is an infection of the hair follicle with purulent material extending into the subcutaneous tissue and forming a small abscess.

12. **What pathogen usually causes folliculitis? What less common pathogen do you need to remember?**

    Folliculitis is most commonly caused by *S. aureus*. Think *Pseudomonas* in the setting of inadequately chlorinated hot tubs or swimming pools. *Candida* folliculitis can occur in immunocompromised patients or after broad-spectrum antibiotic use.

13. **How is folliculitis treated?**

    Most cases of folliculitis resolve on their own. Advise patients to use warm compresses and avoid shaving in the affected area. For persistent cases, prescribe topical mupirocin. Systemic antibiotics are not usually warranted.

14. **What is an abscess? What is the most common pathogen? How is an abscess treated?**

    An abscess is a collection of pus within the dermis and deeper skin tissues. *S. aureus*, particularly MRSA, is the most common cause. I and D is the main treatment modality. The data are unclear as to whether antibiotics provide any additional benefit following I and D.

15. **What causes scabies? How do you recognize it?**

    Scabies is caused by the mite *Sarcoptes scabei*, which tunnels into and leaves visible burrows on the skin, classically in the finger web spaces and on the flexor surface of the wrists. You should know what these burrows look like. Facial involvement is sometimes seen in infants. Patients have severe pruritus, and scratching can lead to secondary bacterial infection.

16. How do you diagnose and treat scabies?

Diagnosis is made by scraping a mite out of a burrow and viewing it under a microscope. Treat scabies with permethrin cream applied to the whole body. Remember to treat all contacts (e.g., the whole family). Do *not* use lindane unless permethrin is not an option. Lindane used to be the treatment of choice but can cause neurotoxicity, especially in young children. After treatment, the dead mites burrowed in the skin can continue to cause pruritus for weeks.

17. How do you recognize and treat tinea versicolor?

Tinea versicolor (also known as pityriasis versicolor) is a *Pityrosporum* fungal infection that most commonly appears as multiple patches of various sizes and colors (brown, tan, and white) on the torso of young adults. It often becomes noticeable in the summer because the affected areas fail to tan and look white. Diagnose from lesion scrapings (KOH preparation). Treat with selenium sulfide shampoo or topical imidazoles.

18. What causes lice? How are lice treated?

Lice (pediculosis) can involve the head (caused by *Pediculus capitis*; common in school-aged children), body (caused by *Pediculus corporis*; unusual in individuals with good hygiene), or pubic area (crabs; caused by *Phthirus pubis* and transmitted sexually). Infected areas tend to itch. Diagnosis is made by seeing the lice on hair shafts. Treat with permethrin cream (preferred over lindane because of the neurotoxicity of lindane) and decontaminate sources of reinfection (wash or sterilize combs, hats, bed sheets, clothing).

19. What causes warts? How are they treated?

Warts are caused by human papillomavirus (HPV). They are infectious and are most commonly seen in older children, classically on the hands. The most common serotypes are 6 and 11. Multiple treatments are available, including salicylic acid, liquid nitrogen, and curettage. Genital warts are also caused by HPV. Approximately 15 of the HPV serotypes are considered to be high-risk types for the development of cervical cancer; serotypes 16 and 18 are associated with the majority of cases of cervical cancer.

20. Define molluscum contagiosum. How do you recognize it? How is it treated?

Molluscum contagiosum is a poxvirus infection that is common in children but may also be transmitted sexually. Diagnosis is made according to the characteristic appearance of the lesions (skin-colored, smooth, waxy papules with a central depression [umbilicated] that are roughly 0.5 cm) or by looking at contents of the lesion, which include cells with characteristic inclusion bodies. The usual treatment is freezing or curettage.

21. True or false: A child with genital molluscum is probably a victim of sexual abuse.

False. A child who has genital molluscum may or may not have contracted the disease from sexual contact. The more common mechanism is autoinoculation, in which the child has a lesion on the hand that spreads to the genital area from scratching. Do *not* automatically assume child abuse, although it must be ruled out.

22. Outline the classic description and natural course of pityriasis rosea.

Pityriasis rosea is typically seen in young adults. Look for a herald patch (slightly erythematous, scaly, ring-shaped or oval patch classically seen on the trunk), followed 1 week later by many similar lesions that tend to itch (Fig. 8-21). Look for lesions on the back with a long axis that parallels the Langerhans skin cleavage lines, typically in a Christmas tree pattern. The condition usually remits spontaneously in 1 month. Think about syphilis in the differential diagnosis. Treat with reassurance.

23. How do you recognize measles (rubeola) infection in a child?

Look for a lack of immunization. Pathognomonic Koplik spots (tiny white spots on the buccal mucosa) are seen 3 days after a high fever, cough, runny nose, and conjunctivitis with or without photophobia. Remember the three Cs of measles: conjunctivitis, cough, and coryza. On the next day, a maculopapular rash begins on the head and neck and spreads downward to cover the trunk (cephalocaudal progression, like a bucket of paint being dumped over the head and dripping down to the feet). Treat supportively.

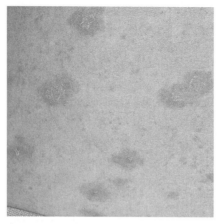

Figure 8-21. Pityriasis rosea. Both small oval plaques and multiple small papules are present. See Plate 22. (*From Habif TP. Clinical dermatology, 5th ed. Philadelphia: Mosby, 2009, Fig. 8-44.*)

24. **Describe the complications of measles.**
Complications include giant cell pneumonia, especially in very young and immunocompromised patients; otitis media; and encephalitis, either acute or late (**subacute sclerosing panencephalitis,** which usually occurs years later and is almost invariably fatal unless caught very early in the course, in which case treatment with lifelong interferon is a possibility).

25. **How do you recognize a rubella infection in children? What are the complications?**
Rubella is milder than measles. Signs and symptoms include low-grade fever, malaise, and tender swelling of the suboccipital and postauricular nodes; arthralgias are common. After a 2- to 3-day prodrome, a faint maculopapular rash appears on the face and neck and spreads to the trunk (cephalocaudal progression), just as in measles. Complications include encephalitis and otitis media.

26. **Why is rubella infection an important disease?**
Rubella is important mainly because infection in pregnant mothers can cause severe birth defects in the fetus. Screen all women of reproductive age, and immunize those without evidence of rubella antibodies before pregnancy to avoid this complication. Remember, however, that the vaccine is contraindicated in pregnant women.

27. **How do you recognize roseola infantum (exanthem subitum)? What causes it?**
Roseola infantum is often easy to recognize because of the progression: high fever (may be >104° F [40° C]) with no apparent cause for 4 days, which may result in febrile seizures, followed by an abrupt return to normal temperature just as a diffuse macular/maculopapular rash appears on the chest and abdomen. The disease is rare in children older than 3 years. It is caused by HHV type 6 (a DNA herpes family virus).

28. **How do you recognize erythema infectiosum (fifth disease) in children? What causes it?**
Look for the classic slapped-cheek rash (Fig. 8-22; confluent erythema over the cheeks looks like someone slapped the child across the face) accompanied by mild constitutional symptoms (e.g., low fever, malaise). One day later, a maculopapular rash appears on the arms, legs, and trunk. The disease is caused by parvovirus B19, the same virus that causes aplastic crisis in sickle cell disease.

29. **How do you recognize chickenpox? What causes it?**
The description and progression of the rash should lead you to the diagnosis: discrete macules (usually on the trunk) turn into papules, which turn into vesicles that rupture and crust over. Such changes occur within 1 day. Because the lesions appear in successive crops, the rash will be in different stages of progression in different areas. The cause is the varicella virus.

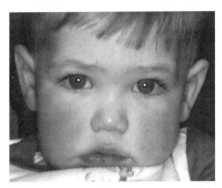

Figure 8-22. Slapped-cheek appearance of erythema infectiosum. See Plate 23. *(From Baren JM, Rothrock SG, Brennan J, Brown L. Pediatric emergency medicine, 1st ed. Philadelphia: Saunders, 2007, Fig. 123-5.)*

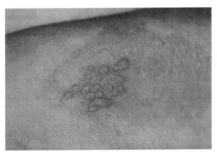

Figure 8-23. Herpes zoster. Grouped vesicopustules on an erythematous base. See Plate 24. *(From Marx J, Hockberger R, Walls R. Rosen's emergency medicine: concepts and clinical practice, 7th ed. Philadelphia: Mosby, 2009, Fig. 118-28. Courtesy David Effron, MD).*

30. **How can you make a definitive diagnosis of chickenpox? At what point is a patient with chickenpox no longer infectious?**

A Tzanck smear of tissue from the base of a vesicle shows multinucleated giant cells. A presumptive diagnosis can be made if the rash is classic. Infectivity ceases only when the last lesion crusts over.

31. **What are the complications of chickenpox?**

A major complication is infection of the lesions with streptococci or staphylococci, which cause erysipelas, cellulitis, and/or sepsis. The patient should be instructed to keep clean to avoid infection. Other complications include pneumonia (especially in very young children, adults, and immunocompromised patients), encephalitis, and (if given aspirin) **Reye syndrome.** Do not give aspirin to a child with a fever unless you have a diagnosis that requires its use, such as Kawasaki disease. The varicella-zoster virus can reactivate years later to cause herpes zoster (also known as shingles; Fig. 8-23), a rash that develops in a dermatomal distribution, often with preceding pain and paresthesias. A child who has not been immunized or exposed to chickenpox can catch the disease from someone with shingles.

32. **Describe the treatment and prophylaxis for chickenpox.**

In most cases, no treatment is needed except supportive care (e.g., acetaminophen, fluids, avoidance of infecting others). Acyclovir can be used in severe cases. Routine vaccination with the varicella vaccine is now recommended for all children in the United States. Varicella-zoster immune globulin is available for prophylaxis in patients with debilitating illness (e.g., leukemia, AIDS) if you see them within 4 days of exposure and for newborns of mothers with chickenpox. Intravenous immunoglobulin can be given if varicella-zoster immune globulin is not available.

33. **What is scarlet fever? What causes it? How is it recognized and treated?**

Scarlet fever is a febrile illness with a rash caused by certain *Streptococcus* species. Look for a history of untreated streptococcal pharyngitis; only streptococcal species that produce erythrogenic toxin can cause scarlet fever. Pharyngitis is followed by a sandpaper-like rash on the abdomen and trunk with classic circumoral pallor and strawberry tongue. The rash tends to desquamate once the fever subsides. Oral penicillin V is the treatment of choice for streptococcal pharyngitis to prevent rheumatic fever. Alternative therapies include amoxicillin, cephalosporins, macrolides, and clindamycin.

34. **What are the diagnostic criteria for Kawasaki disease (mucocutaneous lymph node syndrome)?**

This rare disease is seen in patients younger than 5 years on the Step 3 exam. The diagnostic criteria include fever for more than 5 days (mandatory for diagnosis); bilateral conjunctival injection; changes in the lips, tongue, or oral mucosa (e.g., strawberry tongue, fissuring, injection); changes in the extremities (e.g., skin desquamation, edema, erythema); polymorphous truncal rash, which usually begins 1 day after the fever starts; and cervical lymphadenopathy. Also look for arthralgia or arthritis. Remember the mnemonic CRASH and burn: conjunctivitis, rash, adenopathy, strawberry tongue, and hands/feet desquamation, and burn (fever for 5 days).

35. **What are the most feared complications of Kawasaki disease? How do you prevent them?**

The most feared complications involve the heart (coronary artery aneurysms, congestive heart failure, arrhythmias, myocarditis, and even myocardial infarction). Include Kawasaki disease in the differential diagnosis of any child who has a myocardial infarction. If Kawasaki disease is suspected, give aspirin and intravenous immunoglobulins. Both have been proven to reduce cardiac lesions. Kawasaki disease is one of the few indications for aspirin in a child. Follow the child with echocardiography to detect heart involvement.

TRAUMA AND TOXIC EFFECTS

1. **List the classic drugs that cause photosensitivity of the skin.**

Tetracyclines, phenothiazines, and birth control pills.

2. **When and where are keloid scars seen?**

Keloid scars are overgrowths of scar tissue that occur after an injury; they are seen most frequently in blacks. They are usually slightly pink and classically appear on the upper back, chest, and deltoid area. Also look for keloid scar development after ear piercing (Fig. 8-24). Do not excise these lesions because this may worsen scarring.

3. **What are the three causes of burns? How should all burns be managed initially?**

Burns may be thermal, chemical, or electrical. Initial management of all burns includes abundant intravenous fluids (first choice, lactated Ringer solution; back-up choice, normal

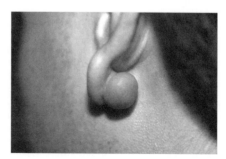

Figure 8-24. Keloid scar on the earlobe after piercing. See Plate 25. (*From Kliegman RM. Nelson textbook of pediatrics, 19th ed. Philadelphia: Saunders, 2011, Fig. 651-1.*)

saline; know that there is a formula for how to replace fluids called the Parkland formula, but the specific equation is not important to know), removal of all clothes and other smoldering items on the body, copious irrigation of chemical burns, and, of course, the ABCs (airway, breathing, circulation). You should adopt a low threshold for intubation. In the setting of burns related to a fire, give 100% oxygen until significant carboxyhemoglobin from carbon monoxide inhalation is ruled out.

4. **How is burn severity classified? Describe the management of each class.**
   Burn-depth terminology no longer includes the use of first-, second-, and third-degree burns. Burn severity is now classified as superficial, superficial partial-thickness, deep partial-thickness, and full-thickness burns.
   Superficial burns are erythematous without blister formation and involve only the epidermis; pain is localized.
   Superficial partial-thickness burns are painful, warm, and moist with blister formation and involve the epidermis and superficial papillary dermis.
   Deep partial-thickness burns have skin that is mottled, waxy, and white in appearance with ruptured blisters. Pain sensation is absent, but pressure sensation is intact.
   Full-thickness burns involve both the epidermis and dermis, have a white to gray leathery appearance, and do not blanch with pressure.

5. **How are chemical burns managed? Which is worse, acid or alkali burns?**
   All chemical burns should be treated with copious irrigation from the nearest source (e.g., tapwater) because the sooner you dilute the chemical, the less damage will be done. Alkali burns are worse than acidic burns because alkaline substances penetrate more deeply.

6. **What is burned skin prone to develop?**
   Burned skin is much more prone to infection, usually by *S. aureus* or *Pseudomonas aeruginosa.* For pseudomonal infection, look for a fruity smell and/or blue-green appearance. Prophylactic antibiotics are given topically only. Give a tetanus booster to all burn patients unless they have recently received one (within the past 5 years).

7. **Distinguish between frostnip and frostbite. How are they managed?**
   In **frostnip,** a mild form of cold injury, the affected skin is cold and painful. In **frostbite,** a more severe form of cold injury, the skin is cold and numb. Treat both with warming of the affected areas, using warm water (not scalding hot) and generalized warming (e.g., blankets).

CHAPTER 9

DISORDERS OF THE ENDOCRINE SYSTEM

1. **What is the difference between a primary and secondary endocrine disorder?**
   In **primary disorders**, the problem is in the gland; the hypothalamic-pituitary axis is functioning appropriately. In primary hypothyroidism, for example, the thyroid gland does not function properly for whatever reason, but the pituitary and hypothalamus respond appropriately. Therefore, thyroid hormone levels are low (as in all cases of hypothyroidism), but thyroid-stimulating hormone (TSH) and thyroid-releasing hormone (TRH) are high (the appropriate response from the pituitary and hypothalamus to low levels of thyroid hormone).

   In **secondary disorders**, the true dysfunction is outside the gland itself. For example, in secondary hypothyroidism, thyroid hormone levels are low, but TSH and/or TRH are also low (inappropriate in the setting of low thyroid hormone). If the pituitary is destroyed or surgically removed, secondary hypothyroidism results from low TSH; the thyroid gland functions well, but no TSH is available to stimulate it. To confuse the picture, the dysfunction may also be completely outside the endocrine axis (e.g., heart failure that causes secondary hyperaldosteronism).

   This concept in endocrine gland dysfunction is quite important. Simple blood tests can localize the problem. You may be able to answer a USMLE question simply by reading through the various values for hormones and hormone-releasing factors and figuring out where in the hypothalamus-pituitary–target gland axis the problem lies.

THYROID DISORDERS

1. **What physical and laboratory findings suggest thyroid cancer? What is the most common type of thyroid cancer? What risk factor is of particular concern for thyroid cancer?**
   Patients often have a single, stony-hard nodule or mass in the thyroid gland that may be rapidly enlarging. The nodule fails to take up radioactive tracer on a nuclear scan (a so-called cold nodule). The most common type is papillary thyroid cancer. Other worrisome findings are hoarseness, which indicates recurrent laryngeal nerve invasion, and an increase in calcitonin level, which indicates the rare medullary thyroid cancer. Patients with medullary thyroid cancer may have multiple endocrine neoplasia (MEN) syndrome. Historically, irradiation to the head or neck is of concern because of its association with thyroid cancer.

2. **How should you evaluate a thyroid mass for possible malignancy?**
   To evaluate a nodule in the thyroid gland, order thyroid function tests. TSH measurement is the best screening test; toxic or functional nodules are unlikely to be cancer. If the TSH level is normal, perform fine-needle aspiration of the mass. If the TSH level is low, then order a nuclear scan. A cold nodule or area of decreased uptake is more suspicious than a nodule with normal or increased uptake. Ultrasound is also commonly used to help evaluate a thyroid mass. If the history is suspicious (radiation to neck, MEN syndrome, hoarseness, stony-hard nodule), perform a biopsy even if the other tests are normal.

3. **What are the common symptoms and signs of hyperthyroidism?**
   Symptoms: nervousness, anxiety, irritability, insomnia, heat intolerance, sweating, palpitations, tremors, weight loss with increased appetite, fatigue, weakness, emotional lability, and diarrhea.
   Signs: enlarged thyroid gland, warm skin, thyroid stare/lid lag, exophthalmos, proptosis, ophthalmoplegia (Graves disease), pretibial myxedema (Graves disease), tremor, tachycardia, and atrial fibrillation. Check the TSH level when a patient has new-onset atrial fibrillation.

4. **What are the most common causes of hyperthyroidism?**
   The most common cause is **Graves disease**, which is characterized by a diffusely enlarged thyroid gland, positive thyroid-stimulating immunoglobulins and antibodies, exophthalmos, proptosis, ophthalmoplegia, and pretibial myxedema. In elderly patients, look for toxic multi-nodular goiter (individual lumps instead of diffuse enlargement of the gland, and hot nodules on a nuclear scan). Other causes include adenoma (single lump that is "hot" on a nuclear scan), subacute thyroiditis (viral infection with **tender, painful** thyroid gland), and factitious hyperthyroidism (in which the patient takes thyroid hormone). Rare, exotic causes include amiodarone (which can cause hypothyroidism or hyperthyroidism), TSH-producing pituitary tumors, thyroid carcinoma, and struma ovarii (an ovarian teratoma that secretes thyroid hormone).

5. **Describe the classic laboratory pattern of primary hyperthyroidism.**
   The TSH level is low, whereas triiodothyronine (T_3) and thyroxine (T_4) are higher than normal.

6. **How is hyperthyroidism treated?**
   Short-term (stabilizing) treatment: Propylthiouracil (PTU) and methimazole/carbimazole can be used as suppressive agents. Beta-blockers are used for hyperadrenergic symptoms (e.g., tachycardia) and in the setting of thyroid storm (severe hyperthyroid state—an emergency). Iodine can also suppress the thyroid gland but is rarely used for this purpose clinically.
   Definitive (curative) treatment: Radioactive iodine ablation of the thyroid gland is typically used. Surgery is preferred in pregnant patients. Hypothyroidism may result from either treatment; if so, it is treated with lifelong thyroid hormone replacement.

7. **What are the symptoms and signs of hypothyroidism?**
   Symptoms: weakness, lethargy, fatigue, cold intolerance, weight gain with anorexia, constipation, loss of hair, hoarseness, menstrual irregularity (menorrhagia is classic), myalgias and arthralgias, memory impairment, and dementia. Always rule out hypothyroidism as a cause of dementia.
   Signs: bradycardia; dry, coarse, cold, and pale skin; periorbital and peripheral edema; coarse, thin hair; thick tongue; slow speech; decreased reflexes; hypertension; carpal tunnel syndrome and paresthesias; vitiligo, pernicious anemia, and diabetes (remember the autoimmune association between these three conditions and Hashimoto disease); and coma (severe disease).
   In children, congenital hypothyroidism may occur (mental, motor, and growth retardation).

8. **What are the common causes of hypothyroidism?**
   The most common known cause is Hashimoto thyroiditis. Among affected individuals, women of reproductive age outnumber men by 8:1. Histology reveals lymphocytes in the thyroid gland, as well as antithyroid and antimicrosomal antibodies. Other autoimmune diseases may coexist. The associated goiter is nontender. The second most common cause is iatrogenic after treatment of hyperthyroidism. Other less common causes include iodine deficiency, amiodarone, lithium, and secondary hypothyroidism caused by pituitary or hypothalamic failure (look for low TSH), such as in Sheehan syndrome (hypopituitarism caused by pituitary necrosis from blood loss and hypovolemic shock during and after childbirth).

9. **Describe the laboratory findings in primary hypothyroidism.**
   Elevated TSH, decreased T_3 and T_4, antithyroid and antimicrosomal antibodies (if caused by Hashimoto thyroiditis), hypercholesterolemia, and anemia (which may be caused by chronic disease or coexisting pernicious anemia).

10. **Why is free T_4 (or free T_4 index) better than total T_4 for measuring thyroid hormone activity?**
    Free T_4 (free T_4 index) measures the active form of thyroid hormone. Many conditions cause a change in the amount of thyroid-binding globulin (TBG) and thus change total T_4 levels in the absence of hypothyroidism or hyperthyroidism. Common examples include pregnancy, estrogen therapy, and oral contraceptive pills, all of which increase TBG. Nephrotic syndrome, cirrhosis, and corticosteroid treatment all decrease TBG. T_3 resin uptake is an older test that is not worth the effort to learn for the Step 3 exam, but if you are asked, it should rise or fall in the same way as free T_4. Although an oversimplification, this principle should serve you well in the exam.

11. **How is hypothyroidism treated?**
    With T_4 or thyroxine. T_3 should not be used. In elderly patients, it is important to "start low and go slow," because overtreatment can be dangerous.

12. **What is sick euthyroid syndrome?**
    Any patient with any illness may have temporary derangements in thyroid function that resemble hypothyroidism. TSH ranges from normal to mildly elevated, and serum T_4 ranges from normal to mildly decreased. Clinical circumstances and physical findings are the best guides to whether the patient has true hypothyroidism. In patients with sick euthyroid syndrome, simply treat the underlying illness. If the diagnosis is in doubt, either remeasure thyroid parameters after the patient recovers (preferred) or try an empirical dose of levothyroxine (if the patient does not respond to treatment of the underlying illness).

13. **True or false: Hypothyroidism can cause elevated cholesterol.**
    True. Thyroid hormone replacement corrects the elevated cholesterol.

14. **What are the different types of thyroiditis? What are the presenting symptoms?**
    Thyroiditis can present as an acute illness with significant thyroid pain (e.g., subacute thyroiditis and infectious thyroiditis) or as a condition with no evidence of thyroid inflammation in which there is only thyroid dysfunction or goiter.
    Subacute thyroiditis manifests in the hyperthyroid phase as neck pain, a tender goiter, and elevated T_4 and/or T_3 levels. Patients typically go from a hyperthyroid to a hypothyroid state to recovery.
    Infectious thyroiditis may be acute or chronic. Acute infections are most commonly caused by *Staphylococcus* and *Streptococcus* and frequently involve abscess formation. Acute infections present with fever, rapid-onset neck pain, and tenderness that usually is unilateral. Thyroid ultrasound can differentiate subacute thyroiditis from infectious thyroiditis. Treat with intravenous antibiotics. Chronic infections are often bilateral, usually have less thyroid pain and tenderness than acute infections, and are typically caused by organisms such as mycobacteria, fungi and *Pneumocystis*. Needle aspiration is required to identify the causative organism.
    Other causes of thyroiditis that are unlikely to appear in the USMLE include painless thyroiditis (painless but with transient hyperthyroidism then sometimes hypothyroidism before recovery), postpartum thyroiditis (similar to painless thyroiditis but within 1 year of childbirth), drug-induced thyroiditis (look for lithium, amiodarone, or interferon-alpha), radiation thyroiditis, and fibrous thyroiditis.

DIABETES MELLITUS

1. **Outline the current recommendations for diabetes mellitus screening.**
   Universal screening is not generally recommended. Screening is more accepted, but not universal, in patients who are obese, older than 45 years, or who have a family history of diabetes and members of certain minority groups (blacks, Hispanics, Pima Indians). Screening in pregnancy is mandatory!

2. **Define diabetes.**
   Diabetes is defined as (1) a glucose level greater than or equal to 126 mg/dL after an overnight (or 8-hour) fast on two separate occasions or (2) a random glucose level greater than 200 mg/dL or (3) a hemoglobin A_{1C} (Hb A_{1C}) level of greater than or equal to 6.5% on two separate occasions. If the patient has classic symptoms of diabetes (see the next question), one test is sufficient to make the diagnosis. In an asymptomatic patient, it is best to repeat the test. An oral glucose tolerance test is common in pregnancy; otherwise, it is rarely used because of poor reproducibility and poor patient compliance. With a glucose tolerance test, diabetes is diagnosed when glucose levels in the blood reach or exceed 200 mg/dL within 2 hours of receiving a 75-g oral dose of glucose.

3. **What are the classic presenting symptoms of new-onset diabetes?**
   Polyuria, polydipsia, and polyphagia (pee a lot, drink a lot, and eat a lot). You should also be suspicious if patients present with candidal infections (e.g., thrush or vaginal yeast infection), weight loss (as a result of excessive urination), or blurry vision. Prolonged hyperglycemia causes the lenses in the eyes to swell, and the patient may become myopic. Older

patients may even claim that they no longer need their reading glasses (i.e., presbyopia is temporarily corrected by lens swelling).

4. **What are the classic differences between type 1 and type 2 diabetes?**

	TYPE 1 (10% OF CASES)	TYPE 2 (90% OF CASES)
Age at onset	Most commonly <30 yr	Most commonly >30 yr
Associated body habitus	Thin	Obese
Development of ketoacidosis	Yes	No
Development of hyperosmolar state	No	Yes
Level of endogenous insulin	Low to none	Normal to high (insulin resistance)
Twin concurrence	<50%	>50%
HLA association	Yes	No
Response to oral hypoglycemics	No	Yes
Antibodies to insulin	Yes (at diagnosis)	No
Risk of diabetic complications	Yes	Yes
Islet cell pathology	Insulitis (loss of most B cells)	Normal number, but with amyloid deposits

HLA, Human leukocyte antigen.

Remember, however, that these findings may overlap.

5. **What are the goals of diabetes treatment in terms of glucose levels?**
The goals are to keep postprandial glucose levels less than 180 mg/dL and fasting glucose levels at 70 to 130 mg/dL. Attempts at stricter control may result in hypoglycemia; watch for symptoms of sympathetic nervous system activation and mental status changes.

6. **What is a good measure of long-term diabetes control?**
Hb A_{1C} is a measure of average control of blood glucose over the previous 2 to 3 months. The current recommendation is to keep the Hb A_{1C} level below 7% in most patients. Less stringent Hb A_{1C} goals (such as <8%) may be appropriate for patients with a history of severe hypoglycemia, limited life expectancy, advanced microvascular or macrovascular complications, and extensive comorbid conditions.

Hb A_{1C} measurement is a good way to catch patients with nocturnal hyperglycemia or less-than-honest patients who falsely record low glucose test readings. A rough rule of thumb is that Hb A_{1C} times 20 equals the average blood glucose level.

7. **When a nondiabetic patient has hypoglycemia, how can you distinguish between a factitious disorder (exogenous insulin) and an insulinoma (endogenous insulin)?**
Measure the **C-peptide level.** C-peptide is produced when the body makes insulin, but it is absent in prescription insulin preparations. Therefore, C-peptide is high for an insulinoma and low for factitious disorder. This is a classic USMLE question. Endogenous insulin has C-peptide, so overdoses of sulfonylurea medications will also cause increased C-peptide levels; investigate this possibility with a urine sulfonylurea screen.

8. **What should you remember before giving intravenous iodinated contrast material to a diabetic patient or a patient with renal insufficiency?**
Diabetic patients and patients with renal insufficiency are prone to acute renal failure induced by intravenously administered iodinated contrast agents used for intravenous pyelography (IVP), conventional angiography, and computed tomography (CT). You need to weigh carefully the risk-to-benefit ratio of using intravenous contrast agents. If you choose to give contrast, first hydrate the patient well with intravenous fluids to avoid renal shutdown. Acetylcysteine and bicarbonate have been traditionally used to try to decrease the risk of contrast nephropathy in patients at high risk, but newer studies indicate that fluids are the

only intervention that helps. The concerns about intravenous iodinated contrast do not apply to oral contrast agents (e.g., barium).

9. **What is diabetic ketoacidosis (DKA)? How is it treated?**
All type 1 diabetics will die without insulin. DKA is what happens before they die. Clinically, look for Kussmaul breathing (deep, rapid respirations), dehydration, hyperglycemia, acidosis (caused by excessive ketone formation), and elevated ketone levels in serum (often associated with a fruity odor of the breath) and urine.

Treatment involves intravenous fluids, insulin, and replacement of electrolytes (especially potassium and phosphate). For the USMLE, do not use bicarbonate to correct acidosis. Remember to search for the cause of DKA, which most commonly is noncompliance with insulin therapy. The second most common cause is an infection. The mortality rate for DKA with current treatment efforts is less than 10%.

10. **What is nonketotic hyperglycemic hyperosmolar state? How is it treated?**
This state occurs in type 2 diabetics who go without adequate treatment before they die. Hyperglycemia and increased serum osmolarity are present in the absence of ketones and acidosis. Glucose spilled in the urine acts as a diuretic, so patients are severely dehydrated; the first three treatments are thus "fluids, fluids, and fluids" (i.e., intravenous hydration with normal saline). Insulin and electrolyte replacement are also required. The mortality rate can approach 50% if mental status changes are present at the time of diagnosis.

11. **What are the common long-term complications of diabetes mellitus?**
    - **Atherosclerosis, coronary artery disease, myocardial infarction.** Diabetic patients often have silent heart attacks (no chest pain because of autonomic neuropathy). Risk factor modification should be regularly assessed, including smoking cessation, blood pressure control, and cholesterol monitoring.
    - **Retinopathy.** Diabetes is the leading cause of blindness in the United States for individuals younger than 50 years. Diabetic patients should be routinely screened for diabetic retinopathy.
    - **Nephropathy.** Diabetes is the leading cause of end-stage renal disease requiring hemodialysis (roughly 30% of cases; hypertension is a close second). Patients should be routinely screened for microalbuminuria and started on an angiotensin-converting enzyme (ACE) inhibitor or angiotensin II receptor blocker (ARB) if present.
    - **Peripheral vascular disease.** Diabetes is a leading cause of limb amputation and may lead to claudication, strokes, and impotence.
    - **Peripheral neuropathy.** This complication causes silent heart attacks, numbness in the feet, and other conditions (see Question 12). Patients should have a foot examination at every visit if peripheral neuropathy is present.
    - **Increased risk of infection.** White blood cells do not function as well in a hyperglycemic environment. This dysfunction coupled to an inability to sense pain and clogged arteries that cannot deliver white cells to the site of an early infection provides a recipe for disaster. Patients should receive pneumococcal vaccination and yearly influenza vaccination.

    All of these complications can be delayed or even prevented by good glucose control.

12. **What problems may result from diabetic peripheral neuropathy?**
    - **Gastroparesis.** Because the stomach does not empty well, patients experience early satiety and vomiting. Treat with motility enhancers, such as metoclopramide.
    - **Charcot joints.** Joints are deformed secondary to lack of sensation. Patients may break a bone and not feel it. The causes are neuropathy and atherosclerosis.
    - **Impotence.** The causes are neuropathy and atherosclerosis.
    - **Cranial nerve palsies** (especially of cranial nerves III, IV, and VI). Patients have diplopia and extraocular muscle paralysis, which should resolve within 8 weeks without treatment.
    - **Orthostatic hypotension.** This problem occurs even when the patient is well hydrated because the arteries do not clamp down when the patient stands up and the heart rate fails to increase appropriately.
    - **Pressure ulcers in the feet.** As with Charcot joints, lack of sensation leads to overuse or failure to rest an injured or tired foot because it is numb and the patient is unaware. All diabetic patients with foot numbness should wear socks and comfortably fitting shoes and inspect their feet regularly. Most cases of foot gangrene in diabetic patients begin as a simple callous or blister.

13. **Describe the treatment for diabetic retinopathy.**

If the retinopathy is proliferative (neovascularization or new, irregular vessel formation), the treatment is **panretinal laser photocoagulation.** A laser beam is used to burn tiny spots around the periphery of the retina, sparing the central retina, to prevent progression to blindness. Focal (limited) laser photocoagulation is generally performed for nonproliferative retinopathy only if symptoms are present (from macular edema). All diabetics should be seen annually by an ophthalmologist to monitor retinal changes.

14. **Describe the onset, peak, and duration of action of each of the insulin preparations.**

INSULIN PREPARATION	ONSET (h)	PEAK (h)	DURATION (h)
Ultrarapid acting			
Insulin aspart	<0.25	1-3	3-5
Insulin lispro	0.25-0.5	0.5-2.5	3-5
Insulin glulisine	0.2-0.5	1.5-2.5	3-4
Rapid acting			
Regular insulin	0.5-1	2-4	5-8
Intermediate to long acting			
NPH insulin	2-3	4-12	12-20
Long-acting			
Insulin glargine	1.5-4	None	24+
Insulin detemir	3-4	3-9	Dose dependent; 6-23

NPH, Neutral protamine Hagedorn.

15. **How do you adjust the dosage of neutral protamine Hagedorn (NPH) or regular insulin for high glucose levels?**

Regular insulin starts to work in 45 minutes; its action peaks around 3 to 4 hours after injection, and the duration of action is 6 to 8 hours. NPH insulin takes 1 to 1.5 hours until onset of action; its action peaks at 6 to 8 hours, and the total duration of action is about 12 to 20 hours. Therefore for insulin adjustments, the following guidelines apply:

- If the patient has high (low) glucose at 7 AM, increase (decrease) NPH insulin at dinner time the night before.
- If the patient has high (low) noon glucose, increase (decrease) the morning dose of regular insulin.
- If the patient has high (low) glucose at 5 PM, increase (decrease) the morning dose of NPH insulin.
- If the patient has high (low) glucose at 9 PM, increase (decrease) the dinner-time dose of regular insulin.

16. **Define the Somogyi effect and the dawn phenomenon.**

The **Somogyi effect** is the reaction of the body to hypoglycemia. If too much NPH insulin is given at dinner time, the glucose level at 3 AM on the next morning will be low (hypoglycemia). The body reacts to hypoglycemia by releasing stress hormones, which cause a high glucose level at 7 AM. The treatment is to decrease evening (NPH) insulin. The **dawn phenomenon** is hyperglycemia caused by normal secretion of growth hormone early in the morning. The glucose level is high at 7 AM and normal or high at 3 AM (no hypoglycemia). The treatment is to increase evening (NPH) insulin.

17. **How do you manage diabetic patients who are not allowed to eat because they are scheduled for surgery?**

Generally, one third to half of the normal dose of insulin is given. Glucose is closely monitored intraoperatively and postoperatively by the anesthesiologist. Regular intravenous insulin can be given to control glucose levels on the basis of blood glucose measurements.

18. **What is the issue with beta-blockers and hypoglycemia in diabetic patients?**
    If you give a beta-blocker to a diabetic patient, you may mask the classic symptoms of hypoglycemia (tachycardia, diaphoresis) that are caused by catecholamine release. You must weigh the risk-to-benefit ratio of using beta-blockers in diabetic patients (as in all patients). If a diabetic patient is having or has had a previous myocardial infarction or has congestive heart failure, the benefits outweigh the risks of treatment.

19. **What are the best oral agents to use in type 1 diabetes?**
    None. Patients with type 1 diabetes require insulin. Currently available oral agents do not work for type 1 diabetic patients.

20. **What is the first treatment for type 2 diabetes?**
    Weight loss, because it may reduce glucose levels by reducing insulin resistance. However, medications are usually needed and oral agents are tried first, typically beginning with metformin. Other agents include insulin secretagogues (glipizide, glimepiride, nateglinide, glyburide, repaglinide), thiazolidinediones (rosiglitazone, pioglitazone), alpha-glucosidase inhibitors (acarbose, miglitol), GLP-1 agonists (exenatide, liraglutide), DPP-4 inhibitors (saxagliptin, sitagliptin, linagliptin), and amylin analogues (pramlintide). The thiazolidinediones are falling out of favor because of the risk of fluid retention and exacerbation of congestive heart failure (rosiglitazone and pioglitazone), the risk of myocardial infarction (rosiglitazone), and the risk of bladder cancer (pioglitazone).
    Many type 2 diabetic patients eventually require insulin, and insulin may be required early if blood glucose or Hb A_{1C} levels are significantly elevated. In fact, current guidelines suggest using basal insulin administration early in therapy (generally after one or two oral agents have been started) to get blood glucose and Hb A_{1C} under control as early as possible.

ADRENAL DISORDERS

1. **What is the significance of adrenal tumors?**
   Most are benign, but they may be functional and can cause primary hyperaldosteronism (Conn syndrome) or hyperadrenalism (Cushing syndrome). Another possibility is pheochromocytoma, which is associated with intermittent severe hypertension, mental status changes, headaches, and diaphoresis.

2. **How can you differentiate a Wilms tumor from a neuroblastoma?**
   Both occur as flank masses in children (peak age around 2 years). Neuroblastomas most commonly arise from the adrenal gland and often contain calcifications, whereas a Wilms tumor arises from the kidney and rarely calcifies, so imaging (CT scan) can usually distinguish the two. In rare cases, neuroblastomas regress spontaneously (for unknown reasons).

3. **What do you need to know about neuroblastoma for the USMLE?**
   Neuroblastomas are a heterogeneous group of tumors that arise from neural crest cells. They can arise anywhere throughout the sympathetic nervous system, with the adrenal gland and abdomen being the two most common sites, in that order. Neuroblastoma metastasizes widely, including to lymph nodes, bone marrow, liver, and skin. Presenting symptoms depend on the location of the tumor and sites of metastases. In the USMLE, look for symptoms and signs such as abdominal pain, an abdominal mass (hepatic or retroperitoneal), anorexia, weight loss, back pain, bone pain, secretory diarrhea, hypertension, and leg edema.
   Laboratory findings may include elevated ferritin and lactate dehydrogenase (LDH). A complete blood count, serum chemistries, and liver and renal function tests should be ordered. Urine or serum catecholamine levels (vanillylmandelic acid [VMA] and homovanillic acid [HVA]) assist in diagnosis. Bone marrow biopsy, bone radiographs, bone scan, abdominal CT or magnetic resonance imaging (MRI) scans, chest x-ray, and head CT scans are used for diagnosis and staging. Tissue biopsy is required for definitive diagnosis.
   Neuroblastomas are treated with surgery, but they may also require chemotherapy and sometimes radiation therapy. Infants younger than 1 year have a better prognosis than older children.

4. What are the symptoms and signs of primary hyperaldosteronism (Conn syndrome)? What are the causes?

Symptoms: weakness and edema.

Signs: hypertension, hypokalemia, hypernatremia, and edema.

Conn syndrome is caused by an aldosterone-secreting adrenal neoplasm. Because it is a primary disease, renin levels are low; the rest of the endocrine axis responds appropriately to gland dysfunction. Order a CT scan of the abdomen to look for an adrenal mass. The treatment is surgical removal of the tumor.

5. What causes secondary hyperaldosteronism?

Secondary hyperaldosteronism is *much more common* than primary disease. It is due to low perfusion of the kidney, as in congestive heart failure; renal artery stenosis (bruit); dehydration; nephrotic syndrome; and cirrhosis. The key mechanism is that the kidney senses hypoperfusion and secretes renin; therefore the renin level is high. Treatment of the underlying disorder (if possible) resolves the hyperaldosteronism. Potassium levels may be normal or even high. Of note, hyperkalemia may be the cause of increased aldosterone release just as hypocalcemia causes increased release of parathyroid hormone. Both are normal physiologic responses.

6. What are the symptoms and signs of Cushing syndrome (increased corticosteroids)?

Symptoms: weight gain, changes in appearance, easy bruising, acne, hirsutism, emotional lability, depression, psychosis, weakness, menstrual changes, sexual dysfunction, insomnia, and memory loss.

Signs: buffalo hump, truncal and central obesity with wasting of extremities, round plethoric facies, purplish skin striae, acne, hirsutism, weakness (especially of the proximal muscles), hypertension, depression, psychosis, peripheral edema, poor wound healing, glucose intolerance or diabetes, osteoporosis, and hypokalemic metabolic alkalosis (due to mineralocorticoid effects of certain corticosteroids). Growth may be stunted in children.

7. What causes Cushing syndrome?

The most common cause is iatrogenic because steroids are prescribed for many different disorders. The second most common cause is Cushing disease (a pituitary adenoma that secretes adrenocorticotropic hormone [ACTH]), which causes roughly 60% of noniatrogenic cases. Among affected individuals, women of reproductive age outnumber men by 5:1. Other causes include ectopic ACTH production (classically by small cell lung cancer, which is more common in men) and adrenal adenomas or carcinomas (more common in children).

8. How is Cushing syndrome diagnosed?

The first test is either 24-hour measurement of free cortisol in urine (free cortisol levels are abnormally elevated) or a dexamethasone suppression test (cortisol levels are not appropriately suppressed several hours after administration of dexamethasone). Measurement of a random cortisol level is an inappropriate test because of wide interpatient and intrapatient variations. **Remember that ACTH is elevated in Cushing disease but is decreased with an adrenal adenoma**. If ACTH is increased, an MRI scan of the brain should be obtained to look for a pituitary adenoma. If ACTH is decreased and the patient has no history of taking steroids, an abdominal CT or MRI scan should be obtained to look for an adrenal tumor. Primary cancer is usually obvious when ectopic ACTH is the cause (e.g., weight loss, hemoptysis with a lung mass on chest radiography in patients with small cell lung cancer). Treatment is based on the cause and usually involves surgery.

9. Define hirsutism. What causes it?

Hirsutism is a male hair growth pattern in women or prepubescent children. The most common cause is familial, genetic, or idiopathic hirsutism, but in the USMLE watch for **polycystic ovary syndrome** (Stein-Leventhal syndrome), Cushing syndrome, and drugs (minoxidil, phenytoin, cyclosporine). If virilization (clitoral enlargement, deepening of the voice, temporal balding) accompanies the hirsutism, consider an androgen-secreting ovarian tumor (e.g., Sertoli-Leydig cell tumor or arrhenoblastoma) or adrenal source (congenital adrenal hyperplasia, Cushing syndrome, or adrenal tumor).

10. **What causes virilization in children?**
In female neonates, congenital adrenal hyperplasia is a likely cause of virilization. The classic example is a female infant born with ambiguous genitalia. However, the patient may also be a male child with precocious puberty. At least 90% of cases are due to **21-hydroxylase deficiency.** Because 21-hydroxylase is involved in the production of both aldosterone and cortisol, children develop signs of hypoadrenalism, with salt wasting, hypotension, hyperkalemia, hyponatremia, hypoglycemia, acidosis, and nausea and vomiting. Abnormally high levels of serum 17-hydroxyprogesterone or urinary 17-ketosteroids (dehydroepiandrosterone [DHEA], DHEA sulfate, and androsterone), along with decreased free cortisol in the serum, confirm the diagnosis. Give corticosteroids to prevent death. In older children, worry about a testosterone-secreting gonadal neoplasm.

11. **What is the classic cause of ambiguous genitalia in the Step 3 exam?**
Adrenogenital syndrome, also known as congenital adrenal hyperplasia. Ninety percent of cases are caused by **21-hydroxylase deficiency.** Patients are female because affected males experience precocious sexual development. Patients with 21-hydroxylase deficiency have salt wasting (low sodium), hyperkalemia, hypotension, and elevated 17-hydroxyprogesterone. Treat with steroids and intravenous fluids immediately to prevent death.

12. **What should you tell the parents of a child with ambiguous genitalia?**
Tell the parents the truth: you do not know the child's gender. No patient with ambiguous genitalia should be assigned a sex until the workup is complete. Karyotyping must be performed.

13. **What are the symptoms and signs of hypoadrenalism (Addison disease)?**
Symptoms: anorexia, weight loss, weakness, apathy.
Signs: hypotension, hyperkalemia, hyponatremia, hyperpigmentation (only if the pituitary is functioning because of melanocyte-stimulating hormone), nausea and vomiting, diarrhea, abdominal pain, mild fever, hypoglycemia, acidosis, eosinophilia, and shock.

14. **What is the most common type of hypoadrenalism?**
Secondary (iatrogenic) hypoadrenalism caused by steroid treatment. Individuals who are taken off long-term steroid therapy may be unable to secrete an appropriate amount of corticosteroids in response to stress for up to 1 year. Watch out for the classic postoperative patient who crashes (with hypotension, shock, and hyperkalemia) shortly after surgery and has a history of a disease requiring steroid therapy within the previous year. You may assess ACTH (usually high) and cortisol levels (inappropriately low) to help make the diagnosis, but do not wait for the results to give steroids. The patient may die. Give prophylactic stress doses of corticosteroids in the setting of an illness, operation, or other stressor to prevent an adrenal crisis.

15. **What are the other causes of hypoadrenalism?**
The most common primary (noniatrogenic) cause is autoimmune (idiopathic) disease. Patients may have other autoimmune diseases, such as hypothyroidism, pernicious anemia, vitiligo, diabetes, or hypoparathyroidism. Other causes include metastatic cancer (especially lung cancer), infection (tuberculosis, fungal infections, opportunistic infections in AIDS and other immunosuppressed states), ketoconazole, and pituitary/hypothalamic failure.

16. **How is hypoadrenalism diagnosed?**
An ACTH stimulation test can be performed. Plasma cortisol is measured, ACTH is administered, and cortisol is remeasured in 1 hour. The cortisol level should rise appropriately, usually 18 µg/dL or doubling of the baseline level, depending on the baseline value. An inappropriate response to ACTH indicates hypoadrenalism. Do not withhold treatment to make a diagnosis if the patient is crashing.

PARATHYROID/PITUITARY DISORDERS

1. **What are the symptoms and signs of hyperparathyroidism?**
The same as those for hypercalcemia ("bones, stones, groans, and psychiatric overtones"; see Question 5 in this section). In primary cases, serum calcium is high, phosphorus is normal to low, and parathyroid hormone (PTH) is increased. In secondary cases, calcium is low.

2. **What causes hyperparathyroidism?**

Ninety percent of primary cases are due to a parathyroid adenoma, which can usually be confirmed with a nuclear medicine scan. Other causes include parathyroid hyperplasia and parathyroid carcinoma. Secondary hyperparathyroidism occurs as a normal physiologic response to low serum calcium levels (e.g., from renal failure). Tertiary hyperparathyroidism occurs when PTH has been elevated for too long (secondary to longstanding hypocalcemia) and continues to be oversecreted even when calcium is normalized with treatment. Put all patients with renal failure on calcium supplements to prevent this complication.

3. **What are the signs and symptoms of hypoparathyroidism?**

The same as those for hypocalcemia (carpopedal spasm, tetany, and prolonged QT interval on electrocardiography [ECG]; see Question 8 in this section). Calcium is low, phosphorus is high, and PTH is low.

4. **What causes hypoparathyroidism?**

The most common cause is accidental removal or damage during thyroid surgery. Watch for tetany after thyroid surgery. Rare causes are genetic. Watch for **DiGeorge syndrome** in children with congenital absence of parathyroid glands, tetany in the first 48 hours of life, an absent thymus gland, immunodeficiency, cardiac anomalies, and midline facial defects.

5. **What are the symptoms and signs of hypercalcemia?**

Symptoms: "bones, stones, groans, and psychiatric overtones." In other words: bone resorption with osteomalacia and osteitis fibrosa cystica; kidney stones; abdominal pain secondary to nausea and vomiting, ileus, nephrolithiasis, peptic ulcer disease, constipation, or pancreatitis (all increased with hypercalcemia); and emotional lability, delirium, depression, and/or psychosis.

Signs: shortened QT interval on ECG, weakness, polyuria, bone changes and kidney stones on radiographs, and renal failure.

6. **What causes hypercalcemia?**

In outpatients, the most common cause is hyperparathyroidism. In hospitalized patients, the most common cause is malignancy. The first test to order is the PTH level, which helps to differentiate hyperparathyroidism (high PTH) from other causes of hypercalcemia such as malignancy, vitamin D intoxication, and thiazide diuretic use (low PTH). Multiple types of cancer can cause hypercalcemia, but the classic USMLE question involves either multiple myeloma or secretion of PTH-like hormone by a squamous cell carcinoma, especially in the lung. Familial hypocalciuric hypercalcemia is characterized by hypercalcemia with low calcium levels in the urine (opposite of other hypercalcemias). Other causes include vitamin A or D intoxication, sarcoidosis or other granulomatous diseases, and excessive calcium intake (milk-alkali syndrome).

7. **What is the treatment for hypercalcemia?**

If the hypercalcemia is asymptomatic or mildly symptomatic with a calcium level of less than 12 mg/dL, immediate treatment is not required. Such patients should be advised to avoid factors that can cause hypercalcemia (e.g., thiazide diuretics, calcium supplements, high-calcium diet, volume depletion).

Severe hypercalcemia (>14 mg/dL) or symptomatic hypercalcemia should be treated with **fluids** as first-line therapy. Calcitonin and bisphosphonates (zoledronic acid or pamidronate) can also be used.

8. **What are the symptoms and signs of hypocalcemia?**

Symptoms: paresthesias (the classic pattern is perioral or distal extremities), muscle aches, dementia, depression, and psychosis.

Signs: prolonged QT interval on ECG, tetany, **Chvostek sign** (tetany elicited by tapping on the facial nerve to cause facial muscle contraction), **Trousseau sign** (carpopedal spasm caused by inflation of a blood pressure cuff or application of a tourniquet), dementia, depression, psychosis, seizures, and papilledema.

9. **What causes hypocalcemia?**

- Hypoparathyroidism (usually after thyroid gland surgery)
- Pseudohypoparathyroidism (genetic end-organ unresponsiveness to PTH with normal PTH levels, shortened metacarpal bones, short stature, and mental retardation)

- DiGeorge syndrome
- Vitamin D deficiency (osteomalacia, rickets)
- Renal failure of any cause and certain renal tubular problems
- Acute pancreatitis (one of the Ranson criteria)
- Secondary to hypomagnesemia

Hypoproteinemia of any cause may lead to low levels of total serum calcium, but levels of ionized calcium (the active form) are normal. In any patient with low serum calcium, the first step is to determine whether the serum albumin level is decreased. If it is, no treatment is required and no symptoms will develop.

10. **How does a prolactinoma typically present?**

Look for the manifestations of elevated prolactin levels:
- Infertility, amenorrhea, or galactorrhea in premenopausal women.
- Postmenopausal women are already amenorrheic and usually do not get galactorrhea. A prolactinoma in postmenopausal women usually becomes large and causes headache or visual changes.
- Men may develop decreased libido, impotence, infertility, or gynecomastia.

Measure the prolactin level if prolactinoma is suspected. If the prolactin level is elevated, an MRI scan of the brain should be performed. Treatment is with a domapine agonist such as cabergoline or bromocriptine. If medical management is unsuccessful or if the prolactinoma is large, transsphenoidal surgery and radiation therapy are indicated.

11. **Give the classic clinical description of a pheochromocytoma. How is it diagnosed?**

Look for wild swings in blood pressure (with some measurements dangerously high), tachycardia, postural hypotension, headaches, sweating, flushing, dizziness, mental status changes, and/or a feeling of impending doom (like a panic attack). The screening test is a 24-hour urine collection for metanephrines, homovanillic acid, and/or vanillylmandelic acid (catecholamine breakdown products that are abnormally elevated in the urine). If levels are high, order an abdominal CT scan to look for an adrenal mass. Surgical tumor removal is the treatment of choice after stabilization with alpha-blockers and then beta-blockers.

12. **Define diabetes insipidus (DI). What are the two types?**

DI involves a lack of antidiuretic hormone (ADH, or vasopressin) effect in the body. Patients with DI secrete inappropriately dilute urine because of a lack of ADH effect and may urinate up to 25 L of urine per day, resulting in dehydration and hypernatremia. Such patients die rapidly if they are unable to drink water. Normally, when the body is dehydrated, ADH causes urine to become highly concentrated through retention of free water. In DI, the urine remains dilute even though the serum osmolarity is quite high as a result of dehydration. The two types are **central** and **nephrogenic.**

13. **What causes central DI?**

Central DI is caused by a lack of ADH production by the posterior pituitary. Although central DI is often idiopathic, look for trauma, neoplasm, or sarcoid/granulomatous disease as the cause. Order a CT or MRI scan of the head if indicated.

14. **What causes nephrogenic DI?**

Nephrogenic DI is due to kidney unresponsiveness to ADH. Look for medications (e.g., lithium and demeclocycline) as the cause.

15. **What diagnostic test can reveal whether DI is central or nephrogenic? How are these conditions treated?**

Give the patient a dose of ADH and measure urine osmolarity. If central DI is the cause, urine osmolarity increases with ADH challenge. In nephrogenic DI, the urine remains inappropriately dilute after the patient is given ADH. Treatment for central DI is ADH replacement (given orally or as a nasal spray). Treatment for nephrogenic DI involves stopping any offending drug and giving a thiazide diuretic; ADH does not help. Although giving a diuretic to a patient with DI seems counterintuitive, it has the paradoxic effect of decreasing urine output.

TRAUMA AND TOXIC EFFECTS

1. **Define hyperthermia. What causes it? How is it managed?**

   Hyperthermia is defined as a body temperature greater than 104° F (40° C). The three primary causes are infections, medications, and heat stroke. If heat stroke is the cause, look for a history of prolonged heat exposure and a high temperature (>104° F [40° C]) without clues to other culprits. Treat with immediate cooling (e.g., wet blankets, ice, cold water). The immediate threats to life are convulsions (treat with diazepam) and cardiovascular collapse. Always rule out infection and medications (especially those with anticholinergic activity such as antihistamines, antipsychotics, and antidepressants) as the cause.

2. **What are the two classic examples of hyperthermia caused by medication?**

   Malignant hyperthermia is a rare idiosyncratic, genetically related reaction to medications, usually caused by inhaled anesthetics (e.g., halothane) or succinylcholine exposure. Treat with dantrolene.

   Neuroleptic malignant syndrome is thought to be related to malignant hyperthermia and is an idiosyncratic, genetically related reaction to an antipsychotic agent. Look for extremely high levels of creatine phosphokinase and mental status changes in a patient taking antipsychotic agents. The first step is to stop the medication. The second step is supportive treatment, especially with lots of intravenous fluids to prevent renal shutdown caused by rhabdomyolysis. The third step, if necessary, is to treat with dantrolene.

   Drug fevers are idiosyncratic reactions to a medication that was typically started within the previous week. They rarely cause fever above 104° F (40° C).

3. **True or false: Alcohol can precipitate hypoglycemia.**

   True. But give thiamine first and then glucose in an alcoholic.

4. **Define hypothermia. How is it managed? What are the complications?**

   Hypothermia is defined as a body temperature of less than 95° F (35° C), usually accompanied by mental status changes and generalized neurologic deficits. If the patient is conscious, you can rewarm the individual slowly with blankets. If the patient is unconscious, consider gastric and bladder lavage with warm water, as well as warm intravenous fluids.

   Monitor the ECG for arrhythmias, which are common in hypothermic patients. You may see the classic **J wave**—a small, positive deflection following the QRS complex. Also monitor electrolytes, renal function, and acid-base status.

5. **True or false: You should not give up resuscitation efforts until the patient is fully warmed in the setting of hypothermic cardiac arrest.**

   True. According to an old saying in medicine, the patient is not considered dead "until warm and dead." Hypothermia can slow body function to a remarkable degree, and there are case reports of resuscitation hours after initial attempts in the field once the body was warmed.

CHAPTER 10

RENAL AND URINARY DISORDERS

LOWER URINARY TRACT

1. **What is nocturnal enuresis? When can it be diagnosed? What are the treatment options?**

   Enuresis is discrete episodes of urinary incontinence during sleep in children who are at least 5 years of age. This is a common issue in children at rates that decrease with age, but prevalence is 5% even at age 10 years. Evaluate with a thorough history and physical examination, as well as urinalysis to rule out conditions such as urinary tract infection (UTI) and diabetes. Advise on the use of a voiding diary. Ultrasound is helpful if there is a history of UTIs or if structural urologic abnormalities are suspected. Estimation of bladder capacity and postvoid residual volume can also be helpful. First-line treatment involves education about the natural course of enuresis, with bladder training, voiding before bedtime, and limiting fluids before bedtime. Enuresis alarms can be used if these behavioral modifications do not work. Desmopressin can be used and is effective in the short term but has high rates of relapse.

2. **What are the presenting symptoms of bladder obstruction? What are the causes? What is the treatment?**

   Look for abdominal pain, a decrease in urine output, and a mass in the lower abdomen (from a distended bladder). Urinalysis is generally benign but may show hematuria. Serum creatinine may be increased. The most common causes are prostatic enlargement, posterior urethral valves, and neurogenic bladder. In women, consider cervical, uterine, and ovarian cancers. (Also be aware that urinary obstruction can occur above the level of the bladder because of conditions such as kidney stones, transitional cell carcinoma, and external compression by tumors). Diagnosis is typically made with ultrasound, although a noncontrast computed tomography (CT) scan is preferred if an obstructing stone is suspected. Treat with bladder decompression using a urethral catheter (unless the patient has had recent urologic surgery). The evidence is mixed on when the catheter can be removed, but about a week is typical. Consider medication such as an alpha-blocker (e.g., terazosin) or a 5-alpha reductase inhibitor (e.g., finasteride) if benign prostatic hyperplasia (BPH) is the cause of the obstruction.

3. **What is neurogenic bladder? What are the causes?**

   Patients with neurogenic bladder have difficulty with bladder control and passing urine because of brain, spinal cord, or peripheral nerve issues. Medications such as oxybutynin may help, but patients often require intermittent catheterization several times per day or may even require an indwelling catheter. Look for a history of spinal cord disease such as spinal cord injury, multiple sclerosis, spina bifida, or syringomyelia, but also consider a brain tumor or peripheral nerve diseases (such as from diabetes) as the cause. Neurogenic bladder may also result as a complication of pelvic surgery. Watch for UTIs as a result of having neurogenic bladder.

4. **What clinical vignette is suspicious for bladder cancer?**

   Persistent, painless hematuria, especially in patients older than 40 years who smoke or work in the rubber or dye industry (exposure to aniline dye). A CT scan to evaluate the upper urinary tract and cystoscopy should be performed to evaluate for potential bladder cancer (as well as other causes of hematuria, including renal cell carcinoma).

UPPER URINARY TRACT

1. **How do you recognize glomerulonephritis? How do you evaluate a possible case of glomerulonephritis?**

   Look for new-onset hypertension, edema, hematuria, and decreased urine output. If glomerulonephritis is suspected, order urinalysis and measurement of serum creatinine, serum albumin, and the urinary protein-to-creatinine ratio to estimate protein excretion in the urine.

   There are many causes of glomerulonephritis (e.g., postinfectious glomerulonephritis, immunoglobulin A [IgA] nephropathy, membranoproliferative glomerulonephritis, rapidly progressive glomerulonephritis, lupus nephritis), but you do not need to be able to differentiate all of them for the Step 3 exam. However, it is helpful to be able to differentiate them into patterns. The findings on urinalysis can point to whether you are dealing with a nephrotic or a nephritic pattern. The nephrotic pattern typically has proteinuria of greater than 3.5 g/day and lipids in the urine, but few cells or casts. The nephritic pattern is characterized by red cells, occasionally white cells, and either the presence or absence of red cell or mixed cellular casts. Serologic testing (e.g., complement levels, antineutrophil cytoplasmic antibody [ANCA], hepatitis B virus [HBV], hepatitis C virus [HCV], antistreptolysin O, cryoglobulin, antiglomerular basement membrane antibodies) may be helpful, but renal biopsy is usually necessary to confirm a diagnosis.

2. **Define nephrotic syndrome. What causes it? How is it diagnosed?**

   Nephrotic syndrome is defined as proteinuria (>3.5 g/day), hypoalbuminemia, edema (the classic pattern is morning periorbital edema), and hyperlipidemia with lipiduria. In children it is usually due to minimal change disease (podocytes with missing "feet" on electron microscopy), which often follows an infection. Measure 24-hour urine protein or a spot urinary protein-to-creatinine ratio to confirm the diagnosis. Treat with steroids. Causes in adults include membranous nephropathy, diabetes, HPV, amyloidosis, lupus erythematosus, and drugs (e.g., penicillamine, captopril).

3. **Define nephritic syndrome. What is the classic cause? How is it treated?**

   Nephritic syndrome is generally defined as oliguria, azotemia (rising blood urea nitrogen [BUN] or creatinine), hypertension, and hematuria. The patient may have some degree of proteinuria but not in the nephrotic range. The classic cause is poststreptococcal glomerulonephritis (PSGN). Treatment is supportive and includes control of hypertension and maintenance of urine output with intravenous fluids and diuretics.

4. **How do you recognize poststreptococcal glomerulonephritis (PSGN)? How is it treated?**

   PSGN occurs most commonly after a streptococcal skin infection but may also occur after pharyngitis. Patients are usually children and generally have a history of infection with a nephritogenic strain of *Streptococcus* species 1 to 3 weeks previously and abrupt onset of edema (especially periorbital), hypertension, hematuria, proteinuria (mild, not in the nephrotic range), hematuria (red blood cell casts), and elevated BUN and creatinine. *Red blood cell casts* on urinalysis confirm the diagnosis of nephritic syndrome. Laboratory tests that support a PSGN diagnosis include proof of recent streptococcal infection (e.g., antistreptolysin O and antiDNAse B titers) and evidence of complement-mediated glomerular inflammation (low C3 and C4 levels). Treat supportively. Control blood pressure and use diuretics for severe edema. Unlike rheumatic fever, treatment of the initial streptococcal infection does not reduce the incidence of PSGN. Nonetheless, any residual infection should be treated with antibiotics. Another nephritic condition, IgA nephropathy (Berger syndrome), can occur within 1 to 2 days of an upper respiratory tract infection or viral pharyngitis and is hence termed *synpharyngitic*. The differentiation in the USMLE would be the delay of only a few days from pharyngitis to nephritic syndrome in IgA nephropathy versus the delay of a few weeks for PSGN.

5. **Define Goodpasture syndrome. What are the presenting symptoms?**

   Goodpasture syndrome (a cause of rapidly progressive glomerulonephritis [RPGN]) is due to the presence of measurable antiglomerular basement membrane antibodies, which cause a linear immunofluorescence pattern on renal biopsy. These antibodies react with and damage both kidneys and lungs. Look for a young man with hemoptysis, dyspnea, and renal failure. Treat with steroids and cyclophosphamide.

6. **Define Wegener granulomatosis. What are the presenting symptoms?**

   Wegener granulomatosis is a vasculitis that also affects the lungs and kidneys. Look for nasal involvement (bloody nose, nasal perforation) or hemoptysis and pleurisy as presenting symptoms, along with renal disease. Patients test positive for **ANCA** titers. Treat with cyclophosphamide and glucocorticoids. Methotrexate is an alternative.

7. **What else should you watch for as a cause of glomerulonephritis?**

   Watch for lupus erythematosus as a cause of glomerulonephritis. Renal failure is a major cause of morbidity and mortality in patients with lupus.

8. **What are the symptoms and signs of acute renal failure?**

   Symptoms: fatigue, nausea and vomiting, anorexia, shortness of breath, mental status changes.

   Signs: increased BUN and creatinine levels, metabolic acidosis, hyperkalemia, tachypnea (caused by acidosis and hypervolemia), and hypervolemia (bilateral rales on lung examination, elevated jugular venous pressure, dilutional hyponatremia).

9. **What are the three broad categories of renal failure?**

   Prerenal, renal/intrarenal, and postrenal.

10. **Define prerenal failure? What are the causes? How do you recognize it?**

    In prerenal failure the kidney is not adequately perfused. The most common cause is hypovolemia (dehydration, hemorrhage). Look for a BUN-to-creatinine ratio greater than 20 and signs of hypovolemia (e.g., tachycardia, weak pulse, depressed fontanelle). Fractional excretion of sodium (FeNa) will be less than 1% (as the body tries to retain sodium). Give intravenous fluids and/or blood. Other common prerenal causes are sepsis (treat the sepsis and give intravenous fluids), heart failure (give digoxin and diuretics), liver failure (hepatorenal syndrome; treat supportively), and renal artery stenosis.

11. **Define postrenal failure. What causes it?**

    In postrenal failure, urine is blocked from being excreted at some point beyond the kidneys (ureters, prostate, urethra). The most common cause is BPH. Patients are men older than 50 years with BPH symptoms (e.g., hesitancy, dribbling, weak stream, nocturia); ultrasound demonstrates bilateral hydronephrosis. Treat with catheterization (suprapubic, if necessary) to relieve the obstruction and prevent further renal damage. Alpha-blockers (e.g., terazosin) or a 5-alpha reductase inhibitor (e.g., finasteride) can improve the symptoms, and surgery should be considered (transurethral resection of the prostate). Other causes are nephrolithiasis (but remember that stones generally have to be bilateral to cause renal failure), retroperitoneal fibrosis (watch for a history of methysergide, bromocriptine, methyldopa, or hydralazine use), and pelvic malignancies.

12. **What is the most common cause of intrarenal failure?**

    Intrarenal failure, which results from a problem within the kidney itself, is most commonly due to **acute tubular necrosis** from various causes.

13. **What do you need to know about intravenous contrast and renal failure?**

    Intravenous contrast can precipitate renal failure, usually in diabetic patients and patients with preexisting renal disease. Avoid contrast in such patients if possible. If you must give intravenous contrast, administer intravenous hydration before and after the contrast is given to decrease the chance of renal failure.

14. **True or false: Muscle breakdown can cause renal failure.**

    True. Myoglobinuria or rhabdomyolysis caused by strenuous exercise (e.g., running marathons), alcohol, burns, muscle trauma, muscle compression (e.g., prolonged immobilization after a fall), heat stroke, and neuroleptic malignant syndrome may cause renal failure. The cellular debris that results from muscle breakdown plugs the renal filtration system. Look for very high levels of creatine phosphokinase (CPK). Urinalysis may reveal red-colored urine that is positive for blood but has no red blood cells (caused by the heme contained in myoglobin). Treat with hydration and diuretics.

15. **What medications commonly cause renal insufficiency or failure?**

    Chronic use of nonsteroidal antiinflammatory drugs (may cause acute tubular necrosis or papillary necrosis), cyclosporine, aminoglycosides, and methicillin.

16. **What are the indications for dialysis in patients with renal failure?**
When renal failure is present, first try to determine the cause and fix it, if possible, to correct the renal failure. Indications for acute dialysis are remembered by the mnemonic AEIOU: metabolic acidosis (roughly, pH <7.25), electrolyte abnormalities (hyperkalemia severe enough to cause arrhythmia), ingestion of dialyzable toxins, volume overload, and uremia (uremic encephalopathy or pericarditis).

17. **What causes chronic renal failure (CRF)?**
Any of the causes of acute renal failure can cause chronic renal failure if the insult is severe or prolonged. Most cases of CRF are due to diabetes mellitus (leading cause) or hypertension (second most common cause). A popular cause on the Step 3 exam is polycystic kidney disease (PKD; see Question 18). Watch for multiple cysts in the kidney, and look for a positive family history (usually autosomal dominant; the autosomal-recessive form presents in children), hypertension, hematuria, palpable renal masses, berry aneurysms in the circle of Willis, and cysts in the liver.

18. **What else do you need to know about PKD?**
There are two types: autosomal-dominant PKD (ADPKD) and autosomal-recessive PKD (ARPKD); the latter is less common because most patients die in utero or shortly after birth because of severe oligohydramnios and associated problems). PKD is characterized by the presence of multiple cysts, usually in both kidneys, which leads to massive enlargement of the kidneys. Extrarenal manifestations include cerebral aneurysms, pancreatic cysts, hepatic cysts, cardiac valvular disease, and aortic root dilatation. ADPKD is responsible for approximately 10% of all cases of end-stage renal disease (ESRD).

19. **How is CRF treated?**
Treat CRF with regular hemodialysis (usually three times per week), water-soluble vitamins (which are removed during dialysis), phosphate restriction and binders (calcium carbonate, calcium acetate, or sevelamer), erythropoietin as needed for anemia, and hypertension control. The only cure is a renal transplant.

20. **When is a kidney transplant considered for patients with renal disease?**
Kidney transplantation is an option for patients with ESRD (glomerular filtration rate <10 mg/min), unless they have active infections or other life-threatening conditions (e.g., AIDS, malignancy). Lupus erythematosus and diabetes are not contraindications to transplantation.

21. **Who makes the best donor for patients who need a kidney transplant?**
Living related donors are best (siblings or parents), especially when human leukocyte antigens (HLAs) are similar, but cadaveric kidneys are more commonly used because of availability. Before transplantation, perform ABO blood typing and lymphocytotoxic (HLA) crossmatching to ensure a reasonable chance of success.

22. **Describe unacceptable kidney donors.**
Unacceptable kidney donors include newborns (most centers set an age <18 years as an exclusion criterion) and patients with a history of generalized or intraabdominal sepsis, malignancy, or any disease with possible renal involvement (e.g., diabetes, hypertension, lupus erythematosus).

23. **Where is the transplanted kidney placed? What happens to the native kidneys?**
A transplanted kidney is placed in the iliac fossa or pelvis (for easy biopsy access in case of later problems, as well as for technical reasons). The recipient's kidneys are usually left in place to reduce the surgical morbidity.

24. **What are the three basic types of rejection after kidney transplantation?**
Hyperacute, acute, and chronic.

25. **What causes hyperacute rejection? What is the classic clinical description?**
Hyperacute rejection is due to preformed cytotoxic antibodies against the donor kidney; it occurs with ABO blood-type mismatch, as well as with other preformed antibodies. In the classic clinical description, the surgery is completed, the vascular clamps are released to allow blood flow, and the transplanted kidney quickly turns bluish black. Treat by removing the kidney.

26. **What causes acute rejection? What are the presenting symptoms? How is it treated?**
    Acute rejection is T-cell mediated. It occurs *days to weeks* after the transplant with fever, oliguria, weight gain, tenderness and enlargement of the graft, hypertension, and/or laboratory test derangements. Increases in creatinine are more reliable than increases in BUN in identifying the condition. Treatment involves pulse corticosteroids, anti–T-cell antibody therapies, (polyclonal antibodies, OKT3), other antibody therapies (basiliximab, daclizumab), and other immunosuppressants (tacrolimus, mycophenolate, cyclosporine). **Accelerated rejection** occurs over the *first few days* and is thought to reflect reactivation of previously sensitized T cells.

27. **What causes chronic rejection? What are the presenting symptoms? How is it treated?**
    Chronic rejection can be mediated by T cells or antibodies. The symptoms of this late cause (months to years after transplantation) of renal deterioration include a gradual decline in kidney function, proteinuria, and hypertension. Treatment is supportive and not effective, but the graft may last for several years before it gives out completely. A new kidney can be transplanted if this occurs.

28. **How do you distinguish the nephrotoxicity of cyclosporine from rejection?**
    Cyclosporine is a well-known cause of nephrotoxicity that can be difficult to clinically distinguish from graft rejection. When in doubt, a percutaneous needle biopsy of the graft should be performed if the patient is taking cyclosporine, because in most cases the two can be distinguished histologically. Renal ultrasound also helps. In a practical context, if you increase the immunosuppressive dose, acute rejection should decrease, whereas cyclosporine toxicity stays the same or worsens.

29. **How do you differentiate among the common pediatric hematologic disorders that affect the kidney?**

	HUS	**HSP**	**TTP**	**ITP**
Most common age	Children	Children	Young adults	Children or adults
Previous infection	Diarrhea (O157:H7 *E. coli*)	URI	None	Viral (especially in children)
Red blood cell count	Low	Normal	Low	Normal
Platelet count	Low	Normal	Low	Low
Peripheral smear	Hemolysis (schistocytes)	Normal	Hemolysis (schistocytes)	Normal
Kidney effects	ARF, hematuria	Hematuria	ARF, proteinuria	None
Treatment	Supportive*	Supportive*	Plasmapheresis, NSAIDs; no platelets[†]	Steroids, IVIG, anti-D immunoglobulin, rituximab;[‡] splenectomy if drugs fail
Key differential points	Age, diarrhea	Rash, abdominal pain, arthritis, melena	CNS changes, age	Antiplatelet antibodies

ARF, Acute renal failure; CNS, central nervous system; E. coli, *Escherichia coli*; HSP, Henoch-Schönlein purpura; HUS, hemolytic uremic syndrome; ITP, idiopathic thrombocytopenia; IVIG, intravenous immunoglobulin; NSAIDs, nonsteroidal antiinflammatory drugs; TTP, thrombotic thrombocytopenic purpura; URI, upper respiratory tract infection.

*In HUS and HSP, patients may need dialysis and transfusions.
[†]Do not give platelet transfusions to patients with TTP; clots may form.
[‡]Give steroids only if the patient is bleeding or platelet counts are very low (<20,000 cells/μL).

30. **Which is more likely to be seen on a plain abdominal radiograph: kidney stones or gallbladder stones?**

Kidney stones (85%), which more commonly calcify, are more likely to be seen than gallstones (15%).

31. **What are the signs and symptoms of renal stones? How are they diagnosed and treated?**

A kidney stone (nephrolithiasis) generally causes severe, intermittent, unilateral flank and/ or groin pain when the stone dislodges and gets stuck in the ureter (ureterolithiasis). Most stones can be seen on abdominal radiographs and are composed of calcium. A noncontrast CT scan is the imaging modality of choice for stone detection if clinical suspicion is high, but plain abdominal radiographs are negative. Symptomatic urolithiasis should be treated with abundant hydration and pain control (to see if the stone will pass). If the stone does not pass, it needs to be removed surgically (preferably endoscopically) or by lithotripsy.

32. **What causes kidney stones?**

Nephrolithiasis is often idiopathic, but on the Step 3 exam watch for one of the following underlying disorders that predispose to the development of kidney stones:

Hypercalcemia as a result of hyperparathyroidism or malignancy (calcium stones).

Infection from ammonia-producing organisms (*Proteus* species, staphylococci). Look for **staghorn calculi** (large stones composed of magnesium, ammonia, and phosphate [struvite] that fill the renal calyceal system).

Hyperuricemia from uric acid stones caused by gout or leukemia treatment (allopurinol and intravenous hydration are given before leukemia chemotherapy to prevent this complication).

Cystinuria or **aminoaciduria** should be suspected if the stone is made of cystine or occurs in a patient who suffers from repetitive stone formation.

Note: Send any recovered stones to the laboratory for analysis to determine the type of stone.

33. **How is renal cell carcinoma diagnosed and treated?**

Painless hematuria (gross or microscopic) is the most typical presenting sign. Patients rarely have the classic triad of hematuria, flank pain, and a palpable flank mass. A CT scan (preferred over intravenous pyelography) is a good initial diagnostic test. The treatment for disease confined to the kidney or with extension limited to renal vein invasion (classic) is surgical resection. For other organ invasion or distant metastatic disease (usually to the lung or bone), immunotherapy (e.g., interleukin-2) is the preferred treatment.

34. **Describe the classic findings for nephrolithiasis.**

Nephrolithiasis (kidney stones) can cause severe flank pain that often radiates to the groin and is colicky in nature. It may cause hematuria (gross or microscopic), and an abdominal radiograph often reveals the stone (85% of stones are radiopaque). A noncontrast helical CT scan is the diagnostic test of choice.

35. **What are the different types of stones? What causes them?**

Roughly 75% to 85% of stones contain calcium. Look for hypercalcemia (usually caused by hyperparathyroidism) or small bowel bypass, which increases oxalate absorption and thus calcium stone formation. Roughly 10% to 15% of stones are struvite (magnesium-ammonium-phosphate) stones, which are caused by UTI (usually with *Proteus* species). The classic example is a staghorn calculus (a stone that fills the entire calyceal system). About 5% to 10% of stones are composed of uric acid. Look for gout or leukemia. The remaining 1% to 3% are cystine stones, which suggest hereditary cystinuria.

36. **How is nephrolithiasis treated?**

The cornerstones of nephrolithiasis treatment are large amounts of fluid hydration, narcotics for pain, and observation, because most stones pass spontaneously. There is some evidence that alpha-blockers such as terazosin or tamsulosin will facilitate stone passage by relaxing smooth muscle in the genitourinary tract. Stones 4 mm or less in diameter pass spontaneously. Stones 4 to 10 mm in diameter may or may not pass. Spontaneous passage is unlikely for stones greater than or equal to 10 mm in diameter. If a stone does not pass, treat with lithotripsy, uteroscopy with stone retrieval, or open surgery (last resort).

FLUID, ELECTROLYTE, AND ACID-BASE DISORDERS

1. **Define the syndrome of inappropriate antidiuretic hormone secretion (SIADH). How is it diagnosed?**
   The name says it all: ADH is released inappropriately. SIADH is a consideration in patients with hyponatremia and normal volume status (euvolemic). In SIADH, serum osmolarity is low but urine osmolarity is high (inappropriate urine concentration). Look for the low values for all electrolytes and laboratory tests (the classic example is uric acid) because of dilution of serum with free water secondary to inappropriate ADH.

2. **What causes SIADH?**
   Central nervous system causes: stroke, hemorrhage, infection, trauma.
   Medications: narcotics, oxytocin (watch for pregnant patients), chlorpropamide, antiepileptic agents.
   Trauma: pain is a powerful stimulus for ADH. Watch for SIADH development in a postoperative patient who is in pain and receiving fluids (and often narcotics).
   Lung problems: simple pneumonia or ADH-secreting small cell cancer of the lung.

3. **How is SIADH treated?**
   Treat with water restriction. Stop intravenous fluids and restrict oral fluid intake. For Step 3 exam purposes, do not give hypertonic saline unless the patient has active seizures before your eyes. You may cause brainstem damage or central pontine myelinolysis if correction of the sodium level is too rapid. **Demeclocycline** is sometimes used to treat SIADH if water restriction fails because it induces nephrogenic diabetes insipidus, which allows the patient to get rid of free water.

4. **What do you need to know about diabetes insipidus?**
   Think of diabetes insipidus as the opposite of SIADH. There is a lack of ADH (vasopressin) effect in the body. Diabetes insipidus may lead to dehydration and hypernatremia. There are two types: central and nephrogenic. See Chapter 9 on endocrinology for a more in-depth discussion.

5. **What may cause a false laboratory report of hyperkalemia?**
   Hemolysis of the blood sample. Repeat the test if a high value does not make sense (e.g., high level with no electrocardiogram changes or symptoms).

6. **What can cause false hyponatremia (pseudohyponatremia)?**
   Pseudohyponatremia may be caused by hyperglycemia, hyperproteinemia (e.g., multiple myeloma), or hyperlipidemia. The hyponatremia resolves on correction of the glucose, lipid, or protein level.

7. **What may result from rapid correction of hyponatremia?**
   Brainstem damage (**central pontine myelinolysis**). For this reason you should generally not give hypertonic saline to correct hyponatremia except in severe or symptomatic cases, and then it should be given in limited quantities.

8. **What effect do serum acidosis and serum alkalosis have on potassium and calcium levels?**
   Alkalosis may cause hypokalemia and symptoms of hypocalcemia (perioral numbness, tetany) caused by cellular shift, whereas acidosis may cause hyperkalemia via the same mechanism. Correction of acid-base status will correct the potassium and calcium derangements.

9. **What is the relationship between low calcium and potassium levels and low levels of magnesium?**
   Hypokalemia and/or hypocalcemia may be due to hypomagnesemia. In addition, if hypomagnesemia is present, it is often impossible to correct the hypokalemia or hypocalcemia until you correct the hypomagnesemia. If a patient has hypokalemia that does not correct on administration of potassium supplements, check the magnesium level.

10. **Which two electrolytes are classically depleted in the setting of diabetic ketoacidosis or a diabetic hyperosmolar hyperglycemic state?**
    Potassium and phosphorus.

11. **What does a BUN-to-creatinine ratio greater than 20 generally imply?**
Dehydration.

12. **What metabolic derangements are seen in CRF?**
   - Azotemia (high levels of BUN and creatinine)
   - Metabolic acidosis
   - Hyperkalemia
   - Fluid retention (may cause hypertension, edema, congestive heart failure, and pulmonary edema)
   - Hypocalcemia and hyperphosphatemia (impaired vitamin D production; bone loss leads to renal osteodystrophy)
   - Anemia (caused by lack of erythropoietin; give synthetic erythropoietin to correct)
   - Anorexia, nausea, vomiting (from buildup of toxins)
   - Central nervous system disturbances (mental status changes and even convulsions or coma from toxin buildup)
   - Bleeding (caused by disordered platelet function)
   - Uremic pericarditis (a friction rub may be heard)
   - Skin pigmentation and pruritus (skin turns yellowish-brown and itches because of metabolic byproducts)
   - Increased susceptibility to infection (because of decreased cellular immunity)

INFECTIONS

1. **What are the symptoms of cystitis? What are the typical findings for urinalysis?**
Look for dysuria, urgency, frequency, and sometimes hematuria. Consider urethritis as the cause of symptoms in sexually active patients. Renal or bladder stones can also lead to similar symptoms. The presence of leukocyte esterase and nitrite on a dipstick test can help in diagnosing a UTI but false negatives and false positives can occur (although a positive nitrite test almost guarantees a UTI, when present). White blood cells (WBCs) are usually present on urinalysis, and their absence should make you question your diagnosis. A routine urine culture is not necessary but may be indicated if the diagnosis is in doubt, if symptoms persist or recur, or if a complicated infection is suspected.

2. **What are the most likely organisms?**
UTIs are usually caused by *Escherichia coli* (75% to 85% of cases) but may also be caused by *Staphylococcus saprophyticus, Proteus, Pseudomonas, Klebsiella, Enterobacter,* and/or *Enterococcus* species (or other enteric organisms). Patients who acquire a UTI in hospital or from a chronic, indwelling Foley catheter are more likely to have organisms other than *E. coli.*

3. **What factors increase the likelihood of UTIs?**
Female gender and conditions that promote urinary stasis (BPH, pregnancy, stones, neurogenic bladder, vesicoureteral reflux) or bacterial colonization (indwelling catheter, fecal incontinence, surgical instrumentation) predispose to UTIs.

4. **What is the usual treatment for cystitis?**
The preferred treatment is a 3-day course of trimethoprim-sulfamethoxazole or a fluoroquinolone. A 5-day course of nitrofurantoin may be used but is contraindicated if the creatinine clearance is less than 60 mL/min (which occurs in many older patients). Other options include amoxicillin-clavulanate, cefdinir, and cefpodoxine. The choice of antibiotic should be guided by local resistance patterns.

5. **Why are UTIs in children of special concern?**
In children, a UTI is cause for concern because it may be the presenting symptom of a genitourinary malformation. The most common examples are vesicoureteral reflux and posterior urethral valves. A urine culture should be obtained. Order an ultrasound and either a voiding cystourethrogram (VCUG) or radionuclide cystogram (RNC) to evaluate the urinary tract in any child between 2 months and 2 years of age with a first UTI. Recommendations for imaging in older children are less clear-cut.

6. True or false: You should treat asymptomatic bacteriuria in most patients.

False. The exception is a pregnant patient, in whom asymptomatic bacteriuria is treated because of the high risk of progression to pyelonephritis. Use antibiotics that are safe in pregnancy, such as penicillins.

7. How do you differentiate pyelonephritis from cystitis? How is pyelonephritis diagnosed? How is it treated?

Look for an acutely ill patient (e.g., fever, tachycardia, hypotension) with costovertebral angle (CVA) tenderness. The urinalysis is similar to that for cystitis, but WBC casts may also be present. A urine culture should be obtained. Do not forget to perform a pregnancy test in women of childbearing age.

Uncomplicated and mild to moderate pyelonephritis (i.e., a patient who is not significantly ill) may be treated on an outpatient basis with a fluoroquinolone such as ciprofloxacin or levofloxacin. Complicated or moderate to severe pyelonephritis should be treated on an inpatient basis with intravenous antibiotics such as a fluoroquinolone, ceftriaxone, or ampicillin-sulbactam. Obtain blood cultures on admission. Once the patient improves clinically, treatment can be completed as an outpatient with a 10- to 14-day course of antibiotics. If the patient does not improve, perform a CT or ultrasound scan to look for a perinephric abscess or renal calculus. Note that nitrofurantoin does not have any renal penetration and is therefore never an appropriate treatment for pyelonephritis.

TRAUMA AND TOXIC EFFECTS

1. What are the important renal sequelae of electrical burns?

Because most of the tissue destruction due to electrical burns is internal, sequelae include muscle necrosis, myoglobinuria, acidosis, and renal failure. Use large amounts of intravenous hydration to prevent renal shutdown. The immediate life-threatening risk with electricity exposure and burns (including lightning and a child who puts his or her finger in an electrical outlet) is cardiac arrhythmia. Perform electrocardiography.

DISEASES AND DISORDERS OF THE FEMALE REPRODUCTIVE SYSTEM

CHAPTER 11

BREAST

1. **When a woman has a nipple discharge, what historic points are important?**

   A history of using oral contraceptive pills, hormone therapies, or antipsychotic medications or symptoms suggestive of hypothyroidism, which can all cause a nipple discharge. The color of the discharge and whether it is unilateral or bilateral is also very important. For example, if a nipple discharge is bilateral and nonbloody, it is not due to breast cancer but may be due to a prolactinoma (check the prolactin level) or endocrine disorder (check a thyroid-stimulating hormone level). Alternatively, when a nipple discharge is unilateral and bloody (nipple discharge secondary to carcinoma generally contains hemoglobin) and/or is associated with a mass, this should raise concern about possible breast cancer. Perform a biopsy of any mass if present.

2. **What are the most likely causes of a breast mass in a woman younger than 35 years?**

   Fibrocystic disease: bilateral, multiple, cystic lesions that are tender to the touch, especially premenstrually. This is the most common of all breast diseases. In general, no workup is needed other than routine follow-up. Oral contraceptive pills, progesterone, or danazol may help to relieve symptoms.

   Fibroadenoma: a painless, discrete, sharply circumscribed, unilateral, rubbery, mobile mass. This is the most common benign tumor of the female breast. Patients may be observed for one or more menstrual cycles in the absence of symptoms. Because tumors are estrogen dependent, pregnancy and oral contraceptive pills may stimulate growth, whereas menopause causes regression. Excision is curative but is not required except for cosmetic reasons.

   Mastitis/abscess: typically in the first few postpartum months, lactating women may develop a painful, swollen, erythematous breast(s). The nipple may be cracked or fissured (which can be treated with lanolin ointment to protect it). The patient should be treated with analgesics (e.g., acetaminophen, ibuprofen) and instructed to continue breastfeeding from the affected breast(s) even though it is painful (use a breast pump to empty the breast if needed) to prevent further milk duct blockage and abscess formation. An antistaphylococcal antibiotic (e.g., dicloxacillin or cephalexin) should be given for more than mild symptoms. If there is a risk of methicillin-resistant *Staphylococcus aureus* (MRSA) or if MRSA is cultured, use trimethoprim-sulfamethoxazole or clindamycin. If a fluctuant mass develops or there is no response to antibiotics within a few days, an abscess is probably present and must be drained.

   Fat necrosis: patients have a history of trauma in the area of the mass.

3. **True or False: Mammography should be performed for any suspicious breast lesion in a woman younger than 30 years.**

   False. Mammography is usually not done in women under age 30 because breast tissue is often too dense to discern a mass. If you are suspicious of breast cancer, which is very rare in this age group, proceed to ultrasound imaging or directly to biopsy.

4. **What are the likely causes of a breast mass in a woman older than 35 years?**

   Fibrocystic disease: as mentioned previously, but aspiration of cyst fluid and baseline mammography are recommended. If the cyst fluid is nonbloody and the mass resolves after aspiration, the patient needs only reassurance and follow-up (with a baseline mammogram). If the fluid is bloody or the cyst recurs quickly, perform a biopsy to rule out cancer.

Fibroadenoma: order a baseline mammogram. Observe briefly if the mass is small and seems benign clinically *and* if the woman is premenopausal and has no risk factors for breast cancer. Otherwise, perform a biopsy. Phyllodes tumors (the minority are malignant) may masquerade as fibroadenoma.

Fat necrosis: as mentioned previously.

Mastitis/abscess: as mentioned previously.

Breast cancer: on the Step 3 exam, you may not get the classic presentation of nipple retraction and/or *peau d'orange* in a nulliparous woman with a strong family history. For a woman aged 35 years or older, you will never be faulted for performing a biopsy of any mass. In the absence of a classic benign presentation (e.g., trauma to the breast with fat necrosis or bilateral masses with premenstrual syndrome mastalgia), always consider biopsy. Also order baseline mammography.

5. **True or False:** If a patient is postmenopausal or older than 50 years and develops a new breast mass, you should assume cancer until proven otherwise.
   True. The risk of breast cancer begins to increase sharply and the incidence of benign disorders begins to decrease sharply in this age group. Most benign disorders are caused by reproductive hormones that women in this age group lack.

6. **True or False:** Mammography is best used as a tool to evaluate a palpable breast mass.
   False. Mammography is best used as a tool to detect nonpalpable breast masses (as a screening tool). A suspicious lesion found on mammography should be biopsied, even if it seems benign or is inapparent on physical examination. In addition, a clinically suspicious mass should be biopsied unless imaging demonstrates unequivocally benign findings (e.g., a cyst).

UTERUS

1. What are fibroids? How common are they? How often do they become malignant?
   Fibroids (i.e., leiomyomas) are benign uterine tumors. They are the most common tumors in women and the most common indication for hysterectomy (when they grow too large or cause symptoms). Up to 40% of women have fibroids by the age of 40 years. Malignant transformation to a leiomyocsarcoma is quite rare (<1%).

2. Explain the relationship between uterine leiomyomas and hormones. What are the symptoms of leiomyomas? What is the treatment?
   Leiomyomas of the uterus are estrogen dependent. Therefore you may see rapid growth during pregnancy or with the use of oral contraceptive pills, and regression may occur after menopause. Leiomyomas may cause infertility, pain, and menorrhagia or metrorrhagia. Anemia caused by leiomyoma is an indication for hysterectomy. In rare cases a patient may have a polyp protruding through the cervix. Dilation and curettage are needed to rule out endometrial cancer in women who develop leiomyoma after the age of 35 years.
   Treatment is usually surgical (use of levonorgestrel-releasing intrauterine devices is increasing, although randomized trials are lacking). Myomectomy can sometimes maintain or even restore fertility; the alternative is hysterectomy.

3. Define endometriosis. What are the symptoms and signs?
   Endometriosis involves endometrial glands located outside the uterus (ectopic). Patients are usually nulliparous and older than 30 years with the following symptoms: **dysmenorrhea** (painful menstruation), **dyspareunia** (painful intercourse), **dyschezia** (painful defecation), and/or perimenstrual spotting. The most common site for ectopic endometrial glands is the ovaries; look for tender adnexa in an afebrile patient. Other sites include the broad (uterosacral) ligament and peritoneal surface. Nodularities on the broad ligament are classic findings on physical examination; the classic sequela is a retroverted uterus.

4. How is endometriosis diagnosed and treated?
   The gold standard of diagnosis is laparoscopy with visualization of the endometriosis. Treat first with birth control pills (if acceptable to the patient); danazol and gonadotropin-releasing

hormone agonists (e.g., leuprolide) are second-line agents. Surgery and cautery can be used to destroy the endometriomas, a procedure that often improves fertility. In an older patient, consider hysterectomy and bilateral salpingo-oophorectomy for severe symptoms.

5. **What is the most likely cause of infertility in a menstruating woman older than 30 years without a history of pelvic inflammatory disease (PID)?**
Endometriosis.

6. **Define adenomyosis. What is the classic presentation? What is the treatment?**
Adenomyosis is endometrial glands within the uterine musculature. Patients are usually older than 40 years with dysmenorrhea and menorrhagia and a large, boggy uterus on physical examination. Perform dilation and curettage first to rule out endometrial cancer. Consider hysterectomy to relieve severe symptoms; gonadotropin-releasing hormone agonists may also relieve symptoms.

7. **What is the rule of thumb for postmenopausal vaginal bleeding?**
Postmenopausal vaginal bleeding is cancer until proven otherwise. Endometrial cancer is the most common type to present in this fashion; it is also the fourth most common cancer overall in women. Perform an endometrial biopsy (generally preferred) or transvaginal ultrasound for any woman with postmenopausal bleeding (as well as a Papanicolaou [Pap] smear).

8. **List the main risk factors for endometrial cancer.**
   • Obesity
   • Nulliparity
   • Late menopause
   • Diabetes, hypertension, and gallbladder disease (probably related to obesity)
   • Chronic, unopposed estrogen stimulation (e.g., polycystic ovary syndrome [PCOS], estrogen-secreting neoplasm [granulosa–theca cell tumor], and estrogen replacement therapy without progesterone)

9. **What is the most common type of endometrial cancer? How is it treated?**
Most uterine cancers are adenocarcinomas and spread by direct extension. Treat with surgery and radiation.

10. **What commonly prescribed medication reduces the risk of endometrial cancer?**
Oral contraceptive pills, which also decrease the risk of ovarian cancer.

OVARY, FALLOPIAN TUBE, AND BROAD LIGAMENT

1. **What are the presenting symptoms for torsion of the ovary and fallopian tube?**
The classic presentation for ovarian torsion is acute pelvic pain in a woman with an adnexal mass, either with or without nausea and vomiting. However, the presenting signs and symptoms can be nonspecific (e.g., abdominal pain, fever, abnormal genital tract bleeding), so maintaining a high index of suspicion is important. Ovarian torsion is one of the most common gynecologic emergencies and may affect both adult and pediatric patients, although it occurs most commonly in the reproductive years.

2. **What are the risk factors for ovarian torsion? How is it diagnosed?**
The main risk factor for torsion is an ovarian mass, but pregnancy also increases the risk, and torsion may occur with a normal ovary. Prompt diagnosis is important to preserve ovarian/tubal function. Order a pregnancy test, complete blood count (CBC), and electrolyte panel. Pelvic ultrasound is the imaging modality of choice when torsion is suspected.

3. **How is ovarian torsion managed?**
With prompt surgery to preserve ovarian function and prevent other adverse events such as hemorrhage and peritonitis.

4. **What are the various causes of ovarian and fallopian tube masses?**
Ovarian masses may be caused by physiologic cysts (i.e., follicular cyst or corpus luteum cyst), benign neoplasms (e.g., dermoid cyst), ovarian cancer, or metastatic disease. Fallopian tube masses may be an ectopic pregnancy, fallopian tube malignancy, or hydrosalpinx.

5. What should you think about when evaluating an adnexal mass?

Adnexal masses are common, and the goal of evaluation is to determine the most likely cause. The likelihood of different types of adnexal mass depends on the anatomic location and the age and reproductive status of the patient. In children, ovarian torsion and ovarian malignancy are the most likely causes of an adnexal mass. In premenopausal women, most masses are benign and are associated with the menstrual cycle (e.g., follicular cysts), but always consider ectopic pregnancy. In postmenopausal women, malignancy must be ruled out.

6. How is an adnexal mass evaluated?

After taking a history and performing a physical examination, order a pregnancy test, CBC, and pelvic ultrasound. Most diagnoses can be established on the basis of these studies. If there is a clinical suspicion of malignancy (based on the ultrasound, age/menopausal status, risk factors, and laboratory results), surgical exploration is needed to make a definitive diagnosis.

7. What is premature ovarian failure? What are the presenting symptoms?

Premature ovarian failure, also called premature menopause or, more recently, 46,XX primary ovarian insufficiency, is a spectrum disorder with a continuum of impaired ovarian function. The condition involves the development of hypergonadotropic hypogonadism before 40 years of age in a woman with a normal karyotype. Premature ovarian failure is characterized by oligomenorrhea and/or amenorrhea, elevated serum gonadotropin, and low serum estradiol concentrations. Symptoms of estrogen deficiency are typically present (e.g., hot flashes and vaginal dryness). Ovarian function occurs intermittently in many of these women, so pregnancy can occur. Additional information about the evaluation of secondary amenorrhea is discussed in more detail later in the chapter.

CERVIX

1. What is the best available screening method to reduce the incidence and mortality of cervical cancer?

A Pap smear. All female patients should have a Pap smear if one is due, even if they are attending for a totally unrelated complaint. Screening should start at the age of 21 years. The frequency of screening depends on whether human papillomavirus (HPV) testing is also being used, the patient's age, and results of previous Pap smears. See the table on cancer screening in Chapter 1 for additional details.

2. What should you do if a Pap smear is abnormal?

The follow-up for an abnormal Pap smear depends on the cervical cytologic results. Low-grade lesions may be evaluated with HPV testing and colposcopy/endocervical curettage, if needed. High-grade lesions require colposcopy with biopsy and/or loop electrosurgical excision (LEEP). Invasive cancer requires surgery (at least a hysterectomy) and may include radiation with cisplatin-based chemotherapy.

3. List the main risk factors for cervical cancer.
- Age younger than 20 years on first coitus, pregnancy, or marriage
- Multiple sexual partners (role of HPV and possibly herpes virus)
- Coitus with a promiscuous partner
- Smoking
- Low socioeconomic status
- High parity (which protects against endometrial and breast cancer)

4. Where does cervical cancer begin? How does it present? How is it treated?

Invasive cervical cancer begins in the transformation zone, and the presenting symptoms are usually vaginal bleeding or discharge (postcoital bleeding, intermenstrual spotting, or abnormal menstrual bleeding). Treat with surgery and/or radiation.

5. What do you need to know about diethylstilbestrol (DES) and cancer?

Maternal exposure to DES during pregnancy increases a daughter's risk of developing clear cell cancer of the cervix and/or vagina.

VAGINA/VULVA

1. **What is indicated by a "bunch of grapes" protruding from a pediatric vagina?**
   Sarcoma botryoides, a malignant tumor (a type of embryonal rhabdomyosarcoma).

2. **What causes vaginitis or discharge in prepubescent girls?**
   Most cases are nonspecific or physiologic, but look for a vaginal foreign body, sexual abuse (especially if a sexually transmitted disease is present), or candidal infection. A candidal infection may be a symptom of diabetes; check the serum glucose level and/or the urine for glycosuria.

3. **How do you recognize and treat an imperforate hymen?**
   Imperforate hymen classically presents at menarche with hematocolpos (blood in the vagina) that cannot escape; thus the hymen bulges outward. Treatment is surgical opening of the hymen.

MENSTRUAL DISORDERS

1. **What is dysmenorrhea? How is it diagnosed? How is it treated?**
   Dysmenorrhea is pain that precedes and/or occurs during menstruation and interferes with daily activities. The pain can be sharp, dull, throbbing, burning, or shooting. Dysmenorrhea is a clinical diagnosis that requires a thorough history, physical examination, and sometimes additional tests (e.g., Pap test, pelvic ultrasound, testing for gonorrhea/chlamydia). Nonsteroidal antiinflammatory drugs (NSAIDs) help in many cases of dysmenorrhea. Hormonal contraceptives are also helpful.

2. **What is premenstrual dysphoric disorder? How is it treated?**
   Premenstrual dysphoric disorder is a severe form of premenstrual syndrome (PMS) occurring in a predictable, cyclic pattern just before menstruation and resolving shortly after menstruation. Mood symptoms predominate and include feelings of sadness or despair, irritability, anxiety, anhedonia, trouble concentrating, fatigue, and difficulty in sleeping. Other signs and symptoms may include food cravings, bloating, breast swelling/tenderness, and headaches. Selective seretonin reuptake inhibitors are the first-line treatment for premenstrual dysphoric disorder. Fluoxetine, sertraline, paroxetine, and escitalopram are approved by the Food and Drug Administration (FDA) for this indication.

3. **What is the first test to order for any woman of reproductive age with abnormal uterine bleeding?**
   A pregnancy test.

4. **Define dysfunctional uterine bleeding (DUB). When is it physiologic?**
   DUB is abnormal uterine bleeding not associated with a tumor, inflammation, or pregnancy. It is the most common cause of abnormal uterine bleeding and is a diagnosis of exclusion. More than 70% of cases are associated with anovulatory cycles (unopposed estrogen). The age of the patient is important because after menarche and immediately before menopause, DUB is extremely common and, in fact, is considered physiologic. Most other women have polycystic ovary syndrome (PCOS), the most common nonphysiologic cause of DUB.

5. **Why is dilation and curettage performed in women older than 35 years with DUB? What test should be ordered for all women with DUB (regardless of age)?**
   Dilation and curettage is performed to rule out endometrial cancer. Hemoglobin and hematocrit tests (or CBC) should be ordered for all women with DUB to make sure that the patient is not anemic from excessive blood loss.

6. **What causes DUB other than PCOS? How is DUB treated?**
   Causes of DUB include infections, endocrine disorders (thyroid, adrenal, pituitary/prolactin), coagulation defects, and estrogen-producing neoplasms. In the absence of treatable pathology, treat first with NSAIDs, which are first-line agents for DUB and dysmenorrhea. Oral contraceptive pills are also a first-line agent for menorrhagia and DUB if the patient does not wish to become pregnant and menstrual cycles are irregular. Monotherapy with progesterone is used for severe bleeding.

7. **Distinguish between primary and secondary amenorrhea.**
A patient with primary amenorrhea has never menstruated, whereas a patient with secondary amenorrhea used to menstruate but menstruation has stopped.

8. **Until proven otherwise, what is the cause of secondary amenorrhea in a previously menstruating woman of reproductive age?**
Pregnancy. Always order a human chorionic gonadotropin (hCG) test to rule out pregnancy as the first step in your evaluation of secondary amenorrhea.

9. **True or False: Excessive exercise may cause amenorrhea.**
True. It is not uncommon to find amenorrhea (or hypomenorrhea) in female athletes who train hard. The condition results from exercise-induced depression of gonadotropin-releasing hormone.

10. **What are other common causes of secondary amenorrhea?**
   • PCOS
   • Anorexia
   • Endocrine disorders (headaches, galactorrhea, and visual field defects may indicate a pituitary tumor)
   • Antipsychotic agents (because of increased prolactin)
   • Previous chemotherapy (causes premature ovarian failure and menopause)
   Although not considered secondary amenorrhea, **menopause** should be kept in mind as a cause for cessation of menstruation.

11. **After ruling out pregnancy, if the cause of secondary amenorrhea is not obvious from the history and physical examination, what is the next step in your evaluation?**
Administer progesterone to assess the patient's estrogen status. If vaginal bleeding develops within 2 weeks of administering progesterone, the patient has sufficient estrogen. In this case, check the luteinizing hormone (LH) level. If it is high, consider PCOS. If it is low or normal, check the levels of prolactin and thyroid-stimulating hormone (TSH). The high thyrotropin-releasing hormone (TRH) level in hypothyroidism causes high prolactin levels because TRH is a stimulus for prolactin release; high TRH will cause high TSH (as long as the anterior pituitary is functioning), so most physicians order TSH measurement. If the prolactin level is high with a normal TSH level, order a magnetic resonance imaging (MRI) scan of the brain to rule out pituitary prolactinoma. If the prolactin level is normal, look for low levels of gonadotropin-releasing hormone, which may be induced by drugs, stress, or exercise. In these patients, clomiphene can be used in an attempt to facilitate pregnancy.

12. **What if the patient fails to have vaginal bleeding after receiving progesterone?**
If the patient has no vaginal bleeding, estrogen levels are inadequate. Check the follicle-stimulating hormone (FSH) level next. If it is elevated, premature ovarian failure is the problem; check for autoimmune disorders, karyotype abnormalities, and a history of chemotherapy. If the FSH level is low or normal, the problem may be a brain tumor (e.g., craniopharyngioma). Order an MRI scan of the brain. Clomiphene is ineffective in these patients.

13. **At what age can primary amenorrhea be diagnosed? What is the first step in evaluation?**
A diagnosis of primary amenorrhea is made when a girl has not menstruated by the age of 16 years. Patients should also be evaluated in the absence of secondary sexual characteristics by the age of 14 years or in the absence of menstruation within 2 years of developing secondary sex characteristics (breast development, axillary and pubic hair). The first step is to rule out pregnancy.

14. **In a patient older than 14 years with no secondary sexual characteristics or development, what is the most likely cause of amenorrhea?**
The most likely cause in this setting is a congenital problem. In a phenotypically normal female with normal breast development but no axillary or pubic hair, think of **androgen insensitivity syndrome.** In such patients the uterus is absent. In the presence of normal

breast development and a uterus, the first step is to measure the prolactin level to rule out pituitary adenoma. If the prolactin level is high, order an MRI scan. If it is normal, administer progesterone and follow the same procedure as for the evaluation of secondary amenorrhea.

15. **When in doubt, what is the best way to evaluate any type of amenorrhea?**
First, order a pregnancy test. If it is negative, administer progesterone. Further testing depends on the results of the progesterone challenge (bleeding or no bleeding). A TSH level and/or a prolactin level should also be measured, especially in the case of symptoms of hypothyroidism or a pituitary tumor.

MENOPAUSE

1. **When does menopause occur? What are the symptoms and signs?**
The average age at menopause is approximately 51 years. Patients have irregular menstrual cycles or amenorrhea, hot flashes and mood swings, and an elevated FSH level. Patients also may complain of dysuria, dyspareunia, incontinence, and/or vaginal itching, burning, or soreness. Vaginal symptoms are often due to atrophic vaginitis; look for thin, dry, and atrophic vaginal mucosa with increased parabasal cells on cytology. Topical estrogen improves vaginal symptoms, but other symptoms require oral therapy.

2. **What is the current state of hormone replacement therapy?**
Hormone replacement therapy is currently recommended in the short term for management of moderate to severe vasomotor flushing. Long-term use for prevention of disease (such as osteoporosis and cardiovascular disease) is no longer recommended on the basis of results from the Women's Health Initiative and the HERS trial.

3. **Which women are candidates for hormone replacement therapy?**
Hormone replacement therapy (i.e., estrogen with or without progesterone) is now controversial and is probably best used only as a means of symptom relief. Observation during therapy is necessary, because estrogen and progesterone are not harmless. Every woman should make the decision for herself after weighing the risks and benefits.

4. **What are the known benefits of estrogen therapy?**
   - Decreases in the risk of osteoporosis and fractures
   - Reduced hot flashes and genitourinary symptoms of menopause (dryness, urgency, atrophy-induced incontinence, frequency)
   - Decreased risk of colorectal cancer (according to the Women's Health Initiative, when combined estrogen and progesterone therapy is used)

5. **What are the known risks of estrogen therapy?**
   - Increased risk of endometrial cancer (eliminated by coadministration of progesterone)
   - Small increase in the risk of coronary heart disease with combined estrogen and progesterone therapy, although the risk is not increased in women who are 50 to 59 years of age or within 10 years since menopause occurred
   - Increased risk of venous thromboembolism
   - Increased risk of breast cancer (when combined estrogen and progesterone therapy is used, according to the Women's Health Initiative; there was a slightly decreased risk of breast cancer with estrogen only, although this decrease was not statistically significant)
   - Increased risk of stroke (for either estrogen only or combined estrogen and progesterone therapy, according to the Women's Health Initiative)
   - Increased risk of gallbladder disease

6. **What are the most common side effects of estrogen therapy?**
   - Endometrial bleeding
   - Bloating
   - Breast tenderness
   - Headaches
   - Nausea

7. **What are the absolute contraindications to estrogen therapy?**
   - Unexplained vaginal bleeding
   - Active liver disease
   - History of thromboembolism
   - Coronary artery disease
   - History of endometrial or breast cancer
   - Pregnancy

8. **What are the relative contraindications to estrogen therapy?**
   - Seizure disorder
   - Hypertension
   - Uterine leiomyomas
   - Familial hyperlipidemia
   - Migraine headaches
   - Thrombophlebitis
   - Endometriosis
   - Gallbladder disease

9. **What tests are often performed before estrogen therapy is started?**
   The classic tests are endometrial biopsy, ultrasound, or dilation and curettage to rule out endometrial hyperplasia and/or cancer and evaluate any unexplained bleeding, even if the patient is on therapy, unless she has had a normal evaluation within the previous 6 months.

10. **What is postmenopausal vaginal bleeding? What do you need to do to evaluate postmenopausal vaginal bleeding?**
    Vaginal bleeding starting 12 months or more after the cessation of menses or unscheduled bleeding in a postmenopausal woman who has been taking hormone replacement therapy for 12 months or more. All women with postmenopausal vaginal bleeding require evaluation for potential malignancy (i.e., endometrial cancer, premalignant atypical endometrial hyperplasia, and cervical cancer). Evaluation includes a Pap smear and either an endometrial biopsy or transvaginal ultrasound. If ultrasound is performed and the endometrial lining is thicker than 4 mm or is otherwise abnormal, endometrial biopsy is required.

11. **True or false: Women without a uterus do not need to take progesterone with estrogen.**
    True. The main reason for giving progesterone with hormone replacement therapy is to eliminate the increased risk of endometrial cancer that accompanies unopposed estrogen therapy. If a woman has no uterus, then she has no need for progesterone.

PELVIC RELAXATION AND URINARY DISORDERS

1. **What causes pelvic relaxation or vaginal prolapse? What are the symptoms and signs?**
   Pelvic relaxation is due to weakening of the pelvic supporting ligaments. Look for a history of several vaginal deliveries, a feeling of heaviness or fullness in the pelvis, backache, worsening of symptoms on standing, and resolution of symptoms on lying down.

2. **What types of pelvic relaxation are seen clinically? How are they treated?**
   Cystocele: the bladder bulges into the *upper anterior vaginal wall*. Common symptoms include urinary urgency, frequency, and/or incontinence.
   Rectocele: the rectum bulges into the *lower posterior vaginal wall*. Watch for difficulty with defecation.
   Enterocele: loops of bowel bulge into the *upper posterior vaginal wall*.
   Urethrocele: the urethra bulges into the *lower anterior vaginal wall*. Common symptoms include urinary urgency, frequency, and/or incontinence.
   Conservative treatment for all types of pelvic relaxation involves pelvic strengthening exercises and/or a pessary (artificial device to provide support). Surgery is used for refractory or severe cases or if the patient desires this approach.

FEMALE FERTILITY/INFERTILITY

1. **Other than abstinence, what are the most effective forms of birth control (when used properly)?**
   The most effective forms of birth control are sterilization (e.g., tubal ligation and vasectomy), implants (etonogestrel implant), or an intrauterine device (IUD). These are closely followed in effectiveness by injectable hormone depot preparations (medroxy progesterone), then birth control pills/patch and a hormonal vaginal ring.

2. **Which forms of birth control prevent most sexually transmitted diseases?**
   Abstinence and condoms.

3. **What are the major problems with intrauterine devices?**
   They increase the risk of ectopic pregnancy and PID (watch for *Actinomyces* species as the cause). For these reasons, IUDs are most appropriate for older, monogamous women. Of note, the increased risk of ectopic pregnancy means that *if a woman with an IUD becomes pregnant*, there is a higher risk that such a pregnancy will be ectopic. However, pregnancy in a patient with an IUD is rare.

4. **What are the absolute contraindications to oral contraceptive pills?**
   - Venous thromboembolism, current or past (deep venous thrombosis or pulmonary embolism)
   - Cerebrovascular disease (stroke)
   - Coronary artery disease
   - Complicated valvular heart disease
   - Diabetes with complications
   - Breast cancer
   - Pregnancy
   - Lactation (within 6 weeks after delivery)
   - Liver disease
   - Headaches with focal neurologic symptoms
   - Major surgery with prolonged immobilization
   - Age older than 35 years and smoking 15 or more cigarettes per day
   - Hypertension (blood pressure >160/100 mm Hg or with concomitant vascular disease)

5. **What are the relative contraindications to oral contraceptive pills?**
   - Less than 21 days since delivery
   - Lactation (6 weeks to 6 months)
   - Undiagnosed vaginal or uterine bleeding
   - Age older than 35 years and smoking 15 or fewer cigarettes per day
   - History of breast cancer but no recurrence in the previous 5 years
   - Interacting drugs (certain anticonvulsants, rifampin)
   - Gallbladder disease
   - Headaches without an aura, age 35 years or older
   - Hypertension (well-controlled or systolic blood pressure of 140 to 159 mm Hg or diastolic blood pressure of 90 to 99 mm Hg)

6. **What is the relationship between oral contraceptive pills and hypertension?**
   Oral contraceptive pills are one of the most common causes of secondary hypertension. Any patient taking birth control pills for whom an increase in blood pressure is noted should discontinue the pills and have her blood pressure rechecked at a later date.

7. **What do you need to know about oral contraceptive pills and surgery?**
   Because of the risks of thromboembolism, oral contraceptive pills should be stopped 1 month before elective surgery and should not be restarted until 1 month after surgery.

8. **What are the side effects of oral contraceptive pills?**
   The side effects include glucose intolerance (check for diabetes mellitus annually in women at high risk), depression, edema, weight gain, bloating cholelithiasis, **benign liver adenomas,** melasma (called *the mask of pregnancy*), nausea, vomiting, headache, hypertension, and drug

interactions. Drugs such as rifampin and antiepileptic agents may induce metabolism of oral contraceptive pills and reduce their effectiveness.

9. **What is the relationship between oral contraceptive pills and breast and cervical cancers?**

Oral contraceptive pills have little if any effect on the risk of developing breast cancer. The incidence of cervical neoplasia may be increased in users of birth control pills, but this effect may also be due to the confounding factor of a higher frequency of sexual relations or a greater number of partners compared with those who do not use oral contraceptives. None-theless, users of birth control pills should have regular Pap smears.

10. **What is the relationship between oral contraceptive use and ovarian and endo-metrial cancers?**

It has been shown that oral contraceptive pills reduce the incidence of ovarian cancer by 50%; they also reduce the incidence of endometrial cancer.

11. **What are the other beneficial effects of oral contraceptive pills?**

They decrease the incidence of menorrhagia, dysmenorrhea, benign breast disease, functional ovarian cysts (often prescribed for the previous four effects), premenstrual tension, iron-deficiency anemia, ectopic pregnancy, and salpingitis.

12. **True or false: Women who smoke cannot take birth control pills.**

True—if the woman is older than 35 years and smokes. The risk of thromboembolism is sharply increased in women older than 35 years who smoke and take combination birth con-trol pills. Postmenopausal women, however, can take estrogen therapy regardless of smoking status.

13. **What is the most likely cause of infertility in a normally menstruating woman younger than 30 years?**

PID.

14. **What is the most likely cause of infertility in a woman younger than 30 years with abnormal menstruation?**

PCOS.

15. **Define PCOS. How do you recognize it?**

PCOS is an endocrine imbalance characterized by androgen excess and an LH-to-FSH ratio greater than 2:1. Patients also frequently develop enlarged ovaries with multiple peripherally oriented cysts, which can be seen on ultrasound. In the Step 3 exam, watch for an over-weight woman who has acne, hirsutism, amenorrhea, and/or infertility.

16. **How is PCOS treated? With what risk is it associated?**

Treat with oral contraceptive pills or cyclic progesterone. If the patient wishes to become pregnant, you can use **clomiphene** to induce ovulation. Chronic unopposed estrogen (i.e., not enough progesterone and hence infrequent menses) increases the risk of **endometrial cancer** in affected patients. Spironolactone can be used to treat hirsutism associated with PCOS. Metformin is sometimes used to treat the insulin resistance associated with PCOS and to help restore ovulation. However, metformin is not FDA approved for this use, and oral contraceptive pills or cyclic progesterone are the preferred agents for endometrial protection.

17. **Is infertility usually a male or a female problem?**

Two thirds of cases are due to a female problem, and one third to a male problem.

18. **Assuming that the history and physical examination offer no clues, what is the first step in evaluating a couple for infertility?**

Semen analysis, which is cheap, easy, and noninvasive. Remember this is counterintuitive because the issue is more often with the female, but it is much easier to test the man than the woman.

19. **What is the next step after semen evaluation?**

Documentation of ovulation. The history may suggest an ovulatory problem (irregular men-strual cycle length, duration, or amount of flow; lack of premenstrual syndrome symptoms).

Basal body temperature, luteal-phase progesterone levels, and/or endometrial biopsy can be evaluated to check for ovulation.

20. **What radiologic test is commonly used to examine the fallopian tubes and uterus? What points in the history may lead you to suspect a uterine or tube problem?**
    Hysterosalpingography is commonly used to examine the uterus and tubes. The history may suggest a tubal problem (PID, previous ectopic pregnancy) or a uterine problem (previous dilation and curettage that caused intrauterine synechiae; a history of fibroids; or symptoms of endometriosis).

21. **What test is the last resort in the workup for infertility?**
    Laparoscopy can be performed as a last resort or if the patient has a history suggestive of endometriosis. Lysis of adhesions and destruction of endometriosis lesions often restore fertility.

22. **Which two medications can be used to try to restore female fertility? In what situations are they effective?**
    Medical therapy usually consists of clomiphene citrate to induce ovulation, but this approach requires adequate production of estrogen. If the woman is hypoestrogenic, use human menopausal gonadotropin (hMG), which is a combination of FSH and LH. If medications fail, in vitro fertilization can be attempted.

23. **What is the main risk associated with medical induction of ovulation?**
    Multiple-gestation pregnancy.

NEOPLASMS

1. **Over the course of their lifetime, how many women in the United States will develop breast cancer?**
   Roughly 1 in 8.

2. **What are the risk factors for breast cancer?**
   A personal history of breast cancer (major risk factor); female sex; family history in first-degree relatives; age older than 40 years (rare before age 30 years; the incidence steadily increases with age); early menarche, late menopause, late first pregnancy, or nulliparity (more menstrual cycles represents higher risk); atypical hyperplasia of the breast; radiation exposure before the age of 30 years; inherited gene mutations (e.g., *BRCA1*, *BRCA2*); dense breast tissue; a high-fat diet; DES exposure; recent oral contraceptive use; combined postmenopausal hormone replacement therapy; excessive alcohol consumption; obesity; and possibly a lack of history of breastfeeding.

3. **What classic signs and symptoms indicate that a breast mass is cancer until proven otherwise?**
   - Fixation of the breast mass to the chest wall or overlying skin
   - Satellite nodules or ulcers on the skin
   - Lymphedema (*peau d'orange*)
   - Matted or fixed axillary lymph nodes
   - Inflammatory skin changes (red, hot skin with enlargement of the breast caused by inflammatory carcinoma)
   - Prolonged unilateral scaling erosion of the nipple with or without discharge (may be Paget disease of the nipple)
   - Microcalcifications on mammography
   - Any new breast mass in a postmenopausal woman

4. **What is the conservative approach to ensure that you do not miss a breast cancer?**
   When in doubt, biopsy every palpable breast mass in women older than 35 years that is not clearly a cyst (ultrasound is needed to make the determination), especially if the patient has any of the risk factors mentioned in the previous question. If the Step 3 question does not

want you to biopsy the mass, it will give definite clues that the mass is not a cancer (e.g., bilateral lumpy breasts that become symptomatic with every menses and have no dominant mass, patient younger than 30 years).

5. **What should you do for a breast mass in a woman younger than 30 years?**
   In women younger than 30 years, breast cancer is rare. For a discrete breast mass in this age group, you should think of fibroadenoma. Consider ultrasound of the breast and observe the patient over a few menstrual cycles before considering biopsy unless the ultrasound is suspicious. Fibroadenomas are usually roundish, feel rubbery, and are freely movable.

6. **What is the most common histologic type of breast cancer?**
   Invasive (infiltrating) ductal carcinoma accounts for about 70% of breast cancers.

7. **What is the role of mammography in deciding whether to biopsy a breast mass?**
   When a palpable breast mass is detected, the decision to perform a biopsy is made on *clinical* grounds. A mammogram that looks benign should not deter you from performing a biopsy if you are clinically suspicious. However, a lesion that is detected on mammography and looks suspicious should be biopsied, even if it is not palpable. Needle localization biopsy can be used.

8. **True or False: Mammography should not be performed in women younger than 30 years.**
   True in most cases. The breast tissue is too dense for current techniques to be of value. Mammograms for women younger than 30 years are rarely helpful.

9. **How does tamoxifen affect breast cancer? What other therapies may be used?**
   Tamoxifen (often with endocrine therapy) improves outcomes in premenopausal women with estrogen-receptor–positive breast cancer. Tamoxifen also decreases the risk of breast cancer in women at high risk of developing the disease.
   Raloxifene is as effective as tamoxifen in reducing breast cancer risk in postmenopausal women at increased risk of the disease. However, raloxifene did not reduce the risk of noninvasive breast cancers, such as ductal carcinoma in situ (DCIS) and lobular carcinoma in situ (LCIS).
   Aromatase inhibitors (e.g., anastrozole, exemestane, and letrozole) are used for the treatment of hormone-sensitive breast cancer in postmenopausal women. Aromatase inhibitors are generally not used in premenopausal women.
   Trastuzumab is used after surgery and chemotherapy for HER-2/neu (also known as ERBB2) breast cancer and targets the HER-2 protein.

10. **True or False: Mastectomy and breast-conserving surgery with radiation are considered equal in efficacy.**
    True. In either case, perform axillary node dissection (or a sentinel node biopsy) to determine spread to the nodes. If the nodes are positive for cancer, give chemotherapy.

11. **How does ovarian cancer classically present? How are ovarian masses evaluated?**
    Female patients classically present late with weight loss, pelvic mass, ascites, and/or bowel obstruction. Any ovarian enlargement in a postmenopausal female is cancer until proven otherwise. In women of reproductive age, most ovarian enlargements are benign. Ultrasound is a good first test to evaluate an ovarian lesion.

12. **How is ovarian cancer treated? What is the cell of origin? What is the most common type of ovarian cancer?**
    Ovarian cancer is usually treated with debulking surgery and chemotherapy. The prognosis is usually poor because of late presentation. Most ovarian cancers arise from the ovarian epithelium. Serous cystadenocarcinoma is the most common type; histopathologic studies classically reveal psammoma bodies. Mucinous cystadenocarcinoma is also common. When clinicians use the term ovarian cancer without a qualifier, they are talking about epithelial malignancies (i.e., cystadenocarcinomas).

13. List the three commonly tested germ-cell tumors. What clues suggest their presence?
   1. **Teratoma/dermoid cysts** (most common and most tested type). Look for a tumor description that includes skin, hair, and/or teeth or bone; the tumor may show up as calcifications on a radiograph.
   2. **Sertoli-Leydig cell tumors,** which cause virilization (hirsutism, receding hairline, deepening voice, clitoromegaly).
   3. **Granulosa/theca cell tumors,** which cause feminization and precocious puberty.
   Female patients with germ cell tumors of the ovary are classically younger than 30 years.

14. What commonly used medication reduces the risk of ovarian cancer?
   Oral contraceptives 5, which also reduce the incidence of endometrial cancer.

INFECTIONS

1. What is PID? How do you recognize it on the Step 3 exam?
   PID is typically due to an ascending sexually transmitted infection of the upper female genital tract that may involve the endometrial cavity (endometritis), fallopian tubes (salpingitis), ovaries (oophoritis), parametrial tissues/ligaments (parametritis), and/or peritoneal cavity (peritonitis). According to the newest Centers for Disease Control (CDC) recommendation, PID should be diagnosed and treated if a young, sexually active woman (or older woman at risk of sexually transmitted infections) has pelvic or lower abdominal pain, no other cause can be found, and the patient has at least one of the following: (1) cervical motion tenderness, (2) uterine tenderness, or (3) adnexal tenderness. This approach has high sensitivity: the risk associated with treatment when you are wrong is low (risk of antibiotic administration), but the risk of missing and not treating PID is high (permanent infertility).

2. How is PID treated? What are the common sequelae?
   Treat PID with more than one antibiotic to cover multiple organisms, especially *Neisseria gonorrhoeae* and *Chlamydia trachomatis* (the most common organisms). Several different regimens are recommended by the CDC, but the following are good choices: ceftriaxone plus doxycycline for outpatients; cefoxitin or cefotetan plus doxycycline for inpatients to cover multiple organisms. Also consider *Escherichia coli*, anaerobes, and, with a history of IUD use, *Actinomyces israelii*.
   Common sequelae include infertility caused by scarring of the fallopian tubes and progression to a tuboovarian abscess (palpable on examination, may respond to antibiotics alone) that may rupture. Treat a rupture with emergent laparotomy and excision of the affected tube (unilateral disease) or total abdominal hysterectomy and bilateral salpingo-oophorectomy for bilateral disease.

3. Cover the right-hand columns in the following table and specify the findings and treatment for the vaginal infections listed.

ORGANISM	FINDINGS	TREATMENT
Candida species	Cottage cheese appearance, pseudohyphae on KOH preparation, history of diabetes, antibiotic treatment, or pregnancy	Topical or oral antifungal
Trichomonas vaginalis	Bugs can be seen swimming under microscope; pale green, frothy, watery discharge; "strawberry" cervix	Metronidazole
Gardnerella vaginalis	Malodorous discharge; fishy smell on KOH preparation, clue cells	Metronidazole

Continued

ORGANISM	FINDINGS	TREATMENT
Human papillomavirus	Venereal warts, koilocytosis on Pap smear	Many (acid, cryotherapy, laser therapy, podophyllin)
Herpes virus	Multiple shallow, painful ulcers; recurrence and resolution	Acyclovir, valacyclovir
Syphilis (stage I)	Painless chancre, spirochete on dark-field microscopy	Penicillin
Syphilis (stage II)	Condyloma lata, maculopapular rash on palms, serology	Penicillin
Chlamydia trachomatis	Most common STD; dysuria, positive culture and antibody tests	Doxycycline or azithromy-cin*
Neisseria gonorrhoeae	Mucopurulent cervicitis; gram-negative organism on Gram stain	Ceftriaxone
Molluscum	Characteristic appearance of lesions, intracellular inclusions	Curettage, cryotherapy, or electrocauterization/ coagulation
Pediculosis	Crabs; look for itching; lice can be seen on pubic hairs	Permethrin cream (or malathion)

KOH, Potassium hydroxide; STD, sexually transmitted disease.

*Chlamydia can be treated with erythromycin if the patient is pregnant. If compliance is an issue (alcoholic, drug abusing, homeless, or unreliable patient), give azithromycin 1 g orally in a single dose so that you can watch the patient take it. **Patients with gonorrhea should be treated for presumed chlamydial coinfection (but the opposite is not true).**

4. True or False: For all of the infections listed in the previous table, you should seek out and treat the patient's sexual partners.
   False. Infections with *Candida* and *Gardnerella* species are not typically sexually transmitted diseases; they are usually caused by disturbances in the normal vaginal flora. You should treat the patient's sexual partners and give counseling (e.g., condom use) for the other infections, which are sexually transmitted.

5. True or False: Patients with gonorrhea are usually treated for presumed chlamydial infection.
   True. A common current treatment strategy is to give both ceftriaxone (for gonorrhea) and doxycycline (for *Chlamydia*) to patients with gonorrhea. The reverse is not true; do *not* automatically give gonorrhea treatment to patients with chlamydial infection.

6. Which group of patients should always be screened for syphilis?
   Pregnant women. Early treatment can prevent birth defects.

7. True or false: Sexually active teenage girls need screening for chlamydial infection and gonorrhea.
   True. There are high numbers of reported cases of *Chlamydia* infection and gonorrhea in younger women. The CDC recommends annual screening for *Chlamydia* among all sexually active females aged 25 years and younger. The CDC also recommends screening of high-risk sexually active females for gonorrhea.

CHAPTER 12

PREGNANCY, LABOR AND DELIVERY, THE FETUS, AND THE NEWBORN

PREGNANCY COMPLICATIONS

1. True or false: A high-normal blood urea nitrogen (BUN) or creatinine level during pregnancy often indicates renal disease.
   True. BUN and creatinine decrease significantly in pregnancy after the first trimester in women with normal renal function.

2. What is a hydatidiform mole? What are the clues to its presence?
   A hydatidiform mole is one form of gestational trophoblastic neoplasia in which the products of conception basically become a tumor. Look for the following clues:
   • Preeclampsia before the third trimester
   • A human chorionic gonadotropin (hCG) level that does not return to zero after delivery (or abortion/miscarriage) or that rapidly rises during pregnancy
   • First- or second-trimester bleeding with possible expulsion of "grapes" from the vagina (the gross appearance of the tumor resembles a bunch of grapes) and excessive nausea/hyperemesis
   • Uterine size/date discrepancy
   • A so-called snow-storm pattern on ultrasound

3. Distinguish between complete and partial hydatidiform moles. How are hydatidiform moles treated?
   Complete moles have a karyotype of 46,XX (with all chromosomes from the father) and no fetal tissue. **Incomplete moles** usually have a karyotype of 69,XXY with fetal tissue in the tumor.
   Treat hydatidiform moles with uterine dilation and curettage. Then follow with serial measurement of hCG levels until they fall to zero. If the hCG level does not fall to zero or if it rises, the patient has either an invasive mole or a choriocarcinoma (increasingly aggressive forms of gestational trophoblastic neoplasia) and needs chemotherapy (usually methotrexate or dactinomycin, both of which are extremely effective).

4. How is intrauterine growth retardation (IUGR) defined? What causes it?
   IUGR is defined as fetal size below the tenth percentile for age. Causes are best understood in broad terms as maternal (e.g., smoking, alcohol or drugs, lupus erythematosus), fetal (e.g., TORCH infections [toxoplasmosis, other agents, rubella, cytomegalovirus, herpes simplex], or placental (e.g., hypertension, preeclampsia). TORCH infections are discussed in more detail at the end of this chapter.

5. List the teratogenic effects of maternal diabetes mellitus. What is the best way to reduce these complications?
   • Cardiovascular malformations
   • Cleft lip and/or palate
   • Caudal regression (lower half of the body is incompletely formed)
   • Neural tube defects
   • Left-sided colon hypoplasia/immaturity
   • Macrosomia (most common and classic)
   • Microsomia (can occur if the mother has longstanding diabetes)
   Tight control of glucose during pregnancy dramatically reduces these complications.

6. What other problems does maternal diabetes cause in pregnancy?
   In the mother, diabetes can result in polyhydramnios and preeclampsia (as well as the complications of diabetes). Problems in infants born to a diabetic mother (other than birth defects) include an increased risk of respiratory distress syndrome and postdelivery hypoglycemia (from fetal islet cell hypertrophy caused by maternal and thus fetal hyperglycemia).

189

After birth, the infant is cut off from the mother's glucose supply, and the hyperglycemia resolves, but the infant's islet cells still overproduce insulin and cause hypoglycemia. Treat with intravenous glucose.

7. **True or false: Oral hypoglycemic agents should not be used during pregnancy.**
True. Use insulin to treat diabetes if diet and exercise cannot control glucose levels. Oral hypoglycemic agents, unlike insulin, may cross the placenta and cause fetal hypoglycemia.

8. **True or false: In terms of surgery, the usual rule of thumb is to treat disease in a pregnant woman the same as you would treat it in a nonpregnant woman.**
The answer to this question depends on the circumstances. It is definitely true in the case of an acute surgical emergency. Pregnant women can develop appendicitis, for which the presenting symptom may be right upper quadrant pain because of displacement of the appendix by the pregnant uterus. Just as in nonpregnant patients, laparotomy or laparoscopy is perfectly appropriate when the diagnosis is uncertain and the patient has signs of peritoneal involvement.

For semiurgent conditions (e.g., ovarian neoplasm), it is best to wait until the second trimester to perform surgery (when the pregnancy is most stable). Purely elective cases are avoided during pregnancy.

9. **What is the preferred method of anesthesia in obstetric patients? Why?**
Epidural anesthesia is the preferred method in obstetric patients. General anesthesia involves a higher risk of aspiration and resultant pneumonia because the gastroesophageal sphincter is relaxed in pregnancy and patients usually have not refrained from eating before going into labor. There also is concern about the effect of general anesthetic agents on the fetus. Spinal anesthesia can interfere with the mother's ability to push and is associated with a higher incidence of hypotension than with epidural anesthesia.

10. **True or false: Preeclampsia and eclampsia are risk factors for the development of hypertension in the future.**
False.

11. **What are the risk factors for developing an ectopic pregnancy?**
The major risk factor for ectopic pregnancy is a previous history of pelvic inflammatory disease (PID) (tenfold increase in ectopic pregnancy rate). Other risk factors include a previous ectopic pregnancy, history of tubal sterilization or tuboplasty, pregnancy that occurs when an intrauterine device is in place, and a history of diethylstilbestrol (DES) exposure, which can cause tubal abnormalities in women who were exposed in utero.

12. **What are the classic symptoms and signs of a ruptured ectopic pregnancy?**
A recent history of amenorrhea with current vaginal bleeding and abdominal pain. Patients also have a positive hCG pregnancy test. If you palpate an adnexal mass, it may be an ectopic pregnancy or a corpus luteum cyst.

13. **What should you do if you suspect an ectopic pregnancy?**
Order an ultrasound to look for a gestational sac or fetus. When the diagnosis is in doubt and the patient is doing poorly (e.g., hypovolemia, shock, severe abdominal pain, rebound tenderness), perform laparoscopy for a definitive diagnosis and treatment, if necessary. Culdocentesis is rarely performed in a stable patient to check for blood in the pouch of Douglas (with a ruptured ectopic pregnancy) because it has a high false-negative rate.

14. **How is symptomatic ectopic pregnancy managed?**
With surgery. A tubal pregnancy, if stable and of less than 3 cm in diameter, can be treated with salpingostomy and removal of the products of conception. The tube is left open to heal on its own; this strategy retains normal tubal function and fertility. If the patient is unstable or the ectopic pregnancy has ruptured or is greater than 3 cm in diameter, salpingectomy is required. In rhesus (Rh)-negative patients, give RhoGAM after treatment. Methotrexate (causes fetal demise) is an alternative treatment for small (<3 cm) unruptured tubal pregnancies.

15. **What are the diagnostic signs and symptoms of preeclampsia? When does it occur?**
Preeclampsia causes **hypertension,** defined as a greater than 30-point increase in systolic or a greater than 15-point increase in diastolic blood pressure over baseline. Other signs and symptoms include **proteinuria** (protein score of 2+ or more on urinalysis), oliguria, edema of

the hands or face, headache, visual disturbances, or the HELLP syndrome (**h**emolysis, **e**levated **l**iver enzymes, **l**ow **p**latelets, and right upper quadrant or epigastric pain). Preeclampsia usually occurs in the third trimester.

16. **What are the main risk factors for preeclampsia? How is it treated?**
    The risk factors (in decreasing order of importance) include chronic renal disease, chronic hypertension, family history of preeclampsia, multiple gestations, nulliparity, extremes of reproductive age (the classic patient is a young woman with her first child), diabetes, and black race. The definitive treatment is delivery. This is the treatment of choice if the patient is at term. In a preterm patient with mild disease, hypertension can be treated with hydralazine, labetalol, or methyldopa. Advise bed rest and observe. If the patient has severe disease (defined as oliguria, mental status changes, headache, blurred vision, pulmonary edema, cyanosis, HELLP syndrome, blood pressure >160/110 mm Hg, or progression to eclampsia [seizures]), deliver the infant once the mother is stabilized. Otherwise, both mother and infant may die.

17. **True or false: The combination of hypertension and proteinuria during pregnancy means preeclampsia until proven otherwise.**
    True.

18. **When is edema normal during pregnancy? When is it not?**
    Mild ankle edema is normal in pregnancy, but moderate to severe edema of the ankles or edema of the hands is likely to be preeclampsia.

19. **What should you consider if preeclampsia develops before the third trimester?**
    The possibility of gestational trophoblastic disease (i.e., hydatidiform mole or choriocarcinoma).

20. **Distinguish between preeclampsia and eclampsia. How can eclampsia be prevented?**
    Preeclampsia plus seizures equals eclampsia. Eclampsia can be prevented by regular prenatal care so that you catch the disease in the preeclamptic stage and treat appropriately.

21. **What should you use to treat seizures in eclampsia? What are the toxic effects?**
    Magnesium sulfate is the treatment of choice for preeclamptic seizure prophylaxis and for eclamptic seizures; it also lowers blood pressure. Toxic effects include hyporeflexia (first sign of toxicity), respiratory depression, central nervous system depression, coma, and death. If toxicity occurs, the first step is to stop the magnesium infusion.

22. **True or false: When eclampsia occurs, you must deliver the infant immediately, regardless of maternal status.**
    False. Do *not* try to deliver the infant until the mother is stable (e.g., do not perform a cesarean section while the mother is having seizures).

23. **Why are preeclampsia and eclampsia so important?**
    Preeclampsia and eclampsia cause uteroplacental insufficiency, IUGR, fetal demise, and increased maternal morbidity and mortality rates.

24. **What are the problems with preexisting maternal hypertension in pregnancy?**
    Preexisting hypertension (present before conception) increases the risk of IUGR and preeclampsia.

25. **True or false: The initial workup for third-trimester bleeding, like most conditions, requires a history and thorough physical examination, including a good pelvic examination.**
    False. You should record a history and perform a partial physical examination, but an ultrasound scan should *always* be obtained before a pelvic examination is performed.

26. **Describe the initial management of third-trimester bleeding.**
    For all cases of third-trimester bleeding, start intravenous fluids, give blood if needed, start the patient on oxygen, and start fetal and maternal monitoring. Then order a complete blood count (CBC), coagulation profiles, ultrasound, and a drug screen (if drug use is suspected, because cocaine causes placental abruption). Give RhoGAM if the mother is Rh negative.

A Kleihauer-Betke test can quantify fetal blood in the maternal circulation and can be used to calculate the dose of RhoGAM.

27. **Define hyperemesis gravidarum. How do you recognize and treat it?**
Hyperemesis gravidarum is intractable nausea and vomiting leading to dehydration and possible electrolyte disturbances. It occurs in the first trimester, usually in younger patients in their first pregnancy who have underlying social stressors or psychiatric problems. Treat with supportive care, as well as small, frequent meals and antiemetic medications such as pyridoxine-doxylamine, diphenhydramine, meclizine, dimenhydrinate, prochlorperazine, metoclopramide, and ondansetron. Patients may need intravenous fluids and correction of electrolyte abnormalities.

28. **Define cholestasis of pregnancy. How is it treated?**
Cholestasis of pregnancy involves itching (often severe) and/or abnormal liver function tests, usually in the second and third trimester. In rare cases, jaundice may coexist. The only known definitive treatment is delivery, but ursodeoxycholic acid or cholestyramine may help with symptoms.

29. **What is acute fatty liver of pregnancy? How is it treated?**
Acute fatty liver of pregnancy is a more serious disorder than cholestasis. It occurs in the third trimester or after delivery and usually progresses to hepatic coma. Treat with intravenous fluids, glucose, and fresh frozen plasma to correct coagulopathies. Vitamin K does not work, because the liver is in temporary failure. If the patient survives with supportive care, liver dysfunction usually resolves on its own with time.

30. **What are the maternal and fetal complications of multiple gestations (e.g., twin pregnancy)?**
Maternal complications include anemia, hypertension, premature labor, postpartum uterine atony, postpartum hemorrhage, and preeclampsia.
Fetal complications include polyhydramnios, malpresentation, placenta previa, abruptio placentae, velamentous cord insertion/vasa previa, premature rupture of the membranes, prematurity, umbilical cord prolapse, IUGR, congenital anomalies, and increased perinatal morbidity and mortality.
The higher the number of fetuses, the higher is the risk of most of the conditions mentioned for both mother and offspring.

31. **How are multiple gestations delivered?**
For vertex-vertex twin presentations (both infants are head first), you can try vaginal delivery for both infants; but for any other twin presentation combination or for more than two infants, perform a cesarean section.

32. **List the top three causes of maternal mortality in the United States.**
   - Pulmonary embolus
   - Hypertension/pregnancy-induced hypertension (preeclampsia/eclampsia)
   - Hemorrhage
The maternal mortality rate increases with age and is higher among black women.

UNCOMPLICATED PREGNANCY

1. **When does a standard home pregnancy test become positive?**
Roughly 2 weeks after conception (about the time the woman realizes that her period is late).

2. **List the symptoms and signs of pregnancy.**
   - Amenorrhea
   - Morning sickness
   - Weight gain
   - Hegar sign (softening and compressibility of the lower uterine segment)
   - Chadwick sign (dark discoloration of the vulva and vaginal walls)
   - Linea nigra
   - Melasma (also known as chloasma or the mask of pregnancy)
   - Auscultation of fetal heart tones

- Gestational sac or fetus seen on ultrasound
- Uterine contractions
- Palpation/ballottement of fetus

3. **What are the normal changes and complaints in pregnancy?**
   Normal changes in pregnancy include nausea or vomiting (morning sickness), amenorrhea, a heavy (possibly even painful) feeling in the breasts, increased pigmentation of the nipples and areolae, Montgomery tubercles (sebaceous glands in the areola), backache, linea nigra, melasma (chloasma), striae gravidarum, and mild ankle edema. Heartburn and increased frequency of urination are also common problems.

4. **What commonly used drugs are generally considered safe in pregnancy?**
   A short list of drugs that are generally safe in pregnancy includes acetaminophen, penicillins, cephalosporins, erythromycin, nitrofurantoin, histamine-2 receptor blockers, antacids, heparin, hydralazine, methyldopa, labetalol, insulin, and docusate.

5. **True or false: Levels of hCG roughly double every 2 days in the first trimester.**
   True. An hCG level that stays the same or increases only slowly on serial testing indicates a fetus in trouble (e.g., threatened abortion, ectopic pregnancy) or fetal demise. A rapidly increasing hCG level or one that does not decrease after delivery may indicate a hydatidiform mole or choriocarcinoma.

6. **When can ultrasound detect an intrauterine gestational sac? Why do you need to know this information?**
   At roughly 5 weeks after the last menstrual period (or when hCG is >2000 mIU), evidence of intrauterine pregnancy can be detected by transvaginal sonography. A definite fetus and fetal heartbeat can be detected by transvaginal ultrasound at 5 to 6 weeks of gestation. Use this information when trying to determine the possibility of an ectopic pregnancy. For example, if the patient's last menstrual period was 4 weeks ago, and a pregnancy test is positive, you cannot rule out an ectopic pregnancy with ultrasound. If, however, the patient's last menstrual period was 10 weeks ago with a positive pregnancy test and an ultrasound of the uterus does not show a gestational sac, be suspicious of an ectopic pregnancy.

7. **Which vitamin should all pregnant women take? Why?**
   Give all pregnant patients folate to prevent neural tube defects. Ideally, all women of reproductive age should take folate because it is most effective in the first trimester, before most women know that they are pregnant. Iron supplements are frequently given to pregnant women to help prevent anemia.

8. **What routine tests should be carried out for all pregnant patients?**
   - **Papanicolaou smear** if this test is due for the patient. Pregnancy does not change the frequency of screening.
   - **Urinalysis** at the first visit and every visit thereafter (to screen for proteinuria, preeclampsia, and bacteriuria; not a good screen for diabetes).
   - **Urine culture** obtained at 12 to 16 weeks to screen for asymptomatic bacteriuria.
   - **Hemoglobin and hematocrit** at the first visit to see if the patient is anemic (because pregnancy may worsen anemia). This test should be repeated in the third trimester.
   - **Blood type, Rh type, and antibody screen** at the first visit (for identification of possible isoimmunization).
   - **Syphilis test** at the first visit (mandated in most states) and subsequent visits (for high-risk patients).
   - **Rubella antibody screen.** If the patient is found to be nonimmune, counsel her on the benefit of postpartum immunization. Rubella vaccine should not be given during pregnancy.
   - **Glucose screening for gestational diabetes** at the first visit for patients with risk factors for diabetes mellitus (obesity, positive family history, or age over 30 years); otherwise, screen at 24 to 28 weeks. Use fasting serum glucose and serum glucose levels 1 or 2 hours after an oral glucose load (oral glucose tolerance test).
   - **Serum alpha-fetoprotein (AFP)** measured at 15 to 20 weeks, primarily to detect open spina bifida and anencephaly.

- **Hepatitis B antigen testing** to prevent perinatal transmission.
- **Varicella** testing in all pregnant women to determine immunity to varicella.
- **Thyroid function.** Maternal hypothyroidism may affect fetal neurologic development and can lead to fetal and maternal complications.
- **HIV test.** The American College of Obstetrics and Gynecology (ACOG) advocates an opt-out rather than an opt-in approach to increase screening.
- **Chlamydia screening.** The Centers for Disease Control (CDC) and ACOG advocate testing all pregnant women at the first prenatal visit.
- **Down syndrome screening** should be offered to all pregnant patients. There are multiple screening approaches, as described in Questions 21 to 27 in this section.
- **Beta-hemolytic group B *Streptococcus* (GBS)** screening should be performed at 35 to 37 weeks using a swab of the lower vagina and rectum.
- **Other tests.** A tuberculosis skin test should be performed for women at high risk. Testing for gonorrhea is warranted for women at high risk of this infection. Testing for toxoplasmosis is controversial. If asked, you should order *Chlamydia* and gonorrhea cultures for any pregnant teenager. Testing for sexually transmitted diseases should be repeated in the third trimester for women who continue to be at risk or for women who acquire a risk factor during pregnancy.

9. **Explain Rh incompatibility. In what situations does it occur?**
Rh blood-type incompatibility is of concern because it can lead to hemolytic disease of the newborn. Rh incompatibility occurs when the mother is Rh negative and her infant is Rh positive. The USMLE assumes an understanding of the inheritance of the Rh factor. If both the mother and the father are Rh negative, there is nothing to worry about because their infant will be Rh negative. If the father is Rh positive, the infant has a 50/50 chance of being Rh positive.

10. **True or false: The first child is usually the most severely affected by Rh incompatibility.**
False. Previous maternal sensitization is required for disease to occur. In other words, if a nulliparous Rh-negative mother has never received blood products, her first Rh-positive infant will not be affected by hemolytic disease—except in the rare case of sensitization during the first pregnancy from undetected fetomaternal bleeding, which commonly occurs later in the pregnancy and in most instances can be prevented by RhoGAM administration at 28 weeks gestation. The second Rh-positive infant, however, will be affected unless RhoGAM was administered at 28 weeks and within 72 hours after delivery for the first pregnancy. Any history of blood transfusion, abortion, ectopic pregnancy, stillbirth, or delivery can cause sensitization.

11. **How much RhoGAM should you give if the maternal Rh antibody titer is extremely high?**
In this setting, RhoGAM is worthless because sensitization has already occurred. RhoGAM administration is a good example of primary prevention. Close fetal monitoring for hemolytic disease is required.

12. **How do you recognize, monitor, and treat hemolytic disease of the newborn?**
Hemolytic disease of the newborn in its most severe form causes fetal hydrops (edema, ascites, pleural and/or pericardial effusions) and death. Amniotic fluid spectrophotometry and ultrasound can help in gauging the severity of fetal hemolysis. Treatment of hemolytic disease involves (1) delivery, if the fetus is mature (check lung maturity with a lecithin-to-sphingomyelin ratio); (2) intrauterine transfusion; and (3) phenobarbital, which helps the fetal liver to break down bilirubin by inducing enzyme expression.

13. **True or false: ABO blood group incompatibility can cause hemolytic disease of the newborn.**
True. ABO blood group incompatibility can cause hemolytic disease of the newborn when the mother is type O and the infant is type A, B, or AB. This condition does not require previous sensitization because immunoglobulin G (IgG) antibodies (which can cross the placenta) occur naturally in mothers with blood type O, but not in mothers with other blood types. The hemolytic disease is usually less severe than for Rh

incompatibility, but the treatment is the same. In rare instances, other minor blood antigens also may cause a reaction.

14. **When should RhoGAM be given?**
To reiterate, give RhoGAM only when the mother is Rh negative and the father is Rh positive or when his blood type is unknown. During routine prenatal care, check for Rh antibodies at the first visit. If the test is positive, do not give RhoGAM—you are too late. Otherwise, give RhoGAM routinely at 28 weeks gestation and immediately after delivery. Also give RhoGAM after an abortion, stillbirth, ectopic pregnancy, amniocentesis, chorionic villus sampling (CVS), and any other invasive procedure that may cause transplacental bleeding during pregnancy.

15. **How do you detect and manage potential hemolytic disease of the newborn?**
If indicated by maternal and potential fetal blood type, check maternal titers of Rh antibody every month, starting in the seventh month of gestation. Give RhoGAM automatically at 28 weeks and within 72 hours after delivery, as well as after any procedures that may cause transplacental hemorrhage.

16. **How do you treat gonorrheal and chlamydial genital infections during pregnancy?**
The treatment for gonorrhea remains unchanged because ceftriaxone is safe during pregnancy. For chlamydial infection, give azithromycin, amoxicillin, or erythromycin base instead of doxycycline or erythromycin estolate.

17. **What do you need to know about vaginal GBS colonization and pregnancy?**
Pregnant women should be tested for vaginal GBS. Women who are carriers should be treated during labor with penicillin G or ampicillin. Earlier treatment (e.g., second trimester) is ineffective because GBS frequently returns and is usually only dangerous during labor and delivery. The reason for treating asymptomatic carriers is to prevent neonatal sepsis and endometritis, both of which are commonly caused by GBS.

18. **What test is used to screen for neural tube defects? At what time during pregnancy is it measured? Explain the significance of a low or high AFP level in maternal serum.**
Maternal AFP is most accurate when measured between 15 and 20 weeks of gestation. A low AFP level may represent **Down syndrome,** fetal demise, or inaccurate dates. A high AFP level may represent **neural tube defects** (e.g., anencephaly, spina bifida), **ventral wall defects** (e.g., omphalocele, gastroschisis), multiple gestation, or inaccurate dates.

19. **What should be done if the AFP is elevated?**
Repeat the test. As many as 30% of maternal serum AFP test results may be elevated but are normal on repeat testing. The initial elevation is not associated with an increased risk of neural tube defects.

20. **What further testing should a patient undergo if AFP remains elevated?**
If AFP remains elevated, the patient is first advised to undergo ultrasound to determine whether a neural tube defect or other anomaly is present. The ultrasound is also used to confirm gestational age, number of fetuses, and fetal viability. Further evaluation with amniocentesis may be required if the ultrasound findings are uncertain or there is a concern for nonvisualized neural tube defects (according to elevated AFP in amniotic fluid or detection of acetylcholinesterase in amniotic fluid). There is a small risk of miscarriage after amniocentesis.

21. **What prenatal tests are available to screen for Down syndrome?**
The first-trimester combined test, integrated tests, sequential testing, contingent testing, the quadruple test, and maternal plasma-based tests. The American College of Obstetricians and Gynecologists (ACOG) recommends that all women be offered screening before 20 weeks of gestation.

22. **What is the first-trimester combined test for Down syndrome? When is it performed?**
The first-trimester combined test is performed at 11 to 13 weeks of gestation. The test involves determination of nuchal translucency (NT) by ultrasound, combined with serum pregnancy-associated plasma protein-A (PAPP-A) and serum hCG. CVS is used for women who test positive in this first-trimester screening.

23. **Describe the integrated test for Down syndrome.**
   The full integrated test includes ultrasound measurement of NT at 10 to 13 weeks of gestation; PAPP-A at 10 to 13 weeks of gestation; and AFP, unconjugated estradiol (uE3), hCG,
   and inhibin A at 15 to 18 weeks of gestation. Results for the full integrated test are not available until the second trimester.
   The serum integrated test is the same as the full integrated test but without the ultrasound
   evaluation of NT. This test is used in areas where expertise in ultrasound measurement of
   NT is not available. Results for the serum integrated test are not available until the second
   trimester.

24. **Describe sequential testing for Down syndrome.**
   Stepwise sequential testing has been developed to provide a risk estimate during the first trimester. The first-trimester portion of the integrated screen is performed. If the tests indicate a very
   high risk of having an affected fetus, CVS is offered. Women whose results do not place them at
   very high risk of having an affected fetus go on to have the second-trimester portion of the screen.

25. **Describe contingent testing for Down syndrome.**
   Contingent testing has not yet been proven efficacious in a prospective clinical trial and
   probably will not be tested on the USMLE; it is mentioned here in case it is or in case you
   are studying for an obstetrics shelf exam. Contingent screening involves three risk cutoffs:
   (1) women at very high risk of having a fetus with Down syndrome after first-trimester
   testing are offered immediate invasive prenatal diagnosis; (2) women at very low risk are
   provided with their risk estimate and require no additional testing; and (3) women at intermediate risk receive second-trimester marker testing.

26. **What is the quadruple test for Down syndrome? For whom is it typically used?
   When is it performed?**
   The quadruple test includes the serum markers AFP, uE3, hCG, and inhibin A. The quadruple test is the best available test for women who attend for prenatal care in the second
   trimester, but it can be used for women who receive earlier prenatal care. It is performed at
   15 to 18 weeks of gestation.

27. **What is the maternal plasma-based test for Down syndrome?**
   This is the newest option that is just becoming widely available and may make many of the
   other tests obsolete in the future. This test, also called cell-free fetal DNA testing, detects
   fetal DNA in the circulation and has a detection rate of greater than 98% and a false-positive
   rate of less than 0.5% for Down syndrome and Edward syndrome (trisomy 18). It is used after
   10 weeks of gestation. Cell-free fetal DNA testing is not yet validated for low-risk women
   but can be used in women with a higher risk of having fetal trisomy (i.e., women who will be
   older than 35 years at the time of delivery, presence of sonographic findings associated with
   fetal aneuploidy, history of previous pregnancy with fetal trisomy, positive screening results
   for tests such as the first-trimester combined test, the integrated test, and the quadruple test).

28. **What is the next step if a woman has a positive screening test for Down
   syndrome?**
   Offer fetal karyotype determination. This is performed on a sample obtained via CVS in the
   first trimester and amniocentesis in the second trimester.

29. **Why is CVS performed instead of amniocentesis in some cases?**
   CVS can be performed at 9 to 12 weeks of gestation (earlier than amniocentesis) and is
   generally reserved for women with previously affected offspring or known genetic disease. It
   offers the advantage of a first-trimester abortion if the fetus is affected. CVS is associated with
   a slightly higher miscarriage rate than that for amniocentesis.

30. **True or false: CVS can detect neural tube defects but not genetic disorders.**
   False. CVS can detect genetic or chromosomal disorders but not neural tube defects.

31. **How is tuberculosis treated in pregnancy?**
   In a similar way as in a nonpregnant patient. Use isoniazid, rifampin, and ethambutol
   if the risk of a drug-resistant organism is low. Pyrazinamide should be used with caution
   because of a lack of data on the risk of teratogenicity. However, pyrazinamide should

be added if a drug-resistant organism is suspected. Streptomycin, which is a rarely used second-line agent, should be avoided. Give vitamin B_6 to pregnant patients treated with isoniazid to avoid a deficiency.

32. **On every prenatal visit, listen to fetal heart tones and evaluate uterine size. When can these factors first be observed? What constitutes a size/date discrepancy?**
    Fetal heart tones can be heard with Doppler ultrasound at 10 to 12 weeks and with a normal stethoscope at 16 to 20 weeks. At 12 weeks of gestation, the uterus enters the abdomen and is palpable at the symphysis pubis; at roughly 20 weeks, it reaches the umbilicus. **Uterine size** is evaluated by measuring the distance from the symphysis pubis to the top of the fundus in centimeters. At roughly 20 to 35 weeks, the measurement in centimeters should equal the number of weeks of gestation. A discrepancy greater than 2 to 3 cm is called a **size/date discrepancy.** Ultrasound should be performed for further evaluation (e.g., IUGR, multiple gestations).

33. **What normal changes in laboratory results during pregnancy may be encountered on the Step 3 exam?**
    - The erythrocyte sedimentation rate becomes markedly elevated; hence this test is essentially worthless in pregnancy.
    - Total thyroxine (T_4) and thyroid-binding globulin increase, but free T_4 remains normal.
    - Hemoglobin increases, but plasma volume increases even more; thus the net result is a decrease in hemoglobin and hematocrit.
    - BUN and creatinine decrease because of an increase in the glomerular filtration rate. BUN and creatinine levels at the high end of the normal range indicate renal disease in pregnancy.
    - Alkaline phosphatase increases markedly.
    - Mild proteinuria and glycosuria are normal in pregnancy.
    - Electrolytes and liver function tests remain normal.

34. **What cardiovascular and pulmonary changes occur in a normal pregnancy?**
    Normal cardiovascular changes: blood pressure decreases slightly, the heart rate increases by 10 to 20 beats/min, the stroke volume increases, and cardiac output increases (by up to 50%).
    Normal pulmonary changes: minute ventilation increases because of an increase in tidal volume, but the respiratory rate remains the same or increases only slightly; the residual volume and carbon dioxide decrease. Collectively these changes cause the physiologic hyperventilation/respiratory alkalosis of pregnancy.

35. **What is the average weight gain during pregnancy? What commonly causes weight gain to be greater or less than the average?**
    The average weight gain in pregnancy is roughly 28 lb (12.5 kg). A greater weight gain may mean maternal diabetes. A smaller weight gain may indicate hyperemesis gravidarum or a psychiatric or major systemic disease.

36. **When is ultrasound most accurate at estimating fetal age?**
    At 7 to 10 weeks the crown-rump length is the most accurate measure for estimating fetal age. At 16 to 20 weeks the biparietal diameter (measured on ultrasound) gives the most accurate estimate.

37. **When should ultrasound be used to evaluate the fetus?**
    The indications for ultrasound are now quite liberal. Order ultrasound for all patients who have a size/date discrepancy greater than 2 to 3 cm or risk factors for pregnancy-related problems (e.g., hypertension, diabetes, renal disease, lupus erythematosus, smoking, alcohol or drug use, and a history of previous pregnancy-related problems). Ultrasound is also used when fetal death, distress, or abortion or miscarriage is suspected (e.g., a baby that stops kicking, vaginal bleeding, or a slow fetal heartbeat on auscultation).

38. **How is fetal well-being evaluated?**
    A **nonstress** test is the easiest initial screen. It is performed with the mother at rest. A fetal heart rate tracing is obtained for 20 minutes. A normal trace has at least two accelerations of heart rate, each at least 15 beats/min above baseline and lasting for at least 15 seconds.

A **biophysical profile** is slightly more involved and includes a nonstress test and measurement of amniotic fluid (to determine whether oligohydramnios or polyhydramnios is present), fetal breathing movements, and general fetal movements.

If the fetus scores poorly on the biophysical profile, the next test is the **contraction stress test,** which looks for uteroplacental dysfunction. Oxytocin is given and a fetal heart trace is monitored. If late decelerations are seen on the fetal heart trace with each contraction, the test is positive. In most cases of a positive contraction stress test, a cesarean section is performed.

39. **True or false: A biophysical profile is often used in high-risk pregnancies in the absence of obvious problems.**
    True. A biophysical profile may be measured once or twice a week from the start of the third trimester until delivery to monitor for potential problems.

40. **True or false: Aspirin should be avoided during pregnancy.**
    True. Use acetaminophen instead. One important exception is in patients with antiphospholipid syndrome, in whom aspirin may improve pregnancy outcome (subcutaneous unfractionated heparin or low-molecular-weight heparin also can be used to treat antiphospholipid syndrome in pregnancy).

41. **Define postterm pregnancy. Why is it a major concern? How is it treated?**
    Postterm pregnancy is a pregancy of more than 42 weeks of gestation. Both prematurity and postmaturity increase perinatal morbidity and mortality rates. For postmaturity, **dystocia** (or difficult delivery) becomes more common because of the increased size of the infant.

    In general, if the gestational age is known to be accurate and the cervix is favorable, labor is induced (with oxytocin, for example). If the cervix is not favorable or the dates are uncertain, twice-weekly biophysical profiles are measured. At 41 weeks, most obstetricians advise induction of labor. A 2012 metaanalysis demonstrated that routine labor induction at greater than 41 weeks resulted in lower perinatal mortality and a lower rate of meconium aspiration syndrome when compared with expectant management.

42. **What two rare disorders are associated with prolonged gestation?**
    Anencephaly and placental sulfatase deficiency.

43. **True or false: Asymptomatic bacteriuria detected on routine urinalysis should be treated during pregnancy.**
    True. Up to 20% of patients develop cystitis or pyelonephritis if untreated. This rate is much higher than in nonpregnant patients, who should not be treated for asymptomatic bacteriuria. In pregnancy, the gravid uterus can compress the ureters and increased progesterone can decrease the tone of the ureters, increasing urinary stasis and the risk of urinary tract infection.

44. **Define abortion.**
    Abortion is the termination (intentional or not) of a pregnancy at less than 20 weeks of gestation or when the fetus weighs less than 500 g. The term *miscarriage* describes a spontaneous abortion.

45. **What are the different terms for an unintentional abortion?**
    Threatened abortion: uterine bleeding without cervical dilation and no expulsion of tissue. Treat with bed rest and pelvic rest (although neither of these actually decrease the incidence of continuing to a complete abortion).
    Inevitable abortion: uterine bleeding with cervical dilation, crampy abdominal pain, and no tissue expulsion.
    Incomplete abortion: passage of some products of conception through the cervix.
    Complete abortion: expulsion of all products of conception from the uterus. Treat with serial testing of the hCG level to make sure that it goes down to zero.
    Missed abortion: fetal death with no expulsion of tissue (in some cases not for several weeks). Treat with dilation and curettage for less than 14 weeks of gestation, or attempt delivery for more than 14 weeks of gestation.
    All of the above terms imply a gestation of less than 20 weeks. Treat all abortions with intravenous fluids (and blood transfusions if necessary), and consider dilation and curettage (once the fetus is confirmed as dead or expelled). Give the mother RhoGAM if she has an Rh-negative blood type.

46. Define induced and recurrent abortions. What do recurrent abortions suggest?

Induced abortion is intentional termination of pregnancy at less than 20 weeks of gestation; it may be elective (requested by the patient) or therapeutic (performed to maintain the health of the mother).

   Recurrent abortion is two or three successive, unplanned abortions. The patient's history and a physical examination may suggest the cause, which may include:

- Infection (*Listeria, Mycoplasma,* or *Toxoplasma* species; syphilis)
- Inherited thrombophilia (factor V Leiden, G20210A gene mutation, antithrombin deficiency, deficiency of protein C or protein S)
- Environmental factors (alcohol, tobacco, drugs)
- Diabetes
- Hypothyroidism
- Systemic lupus erythematosus (especially with positive antiphospholipid/lupus anticoagulant antibodies, sometimes an isolated syndrome without coexisting lupus)
- Cervical incompetence (watch for a history of exposure to DES in the patient's mother during pregnancy and/or a patient with recurrent, painless second-trimester abortions; treat future pregnancies with cervical cerclage)
- Congenital abnormalities of the female reproductive tract (if possible, correct to restore fertility)
- Fibroids (remove them)
- Chromosomal abnormalities (e.g., maternal or paternal translocations)

47. Explain the term *bloody show.* How is it diagnosed?

On cervical effacement, a blood-tinged plug of mucus may be released from the cervical canal and heralds the onset of labor. This normal occurrence is a diagnosis of exclusion in the evaluation of third-trimester bleeding.

48. Define quickening. When does it occur?

Quickening is the term used to describe when the mother first detects fetal movements, usually at 18 to 20 weeks of gestation in a primigravida woman and 16 to 18 weeks of gestation in a multigravida woman.

LABOR, DELIVERY, AND THE POSTPARTUM PERIOD (INCLUDING PLACENTAL ABNORMALITIES)

1. What causes third-trimester bleeding?
- Placenta previa
- Abruptio placentae
- Uterine rupture
- Fetal bleeding
- Cervical or vaginal infections (e.g., herpes simplex virus, gonorrhea, chlamydial or candidal infection)
- Cervical or vaginal trauma (usually from sexual intercourse)
- Bleeding disorders (rare before delivery; more common after delivery)
- Cervical cancer (which may occur in pregnant patients)
- Cervical effacement (bloody show)

2. Why should ultrasound be performed before a pelvic examination for third-trimester bleeding?

In case placenta previa is present. Disturbing the placenta may make the bleeding worse and turn a worrisome case into an emergency.

3. Define placenta previa. What are the presenting symptoms? How is it diagnosed and treated?

True placenta previa occurs when the placenta implants in an area where it covers the cervical opening (os). Predisposing factors include multiparity, increasing maternal age, multiple gestation, and a history of prior placenta previa. Because of this condition, you should *always* perform ultrasound before a pelvic examination for third-trimester bleeding. The bleeding is painless and may be profuse. Ultrasound is 95% to 100% accurate in diagnosing placenta previa. A cesarean section is mandatory for delivery, but patients may be admitted to the hospital for bed and pelvic rest and tocolysis if they are preterm and stable and if the bleeding has stopped.

4. **Define abruptio placentae. What are the presenting symptoms? How is it treated?**
Abruptio placentae is premature detachment of a normally situated placenta. Predisposing factors include hypertension (with or without preeclampsia); trauma; polyhydramnios with rapid decompression after membrane rupture; cocaine or tobacco use; and preterm premature rupture of the membranes (PROM). Patients can have this condition without visible vaginal bleeding; the blood may be contained behind the placenta. Usual symptoms include pain, uterine tenderness, increased uterine tone with a hyperactive contraction pattern, and fetal distress. Abruptio placentae may also cause disseminated intravascular coagulation if fetal products enter the maternal circulation. Ultrasound detects only a small percentage of cases. Treat with intravenous fluids (and blood if needed) and rapid delivery (vaginal route preferred).

5. **What causes fetal bleeding that presents as third-trimester vaginal bleeding?**
Visible fetal bleeding is usually due to vasa previa or velamentous insertion of the cord, which occurs when umbilical vessels present in advance of the fetal head, usually traversing the membranes and crossing the cervical os. The biggest predisposing risk factor is multiple gestation (the higher the number of fetuses, the higher the risk). Bleeding is painless and the mother is completely stable, whereas the fetus shows worsening distress (tachycardia initially, then bradycardia as the fetus decompensates). An Apt test performed on vaginal blood is positive for fetal blood (this test differentiates fetal from maternal blood). Treat with immediate cesarean section.

6. **How do you manage fetal malpresentation?**
External cephalic version can be used to rotate the fetus from the breech to the cephalic position. If this fails, a decision must be made as to whether to attempt a vaginal delivery or perform a cesarean section. Although some frank and complete breech fetuses may be delivered vaginally under specific guidelines, it is acceptable to perform a cesarean section for any breech presentation. For a shoulder presentation or an incomplete/footling breech presentation, cesarean section is mandatory. For face and brow presentations, watchful waiting is best, because most cases convert to a vertex presentation; if they do not convert, perform a cesarean section.

7. **Distinguish between true labor and false labor.**
In true labor, normal contractions occur at least every 3 minutes, are fairly regular, and are associated with cervical changes (effacement and dilation). In false labor (Braxton-Hicks contractions), contractions are irregular and no cervical changes occur.

8. **Define preterm labor. How is it treated?**
Preterm labor is labor for a gestation of between 20 and 37 weeks. Put the mother in the lateral decubitus position, order pelvic rest, and give oral or intravenous fluids and oxygen. In some cases these maneuvers stop the contractions. If they fail, you can give a tocolytic agent (beta$_2$ agonist or magnesium sulfate) if no contraindications (heart disease, hypertension, diabetes, hemorrhage, ruptured membranes, cervix dilation of >4 cm) are present. The mother can be managed as an outpatient with an oral tocolytic agent once she is stable. Give steroids to promote fetal lung maturity (discussed in more detail in Questions 14 to 16) for preterm labor that occurs between 24 and 34 weeks of gestation.

9. **What are tocolytic agents? When is it not appropriate to give them?**
Tocolytic agents stop uterine contractions. Common examples are beta$_2$ agonists (terbutaline, ritodrine) and magnesium sulfate. Do not give a tocolytic agent to the mother in the presence of preeclampsia, severe hemorrhage, chorioamnionitis, IUGR, fetal demise, or fetal anomalies incompatible with survival.

10. **Define PROM. How is it diagnosed?**
PROM is rupture of the amniotic sac before the onset of labor. Diagnosis of rupture of membranes (whether premature or not) is based on the patient's history, a sterile speculum examination, and/or a positive nitrazine test. The sterile speculum examination shows

pooling of amniotic fluid and a ferning pattern when the fluid is placed on a microscopic slide and allowed to dry. Nitrazine paper turns blue in the presence of amniotic fluid. Ultrasound should be performed in cases of PROM to assess the amniotic fluid volume, gestational age, and any anomalies that may be present.

11. **What usually follows membrane rupture? What should you do if it does not occur?**
Spontaneous labor usually follows membrane rupture; for this reason, amniotomy may be performed in an attempt to induce labor if the membrane does not rupture spontaneously. If labor does not occur within 6 to 8 hours of membrane rupture, and the mother is at full term and the cervix is favorable, labor should be induced.

Labor is induced because the main risk of PROM is infection, which may occur in the mother (chorioamnionitis) and/or infant (neonatal sepsis, pneumonia, meningitis). The usual culprits are GBS, *Escherichia coli,* or *Listeria* species.

12. **Define preterm PROM (PPROM). How is it managed?**
PPROM is premature rupture of membranes before 36 to 37 weeks of gestation. The risk of infection increases with the length of time after membrane rupture. Order a culture and Gram stain of the amniotic fluid. If the results are negative, treatment simply involves pelvic and bed rest with frequent follow-up. If the culture is positive for GBS, treat the mother with penicillin G or ampicillin, even if she is asymptomatic.

13. **What is fetal fibronectin? When is a test for this substance useful? Is the test more helpful when positive or negative?**
Fetal fibronectin (an extracellular matrix protein that helps attach the amniotic membrane to the uterine lining) can be detected in the vaginal secretions of some women with signs and symptoms of preterm labor. The test is most helpful when negative between 22 and 34 weeks of gestation, because it indicates a very low likelihood of delivery in the 2 weeks that follow. In such cases a more conservative, observational approach can be used. When fetal fibronectin is positive in this setting, the woman is at higher risk of delivery in the next 2 weeks, and a more aggressive approach to tocolysis and hastening of fetal lung maturity is typically adopted.

14. **When should fetal lung maturity be evaluated?**
Evaluation of fetal lung maturity is indicated before elective deliveries that are, or may be, at less than 39 weeks of gestation. Testing is not necessary for well-documented pregnancies of 39 or more weeks of gestation or pregnancies of less than 32 weeks of gestation (because fetal lung maturity is unlikely), or when a delay in delivery because of fetal lung immaturity will place the mother or fetus at significant risk.

15. **What tests can be used to assess fetal lung maturity?**
   • Lamellar body count
   • Lecithin/sphingomyelin ratio
   • Phosphatidylglycerol
   • Surfactant/albumin ratio
   • Optical density at 650 nm
   • Foam stability index
For the purposes of the USMLE, it is not necessary to know the details of these tests. No test performs better than any other. All of these tests are better at predicting the absence, rather than the presence, of respiratory distress.

16. **What is the role of steroids in preterm labor?**
Steroids are often given with tocolytic agents (at 24 to 34 weeks of gestation) to hasten fetal lung maturity and thus decrease the risk of respiratory distress syndrome in the neonatal period.

17. **What problems may be encountered when oxytocin is used to augment labor?**
On the Step 3 exam, watch for uterine hyperstimulation (painful, overly frequent, and poorly coordinated uterine contractions), uterine rupture, fetal heart-rate decelerations, and water intoxication/hyponatremia (caused by the antidiuretic hormone effect of oxytocin). Treat all of these complications first by discontinuing the oxytocin infusion, for which the half-life is less than 10 minutes.

18. **What problems are associated with the use of intravaginal prostaglandin and amniotomy?**

   Prostaglandin E2 (dinoprostone) or misoprostol may be used locally to induce cervical effacement (a process sometimes called ripening) and is highly effective in combination with (or before) oxytocin administration. It also may cause uterine hyperstimulation. **Amniotomy** (creating a manual opening in the amniotic membrane) also hastens labor but exposes the fetus and uterine cavity to possible infection if labor does not occur promptly.

19. **What are the contraindications to labor induction or augmentation?**

   The list is almost the same as the list of contraindications to vaginal delivery: placenta or vasa previa, umbilical cord prolapse, prior classic (vertical) cesarean section, transverse fetal position, active genital herpes, cephalopelvic disproportion, and cervical cancer.

20. **What does a basic fetal heart trace show?**

   The fetal heart rate and the uterine contraction pattern over time.

21. **In fetal heart monitoring, what is the difference between early decelerations, late decelerations, and variable decelerations?**

   For **early decelerations** (Fig. 12-1), the peaks match up (nadir of fetal heart deceleration and peak of uterine contraction). This pattern signifies **head compression** (probably a vagal response) and is normal.

   Variable decelerations (Fig. 12-2) are so called because fetal heart rate deceleration varies in relation to uterine contractions. This is the type of deceleration pattern most commonly encountered and signifies **cord compression.** If it is observed, place the mother in the lateral decubitus position, administer oxygen via a face mask, and stop any oxytocin infusion. If the fetal bradycardia is severe (less than 80 to 90 beats/min) or fails to resolve, check the fetal oxygen saturation or scalp pH.

   Late decelerations (Fig. 12-3) occur when a fetal heart rate deceleration occurs after a uterine contraction. This pattern signifies **uteroplacental insufficiency** and is the most worrisome. If it is observed, first place the mother in the lateral decubitus position, give oxygen via a face mask, and stop any oxytocin infusion. Next, give a tocolytic agent (beta$_2$ agonist such as ritodrine or magnesium sulfate) if the mother is not in active labor and intravenous fluids (if the mother is hypotensive). If these late decelerations persist, measure the fetal oxygen saturation or scalp pH. Consider preparing the patient for operative delivery.

22. **What other patterns of fetal distress may be seen on a fetal heart tracing? What is a normal fetal heart rate?**

   Loss of short-term (beat-to-beat) variability, loss of long-term variability (or normal baseline changes in heart rate over 1 min), and prolonged fetal tachycardia (>160 beats/min). The normal fetal heart rate is 120 to 160 beats/min.

23. **What if the question gives you a value for fetal oxygen saturation or scalp pH?**

   Any fetal scalp pH less than 7.2 or an abnormally decreased oxygen saturation is an indication for immediate cesarean delivery. If the pH is greater than 7.2 or oxygenation is normal, you can generally continue to observe the mother and fetus.

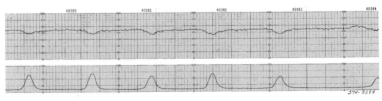

Figure 12-1. Early decelerations are caused by compression of the fetal head. They are shallow, symmetric, uniform decelerations that begin early in the contraction, have a nadir coincident with the peak of the contraction, and return to the baseline by the time the contraction is over. (*From Gabbe SG, Niebyl JR, Simpson JL. Obstetrics: normal and problem pregnancies, 5th ed. Philadelphia: Churchill Livingstone, 2007, Fig. 15-13.*)

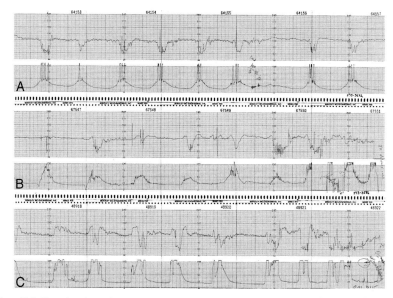

Figure 12-2. Examples of typical variable decelerations. Variable decelerations are often recognized by the accelerations that precede and follow the decelerations. *(From Gabbe SG, Niebyl JR, Simpson JL. Obstetrics: normal and problem pregnancies, 5th ed. Philadelphia: Churchill Livingstone, 2007, Fig. 15-18.)*

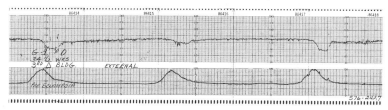

Figure 12-3. Late decelerations in a case complicated by third-trimester bleeding. Note the presence of persistent late decelerations with only three contractions in 20 minutes, as well as the apparent loss of variability of the fetal heart rate. The rise in baseline tone of the uterine activity channel cannot be evaluated with the external system. *(From Gabbe SG, Niebyl JR, Simpson JL. Obstetrics: normal and problem pregnancies, 5th ed. Philadelphia: Churchill Livingstone, 2007, Fig. 15-14.)*

24. Define the characteristics and duration of the normal stages of labor.

STAGE	CHARACTERISTICS	NULLIGRAVIDA	MULTIGRAVIDA
First stage	Onset of true labor to full cervical dilation	<20 h	<14 h
Latent phase	From 0 to 3-4 cm dilation (slow, irregular)	Highly variable	Highly variable
Active phase	From 3-4 cm to full dilation (rapid, regular)	>1 cm/h dilation	>1.2 cm/h dilation
Second stage	From full dilation to birth of baby	30 min-3 h	5-30 min
Third stage	Delivery of baby to delivery of placenta	0-30 min	0-30 min
Fourth stage	Placental delivery to maternal stabilization	Up to 48 h	Up to 48 h

25. Give the order of fetal positions during normal labor and delivery.
    1. Descent
    2. Flexion
    3. Internal rotation
    4. Extension
    5. External rotation
    6. Expulsion

26. **In the fetal circulation, where are the highest and lowest oxygen concentrations?**
    The highest oxygen concentration in the fetal circulation is in the umbilical vein (blood coming from the mother), and the lowest is in the umbilical arteries. Remember also that the oxygen concentration is higher in blood going to the upper extremities than in blood going to the lower extremities.

27. **What changes occur in the circulation as an infant goes from intrauterine to extrauterine life?**
    The first breaths inflate the lungs and cause decreased pulmonary vascular resistance, which increases blood flow to the pulmonary arteries. This and the clamping of the cord increase left-sided heart pressure, causing functional closure of the foramen ovale. The increased oxygen concentration shuts off prostaglandin production in the ductus arteriosus, causing gradual closure.

28. **Distinguish between a protraction disorder and an arrest disorder. What should you do when either occurs?**
    A **protraction disorder** occurs once true labor has begun if the mother takes longer than the table in Question 24 indicates, but labor nonetheless is progressing slowly. An **arrest disorder** (failure to progress) occurs once true labor has begun if no change in dilation is seen over 2 hours or no change in descent is seen over 1 hour.
    In either situation, first rule out an abnormal position and cephalopelvic disproportion. If neither is present, the mother can be treated with labor augmentation (e.g., oxytocin, prostaglandin). If these steps fail, manage expectantly and perform a cesarean section at the first sign of trouble.

29. **What is the most common cause of protraction or arrest disorder?**
    Cephalopelvic disproportion, which is a disparity between the size of the infant's head and the size of the mother's pelvis. Labor augmentation is contraindicated in this setting.

30. **What should you do if shoulder dystocia or impaction occurs during a vaginal delivery?**
    The first step is to try the McRoberts maneuver. Have the mother sharply flex her thighs against her abdomen, which may free the impacted shoulder. Other maneuvers include applying suprapubic pressure, a Woods screw maneuver (rotates the fetus so the anterior shoulder emerges from behind the maternal symphysis), delivery of the posterior arm, and fracture of the clavicle (risky). If these maneuvers fail, the options are limited. A cesarean section is usually the procedure of choice (after pushing the infant's head back into the birth canal).

31. **What are the signs of placental separation during delivery?**
    The signs of placental separation include a fresh show of blood from the vagina, lengthening of the umbilical cord, and a rising fundus that becomes firm and globular.

32. **What is an APGAR score? When is it measured?**
    The APGAR score is a general measure of well-being in newborns. It is commonly assessed at 1 and 5 minutes after birth if values are normal. If the score is less than 7, continue to assess every 5 minutes until the infant reaches a score of 7 or more (while resuscitating the child as needed). There are five APGAR score categories, with a maximum score of 2 points per category and a possible total of 10 points. Remember the APGAR mnemonic: **a**ppearance (skin color), **p**ulse (heart rate), **g**rimace (reflex irritability), **a**ctivity (muscle tone), and **r**espiration (breathing).

Category	NUMBER OF POINTS GIVEN		
	0	1	2
Color	Pale, blue	Body pink, extremities blue	Completely pink
Heart rate	Absent	<100 beats/min	>100 beats/min
Reflex irritability*	None	Grimace	Grimace and strong cry, cough, sneeze
Muscle tone	Limp	Some flexion of extremities	Active moan
Respiratory effort	None	Slow, weak cry	Good, strong cry

*Reflex irritability is usually measured as the infant's response to stimulation of the sole of the foot or catheter insertion into the nose.

33. **True or false: The APGAR score is important because it is the first assessment of how a child is doing.**
False. Do not wait until the 1-minute mark to evaluate the infant. You may have to suction or intubate the infant seconds after delivery.

34. **Which vitamin is given to all newborns?**
Vitamin K is given as prophylaxis against hemorrhagic disease of the newborn.

35. **True or false: After cesarean section, a patient may have a vaginal delivery in the future.**
The answer depends on the circumstances. After a classic (vertical) uterine incision, patients must have cesarean sections for all future deliveries because of the increased rate of uterine rupture during vaginal delivery. After a lower (horizontal) uterine incision (the incision of choice), a patient may deliver future pregnancies vaginally with only a slightly increased (i.e., acceptable) risk of uterine rupture.

36. **Define lochia. When is it a problem?**
For the first several days after delivery, some vaginal discharge (known as lochia) is normal. It is red for the first few days and gradually turns white or yellowish white by day 10. If the lochia smells foul, suspect endometritis.

37. **What treatment may be given to a woman who does not want to breastfeed?**
Because the breasts can be become engorged with milk and thus quite painful, you may prescribe a tight-fitting bra, ice packs, and analgesia to reduce symptoms. Medications for suppression of lactation (e.g., bromocriptine and estrogens or oral contraceptive pills) are generally no longer recommended because of the risk of thromboembolism and stroke.

38. **List the common contraindications to breastfeeding.**
   • Use of alcohol or illicit drugs (with a few caveats that will not be tested on the USMLE)
   • HIV infection (although the World Health Organization recommends breastfeeding in developing countries if replacement feeding is not possible)
   • Some medications, including antineoplastic agents, antimetabolic agents (cyclophosphamide, mercaptopurine), some anticonvulsants (topiramate), and amiodarone

39. **When does mastitis occur? How do you recognize and treat it?**
Mastitis (inflammation of the breast) usually develops in the first 2 months after delivery. Breasts are red, indurated, and painful, and nipple cracks or fissuring may be seen. *Staphylococcus aureus* is the usual cause. Treat with analgesics (e.g., acetaminophen, ibuprofen), warm and/or cold compresses, and continued breastfeeding from the affected breast(s) even if painful (use a breast pump to empty the breast if needed) to prevent further milk duct blockage and abscess formation. An antistaphylococcal antibiotic (e.g., cephalexin, dicloxacillin) is usually given for more than mild symptoms. If a fluctuant mass develops or there is no response to antibiotics within a few days, an abscess is probably present and must be drained.

40. **What are the major causes of maternal mortality associated with childbirth?**
In decreasing order: pulmonary embolism, pregnancy-induced hypertension (preeclampsia or eclampsia), and hemorrhage.

41. **How do you recognize an amniotic fluid pulmonary embolism?**
Look for a recently postpartum mother who develops sudden shortness of breath, tachypnea, chest pain, hypotension, and disseminated intravascular coagulation. Treatment is supportive.

42. **What factors predispose to uterine rupture? What are the symptoms? How is it treated?**
Predisposing factors include previous uterine surgery (especially a prior caesarian section with vertical incision), trauma, oxytocin, grand multiparity (several previous deliveries), excessive uterine distention (e.g., multiple gestation, polyhydramnios), abnormal fetal position, cephalopelvic disproportion, and shoulder dystocia. Uterine rupture is very painful, has a sudden and dramatic onset, and is often accompanied by maternal hypotension or shock. Other classic signs are the ability to feel fetal body parts on abdominal examination and a change in the abdominal contour. Maternal distress is usually more pronounced than fetal distress (unlike abruptio placentae, in which fetal distress is greater). Treat with immediate laparotomy and delivery. Hysterectomy is usually required after delivery.

43. **Define postpartum hemorrhage. What are the common causes?**
Postpartum hemorrhage is defined as a blood loss greater than 500 mL during vaginal delivery or greater than 1 L during cesarean section. The most common cause is **uterine atony** (75% to 80% of cases). Other causes include lacerations, retained placental tissue, coagulation disorders, low placental implantation, and uterine inversion. Retained placental tissue results from placenta accreta (penetration of the placenta through the endometrium into the myometrium), placenta increta (deeper penetration of the placenta into the myometrium), or placenta percreta (penetration of the placenta through the myometrium to the uterine serosa. In all three conditions, the placenta grows more deeply into the uterine wall than it should. The major risk factor for this condition is previous uterine surgery or cesarean section, and the usual treatment is hysterectomy.

44. **What causes uterine atony? How is it treated?**
Uterine atony is caused by overdistention of the uterus (because of multiple gestation, polyhydramnios, or macrosomia), prolonged labor, oxytocin administration, grand multiparity (a history of five or more deliveries), and precipitous labor (too fast or less than 3 hours). Treat with a dilute oxytocin infusion, and use bimanual compression to massage the uterus while the oxytocin infusion is running. If this approach fails, use ergonovine (contraindicated for maternal hypertension), prostaglandin F$_2$-alpha, or misoprostol. If these strategies also fail, the patient may need a hysterectomy; ligation of the uterine vessels can be attempted if the patient wants to retain fertility.

45. **What is the treatment for retained products of conception?**
For retained products of conception (which is probably the most common cause of a *delayed* postpartum hemorrhage), remove the placenta manually to stop the bleeding. Next try curettage in the operating room under anesthesia. If the patient has placenta accreta, placenta increta, or placenta percreta, hysterectomy is usually necessary to stop the bleeding.

46. **What causes uterine inversion? How is it treated?**
When the uterus inverts, it can usually be seen outside the vagina. It is usually iatrogenic, a result of *pulling too hard on the cord*. If inversion occurs, put the uterus back in place manually; you may need to use anesthesia because of pain. Give intravenous fluids and oxytocin.

47. **Define postpartum fever. What are the common causes?**
Postpartum fever is a temperature greater than 100.4° F (38° C) for at least 2 consecutive days and is classically due to endometritis. However, do not forget easy causes of postpartum fever, such as a urinary tract infection or atelectasis/pneumonia. Pulmonary problems are especially common after a cesarean section. Other causes include a pelvic abscess and pelvic thrombophlebitis.

48. **What is the most common cause of endometritis (puerperal fever)? How do you recognize and treat it?**
Watch for endometritis, an infection of the endometrial lining, as a cause of postpartum fever. The hallmark is uterine tenderness and the most common cause is *Streptococcus* species. Treat with clindamycin plus gentamicin after local cultures have been carried out.

49. **What are the presenting symptoms of chorioamnionitis and how is it treated?**
Patients with chorioamnionitis have a fever and a tender, irritable uterus, usually after delivery. Antepartum chorioamnionitis may occur in patients with PROM. Order a culture and Gram stain of the cervix and amniotic fluid, and treat the patient with antibiotics such as ampicillin plus gentamicin while awaiting the culture results.

50. **What should you do if a patient has postpartum fever?**
Look for clues in the history and physical examination. For example, for a patient with a history of PROM and a tender uterus on examination, endometritis is almost certainly the cause of the fever. Next, order cultures of the endometrium, vagina, blood, and urine. Start empiric antibiotic treatment if indicated. Clindamycin plus gentamicin is a good choice; add "big-gun" antibiotics if the patient is crashing.

51. **What should you do if postpartum fever does not improve with antibiotics?**
If a postpartum fever does not resolve with broad-spectrum antibiotics, there are two main possibilities: progression to a pelvic abscess or pelvic thrombophlebitis. A computed tomography (CT) scan will show any pelvic abscess, which should be drained, and sometimes demonstrates thrombophlebitis. Pelvic thrombophlebitis has symptoms of a persistent spiking fever, a lack of response to antibiotics, and no abscess on CT. Give heparin or low-molecular-weight heparin as a cure (and for diagnosis in retrospect).

52. **What should you consider if a postpartum patient goes into shock without evident bleeding?**
   - Amniotic fluid embolism
   - Uterine inversion
   - Concealed hemorrhage (e.g., uterine rupture with bleeding into the peritoneal cavity)

FETUS AND NEWBORN

1. **Define stillbirth.**
A stillbirth (fetal death) is a prenatal or natal (during delivery) death after 20 weeks of gestation.

2. **Name the major cause of neonatal mortality. What is the neonatal mortality rate in the United States?**
The major cause of neonatal mortality is prematurity. The neonatal mortality rate in the United States is roughly 6 in 1000 births (higher in blacks).

3. **List the top three causes of infant mortality in the United States.**
   - Congenital abnormalities
   - Prematurity/low birth weight
   - Sudden infant death syndrome

4. **True or false: Roughly 85% of cases of mental retardation are mild.**
True. Patients with mild mental retardation can have a reasonable level of independence, with assistance or guidance during periods of stress.

5. **What are the common causes of mental retardation?**
Although mental retardation is usually idiopathic, look for fetal alcohol syndrome (the leading preventable cause of mental retardation), Down syndrome (leading overall known cause of mental retardation), and fragile X syndrome (in males).

6. **What screening tests are commonly performed for metabolic and congenital disorders?**
States vary widely in their policies regarding newborn screening. All states screen for hypothyroidism and phenylketonuria at birth; screens must be performed within the first month of life. Most states screen for galactosemia and hemoglobinopathies such as sickle cell disease. Some states include screening for homocystinuria, maple syrup urine disease, congenital adrenal hyperplasia, cystic fibrosis, biotinidase deficiency, tyrosinemia, and toxoplasmosis. If any of these screens are positive, the first step is to order a confirmatory test to make sure that the screening test gave you a true-positive result.

7. **How many vessels does a normal umbilical cord have? What disorder should you suspect if one of the vessels is absent?**
The umbilical cord is checked at birth for the presence of the normal three vessels: two arteries and one vein. If only one artery is present, consider the possibility of congenital renal malformations.

8. **Which gastrointestinal malformation causes primarily respiratory problems?**
Diaphragmatic hernia, which is more common in males. Ninety percent are on the left side. The main point to know is that bowel herniates into the thorax through the diaphragmatic defect, compressing the lung and impeding lung development (pulmonary hypoplasia develops). Patients present with respiratory distress and have bowel sounds in the chest and bowel loops in the thorax on chest radiographs. Treat with surgical correction of the diaphragm.

9. **What is the first step in evaluating neonatal jaundice? Why is jaundice of concern in a neonate?**
The first step is to determine whether the jaundice is physiologic or pathologic. Measure total, direct, and indirect bilirubin. The main concern is **kernicterus,** which is due to high levels of unconjugated bilirubin with subsequent deposition in the basal ganglia. Look for poor feeding, seizures, flaccidity, opisthotonos, and apnea in the setting of severe jaundice.

10. **What causes physiologic jaundice of the newborn? Who gets it?**
Fifty percent of normal infants have physiologic jaundice, and it is even more common in premature infants. Bilirubin is mostly unconjugated because of incomplete maturation of liver function. In full-term infants, bilirubin is less than 12 mg/dL, peaks during days 2 to 4, and returns to normal by 2 weeks. In premature infants, bilirubin is less than 15 mg/dL, peaks during days 3 to 5, and may be elevated for up to 3 weeks.

11. **How is pathologic jaundice recognized? What are the causes?**
In pathologic jaundice, bilirubin levels are higher than those mentioned in the previous question and continue to rise or fail to decrease appropriately. **Any jaundice present at birth is pathologic.** Causes include the following:
Breastfeeding jaundice: occurs in 1 in 10 breastfed infants and is seen in the first week of life. This is essentially an exaggerated physiologic jaundice due to insufficient milk intake, which leads to an inadequate number of bowel movements to remove bilirubin from the body.
Breast milk jaundice: occurs in breastfed infants with peak bilirubin levels of 10 to 20 mg/dL at 2 to 3 weeks of age. Treat with temporary cessation of breastfeeding (switch to bottle feeding) until the jaundice resolves.
Illness: infection or sepsis, hypothyroidism, liver insult, cystic fibrosis, and other illnesses may prolong neonatal jaundice and lower the threshold for kernicterus. The youngest, sickest infants are at greatest risk of hyperbilirubinemia and kernicterus.
Hemolysis: occurs because of Rh incompatibility or congenital red cell diseases that cause hemolysis in the neonatal period. Look for anemia, peripheral smear abnormalities, a positive family history, and higher levels of unconjugated bilirubin.
Metabolic disorders: Crigler-Najjar syndrome causes severe unconjugated hyperbilirubinemia, whereas Gilbert syndrome causes a mild form. Rotor and Dubin-Johnson syndromes cause conjugated hyperbilirubinemia.
Biliary atresia: full-term infants with clay- or gray-colored stools and high levels of conjugated bilirubin. Treat with surgery.
Medications: avoid sulfa drugs in neonates; they displace bilirubin from albumin and may precipitate kernicterus.

12. **How is pathologic jaundice treated?**
Unconjugated hyperbilirubinemia that persists, rises above 15 mg/dL, or rises rapidly is treated with **phototherapy** to convert unconjugated bilirubin to a water-soluble form that can be excreted. A last resort is exchange transfusion, but do not consider this approach unless the level of unconjugated bilirubin is greater than 20 mg/dL.

13. **What should you do if an infant is born to a mother with active hepatitis B?**
    An infant born to a mother with active hepatitis B should receive the first immunization shot and hepatitis B immune globulin at birth.

14. **Describe the effects of alcohol on pregnancy.**
    Alcohol is a definite teratogen and is the most common cause of preventable mental retardation in the United States. You should be able to recognize the classic presentation of a child affected by fetal alcohol syndrome: mental retardation, microcephaly, microphthalmia, short palpebral fissures, midfacial hypoplasia, a smooth philtrum, and cardiac defects. No amount of alcohol consumption can be considered safe during pregnancy. Fetal alcohol syndrome rates vary but may affect as many as 1 in 1000 births in the United States.

15. **What is the usual cause of vaginal bleeding in neonates? How is it treated?**
    Vaginal bleeding in neonates is usually physiologic and due to maternal estrogen withdrawal. No treatment is needed because the bleeding resolves on its own.

16. **What causes DiGeorge syndrome? How do you recognize it?**
    DiGeorge syndrome is caused by a chromosomal deletion at 22q11.2. It causes hypoplasia of the third and fourth pharyngeal pouches. Look for hypocalcemia and tetany (from hypocalcemia caused by absent parathyroid glands) in the first 24 to 48 hours of life. The thymus may also be absent or hypoplastic, and congenital heart defects and typical facies are often present.

17. **How do you recognize Down syndrome?**
    Down syndrome (trisomy 21) is the most common known cause of mental retardation in the United States. The biggest risk factor is maternal age (1 in 1500 offspring of 16-year-old mothers and 1 in 25 offspring of 45-year-old mothers). At birth look for hypotonia, a transverse palmar crease, and characteristic facies (Fig. 12-4). Congenital cardiac defects (especially ventricular septal defects) are common, and affected individuals have an increased risk of leukemia, duodenal atresia, and early Alzheimer disease.

18. **What is the second most common known cause of inherited mental retardation?**
    Fragile X syndrome (X-linked recessive). Affected males often have large testicles.

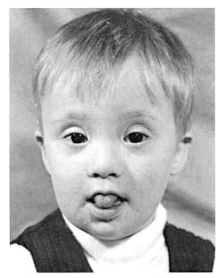

Figure 12-4. Child with Down syndrome. Note the flat facial profile, flat nasal bridge, open mouth, protruding tongue, folded ears, and epicanthic folds. (*From Kliegman RM. Nelson textbook of pediatrics, 19th ed. Philadelphia: Saunders, 2011. Fig. 76-8A.*)

19. **How do you recognize neonatal hypoglycemia? At what concentration is blood glucose considered to be low?**

Signs of neonatal hypoglycemia are nonspecific, but look for jitteriness, hypotonia, lethargy, irritability, tachypnea, apnea/cyanosis, bradycardia, poor feeding, hypothermia, a weak cry, and seizures.

It is challenging and rather controversial to use a specific blood glucose concentration to determine hypoglycemia, but the American Academy of Pediatrics defines neonatal hypoglycemia as blood glucose of less than 47 mg/dL.

20. **What are risk factors for neonatal hypoglycemia?**

Prematurity, being large or small for gestational age, infants of diabetic mothers, and infants of mothers who were treated with oral hypoglycemic or beta-adrenergic agents.

21. **What is the management of neonatal hypoglycemia?**

Treatment is stepwise, depending on whether signs and symptoms are present and on how the infant responds to each intervention. Start with feeding breast milk for asymptomatic infants. The next step is an intravenous glucose infusion. Glucocorticoids are next, followed by glucagon, if necessary.

22. **What presentation suggests galactosemia?**

Congenital cataracts and neonatal sepsis with vomiting after breastfeeding. Patients should avoid galactose- and lactose-containing foods.

23. **Define macrosomia. What is the likely cause?**

Macrosomia is defined as a newborn that weighs more than 4 kg (roughly 9 lb). The cause is maternal diabetes mellitus until proven otherwise.

24. **Cover the right-hand column in the following table and specify the effects of the listed classic teratogens on an exposed fetus.**

AGENT	DEFECTS CAUSED
Thalidomide	Phocomelia (absence of long bones and flipper-like appearance of the hands)
Antineoplastic drugs	Many
Tetracycline	Yellow or brown teeth
Aminoglycosides	Deafness
Valproic acid	Spina bifida, hypospadias
Progesterone	Masculinization of female fetus
Cigarettes	Intrauterine growth retardation, low birth weight, prematurity
Oral contraceptive pills	VACTERL syndrome
Lithium	Cardiac (Ebstein) anomalies
Radiation	Intrauterine growth retardation, central nervous system defects, eye defects, malignancy (e.g., leukemia)
Alcohol	Fetal alcohol syndrome
Phenytoin	Craniofacial, limb, and cerebrovascular defects; mental retardation
Warfarin	Craniofacial defects, intrauterine growth retardation, central nervous system malformation, stillbirth
Carbamazepine	Fingernail hypoplasia, craniofacial defects
Isotretinoin*	Central nervous system, craniofacial, ear, and cardiovascular defects

AGENT	DEFECTS CAUSED
Iodine	Goiter, neonatal hypothyroidism
Cocaine	Cerebral infarcts, mental retardation
Diazepam	Cleft lip and/or palate
Diethylstilbestrol	Clear cell vaginal cancer, adenosis, cervical incompetence

VACTERL, Vertebral anomalies, imperforate anus, cardiac anomalies, tracheoesophageal fistula, renal anomalies, limb anomalies.
*Vitamin A is generally considered teratogenic when recommended intake levels are exceeded.

25. **Which vitamin is a known teratogen?**
Vitamin A. Female patients taking one of the vitamin A analogs as treatment for acne must have a negative pregnancy test before the medication is started and should be counseled about the risks of teratogenicity. Some form of birth control should be used, and periodic pregnancy tests should be offered.
   Isotretinoin is such a significant teratogen that access to this medication is very restricted. All patients and prescribers must be in a special program designed to eliminate fetal exposure to isotretinoin. There are strict qualification criteria, including monthly pregnancy testing, and two forms of contraception are recommended.

26. **Define oligohydramnios. What causes it? Why is it worrisome?**
Oligohydramnios is a deficiency of amniotic fluid (<500 mL or an amniotic fluid index of <5). Causes include IUGR, PROM, postmaturity, and renal agenesis (Potter disease). Oligo-hydramnios may cause fetal problems, including pulmonary hypoplasia, cutaneous or skeletal abnormalities caused by compression, and hypoxia caused by cord compression.

27. **Define polyhydramnios. What causes it? Why is it worrisome?**
Polyhydramnios is an excess of amniotic fluid (>2 L or an amniotic fluid index of >25). Causes include maternal diabetes, multiple gestation, neural tube defects (anencephaly, spina bifida), gastrointestinal anomalies (omphalocele, esophageal atresia), and hydrops fetalis. Polyhydramnios can cause maternal problems, including postpartum uterine atony (with resultant postpartum hemorrhage) and maternal dyspnea (an overdistended uterus compromises pulmonary function).

28. **Distinguish between caput succedaneum and cephalohematoma. How are these conditions treated?**
Both conditions are noted in newborns after vaginal delivery. Caput succedaneum is diffuse swelling or edema of the scalp that crosses the midline, is benign, and requires no further investigation or treatment. Cephalohematomas are subperiosteal hemorrhages that are sharply limited by sutures and do not cross the midline. Cephalohematomas are usually benign and self-resolving, but in rare cases they may indicate an underlying skull fracture. Order a radiograph or CT scan to rule out fracture if given the option.

29. **What should you know about infant respiratory distress syndrome?**
Infant respiratory distress syndrome is due to atelectasis from a deficiency of surfactant; it is seen almost exclusively in premature infants and infants of diabetic mothers. Look for rapid, labored respirations; substernal retractions; cyanosis; grunting; and/or nasal flaring. Arterial blood gas results show hypoxemia and hypercarbia; radiography reveals diffuse atelectasis (described as diffuse, granular infiltrates). Treat with oxygen, give a surfactant, and intubate if necessary. Complications include intraventricular hemorrhage and pneumothorax or bronchopulmonary dysplasia (complications of acute or chronic mechanical ventilation).

30. **What prenatal tests help to indicate whether respiratory distress syndrome will occur?**
Measurement of amniotic fluid in the pregnant mother can indicate whether the fetus is producing adequate surfactant. A lecithin-to-sphingomyelin ratio of greater than 2:1 or the presence of **phosphatidylglycerol** in the amniotic fluid indicates fetal lung maturity and a low

likelihood of infant respiratory distress syndrome. The fluorescence polarization test reflects the ratio of surfactant to albumin in amniotic fluid and is a direct measure of surfactant concentration. An elevated ratio indicates fetal lung maturity.

31. **Define diaphragmatic hernia. How is it recognized clinically?**
    A defect in the diaphragm allows the bowel to herniate into the chest. Diaphragmatic hernia is mentioned in the pulmonary section because the presenting symptom is respiratory difficulty, not gastrointestinal problems. Herniated bowel pushes on the developing lung and causes lung hypoplasia on the affected side. Look for a scaphoid abdomen and bowel sounds in the chest. Herniated bowel can be seen on chest radiographs; 90% of cases are left sided.

32. **How do you recognize and diagnose a tracheoesophageal fistula? How is it treated?**
    The most common type (85% of cases) of tracheoesophageal fistula is an esophagus with a blind pouch proximally and a fistula between a bronchus/carina and the distal esophagus (Fig. 12-5). Look for a neonate with excessive oral secretions, coughing or cyanosis on attempted feeding, abdominal distention, and aspiration pneumonia. The diagnosis is made on the basis of an inability to insert a nasogastric tube; alternatively, an injection of air via a nasogastric tube under x-ray (i.e., fluoroscopy) guidance shows only the proximal esophagus. Treatment is early surgical correction.

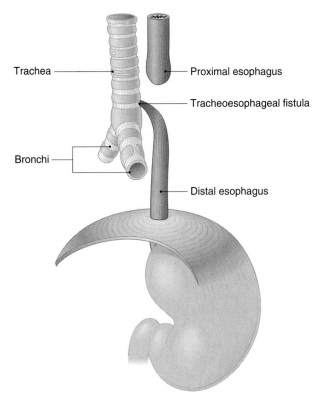

Figure 12-5. Tracheoesophageal fistula. Diagram of the most common type of esophageal atresia and tracheo-esophageal fistula. (*From Gilbert-Barness E. Potter's pathology of the fetus, infant and child, 2nd ed. Philadelphia: Mosby, 2007. Fig. 25-6).*

PERINATAL INFECTIONS

1. **What are the three common causes of neonatal conjunctivitis?**
   Chemicals, *Neisseria gonorrhoeae,* and *Chlamydia trachomatis.*

2. **What causes chemical conjunctivitis? How do you recognize it?**
   Chemical conjunctivitis is caused by the silver nitrate (or erythromycin) drops that are given to all newborns to prevent gonorrheal conjunctivitis. The drops may cause chemical conjunctivitis (with no purulent discharge) that appears within 12 hours of administration and resolves within 48 hours. Chemical conjunctivitis is always the best guess if conjunctivitis develops in the first 24 hours of life.

3. **How can you distinguish gonorrheal from chlamydial conjunctivitis?**
   In cases of suspected **gonorrheal conjunctivitis,** look for symptoms of gonorrhea in the mother. The infant has an extremely purulent discharge starting between 2 and 5 days after birth. Infants who were given prophylactic drops should not develop gonorrheal conjunctivitis. Treatment involves systemic ceftriaxone or cefotaxime.
   In cases of **chlamydial (inclusion) conjunctivitis,** the mother often reports no symptoms. The infant has mild to severe conjunctivitis beginning between 5 and 14 days after birth. Oral erythromycin is recommended for chlamydial conjunctivitis and pneumonia; topical therapy for chlamydial conjunctivitis is not effective.

4. **If you forget everything else about neonatal conjunctivitis, what point should you remember to help you distinguish among the three causes discussed?**
   The varying time frames during which they occur.

5. **What is the definition of neonatal sepsis? What pathogens typically cause neonatal sepsis? What are the risk factors?**
   Neonatal sepsis is a syndrome that manifests as systemic signs of infection and/or isolation of a bacterial pathogen in the bloodstream of an infant 28 days old or younger. Early-onset sepsis usually is due to vertical transmission from amniotic fluid or during vaginal delivery from bacteria colonizing or infecting the mother's lower genital tract. Late-onset sepsis comes either from maternal vertical transmission or from contact with care providers or environmental sources. GBS and *E. coli* are the most common causes. *Listeria monocytogenes* is another cause of sepsis but is rare and is usually seen during outbreaks of listeriosis. *S. aureus* is an emerging pathogen; enterococci and other gram-negative rods can also cause neonatal sepsis.

6. **What are the maternal and neonatal risk factors for neonatal sepsis?**
   Intrapartum maternal fever, delivery at less than 37 weeks of gestation, chorioamnionitis, a 5-minute APGAR score of 6 or less, evidence of fetal distress, maternal GBS colonization, and a duration of 18 hours or longer since membrane rupture.

7. **What are the clinical manifestations of neonatal sepsis?**
   The signs and symptoms are subtle and nonspecific, so be careful. Look for temperature instability, jaundice, respiratory distress, hepatomegaly, anorexia, vomiting, lethargy, cyanosis, and apnea. Also look for abdominal distention, irritability, and diarrhea, although these are less common.

8. **How do you evaluate an infant with suspected neonatal sepsis?**
   Blood culture, CBC, chest x-ray (if respiratory abnormalities are present), and lumbar puncture. Neutropenia is a fairly specific marker for neonatal sepsis. A urine culture should be ordered if the child is older than 6 days.

9. **How do you treat neonatal sepsis?**
   Treat empirically with ampicillin and gentamicin for early-onset sepsis to cover GBS and *E. coli.* Empirical treatment for late-onset neonatal sepsis (infants older than 7 days of age) is ampicillin and gentamicin if the infant is being admitted from the community. For an infant who has been hospitalized since birth, substitute vancomycin for ampicillin to cover antimicrobial-resistant organisms.

10. **What else do you need to know about GBS?**
    GBS, also known as *Streptococcus agalactiae*, is the most common cause of neonatal meningitis or sepsis. The organism is often part of the normal vaginal flora and may be acquired from the birth canal. GBS is penicillin sensitive. Expectant mothers are cultured for GBS; if it is present around the time of delivery, then prophylactic intravenous penicillin (preferred) or intravenous ampicillin is given to the mother to prevent meningitis in the newborn.

11. **What are the TORCH syndromes? What do they cause?**
    TORCH is an acronym for several maternal infections that can cross the placenta and cause intrauterine fetal infections that may result in birth defects. Most TORCH infections can cause mental retardation, microcephaly, hydrocephalus, hepatosplenomegaly, jaundice, anemia, low birth weight, and IUGR. These infections include:
    T = **T***oxoplasma gondii*: look for exposure to cats. Specific defects include intracranial calcifications and chorioretinitis.
    O = **O**ther agents: varicella zoster causes limb hypoplasia and scarring of the skin. Syphilis causes rhinitis, saber shins, Hutchinson teeth, interstitial keratitis, and skin lesions.
    R = **R**ubella: worst in the first trimester (some recommend abortion if the mother has rubella in the first trimester). Always check antibody status on the first visit for patients with a poor immunization history. Look for cardiovascular defects, deafness, cataracts, and microphthalmia.
    C = **C**ytomegalovirus: most common infection of the TORCH group. Look for deafness, cerebral calcifications, and microphthalmia.
    H = **H**erpes: look for vesicular skin lesions (with positive Tzanck smears) and a history of maternal herpes lesions.

12. **What do you need to know about HIV testing and transmission from a mother to her child?**
    In untreated HIV-positive patients, HIV is transmitted to the fetus in roughly 25% of cases. When triple-drug therapy is given to the mother prenatally and zidovudine is given to the infant for 6 weeks after birth, HIV transmission is reduced to roughly 2%. A noninfected infant may still have a positive HIV antibody test at birth because maternal antibodies can cross the placenta. Within 6 to 18 months, however, the test result reverts to negative. This is why infants of infected mothers are tested using a direct HIV DNA polymerase chain reaction test at birth, at 4 to 6 weeks of age, and 2 months after the second test. Babies who have these three negative tests should have an HIV antibody test at 12 and 18 months of age. Cesarean section may reduce HIV transmission to the child.

13. **What should you do if a pregnant woman has genital herpes?**
    A decision is generally made when the mother goes into labor (not beforehand). If, at the time of true labor, the mother has active, visible genital herpes lesions, perform a cesarean section to prevent transmission to the fetus. If, at the time of true labor, the mother has no visible genital herpes lesions, the child can be delivered vaginally.

14. **What should you do for a child if the mother has chronic hepatitis B or chickenpox?**
    If the mother has chronic hepatitis B, give the infant the first hepatitis B vaccine shot and hepatitis B immunoglobulin at birth. If the mother contracts chickenpox in the last 5 days of pregnancy or the first 2 days after delivery, give the infant varicella zoster immunoglobulin.

15. **What subtype of maternal antibody can cross the placenta?**
    IgG is the only type of maternal antibody that crosses the placenta. This may be an important diagnostic point: an elevated neonatal IgM concentration is never normal, whereas an elevated neonatal IgG often represents maternal antibodies.

CHAPTER 13

DISORDERS OF BLOOD

SPLENIC DISORDERS

1. **What do you need to know about splenic rupture?**
   The spleen is the organ most commonly injured in blunt trauma. Patients with splenic rupture, the most severe form of injury, have a history of blunt abdominal trauma, hypotension, tachycardia, shock, and/or the **Kehr sign** (referred pain in the left shoulder). Patients with Epstein-Barr virus infection or infectious mononucleosis and splenomegaly should avoid contact sports to prevent rupture. Make sure that patients needing splenectomy have received the pneumococcal, meningococcal, and *Haemophilus influenzae* (i.e., encapsulated bugs) vaccines. Splenic injury in children (and more mild injury in adults) is often treated nonoperatively if possible to prevent the morbidity of splenectomy and the risk of future infection with encapsulated bacteria.

ANEMIAS AND CYTOPENIAS

1. **Define anemia.**
   Anemia involves a hemoglobin level of less than 12 mg/dL in women or less than 14 mg/dL in men.

2. **What are the symptoms and signs of anemia?**
   Symptoms: fatigue, dyspnea on exertion, light-headedness, dizziness, syncope, palpitations, angina, and claudication.
   Signs: tachycardia, pallor (especially of the sclera and mucous membranes), systolic ejection murmurs (from high flow), and signs of the underlying cause (e.g., jaundice and/or pigment **gallstones** in hemolytic anemia, positive stool guaiac for a gastrointestinal [GI] bleed).

3. **What are the important elements of the history when a patient has anemia?**
   Important points include medications, blood loss (e.g., trauma, surgery, melena, hematemesis, menorrhagia), chronic diseases (anemia of chronic disease), family history (e.g., hemophilia, thalassemia, sickle cell disease, glucose-6-phosphate dehydrogenase (G6PD) deficiency), and alcoholism (which may lead to iron, folate, and B_{12} deficiencies, as well as GI bleeds).

4. **What findings help you in the setting of acute blood loss as a cause of anemia?**
   The important point is that immediately after blood loss the hemoglobin may be normal; it takes at least 3 to 4 hours, often more, for reequilibration. Look for obvious bleeding, pale and cold skin, tachycardia, and hypotension (signs of hypovolemic shock). Transfuse if indicated, even for a normal hemoglobin level, in the acute setting. Consider internal hemorrhage in the setting of trauma and abdominal aortic aneurysm in patients with a pulsatile abdominal mass.

5. **What medications can cause anemia? How?**
   Many medications can cause anemia through various mechanisms. Methyldopa, penicillins, and sulfa drugs can cause red blood cell antibodies with subsequent hemolysis; chloroquine and sulfa drugs cause hemolysis in patients with G6PD deficiency; phenytoin causes megaloblastic anemia through interference with folate metabolism; and chloramphenicol, cancer drugs, and zidovudine cause aplastic anemia and bone marrow suppression. Other drugs are also implicated, but this list should be sufficient for the USMLE.

6. **What test should be ordered first to help determine the cause of anemia?**
   A complete blood count (CBC) with red blood cell (RBC) indices. First, the hemoglobin level must be below normal to diagnose anemia. The mean corpuscular volume (MCV) tells you whether the anemia is microcytic (MCV <80 fL), normocytic (MCV = 80 to 100 fL), or macrocytic (MCV >100 fL).

7. **What test should be ordered next?**
   A peripheral blood smear. Many classic findings can help in making diagnoses:
   - Sickled cells (sickle cell disease; Fig. 13-1)
   - Hypersegmented neutrophils (folate/B_{12} deficiency; Fig. 13-2)
   - Hypochromic and microcytic RBCs (iron deficiency; Fig. 13-3)
   - Basophilic stippling (lead poisoning; Fig. 13-4)
   - Bite cells (classically, G6PD deficiency; other hemolytic anemias; Fig. 13-5)
   - Heinz bodies (G6PD deficiency; see Fig. 13-5)
   - Howell-Jolly bodies (asplenia; Fig. 13-6)
   - Teardrop-shaped RBCs (myelofibrosis; Fig. 13-7)
   - Schistocytes, helmet cells, and fragmented RBCs (intravascular hemolysis; Fig. 13-8)
   - Spherocytes and elliptocytes (hereditary spherocytosis and elliptocytosis; Fig. 13-9)
   - Acanthocytes and spur cells (abetalipoproteinemia; Fig. 13-10)
   - Target cells (thalassemia, liver disease; Fig. 13-11)
   - Echinocytes, including burr cells and acanthocytes (uremia; Fig. 13-12)
   - Polychromasia (from **reticulocytosis**; should alert you to the possibility of hemolysis; Fig. 13-13)

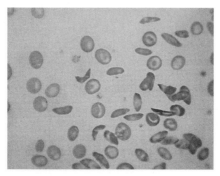

Figure 13-1. Sickle cells show a sickle or crescent shape resulting from polymerization of hemoglobin S. This smear also shows target cells and boat-shaped cells with a lesser degree of polymerization of hemoglobin S than in a classic sickle cell. See Plate 26. (*From Goldman L, Schafer AI. Goldman's Cecil medicine, 24th ed. Philadelphia: Saunders, 2011, Fig. 160-7.*)

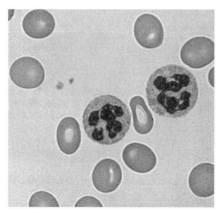

Figure 13-2. Megaloblastic changes of macrocytosis and a hypersegmented neutrophil. See Plate 27. (*From Goldman L, Schafer AI. Goldman's Cecil medicine, 24th ed. Philadelphia: Saunders, 2011, Fig. 170-6.*)

- Rouleaux formation (multiple myeloma; Fig. 13-14)
- Parasites inside RBCs (malaria [Fig. 13-15], babesiosis)
- Iron inclusions in RBCs of the bone marrow (sideroblastic anemia; Fig. 13-16)

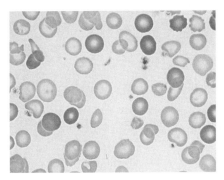

Figure 13-3. Iron-deficiency anemia. Pale red blood cells with an enlarged central area of pallor. See Plate 28. (*From McPherson R, Pincus M. Henry's clinical diagnosis and management by laboratory methods, 21st ed. Philadelphia: Saunders, 2006, Fig. 31-2.*)

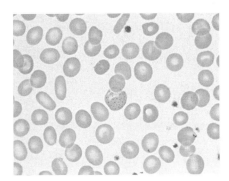

Figure 13-4. Basophilic stippling. Irregular basophilic granules in red blood cells; often associated with lead poisoning and thalassemia. See Plate 29. (*From McPherson R, Pincus M. Henry's clinical diagnosis and management by laboratory methods, 21st ed. Philadelphia: Saunders, 2006, Fig. 29-23.*)

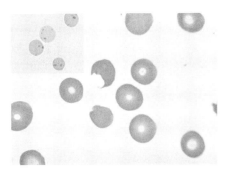

Figure 13-5. Bite cells with Heinz bodies. See Plate 30. (*Courtesy Dr. Robert W. McKenna, Department of Pathology, University of Texas Southwestern Medical School, Dallas, TX.*)

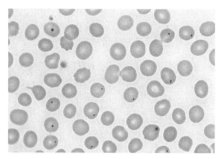

Figure 13-6. Howell-Jolly bodies in peripheral blood erythrocytes. These nuclear remnants indicate a lack of splenic filtrative function. See Plate 31. (*From Orkin SH, et al. Nathan and Oski's hematology of infancy and childhood, 7th ed. Philadelphia: Saunders, 2009, Fig. 14-4.*)

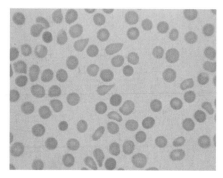

Figure 13-7. Teardrop red blood cells, usually seen in myelofibrosis. See Plate 32. (*From Goldman L, Ausiello D. Cecil medicine, 23rd ed. Philadelphia: Saunders, 2008, Fig. 161-13.*)

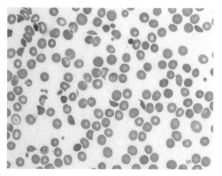

Figure 13-8. Schistocytes and helmet cells. Red blood cell fragments seen in microangiopathic hemolytic anemia and disseminated intravascular coagulation. See Plate 33. (*From McPherson R, Pincus M. Henry's clinical diagnosis and management by laboratory methods, 21st ed. Philadelphia: Saunders, 2006, Fig. 29-19.*)

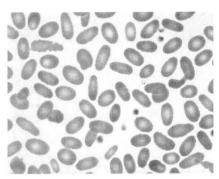

Figure 13-9. Hereditary elliptocytosis. A blood film reveals characteristic elliptical red blood cells. See Plate 34. (*From McPherson R, Pincus M. Henry's clinical diagnosis and management by laboratory methods, 22nd ed. Philadelphia: Saunders, 2011, Fig. 30-16.*)

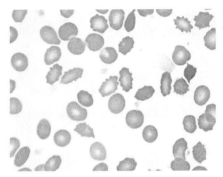

Figure 13-10. Acanthocytes. Irregularly spiculated red blood cells, frequently seen in abetalipoproteinemia or liver disease. See Plate 35. (*From McPherson R, Pincus M. Henry's clinical diagnosis and management by laboratory methods, 21st ed. Philadelphia: Saunders, 2006, Fig. 29-20.*)

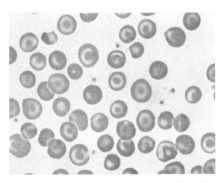

Figure 13-11. Target cells are frequently seen in hemoglobin C disease and liver disease. See Plate 36. (*From McPherson R, Pincus M. Henry's clinical diagnosis and management by laboratory methods, 21st ed. Philadelphia: Saunders, 2006, Fig. 29-18.*)

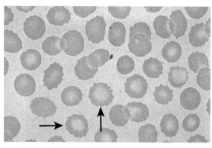

Figure 13-12. Echinocytes, or burr cells (*arrows*), are the hallmark of uremia. See Plate 37. (*From Hoffman R, et al.* Hematology: basic principles and practice, *5th ed. Philadelphia: Churchill Livingstone, 2008, Fig. 156-1.*)

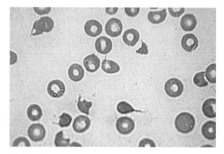

Figure 13-13. Microangiopathic hemolytic anemia demonstrating red blood cell fragments, anisocytosis, polychromasia, and decreased platelets. See Plate 38. (*From Tschudy MM, Arcara KM.* The Harriet Lane handbook, *19th ed. Philadelphia: Mosby, 2011, Plate 7.*)

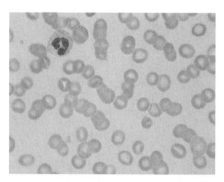

Figure 13-14. Rouleaux formation of stacked red blood cells seen in multiple myeloma. See Plate 39. (*From Goldman L, Ausiello D.* Cecil medicine, *23rd ed. Philadelphia: Saunders, 2008, Fig. 161-19.*)

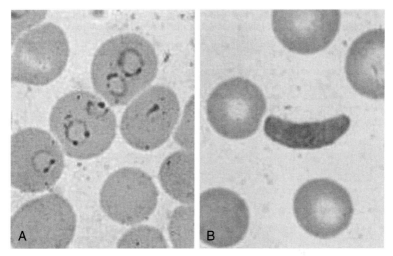

Figure 13-15. Malaria. Peripheral blood film examples of various stages of *Plasmodium falciparum*. See Plate 40. **A,** Small ring forms. **B,** A crescentic gametocyte with centrally placed chromatin. (*From Hoffman R, et al.* Hematology: basic principles and practice, *5th ed. Philadelphia: Churchill Livingstone, 2008, Fig. 159-5.*)

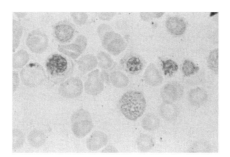

Figure 13-16. Ringed sideroblasts seen in sideroblastic anemia. See Plate 41. (*From Goldman L, Ausiello D.* Cecil medicine, *23rd ed. Philadelphia: Saunders, 2008, Fig. 163-5.*)

8. **What are reticulocytes? Why is a reticulocyte count routinely ordered in an anemia workup?**
    Reticulocytes are immature RBCs. If their count is abnormally decreased in the setting of anemia, the marrow is not responding properly and is the problem. A high reticulocyte count should make you think of hemolysis or blood loss as the cause (the marrow is responding properly and is not the problem).

9. **Which test comes next?**
    At this point, the next test depends on the situation. If you have a complete history and results for the other three tests (CBC with RBC indices, peripheral blood smear, and reticulocyte count), most possibilities will be eliminated, and you can order a confirmatory test. If the answer is still not clear, consider a bone marrow biopsy. For the Step 3 exam, biopsy is unlikely to be necessary unless malignancy is the cause of the anemia.

10. **What are the classic causes of microcytic, normocytic, and macrocytic anemia? Which of these tends to have an inappropriately low reticulocyte count?**

MICROCYTIC	NORMOCYTIC
With normal or elevated reticulocyte count	*With normal or elevated reticulocyte count*
Thalassemia/hemoglobinopathy (e.g., sickle cell disease)	Acute blood loss Hemolytic (multiple causes) Medications (antibody causing)
With low reticulocyte count	*With low reticulocyte count*
Lead poisoning Sideroblastic anemia Anemia of chronic disease (some cases) Iron deficiency	Cancer/dysplasia (e.g., myelophthisic anemia, acute leukemia) Anemia of chronic disease (some cases) Aplastic anemia/medications causing bone marrow suppression Endocrine failure (thyroid, pituitary) Renal failure
MACROCYTIC	
All types have low reticulocyte count	
Folate deficiency Vitamin B_{12} deficiency Medications (methotrexate, phenytoin) Alcohol abuse (interferes with folate use) Cirrhosis, liver disease	

11. **What clues point to hemolysis as the cause of anemia?**
    - Elevated lactate dehydrogenase (LDH)
    - Elevated bilirubin (unconjugated as well as conjugated if the liver is functioning)
    - Jaundice
    - Low or absent haptoglobin (intravascular hemolysis only)
    - Urobilinogen, bilirubin, and hemoglobin in urine (only the conjugated from of bilirubin shows up in urine, and hemoglobin shows up in urine only when haptoglobin has been saturated, as in brisk intravascular hemolysis)
    - Pigmented gallstones or a history of cholecystectomy (usually at a young age)

12. **What is the most common cause of anemia in the United States?**
    Iron deficiency.

13. **Why do people get iron deficiency?**
    Iron deficiency is common in women of reproductive age because of menstrual blood loss. In all patients older than 40 years (men and especially postmenopausal women), it is important to rule out colon cancer as a cause of chronic, asymptomatic blood loss. Increased requirements may also lead to iron deficiency in children and in pregnant or breastfeeding women. Give iron-containing formula or iron supplements to all infants except full-term infants who are exclusively breastfed. Start iron supplementation (iron-fortified cereal or daily iron supplement) at 4 to 6 months for full-term infants and at 2 months for preterm infants. Giving cow's milk before 1 year of age may lead to anemia by causing GI bleeding, so avoidance of cow's milk in the first year is essential. Iron supplements are also commonly given during pregnancy and lactation (because of the increased demand).

14. **What are the classic laboratory abnormalities in iron deficiency anemia? What weird cravings may occur with iron deficiency?**
    Look for low iron and low ferritin levels, elevated total iron-binding capacity (TIBC; also known as transferrin), and low TIBC saturation. In rare cases, patients may develop a craving for ice or dirt (**pica**).

15. **How is iron deficiency treated?**
First you must determine the cause. In a menstruating woman, a presumptive diagnosis of menstrual blood loss is often made. In patients older than 40 years, be sure to test the stool for occult blood and strongly consider colonoscopy to detect occult colon cancer. Postmenopausal vaginal bleeding may also cause anemia and warrants screening for gynecologic cancer. Treat with iron supplements for 3 to 6 months in uncomplicated cases to replete the body's iron stores.

16. **How do you recognize anemia of chronic disease?**
First, look for the presence of a disease that causes chronic inflammation (e.g., rheumatoid arthritis, lupus erythematosus, cancer, tuberculosis). The anemia is either normocytic or microcytic. Serum iron is low but so is TIBC, so the percentage saturation may be near normal. Serum ferritin is elevated (because ferritin is an acute-phase reactant, the level should be increased). Treat the underlying disorder to correct the anemia. Do not give iron.

17. **What are the common causes of thrombocytopenia? What kind of bleeding problems are caused by low platelet counts?**
Common causes of thrombocytopenia include purpura (idiopathic or thrombotic), hemolytic uremic syndrome, disseminated intravascular coagulation (DIC), HIV, splenic sequestration, heparin (including heparin-induced thrombocytopenia; treat by first stopping heparin), other medications (especially quinidine and sulfa drugs), autoimmune disease, and alcohol. Bleeding from thrombocytopenia is in the form of petechiae, nose bleeds, and easy bruising.

18. **Specify the main differences between thrombotic thrombocytopenic purpura (TTP) and idiopathic thrombocytopenic purpura (ITP), including presentation and treatment.**

	TTP	ITP
Most common age	Young adults	Children or adults
Previous infection	None	Viral (especially in children)
Red blood cell count	Low	Normal
Platelet count	Low	Low
Peripheral blood smear	Hemolysis	Normal
Kidney effects	ARF, proteinuria	None
Treatment	Plasmapheresis, NSAIDs; no platelets†	Steroids,* splenectomy if drugs fail
Key differential points	CNS changes, age	Antiplatelet antibodies

ARF, Acute renal failure; CNS, central nervous system; ITP, idiopathic thrombocytopenic purpura; NSAIDs, nonsteroidal antiinflammatory drugs; TTP, thrombotic thrombocytopenic purpura.
*Give steroids only if the patient is bleeding or when platelet counts are very low (<20,000 cells/μL).
†Do not give platelet transfusions to patients with TTP; clots may form.

BLEEDING DISORDERS

1. **How do the following conditions affect coagulation tests?**

CONDITION	PROLONGS	ADDITIONAL INFORMATION
Hemophilia A	PTT	Low levels of factor VIII; normal PT and bleeding time; X linked
Hemophilia B	PTT	Low levels of factor IX; normal PT and bleeding time; X linked
vWF deficiency	Bleeding time and PTT	Normal or low levels of factor VIII; normal PT; autosomal dominant
DIC	PT, PTT, bleeding time	Positive D-dimer or FDPs; postpartum, infection, malignancy; schistocytes and fragmented cells on a peripheral blood smear

CONDITION	PROLONGS	ADDITIONAL INFORMATION
Liver disease	PT, PTT	All factors but VIII are low; stigmata of liver disease; no correction with vitamin K
Vitamin K deficiency	PT, PTT (slight)	Normal bleeding time; low levels of factors II, VII, IX, and X, as well as proteins C and S; look for a neonate who did not receive prophylactic vitamin K; malabsorption, alcoholism, or prolonged antibiotic use (which kills vitamin K–producing bowel flora)

DIC, Disseminated intravascular coagulation; *FDPs*, fibrin degradation products; *PT*, prothrombin time; *PTT*, partial thromboplastin time; *vWF*, von Willebrand factor.

Remember also that uremia causes a qualitative platelet defect and that vitamin C deficiency and chronic corticosteroid therapy can cause a bleeding tendency with normal coagulation test results.

2. How is thalassemia differentiated from iron deficiency?
Both cause microcytic hypochromic anemia, but thalassemia must be differentiated from iron deficiency because iron levels are normal in thalassemia. Iron supplementation is contraindicated in patients with thalassemia because it may cause iron overload. Look for elevations in hemoglobin A2 or hemoglobin F (beta-thalassemia only); target cells, nucleated RBCs, and diffuse basophilia on peripheral blood smears; skull radiographs with a crew-cut appearance; extramedullary hematopoiesis; splenomegaly; and a positive family history. Thalassemia is more common in blacks and individuals of Mediterranean or Asian origin.

3. What diagnostic test confirms a diagnosis of thalassemia? How is it treated?
Diagnosis is made on the basis of hemoglobin electrophoresis. There are four gene loci for the alpha chain of hemoglobin but only two for the beta chain. Patients with alpha-thalassemia are symptomatic at birth or die in utero (fetal hydrops), whereas patients with beta-thalassemia are not symptomatic until 6 months of age.
No treatment is required for minor thalassemia. Patients are often asymptomatic because they are used to living with a lower level of hemoglobin. Thalassemia major is more dramatic and severe. Treat with transfusions as needed and with iron chelation therapy to prevent secondary hemochromatosis.

4. What two clues on the Step 3 exam often point to a diagnosis of sickle cell disease?
A peripheral blood smear and race. Eight percent of African Americans are heterozygous for the sickle cell trait. Know what sickled RBCs look like. Patients usually have a high percentage of reticulocytes (8% to 20%).

5. What are the clinical manifestations and complications of sickle cell disease?
• Aplastic crises (caused by parvovirus B19 infection)
• Bone pain (caused by infarcts; the classic example is avascular necrosis of the femoral head)
• Dactylitis (also known as hand-foot syndrome, seen in children)
• Renal papillary necrosis
• Splenic sequestration crisis
• Autosplenectomy (increased infections with encapsulated bacteria such as *Pneumococcus*, *Haemophilus*, and *Neisseria* species)
• Acute chest syndrome (mimics pneumonia)
• Pigment cholelithiasis
• Priapism
• Stroke

6. How is sickle cell disease diagnosed and treated?
The diagnosis is made on the basis of hemoglobin electrophoresis. Screening is performed at birth, but symptoms usually do not appear until around 6 months of age because of the lack of adult hemoglobin production. Treat patients with prophylactic penicillin until at least 5 years

of age and perhaps longer, beginning as soon as the diagnosis is made. Proper vaccination includes the pneumococcal, meningococcal, and H. *influenzae* vaccines (given to all children anyway), as well as yearly influenza vaccination. Other strategies include folate supplementation, early treatment of infections, and proper hydration.

A sickle cell crisis involves severe pain in various sites caused by RBC sickling. Treat with oxygen, abundant intravenous fluids, and analgesics (do not be afraid to use narcotics). Consider transfusions if symptoms and/or findings are severe.

7. **What are the commonly tested causes of autoimmune hemolytic anemia?**
   - Lupus erythematosus (or medications that cause lupus-like syndromes, such as procainamide, hydralazine, and isoniazid) and other autoimmune disorders
   - Drugs (the classic example is methyldopa, but penicillins, cephalosporins, sulfa drugs, and quinidine have also been implicated)
   - Leukemia or lymphoma
   - Infection (the classic examples are mycoplasmosis, Epstein-Barr virus, and syphilis)

8. **What laboratory test is often positive in patients with autoimmune anemia?**
   The **Coombs test** is positive in most autoimmune anemias. You may also see spherocytes on a peripheral blood smear because of incomplete macrophage destruction (extravascular hemolysis) of RBCs.

9. **What clues point to lead poisoning as a cause of anemia?**
   Lead poisoning causes a hypochromic microcytic anemia, almost always in a child. For acute lead poisoning, look for vomiting, ataxia, colicky abdominal pain, irritability (aggressive behavior, behavioral regression), and encephalopathy, cerebral edema, or seizures. Usually, however, poisoning is chronic and low level with minimal nonspecific symptoms. Watch for basophilic stippling on a peripheral blood smear and elevated free erythrocyte protoporphyrin or lead levels, and consider risk factors for lead exposure (a child who eats paint chips or lives in an old, run-down building).

10. **True or false: Children with risk factors should be screened for lead poisoning.**
    True. Screening of all asymptomatic children via measurement of serum lead levels at 1 and 2 years of age regardless of risk is becoming controversial. However, for children with risk factors, screening is very important because chronic low-level exposure may lead to permanent neurologic sequelae. Screening should start at 6 months in children with risk factors, such as pica (especially of paint chips and dust in old buildings that may have lead paint), residence in an old or neglected building, and/or residence near or family members who work at a lead-smelting or battery-recycling plant. Screen and measure symptomatic exposure in terms of serum lead levels (normal value <10 μg/dL).

11. **How is lead poisoning treated?**
    Treat initially with decreased exposure (best strategy), as well as lead chelation therapy if needed. Use succimer in children and dimercaprol in adults; in severe cases, use dimercaprol plus ethylenediamine tetraacetic acid (EDTA) for children or adults.

12. **How can sideroblastic anemia be recognized on the Step 3 exam? Should the presence of sideroblastic anemia raise concern about other conditions?**
    The typical description is a microcytic hypochromic anemia with increased or normal iron, ferritin, and TIBC (transferrin). This description should immediately steer you away from iron deficiency. Look for polychromatophilic stippling and the classic ringed sideroblasts in bone marrow (know what it looks like). Sideroblastic anemia may be related to myelodysplasia or future blood dyscrasia. Although you will probably not be asked about management, treatment is supportive. In rare cases, the anemia responds to **pyridoxine.** Do not give iron.

13. **Describe the hallmarks of spherocytosis.**
    This normochromic normocytic anemia is associated with spherocytes on a peripheral blood smear, a positive family history (autosomal dominant), splenomegaly, a positive osmotic fragility test, and an increased **mean corpuscular hemoglobin concentration** (the only occasion for which this RBC index is useful for the Step 3 exam). Treatment often involves splenectomy. Spherocytes may also be seen in extravascular hemolysis, but the osmotic fragility test is normal.

14. **Why do patients with chronic renal disease develop anemia? How do you treat it?**
All patients with chronic renal failure develop a normocytic normochromic anemia with a lower reticulocyte count because of a decrease in erythropoietin production. If necessary, give erythropoietin to correct the anemia.

15. **What clues point to a diagnosis of aplastic anemia?**
Although aplastic anemia may be idiopathic, on the Step 3 exam watch for chemotherapy, radiation, malignancy affecting bone marrow (especially leukemias), benzene, and implicated medications (e.g., chloramphenicol, carbamazepine, sulfa drugs, zidovudine, gold). Decreased white blood cell (WBC) and platelet counts accompany the anemia. Treat first by stopping any possible causative medication; then try antithymocyte globulin, colony-stimulating factors (such as erythropoietin, sargramostim, filgrastim, pegfilgrastim), or a bone marrow transplant.

16. **Define myelophthisic anemia. What clues on a peripheral blood smear suggest its presence?**
Myelophthisic anemia is due to a space-occupying lesion in the bone marrow. The common causes are a malignant tumor that destroys bone marrow (most common) and myelodysplasia or myelofibrosis. On a peripheral blood smear, look for marked anisocytosis (different sizes), poikilocytosis (different shapes), nucleated RBCs, giant and/or bizarre-looking platelets, and **teardrop-shaped** RBCs. A bone marrow biopsy may reveal no cells (so-called dry tap if the marrow is fibrotic) or malignant-looking cells.

17. **How do you recognize G6PD deficiency on the USMLE?**
This genetic disorder is an X-linked recessive trait and affects males. It is most common in blacks and individuals of Mediterranean origin. Look for sudden hemolysis or anemia after exposure to fava beans or certain drugs (antimalarial agents, salicylates, sulfa drugs) or after infection. You may see **Heinz bodies** and bite cells on a peripheral blood smear. The diagnosis is made on the basis of an RBC enzyme assay, which should not be performed immediately after hemolysis because of the potential for a false-negative result (all of the older RBCs have already been destroyed, and the younger RBCs are not affected in most patients). Treat with avoidance of precipitating foods and medications; discontinue the triggering medication first.

18. **Name some other causes of anemia.**
    - Endocrine failure (especially the pituitary and thyroid glands; look for endocrine symptoms)
    - Mechanical heart valves (hemolyzed RBCs)
    - DIC, TTP, and hemolytic uremic syndrome (look for schistocytes and RBC fragments on a blood smear and other appropriate findings)
    - Other hemoglobinopathies (the hemoglobin C and E varieties are fairly common)
    - Paroxysmal nocturnal or cold hemoglobinuria
    - *Clostridium perfringens* infection, malaria, and babesiosis (cause intravascular hemolysis and fever)
    - Hypersplenism (associated with splenomegaly and often with low platelet and WBC counts)

19. **When is transfusion indicated for anemia (at what hemoglobin level)?**
Always transfuse on clinical grounds; observe the symptoms. In other words, treat the patient, not the laboratory value. There is no such thing as a trigger value for transfusion. Nevertheless, a hemoglobin level of less than 7 g/dL in the acute setting makes most clinicians nervous, particularly if the patient has heart disease.

20. **What are the most common causes of DIC?**
The most common cause is pregnancy and obstetric complications (roughly 50% of cases), followed by malignancy (33%), sepsis, and trauma (especially head trauma, prostate surgery, and snake bites).

21. **How do you recognize and treat DIC in a classic at-risk patient?**
DIC usually manifests with bleeding diathesis but may have thrombotic tendencies. Look for the classic oozing or bleeding from puncture and intravenous sites and prolonged prothrombin time (PT), partial thromboplastin time (PTT), and bleeding time (BT). DIC is the only disorder on the Step 3 exam that prolongs all three parameters. Other clues include positive D-dimer, increased fibrin degradation products, thrombocytopenia,

decreased fibrinogen, and decreased clotting factors (including factor VIII, which is normal in hepatic necrosis).

Treat the underlying cause (e.g., evacuate the uterus, give antibiotics). You may need to give transfusions with fresh frozen plasma or, in rare cases, heparin (only if thrombosis occurs).

22. **Which clotting tests measure which parts of the coagulation cascade? Which medications affect these tests?**
PT measures the function of the extrinsic clotting pathway (prolonged by warfarin), activated PTT measures the function of the intrinsic clotting pathway (prolonged by heparin), and BT measures platelet function (prolonged by aspirin).

23. **How do specific diseases affect clotting tests? What are the main differential points?**

DISEASE	PT	PTT	BT	PLATELET COUNT	RBC COUNT	OTHER
von Willebrand disease	Normal	High	High	Normal	Normal	Autosomal dominant (look for family history)
Hemophilia A/B	Normal	High	Normal	Normal	Normal	X-linked recessive; A, low factor VIII; B, low factor IX
DIC	High	High	High	Low	Normal/low	Appropriate history, low level of factor VIII
Liver failure	High	High	Normal	Normal/low	Normal/low	Jaundice, normal factor VIII level; do not give vitamin K (ineffective); use FFP
Heparin	Normal	High	Normal	Normal/low	Normal	Watch for thrombocytopenia and thrombosis
Warfarin	High	Normal	Normal	Normal	Normal	Vitamin K antagonist (factors II, VII, IX, and X)
ITP	Normal	Normal	High	Low	Normal	Watch for preceding URI
TTP	Normal	Normal	High	Low	Low	Hemolysis (smear), CNS symptoms (hallucinations, altered mental status, headache, stroke); treat with plasmapheresis; do not give platelets!
Scurvy	Normal	Normal	Normal	Normal	Normal	Fingernail and gum hemorrhages, bone hemorrhages; caused by vitamin C deficiency

BT, bleeding time; CNS, central nervous system; DIC, disseminated intravascular coagulation; FFP, fresh frozen plasma; ITP, idiopathic thrombocytopenic purpura; PT, Prothrombin time; PTT, partial thromboplastin time; RBC, red blood cell; TTP, thrombotic thrombocytopenic purpura; URI, upper respiratory tract infection..

24. **What causes petechiae or platelet-type bleeding in the setting of normal platelet counts?**
Vitamin C deficiency (scurvy) causes bleeding similar to that seen for low platelet counts (splinter and gum hemorrhages, petechiae); perifollicular and subperiosteal hemorrhages are unique to scurvy. Patients have a poor dietary history (the classic example is hot dogs and soda or tea and toast), myalgias and arthralgias, and capillary fragility (bleeding is due to collagen problems in the vessels). Treat with oral vitamin C.
    Other causes include uremia (results in platelet dysfunction), inherited connective tissue disorders (Ehlers-Danlos syndrome, Marfan syndrome), and chronic corticosteroid use (causes capillary fragility).

25. **Which clotting factors are affected by vitamin K? What is the interaction of vitamin K and the liver?**
Vitamin K is needed for hepatic synthesis of factors II, VII, IX, and X as well as proteins C and S. Chronic liver disease (cirrhosis) can cause prolongation of PT and the international normalized ratio (INR) because the liver is unable to synthesize clotting factors, even in the presence of adequate vitamin K levels. In the setting of active bleeding, this problem should be corrected with fresh frozen plasma, although the effects will only be temporary. Vitamin K is ineffective in the setting of severe liver disease.

REACTIONS TO BLOOD COMPONENTS

1 **What are the indications for the use of various blood products?**
Whole blood: used only for rapid, massive blood loss or exchange transfusions (poisoning, TTP).
Packed RBCs: used for routine transfusions for anemia.
Washed RBCs: free of traces of plasma, WBCs, and platelets; good for immunoglobulin A (IgA) deficiency as well as allergic or previously sensitized patients.
Platelets: given for symptomatic thrombocytopenia (usually <10,000 cells/μL). Other general transfusion guidelines include transfusion for less than 20,000 cells/μL in a febrile patient or less than 50,000 cells/μL in a patient for whom surgery is planned.
Granulocytes: used on rare occasions for neutropenia.
Fresh frozen plasma: contains all the clotting factors; used for bleeding diathesis when you cannot wait for vitamin K to take effect (e.g., DIC, severe warfarin poisoning) or when vitamin K will not work (liver failure).
Cryoprecipitate: contains fibrinogen and factor VIII; used in hemophilia, von Willebrand disease, and DIC.

2. **What is the most common cause of a hemolytic transfusion reaction? What blood type can be given in an emergency to avoid a reaction?**
The most common cause of a blood transfusion reaction is laboratory error. Type O negative blood can be used to avoid a reaction when you cannot wait for blood typing or when the blood bank does not have the patient's blood type.

3. **Describe the signs and symptoms of a blood transfusion reaction.**
Look for a **febrile reaction** (e.g., chills, fever, headache, back pain) from antibodies to WBCs; a **hemolytic reaction** (e.g., anxiety or discomfort, dyspnea, chest pain, shock, jaundice) from antibodies to RBCs; or an **allergic reaction** (e.g., urticaria, edema, dizziness, dyspnea, wheezing, and anaphylaxis) to an unknown component in donor serum. Oliguria may be an associated finding.

4. **What should you do if you suspect a transfusion reaction?**
The first step is to *stop the transfusion*. If oliguria is present, treat with intravenous fluids and diuresis (mannitol or furosemide).

5. **What are the other risks of transfusion?**
There is a small but real risk of infection (usually viral infections such as hepatitis B and C, human immunodeficiency virus (HIV), and cytomegalovirus) and hyperkalemia (from hemolysis). For large transfusions (>5 units of packed RBCs), bleeding diathesis may result from dilutional thrombocytopenia and citrate (a blood preservative and calcium chelator that prevents clotting). Look for oozing from puncture or intravenous sites.

MALIGNANT NEOPLASIAS

1. With what conditions is basophilia associated?
Allergies and neoplasm/blood dyscrasia.

2. What are the key differential points for the commonly tested blood dyscrasias?

TYPE	AGE	WHAT TO LOOK FOR IN CASE DESCRIPTION, TRIGGER WORDS
ALL	Children (peak age 3-5 yr)	Pancytopenia (bleeding, fever, anemia), history of radiation therapy, Down syndrome
AML	>30 yr	Pancytopenia (bleeding, fever, anemia), Auer rods, DIC
CML	30-50 yr	White blood cell count greater than 50,000, Philadelphia chromosome, blast crisis, splenomegaly
CLL	>50 yr	Male gender, lymphadenopathy, lymphocytosis, infections, smudge cells, splenomegaly
Hairy cell leukemia	Adults	Blood smear (hairlike projections), splenomegaly
Mycosis fungoides/ Sézary syndrome	>50 yr	Plaquelike, itchy skin rash that does not improve with treatment, a blood smear shows cerebriform nuclei known as butt cells, Pautrier abscesses in epidermis
Burkitt lymphoma	Children	Associated with Epstein-Barr virus (in Africa)
CNS B-cell lymphoma	Adults	Seen in patients with HIV infection, AIDS
T-cell leukemia	Adults	Caused by HTLV-1 virus
Hodgkin disease	15-34 yr	Reed-Sternberg cell, cervical lymphadenopathy, night sweats
Non-Hodgkin lymphoma	Any age	Small follicular type has the best prognosis, the large diffuse type has the worst; primary tumor may be located in the gastrointestinal tract
Myelodysplasia/ myelofibrosis	>50 yr	Anemia, teardrop cells, dry tap on bone marrow biopsy, high MCV and RDW; associated with CML
Multiple myeloma	>40 yr	Bence Jones protein (IgG 50%, IgA 25%), osteolytic lesions, high serum calcium
Waldenström macroglobulinemia	>40 yr	Hyperviscosity, IgM spike, cold agglutinins (Raynaud phenomenon with cold sensitivity)
Polycythemia vera	>40 yr	High hematocrit/hemoglobin, pruritus (especially after hot bath or shower); use phlebotomy
Primary thrombocythemia	>50 yr	Platelet count usually >1,000,000 cells/mL; may have bleeding or thrombosis

ALL, Acute lymphoblastic leukemia; *AML*, acute myelogenous leukemia; *CLL*, chronic lymphocytic leukemia; *CML*, chronic myelogenous leukemia; *CNS*, central nervous system; *DIC*, disseminated intravascular coagulation; *HTLV-1*, human lymphotrophic virus 1; *Ig*, immunoglobulin; *MCV*, mean corpuscular volume; *RDW*, red cell distribution width.

3. **What is the difference between acute leukemia and chronic leukemia?**
For acute leukemia, look for proliferation of minimally differentiated cells such as lymphoblasts and myeloblasts. There should be more than 20% blasts in the bone marrow. Chronic leukemia is marked by proliferation of more differentiated cells such as lymphocytes and myelocytes.

4. **Who tends to get acute lymphocytic leukemia (ALL)? What are the presenting symptoms?**
ALL is most common in children and has a higher incidence in those with Down syndrome. Look for nonspecific symptoms such as fever, lethargy, and a sore throat; start thinking ALL if there is persistence of the fever, bone pain, and/or easy bruising.

5. **How is ALL diagnosed? How is it treated? What is the prognosis?**
Look for an elevated or depressed WBC count, a markedly decreased platelet count, and elevated LDH and uric acid. Lymphoblasts will be seen on a peripheral blood smear. Confirm the diagnosis with a bone marrow biopsy. Order a chest x-ray, a computed tomography (CT) scan, and a lumbar puncture to evaluate for extramedullary involvement/metastases. Treat with chemotherapy. Prognosis is determined by the age of onset and the results of cytogenetic studies. Five-year survival rates are now greater than 85% in children but are lower in adults (30% to 40% overall cure rate).

6. **Who gets acute myelogenous leukemia (AML)? What are the presenting symptoms?**
Most cases of AML occur in adults. Look for symptoms similar to those for ALL, such as easy bruising, fatigue, fever, anemia, and frequent infections. Patients may also have central nervous system involvement, DIC, or gingival hyperplasia.

7. **How is AML diagnosed?**
Look for an increase in myeloid cell lines, as well as decreased leukocyte alkaline phosphatase (LAP) and elevated uric acid levels. A peripheral blood smear will show a predominance of myeloblasts. Look for Auer rods. Confirm the diagnosis with a bone marrow biopsy.

8. **How is AML treated?**
AML is classified into subtypes; treatment depends on the subtype, but chemotherapy (and sometimes bone marrow transplantation) is the key to treatment.

9. **What is chronic lymphocytic leukemia (CLL)? What are the presenting symptoms?**
CLL is a malignancy of mature lymphocytes that is usually seen in patients older than 65 years. CLL is an indolent disease characterized by fatigue, lymphadenopathy, and hepatosplenomegaly. It is sometimes diagnosed incidentally when a CBC reveals lymphocytosis.

10. **How is CLL diagnosed? How is it treated?**
Look for lymphocytosis alone on a CBC with normal hemoglobin, hematocrit, and platelet counts. A peripheral blood smear will show many small lymphocytes. Confirm with a bone marrow biopsy; look for smudge cells and CD5$^+$ expression.
   Asymptomatic patients do not require treatment. If the patient is symptomatic or has advanced-stage CLL, the treatment is radiation therapy (for localized CLL) or chemotherapy (for advanced CLL).

11. **What is chronic myelogenous leukemia (CML)? Who gets it? What are the presenting symptoms?**
CML is a malignancy of myeloid cells that typically occurs in middle-aged adults. It typically remains in a chronic phase for several years and then transforms into an acute leukemia as a blast crisis, which often results in death within a few months.
   CML may be found incidentally on a CBC that reveals leukocytosis. In a symptomatic patient, look for nonspecific symptoms such as fatigue, malaise, fever, weight loss, and night sweats. The symptoms of an acute blast crisis include fever, weight loss, bone pain, and splenomegaly.

12. **How is CML diagnosed?**
Look for a markedly elevated WBC count (often of the order of 150,000 cells/μL) with leuko-cytosis, prominence of myeloid cells with basophilia on a peripheral blood smear, decreased

LAP, and an elevated vitamin B_{12} level. Confirm the diagnosis with demonstration of the Philadelphia chromosome or the BCR-ABL complex via cytogenetic analysis, fluorescence in situ hybridization (FISH) analysis, or reverse transcription polymerase chain reaction (RT-PCR) for blood or bone marrow samples.

13. **How is CML treated?**

Tyrosine kinase inhibitors (e.g., imatinib, dasatinib, or nilotinib) are the initial treatment of choice for most patients with CML. Bone marrow transplantation is an option for some patients in the blast phase.

14. **What is Hodgkin lymphoma? What are the presenting symptoms?**

Hodgkin lymphoma is a malignancy of Reed-Sternberg cells (B-cell origin) for which the typical presentation is cervical lymphadenopathy, as well as the so-called B symptoms: fever (>100.4° F [38° C]), night sweats, and weight loss (>10% over 6 months or less).

15. **How is Hodgkin lymphoma diagnosed? What is the treatment?**

Biopsy an enlarged lymph node to make the diagnosis and look for the presence of Reed-Sternberg cells. Staging is based on the Ann Arbor system and includes a number (I to IV according to the anatomic location of the tumor) and either A or B symptoms, where A indicates the absence of symptoms and B symptoms are as described in the previous question. Treatment is with combination chemotherapy.

16. **What is non-Hodgkin lymphoma? What are the presenting symptoms? How is non-Hodgkin lymphoma diagnosed? What is the treatment?**

Non-Hodgkin lymphoma is a diverse group of malignant neoplasms derived from B-cell progenitors, T-cell progenitors, mature T cells, and sometimes natural killer cells. The symptoms and diagnosis are similar to those for Hodgkin lymphoma. Treatment is with combination chemotherapy.

17. **What are the presenting symptoms for multiple myeloma?**

Multiple myeloma is a malignancy of plasma cells that is typically seen in older adults. Look for back pain, pathologic fractures, fatigue, frequent infections, and signs/symptoms of hypercalcemia. Multiple myeloma needs to be included in the differential diagnosis for a patient with hypercalcemia, anemia, renal failure, or bone pain.

18. **How is multiple myeloma diagnosed?**

Order serum protein electrophoresis (SPEP) to look for monoclonal immunoglobulin and urine protein electrophoresis (UPEP) to look for Bence Jones protein. Other important tests include a CBC, a chemistry screen (including calcium, albumin, creatinine, LDH, and beta$_2$-microglobulin), and serum free monoclonal light-chain analysis. Perform a bone marrow biopsy to confirm the diagnosis (>10% plasma cells) and a full-body skeletal survey to look for osteolytic lesions of the skull and long bones.

19. **How is multiple myeloma treated?**

There are several chemotherapy regimens for the treatment of multiple myeloma that are beyond the scope of the Step 3 exam. However, remember that you will also need to treat the signs, symptoms, and complications of multiple myeloma:

- Hypercalcemia: hydration, steroids, bisphosphonates such as zoledronic acid and pamidronate
- Renal insufficiency: avoid nephrotoxins, maintain hydration, and perform plasmapheresis or hemodialysis as needed
- Bone pain from skeletal lesions: local radiation, bisphosphonates
- Infections: pneumococcal vaccine, yearly influenza vaccine; prophylactic antibiotic administration is controversial
- Anemia: erythropoietin; RBC transfusions as needed
- Hyperviscosity syndrome: plasmapheresis
- Thrombosis: no specific treatment, but be aware that patients with multiple myeloma are at higher risk of both venous thromboembolism and arterial thromboembolism (stroke, transient ischemic attacks, myocardial infarction, peripheral arterial disease)

20. **What are the most common types of cancer in children and young adults (younger than 30 years)?**

Leukemia and lymphoma.

INFECTIONS

1. **With what conditions is eosinophilia associated?**
   - Allergic or atopic diseases (allergic rhinitis, asthma, allergic bronchopulmonary aspergillosis, eczema, urticaria, atopic dermatitis, milk-protein allergy, drug reactions)
   - Parasitic infections
   - Fungal infections
   - HIV infection
   - Malignancies (lymphoma, leukemia, lung cancer, gastric cancer, pancreatic cancer, colon cancer, ovarian cancer)
   - Connective tissue and autoimmune diseases (Churg-Strauss vasculitis, rheumatoid arthritis, lupus, scleroderma, eosinophilic fasciitis, Dressler syndrome, inflammatory bowel disease)
   - Granulomatous disorders (sarcoidosis)
   - Skin disorders (psoriasis, pemphigus)
   - Immune disorders (Wiskott-Aldrich syndrome, hyper-IgE syndrome, IgA deficiency, thymoma)
   - Adrenal insufficiency
   - Pulmonary eosinophilia (Löffler syndrome)
   - Cirrhosis
   - Atheroembolic disease
   - Familial eosinophilia
   - Eosinophilia-myalgia syndrome (from using L-tryptophan)

2. **What are the systemic inflammatory response syndrome (SIRS) criteria?**
   1. Temperature less than 96.8° F (36° C) or greater than 100.4° F (38° C)
   2. Heart rate greater than 90 beats/min
   3. Respiratory rate greater than 24 breaths/min or PCO_2 of less than 32 mm Hg
   4. Leukocyte count greater than 12,000 cells/mL or less than 4000 cells/mL, or greater than 10% bands on a peripheral blood smear.

3. **How do you define SIRS, sepsis, severe sepsis, and septic shock?**
   - SIRS is a serious condition related to systemic inflammation, organ dysfunction, and organ failure, and it can be a sign of sepsis. SIRS can be diagnosed when two of the SIRS criteria are met.
   - Sepsis requires at least two of the SIRS criteria with evidence of an infectious process.
   - Severe sepsis involves the sepsis criteria plus evidence of organ dysfunction or tissue hypoperfusion (manifesting as hypotension, elevated lactate level, acute kidney injury, or decreased urine output).
   - Septic shock is severe sepsis plus persistently low blood pressure that does not respond to fluid resuscitation.

4. **What are the principles for the management of sepsis?**
   Early goal-directed therapy involves adjustments of cardiac preload, afterload, and contractility to balance oxygen delivery with oxygen demand. The main principles for management of sepsis are early initiation of supportive care to correct physiologic abnormalities (e.g., hypotension and hypoxemia) and distinguishing sepsis from SIRS. The standard workup typically includes CBC, lactate, electrolytes, blood urea nitrogen, creatinine, glucose, aspartate aminotransferase, alanine aminotransferase, PT, and PTT tests. Measure arterial blood gas if respiratory failure is a concern. If an infection is present or suspected, identify it and treat it as soon as possible. Studies such as a chest x-ray, urinalysis, urine culture, and blood cultures are usually indicated. Sputum samples, cerebrospinal fluid analysis, and additional imaging such as CT scanning may be required.
   - Stabilize respiration: give oxygen and monitor pulse oximetry. Intubate and provide mechanical ventilation if needed for respiratory failure or a depressed level of consciousness.
   - Assess perfusion: systolic blood pressure of less than 90 mm Hg or mean arterial pressure of less than 70 mm Hg indicates hypotension and inadequate perfusion. Also look for cool vasoconstricted skin, tachycardia, obtundation, or oliguria/anuria. Insert an arterial catheter as needed. An elevated serum lactate level (>1 mmol/L) can indicate organ hypoperfusion, and a level of 4 mmol/L or greater is an independent predictor of septic shock.
   - Establish central venous access: patients with septic shock generally require a central venous catheter to infuse vasopressor agents and for hemodynamic monitoring. Patients

with severe sepsis generally do not require a catheter because they are fluid-responsive and therefore do not need vasopressor agents or invasive hemodynamic monitoring.

- Initial resuscitation: give fluids aggressively (large-volume infusions) in the first 6 hours to increase the central venous pressure (CVP) to 8 to 12 mm Hg, the central venous oxygen saturation to 70%, the mean arterial pressure (MAP) to 65 mm Hg or greater, and urine output to 0.5 mL/kg/hr or greater. The newest sepsis guidelines recommend intravenous fluids at 30 mL/kg for patients for whom there is no contraindication to this strategy.
- Vasopressors: use in patients who remain hypotensive despite adequate fluid resuscitation (e.g., when the CVP is 8 to 12 mm Hg and the MAP remains <65 mm Hg).
- Central venous oxygen: once the CVP and MAP goals are met, if the central venous oxygen saturation is less than 70%, the patient needs an increase in either (1) cardiac output (via dobutamine administration) or (2) oxygen-carrying capacity (via RBC transfusion). If the hemoglobin level is less than 10 g/dL, transfuse; if not, use dobutamine to increase the central venous oxygen saturation to greater than 70%.
- Antibiotics: start intravenous antibiotic therapy immediately after obtaining the appropriate cultures. When choosing the antibiotic, consider the patient's history, Gram stain data, and local resistance patterns. Initial empiric therapy should involve a broad-spectrum antibiotic against gram-positive and gram-negative bacteria. Vancomycin plus either ceftriaxone, piperacillin-tazobactam, or imipenem is a good starting point. If *Pseudomonas* infection is possible, use a regimen such as vancomycin plus ceftazidime plus imipenem.

TOXIC EFFECTS

1. **What is the most important side effect of heparin?**
   Heparin can cause two types of thrombocytopenia. The first is a nonimmune form that is of no clinical consequence and is characterized by a slight fall in platelet count during the first 2 days. The platelet count generally returns to normal with continued heparin administration. The second form is less common but more serious and is called type II heparin-induced thrombocytopenia (HIT). In this immune-mediated disorder, antibodies are formed against the heparin-platelet factor IV complex. In immune-mediated HIT, the platelet count falls by more than 50%, typically 5 to 10 days after heparin therapy is initiated. Immune-mediated HIT can lead to both arterial and venous thrombosis. The diagnosis of HIT is made on clinical grounds but can be confirmed with a functional assay. If HIT is suspected, heparin (and low-molecular-weight heparin) should be discontinued immediately.
   Measure CBCs to monitor platelet counts in patients being treated with heparin.

2. **How are the effects of aspirin, heparin, and warfarin monitored?**
   Heparin is monitored in terms of **PTT,** a measure of the internal coagulation pathway. Warfarin is monitored using **PT,** a measure of the external coagulation pathway. Aspirin prolongs **BT,** a measure of platelet function. Clinically, the effect of aspirin is not monitored via laboratory testing, but be aware that it prolongs the bleeding-time test.

3. **How are the effects of low-molecular-weight heparin monitored?**
   Low-molecular-weight heparin does not affect any of the coagulation parameters mentioned in the previous question, and its effect is not clinically monitored. In rare cases, a special type of factor X assay (anti-Xa) is used to measure its effect.

4. **In an emergency, how can you reverse the effects of heparin, warfarin, and aspirin?**
   Heparin and low-molecular-weight heparin can be reversed with **protamine;** warfarin with fresh frozen plasma (contains clotting factors; immediate effect) and/or vitamin K (takes a few days to work); and aspirin with platelet transfusions and ddAVP.

CHAPTER 14

DISORDERS OF THE MALE REPRODUCTIVE SYSTEM

MALE REPRODUCTIVE SYSTEM

1. **List the relevant characteristics of normal semen**
   - Ejaculate volume greater than 1 mL
   - Sperm concentration greater than 20 million sperm/mL
   - Initial forward motility for more than 50% of sperm
   - Normal morphology for more than 60% of sperm

2. **What do you need to know about breast cancer in men?**
   Breast cancer is about 100 times more common in women than in men and tends to occur at an older age in men than in women. Rates of breast cancer are higher in blacks, who also have a poorer prognosis. Risk factors include family history, obesity, sedentary lifestyle, Jewish ancestry, and prior chest-wall irradiation. Invasive ductal breast cancers account for more than 90% of male breast cancers. The typical presenting sign is a painless, firm, subareolar mass.

3. **How is male breast cancer diagnosed and treated?**
   Mammography is typically performed, but a biopsy is required to confirm the diagnosis and check hormone receptors and HER2 (also known as ERBB2) expression. Simple mastectomy with lymph node evaluation is typically performed. Additional therapies may include chest-wall radiation, tamoxifen, and chemotherapy, depending on the risk of relapse, lymph node involvement, hormone receptor status, and tumor size. Genetic counseling and *BRCA1* and *BRCA2* gene mutation testing gene testing should be strongly considered.

4. **What are the three main risk factors for prostate cancer?**
   Age: Prostate cancer is rare in men younger than 40 years. The incidence increases with age, and about 60% of men older than 80 years have at least microscopic prostate cancer.
   Race: Black greater than white greater than Asian.
   Family history: Men who have a family history of prostate cancer are more likely to develop the disease at a younger age and to die from it than men who do not have a family history.

5. **How do you recognize prostate cancer on the Step 3 exam?**
   Look for patients older than 50 years. Patients often present late because early prostate cancer is asymptomatic. Look for symptoms typical of benign prostatic hyperplasia (urinary hesitancy, dysuria, frequency) with hematuria and/or elevated prostate-specific antigen (PSA). Look for prostate irregularities (nodules) on a rectal examination. Patients may also have back pain from vertebral metastases, which are osteoblastic.

6. **How is prostate cancer treated?**
   Local prostate cancer is treated with surgery (prostatectomy) or local radiation. For metastases, there are several options for hormonal therapy: orchiectomy, gonadotropin-releasing hormone (GnRH) agonists (leuprolide, goserelin, buserelin, triptorelin), an androgen-receptor antagonist (flutamide), and a GnRH antagonists (degarelix). Radiation therapy is used for local disease or pain from bony metastases; standard chemotherapy is usually ineffective.

7. **Define cryptorchidism. When does it occur?**
   Cryptorchidism is arrested descent of the testicle(s) between the renal area and the scrotum. The more premature the infant, the greater the likelihood of cryptorchidism. Many arrested

testes eventually descend on their own within the first year. Intramuscular human chorionic gonadotropin may be used to induce testicular descent. After 1 year, surgical intervention (orchiopexy) is warranted in an attempt to preserve fertility and facilitate future testicular examinations. Affected testes have an increased risk of testicular cancer.

8. **True or false:** It is important to place abdominal testes in the scrotum surgically to decrease the risk of cancer.
   False. Cryptorchidism is a major risk factor for testicular cancer (fortyfold increased risk), but bringing the testis into the scrotum probably does not alter the increased risk. The higher the testicle is found (the further away from the scrotum), and the longer that the undescended testicle is left undescended, the higher the risk of developing testicular cancer and the lower the likelihood of retaining fertility.

9. **What should you know about testicular cancer?**
   It is the most common solid malignancy in adult men younger than 30 years. The main risk factor is **cryptorchidism**. Transillumination and ultrasound help to distinguish a hydrocele, which is filled with fluid and transilluminates, from cancer, which is solid and does not transilluminate. The most common histologic type is seminoma, which is radiosensitive and highly curable. Use ultrasound to make the diagnosis.

10. **What is the usual presenting sign of testicular cancer? Describe the major risk factors and treatment.**
    Testicular cancer usually presents as a painless testicular mass in a young man (15 to 35 years of age). The main risk factor is cryptorchidism. Testicular cancer is generally treated with orchiectomy and radiation; if the disease is widespread, use chemotherapy. Alpha-fetoprotein (AFP) is a marker for yolk sac tumors; human chorionic gonadotropin is a marker for choriocarcinoma. Leydig cell tumors may secrete androgens and cause precocious puberty.

11. **Cover the right-hand columns in the following table and specify the classic differences between testicular torsion and epididymitis. What imaging test can be used to diagnose and distinguish these two conditions?**

	TESTICULAR TORSION	EPIDIDYMITIS
Age	<30 yr (usually prepubertal)	>30 yr*
Appearance	Testis may be elevated into the inguinal canal; swelling	Swollen testis, overlying erythema, urethral discharge/ urethritis, prostatitis
Prehn sign	Pain stays the same or worsens	Pain decreases with testicular elevation
Treatment	Immediate surgery to salvage the testis; surgical orchiopexy for both testes	Antibiotics*

*In men younger than 50 years, epididymitis is commonly due to sexually transmitted disease (chlamydial infection and gonorrhea). Treat accordingly. In men older than 50 years, epididymitis is commonly due to urinary tract infection (e.g., *Escherichia coli*). Treat with trimethoprim-sulfamethoxazole or ciprofloxacin.

Ultrasound is the diagnostic test of choice in the setting of testicular or scrotal pain. It can easily differentiate between these two conditions and visualize testicular tumors (for which pain is sometimes a presenting symptom, although classically they are painless).

12. **What are the presenting symptoms for prostatitis?**
    For acute prostatitis, look for a spiking fever, chills, dysuria, malaise, irritative urinary symptoms (e.g., urgency, frequency, urge incontinence), cloudy urine, and pelvic, perineal, or testicular pain. Pain at the tip of the penis is common. Swelling of the prostate can result in voiding symptoms (e.g., hesitancy and dribbling or even acute urinary retention).

13. **What are the examination findings for prostatitis? What tests should be performed if prostatitis is suspected?**

Look for a tender, firm, edematous prostate gland on digital rectal examination. A urine Gram stain and culture should be performed.

14. **What organisms cause prostatitis? What is the treatment for prostatitis?**

Escherichia coli is responsible for most cases of prostatitis, but *Proteus, Klebsiella, Enterobacter, Serratia,* and *Pseudomonas* species also cause prostatitis. Staphylococci, streptococci, and enterococci have been implicated but are much less common. Treat empirically with trimethoprim-sulfamethoxazole or a fluoroquinolone for about 2 weeks (although some physicians treat for up to 6 weeks). Urine culture results can further guide the choice of therapy.

15. **What are the symptoms and sequelae of benign prostatic hyperplasia (BPH)?**

BPH can cause urinary hesitancy, intermittency, terminal dribbling, decreases in the size and force of the urinary stream, a sensation of incomplete emptying, nocturia, urgency, dysuria, and frequency. BPH may result in acute urinary retention, urinary tract infections, hydronephrosis, and even kidney damage or failure in severe cases.

16. **How is BPH treated?**

Medical therapy, which is started when the patient becomes symptomatic, includes long-acting alpha$_1$-blockers (e.g., terazosin, doxazosin, tamsulosin, alfuzosin, and silodosin) and 5-alpha-reductase inhibitors (finasteride, dutasteride). Transurethral resection of the prostate (TURP) is used for more advanced cases, especially for repeated urinary tract infections, urosepsis, urinary retention, and/or hydronephrosis or kidney damage caused by reflux. Surgical prostatectomy is used in some patients, but is associated with a higher complication rate.

17. **How do you recognize and manage acute urinary retention?**

The presenting symptoms of acute urinary retention are generally abdominal pain; a full, distended bladder that can be palpated on abdominal examination; a history of BPH in men; and a lack of urination in the past 24 hours or longer. The first step is to empty the bladder. If you cannot insert a regular Foley catheter, consider the use of a larger catheter with a firm Coude tip, or alternatively perform a suprapubic tap to drain the bladder. Then address the underlying cause—usually BPH, which in this setting is generally treated with TURP. Neurogenic causes of urinary retention should also be considered including spinal cord compression and multiple sclerosis.

18. **What are the common causes of erectile dysfunction?**

Erectile dysfunction is most commonly caused by vascular problems and atherosclerosis. Medications are also a common culprit (especially antihypertensive and antidepressant agents). Diabetes can cause impotence through vascular (increased atherosclerosis) or neurogenic (diabetic autonomic neuropathy) compromise. Patients undergoing dialysis often have erectile dysfunction. Remember the mnemonic point and shoot: parasympathetic agents mediate erection; sympathetic agents mediate ejaculation.

The history often gives you a clue if the cause of impotence is psychogenic. Look for a normal pattern of nocturnal erections, selective dysfunction (the patient has normal erections when masturbating but not with his partner), and a history of stress, anxiety, or fear.

19. **Distinguish between hydrocele and varicocele.**

A **hydrocele** represents a remnant of the processus vaginalis (remember embryology?) and transilluminates. It generally causes no symptoms and needs no treatment. A **varicocele** is a dilatation of the pampiniform venous plexus (so-called bag of worms, usually on the left). It does not transilluminate, disappears in the supine position, and becomes prominent on standing or if the Valsalva maneuver is performed. Varicoceles may cause infertility or pain. If they are symptomatic, they can be treated surgically.

20. **Define epispadias and hypospadias. How are they treated?**

Both are congenital penile anomalies. In **hypospadias** the urethra opens on the dorsal (under) side of the penis. In **epispadias** the urethra opens on the ventral (top) side of the penis. Epispadias is associated with exstrophy of the bladder. Both conditions are treated with surgical correction.

INFECTIONS

1. **What is the classic cause of orchitis? How is it treated? Does it usually cause infertility?**

   Mumps can cause orchitis, for which the classical presentation is a painful, swollen testis in a postpubertal male. The best treatment is prevention (immunization against the mumps virus). Mumps orchitis rarely causes sterility because it is usually unilateral. Epididymoorchitis is more common and is typically due to spread from adjacent bacterial epididymitis.

2. **What do you need to know about syphilis, HIV, hepatitis B virus (HBV), and hepatitis C virus (HCV)?**

   Syphilis and HIV are discussed in detail in Chapter 15. HBV and HCV are discussed in detail in Chapter 5.

3. **What are the presenting symptoms for genital herpes in men? What causes it?**

   Look for painful vesicles in the anogenital region as a result of infection with human herpes simplex virus (HSV), typically type 2. Other signs and symptoms may include tingling in the genital area, fever, headache, myalgias, and tender inguinal lymphadenopathy.

4. **How do you diagnose genital herpes? What is the treatment?**

   Genital herpes is often a clinical diagnosis, but it can be confirmed by viral polymerase chain reaction (PCR) after unroofing a vesicle. Primary episodes of genital herpes can be treated with acyclovir, famciclovir, or valacyclovir. Treatment of recurrences depends on the frequency of episodes and severity of symptoms. For frequent episodes or severe symptoms, suppressive therapy with any of the above medications may be considered.

5. **What causes infectious urethritis in men? What are the presenting symptoms?**

   Chlamydia and gonorrhea cause most cases of infectious urethritis in sexually active men, but Mycoplasma genitalium, HSV, and Treponema pallidum (syphilis) must also be considered. Dysuria is the most common complaint, but other signs and symptoms include itching, burning, and a urethral discharge. Urethral discharges can range from watery to purulent.

6. **How is urethritis diagnosed?**

   Diagnosis can be made on the basis of symptoms but can also be supported by the presence of a urethral discharge, polymorphonuclear neutrophils on a Gram stain of a urethral swab, positive leukocyte esterase on a urine dipstick, or 10 or more white blood cells per high-power field on urinalysis. Urine PCR for Chlamydia and gonorrhea should be performed in all cases of suspected urethritis.

7. **How is urethritis treated?**

   Empiric treatment for suspected gonococcal urethritis is 250 mg of ceftriaxone intramuscularly and a single oral dose of 1 g of azithromycin, which also treats Chlamydia trachomatis (treatment for Chlamydia is included because it can be asymptomatic). For patients with confirmed nongonococcal urethritis, treat with 1 g of azithromycin orally or 100 mg of doxycycline twice daily for 7 days.

8. **What diseases does human papillomavirus (HPV) infection cause in males? Which HPV subtypes are responsible?**

   Most men who get HPV never develop any signs or symptoms. HPV types 6 and 11 cause 90% of genital warts. Anal cancer is rare, but the incidence is rising; HPV types 16 and 18 cause 70% of anal cancers and precancerous anal lesions. HPV is also implicated in the rising incidence of squamous cell carcinoma of the head and neck.

9. **What is the current recommendation regarding vaccination against HPV in males?**

   The United States Advisory Committee on Immunization Practices (ACIP) recommends routine use of a quadrivalent HPV vaccine series (Gardasil) in males aged 11 or 12 years, although it can be administered to patients as young as 9 years. Vaccination is recommended for males aged 13 to 21 years who have not been vaccinated previously. For males who have sex with males and for immunocompromised males, the ACIP recommends vaccination up to the age of 26 years for those who have not been previously vaccinated.

TRAUMA AND TOXIC EFFECTS

1. What are the signs of urethral injury?

   Urethral injury usually occurs in the context of pelvic trauma. The four hallmark warning signs are a boggy, movable prostate on examination; blood at the urethral meatus; severe pelvic fracture; and scrotal/perineal ecchymosis.

2. True or false: Urethral injury is a contraindication to insertion of a Foley catheter.

   True. Always look for the four warning signs of urethral injury. If even one of these signs is present, do not attempt to insert a Foley catheter. Order a retrograde urethrogram to rule out urethral injury in this setting.

CHAPTER 15

DISORDERS OF THE IMMUNE SYSTEM

IMMUNE DEFICIENCY DISORDERS

1. **What is the most common primary immunodeficiency? How do you recognize it?**
   Immunoglobulin A (IgA) deficiency, which causes recurrent respiratory and gastrointestinal infections. IgA levels are always low, and levels of IgG subclass 2 may be low. Do not give immunoglobulins, which may cause anaphylaxis because of the development of anti-IgA antibodies. Alternatively, if any patient develops anaphylaxis after immunoglobulin exposure, you should think of IgA deficiency.

2. **How do you recognize Bruton agammaglobulinemia?**
   Bruton agammaglobulinemia (X-linked agammaglobulinemia) is an X-linked recessive disorder with low or absent B cells that affects males. Infections begin after the age of 6 months, when maternal antibodies disappear. Look for recurrent lung or sinus infections with *Streptococcus* and *Haemophilus* species.

3. **What is the classic cause of severe combined immunodeficiency? What are the presenting symptoms?**
   Severe combined immunodeficiency may be autosomal recessive or X-linked. The classic cause is **adenosine deaminase deficiency** (autosomal recessive). Patients have B- and T-cell defects and severe infections in the first few months of life. Other symptoms include cutaneous anergy and absent or dysplastic thymus and lymph nodes.

4. **Describe the pathophysiology of chronic granulomatous disease.**
   Chronic granulomatous disease (CGD) is usually an X-linked recessive disorder that affects males. Because of a defect in the activity of the enzyme nicotinamide adenine dinucleotide phosphate (NADPH) oxidase, patients have recurrent infections with catalase-positive organisms (e.g., *Staphylococcus aureus, Pseudomonas* species). The diagnosis is confirmed if the question mentions deficient nitroblue tetrazolium (NBT) dye reduction by granulocytes. This test measures the respiratory burst, which patients with CGD lack. On the USMLE, if you see CGD, look for NBT in the answer.

5. **Complement deficiencies of C5 through C9 cause recurrent infections with which bacterial genus?**
   Neisseria species.

6. **Define chronic mucocutaneous candidiasis.**
   Chronic mucocutaneous candidiasis is a cellular immunodeficiency specific for candidal infection. Patients have thrush and candidal infections of the scalp, skin, and nails, as well as anergy to *Candida* species on skin testing. The condition is often associated with hypothyroidism. The rest of the patient's immune function is intact; no other types of infection are present.

7. **Give the classic description of hyper-IgE syndrome (Job-Buckley syndrome).**
   Patients with hyper-IgE syndrome have recurrent staphylococcal infections (especially of the skin) and have extremely high IgE levels. They also commonly have fair skin, red hair, and eczema.

8. **What is the mechanism of action of the immunosuppressant drugs commonly used in transplant medicine?**
   - Steroids inhibit interleukin-1 production.
   - Methotrexate is a folic acid antagonist, but its precise immunosuppression mechanism is unclear.
   - Cyclosporine inhibits interleukin-2 production.
   - Tacrolimus inhibits signaling through the T-cell receptor.
   - Mycophenolate prevents T-cell activation.

- Azathioprine is an antineoplastic agent that is cleaved to mercaptopurine and inhibits DNA/RNA synthesis (which causes decreased production of B cells and T cells).
- Antithymocyte globulin is an antibody against T cells.
- OKT3 is an antibody to the CD3 receptor on T cells.
- For thalidomide, the mechanism of action is not known.
- Hydroxychloroquine interferes with antigen presentation.
- Basiliximab is a monoclonal antibody against the interleukin-2 receptor.
- Daclizumab is a monoclonal antibody against the interleukin-2 receptor.

9. **What risks are associated with immunosuppression?**
Immunosuppression carries a risk of infection (with common and rare organisms that infect patients with AIDS) and an increased risk of cancer (especially lymphomas and epithelial cell cancers).

HUMAN IMMUNODEFICIENCY VIRUS (HIV)

1. **What sexually transmitted infectious disease should be at the back of your mind when a patient has a sore throat and a mononucleosis-like syndrome?**
HIV infection, because initial seroconversion may present as a mononucleosis-like syndrome (e.g., fever, malaise, pharyngitis, rash, lymphadenopathy).

2. **How is HIV diagnosed? How long after exposure does the HIV test become positive?**
Diagnosis is on the basis of an enzyme-linked immunosorbent assay (ELISA), which, if positive, is confirmed with a Western blot test. All of these tests should be performed before you tell the patient anything. It takes 6 to 12 weeks for antibodies to develop in the majority of patients. Antibodies are present by 6 months in 95% of patients. Therefore, if a patient wants a test because of recent risk-taking behavior, you should retest the patient in 6 months if the initial test is negative.
  Rapid tests are available, but the predictive accuracy varies with the prevalence of HIV infection in the population. Positive tests require confirmatory testing with ELISA and Western blotting. Negative test results are reliable unless the patient is in the window period of acute HIV infection.

3. **Are control tests needed when a purified protein derivative (PPD) tuberculosis test is performed for HIV-positive patients?**
Most authorities no longer recommend control testing (also known as anergy) testing when a PPD test is performed for HIV-positive patients.

4. **Cover the right-hand column in the following table and answer the questions about HIV management on the left.**

QUESTION	ANSWER
After HIV diagnosis, how often should you check the CD4 count?	Every 3-4 mo; every 6 mo for patients who adhere to therapy with sustained viral suppression and have stable clinical status for more than 2-3 yr
When do you start antiretroviral therapy?	As regimens are getting simpler with fewer side effects, treatment thresholds are decreasing. Start treatment when the CD4 count is <350 cells/mL or if there is a history of an AIDS-defining illness. Also initiate treatment in pregnant women, in patients with HIV-associated nephropathy, and in patients with hepatitis B coinfection.

QUESTION	ANSWER
What are the AIDS-defining illnesses?	*Pneumocystis jirovecii* pneumonia Esophageal candidiasis Wasting Kaposi sarcoma Disseminated *Mycobacterium avium* infection Tuberculosis Cytomegalovirus disease HIV-associated dementia Recurrent bacterial pneumonia Toxoplasmosis Immunoblastic lymphoma Chronic cryptosporidiosis Burkitt lymphoma Disseminated histoplasmosis Invasive cervical cancer Chronic herpes simplex virus infection
When do you start PCP prophylaxis?	When the CD4 count is <200 cells/mL or for a history of oropharyngeal candidiasis.
What is the drug of choice for PCP prophylaxis?	Trimethoprim-sulfamethoxazole (Bactrim).
What other agents are used in patients with allergy or intolerance to Bactrim?	Dapsone, aerosolized pentamidine, and atovaquone.
When should you start *Mycobacterium avium* complex (MAC) prophylaxis?	When the CD4 count is <50 cells/mL.
What drugs are used for MAC prophylaxis?	Clarithromycin or azithromycin (rifabutin is an alternative).
True or false: Once the CD4 count is <200 cells/mL, the patient is automatically considered to have AIDS (even without opportunistic infections).	True.
True or false: Give the measles-mumps-rubella vaccine.	True (CD4 count must be >200 cells/mL).
True or false: Give the varicella vaccine.	True, if the patient does not have evidence of immunity (CD4 count must be >200 cells/mL).
True or false: Do not give annual influenza vaccines.	False (give every year to all HIV-infected patients).
True or false: Pneumococcal vaccine should be given.	True. It should be given to all HIV-infected patients, and revaccination every 5 yr should be considered.
True or false: Give hepatitis A vaccine.	True, if the patient has chronic liver disease or is at increased risk of hepatitis A infection.
True or false: Give hepatitis B vaccine.	True.
True or false: PPD testing should be performed annually.	True, if the initial test is negative and the patient is at high risk.
True or false: Oral polio vaccine should be given to patients who are at risk of exposure through travel or work.	False (use inactive polio vaccine injection).

Continued

QUESTION	ANSWER
The risk of which cancer is increased on skin and in the mouth?	Kaposi sarcoma (discussed in more detail in Chapter 8).
The risk of which type of blood cell cancer is increased?	Non-Hodgkin lymphoma (usually primary B-cell lymphomas of the CNS).
What do positive India ink preparations of cerebrospinal fluid indicate?	*Cryptococcus neoformans* meningitis.
What do ring-enhancing lesions in the brain on CT or MRI scans usually mean?	Toxoplasmosis, cysticercosis/*Taenia solium*, or lymphoma.
True or false: HIV may cause thrombocytopenia.	True.
True or false: HIV can cause dementia.	True.
True or false: HIV protects against peripheral neuropathies.	False (HIV can cause them).
True or false: HIV-positive mothers may breastfeed their infants.	False (breast milk transmits HIV).
What is the first-choice agent for CMV retinitis?	Valganciclovir.
What are the second-choice agents for CMV retinitis?	Ganciclovir, foscarnet, and cidofovir.
True or false: Pregnant patients should receive antiretroviral therapy.	True. Three-drug therapy is currently recommended (no different for pregnant females; earlier administration is best).
True or false: Infants born to HIV-positive mothers should take zidovudine (ZDV).	True (for at least 6 wk after delivery).
True or false: Cesarean section increases maternal HIV transmission.	False (it may decrease transmission to the infant).
What is the most likely cause of pneumonia in HIV-positive patients?	*Streptococcus pneumoniae.*
What is the most likely cause of opportunistic pneumonia in HIV-positive patients?	*Pneumocystis jirovecii* (discussed in more detail in Chapter 3).
Name a stain used on sputum to detect PCP.	Silver (Wright-Giemsa or Giemsa).
Name two pathogens that cause chronic diarrhea only in AIDS.	*Cryptosporidium* and *Isospora* species.
True or false: Herpes zoster infection in young adults represents possible HIV infection.	True (suggests immunodeficiency).
True or false: Thrush in young adults may mean HIV infection.	True (also associated with diabetes, leukemia, and steroids).
True or false: A positive HIV antibody test in a newborn is unreliable.	True (maternal antibodies in the neonate can give a false-positive result for the first 6 mo).

CMV, Cytomegalovirus; CNS, central nervous system; CT, computed tomography; MRI, magnetic resonance imaging; PCP, pneumocystis pneumonia; PPD, purified protein derivative.

VASCULAR AND ARTERIAL DISORDERS

1. What is Henoch-Schönlein purpura?
   Henoch-Schönlein purpura is a vasculitis that may involve symptoms of gastrointestinal bleeding and abdominal pain. Look for a history of upper respiratory tract infection, a

characteristic rash on the lower extremities and buttocks, swelling of the hands and feet, arthritis, and/or hematuria and proteinuria. Treat supportively with hydration, rest, and pain relief.

2. **Describe the usual presentation of Kawasaki disease. How is it treated?**
   Kawasaki disease usually affects children younger than 5 years; it is more common in Japanese and female children. Patients have a truncal rash, high fever (which lasts longer than 5 days), conjunctival injection, cervical lymphadenopathy, strawberry tongue, late skin desquamation of the palms and soles, and/or arthritis. Patients may develop coronary vessel vasculitis and subsequent aneurysms, which may thrombose and cause a myocardial infarction. Kawasaki disease should be suspected in any child who has a heart attack. Treat during the acute stage with aspirin and intravenous immunoglobulins to reduce the risk of coronary aneurysm. Kawasaki disease can be remembered by the mnemonic **CRASH and burn:** conjunctivitis, rash, adenopathy, strawberry tongue, and hands/feet desquamation (CRASH; burn is for the 5 days of fever). For complete Kawasaki disease, the patient must have at least four of these five signs in addition to the 5 days of fever. Incomplete (previously called atypical) Kawasaki disease can be diagnosed if the patient has two or three of these signs and laboratory abnormalities that are consistent with Kawasaki disease (e.g., elevated C-reactive protein or erythrocyte sedimentation rate, hypoalbuminemia, anemia). Patients should be screened for coronary aneurysms and other cardiac complications via echocardiography and electrocardiography.

3. **What are the presenting symptoms for Takayasu arteritis?**
   Takayasu arteritis tends to affect Asian women between the ages of 15 and 30 years. It is called "the pulseless disease" because you may not be able to feel the pulse or measure blood pressure on the affected side. The vasculitis affects the aortic arch and its branches. Carotid involvement may cause neurologic signs or stroke, and congestive heart failure is not uncommon. Angiography reveals the characteristic lesions. Treat with steroids.

4. **What autoimmune disorders affect the lungs and kidneys?**
   Wegener granulomatosis and Goodpasture syndrome. These are discussed in more detail in Chapter 10.

MUSCULOSKELETAL/CONNECTIVE TISSUE DISORDERS

1. **What disease classically causes a false-positive result for the rapid plasma reagin (RPR) or Venereal Disease Research Laboratory (VDRL) syphilis test?**
   Systemic lupus erythematosus (SLE). A false-positive result on the RPR or VDRL test is actually one of the diagnostic criteria for SLE.

2. **What other conditions are associated with an increased risk of malignancy?**
   Other diseases with an increased incidence of cancer include dermatomyositis, polymyositis, immunodeficiency syndromes, Bloom syndrome, and Fanconi anemia. Breast, ovarian, and colon cancer have well-known familial tendencies (as well as some other types of cancer), but rarely can a Mendelian inheritance pattern be demonstrated (e.g., *BRCA1* and *BRCA2* genes account for about 5% of breast cancers).

3. **What are the signs and symptoms of dermatomyositis?**
   Dermatomyositis is essentially polymyositis (see the next question) plus skin involvement (a **heliotrope rash around the eyes** with associated periorbital edema is classic). Additional skin findings include a shawl sign (a V-shaped rash around the neck), Gottron papules (scaly eruptions over the metacarpophalangeal and interphalangeal joints of the hands), and mechanic hands (rough, cracked skin on the hands). Patients usually have trouble rising from a chair or climbing steps because of the effects on proximal muscles. Muscle enzymes are elevated, and electromyography is irregular. Muscle biopsy establishes the diagnosis. The incidence of malignancy is higher in affected patients. See Chapter 7 for a complete discussion of dermatomyositis and polymyositis.

4. How do you distinguish among fibromyalgia, polymyositis, and polymyalgia rheumatica?

	FIBROMYALGIA	POLYMYOSITIS	POLYMYALGIA RHEUMATICA
Classic age/sex	Young adult women	Female aged 40-60 yr	Female aged >50 yr
Location	Various	Proximal muscles	Pectoral and pelvic girdles, neck
ESR	Normal	Elevated	Markedly elevated (often >100)
EMG/biopsy	Normal	Abnormal	Normal
Classic findings	Anxiety, stress, insomnia, point tenderness over affected muscles	Elevated CPK, abnormal EMG/biopsy, higher risk of cancer	Temporal arteritis, great response to steroids, very high ESR, elderly patients
Treatment	Antidepressants, NSAIDs, pregabalin, rest	Steroids	Steroids

CPK, Creatine phosphokinase; *ESR*, erythrocyte sedimentation rate; *EMG*, electromyography; *NSAIDs*, nonsteroidal antiinflammatory drugs.

5. **Describe the hallmarks of SLE.**
SLE can cause a malar rash, discoid rash, photosensitivity, kidney damage, arthritis, pericarditis and pleuritis, positive **antinuclear antibody** (ANA), positive **anti-Smith antibody,** positive results on the VDRL and RPR (syphilis) screening tests, positive lupus anticoagulant, blood disorders (thrombocytopenia, leukopenia, anemia, pancytopenia), neurologic disturbances (depression, psychosis, seizures), and oral ulcers. Any of these may be presenting symptoms. Use the ANA titer as a screening test, and confirm with the anti-Smith antibody test. Treat with nonsteroidal antiinflammatory drugs, hydroxychloroquine, corticosteroids, or immunosuppressive/immunomodulating agents (methotrexate, cyclophosphamide, cyclosporine, azathioprine, mycophenolate, tacrolimus, leflunomide, or belimumab).

6. **Describe the hallmarks of scleroderma.**
The hallmarks of scleroderma (also known as progressive systemic sclerosis) are **CREST** symptoms (**c**alcinosis, **R**aynaud phenomenon, **e**sophageal dysmotility with dysphagia, sclerodactyly, and **t**elangiectasia), heartburn, and mask like, leathery facies. Use the ANA test for screening; confirm the diagnosis with the **anticentromere antibody** test (for CREST symptoms only) and the **antitopoisomerase antibody** test (for full-blown scleroderma). Treatment depends on the symptoms. Sclerotic skin lesions can be treated with topical glucocorticoids, calcipotriol, or methotrexate. Systemic therapy depends on the organs affected.

7. **What are the hallmarks of Sjögren syndrome?**
Sjögren syndrome causes dry eyes (keratoconjunctivitis sicca) and dry mouth (xerostomia) and is often associated with other autoimmune diseases. Treat with eye drops and good oral hygiene.

8. **With what is polyarteritis nodosa associated? How is it diagnosed?**
Polyarteritis nodosa is a type of vasculitis classically associated with HBV infection and cryoglobulinemia. Patients present with fever, abdominal pain, weight loss, renal disturbances, and/or peripheral neuropathies. Laboratory abnormalities include elevations in the erythrocyte sedimentation rate and C-reactive protein, leukocytosis, anemia, and hematuria or proteinuria. Patients often have a positive **antineutrophil cytoplasmic antibody** (ANCA) titer. The vasculitis involves medium-sized vessels. Biopsy of an affected organ is the gold standard for diagnosis.

9. **How do you recognize Behçet syndrome on the Step 3 exam?**
Behçet syndrome classically occurs in young men in their 20s and involves painful oral and genital ulcers. Patients may also have uveitis, arthritis, and other skin lesions (especially erythema nodosum). Steroids are the mainstay of therapy.

VACCINATIONS AND CHEMOTHERAPY

1. **What do you need to know about vaccinations?**
   Vaccinations are reviewed in detail in Chapter 1.

ANAPHYLAXIS/IMMUNOLOGIC REACTIONS

1. **List the four classic types of hypersensitivity reaction.**
   - Anaphylactic (type I)
   - Cytotoxic (type II)
   - Immune complex–mediated (type III)
   - Cell-mediated/delayed (type IV)

2. **What causes type I hypersensitivity? Give the classic clinical examples.**
   Type I (anaphylactic) hypersensitivity is due to preformed IgE antibodies that cause release of vasoactive amines (e.g., histamine, leukotrienes) from mast cells and basophils. Examples are anaphylaxis, atopy, hay fever, urticaria, allergic rhinitis, and some forms of asthma. Anaphylaxis may be due to bee stings, food allergy (especially peanuts and shellfish), medications (especially penicillins and sulfa drugs), or latex allergy.

3. **Describe the clinical findings for chronic type I hypersensitivity.**
   Look for eosinophilia, elevated IgE levels, a positive family history, and seasonal exacerbations. Patients may also have allergic "shiners" (bilateral infraorbital edema) and a transverse nasal crease (caused by frequent nose rubbing). Pale, bluish, edematous nasal turbinates with many eosinophils in clear, watery nasal secretions are also classic.

4. **What medication should be avoided in patients with nasal polyps?**
   Do not give aspirin, which may precipitate a severe asthma attack.

5. **What causes type II hypersensitivity? List some classic clinical examples.**
   Type II (cytotoxic) hypersensitivity is due to preformed IgG and IgM antibodies that react with the antigen and cause secondary inflammation. Examples include the following:
   - Autoimmune hemolytic anemia (classically caused by methyldopa, penicillins, or sulfa drugs) or other cytopenias caused by antibodies (e.g., idiopathic thrombocytopenic purpura)
   - Transfusion reactions
   - Erythroblastosis fetalis (rhesus factor incompatibility)
   - Goodpasture syndrome (watch for linear immunofluorescence on kidney biopsy)
   - Myasthenia gravis
   - Graves disease
   - Pernicious anemia
   - Pemphigus vulgaris
   - Hyperacute transplant rejection (as soon as the anastomosis is made at transplant surgery, the transplanted organ deteriorates in front of the surgeon's eyes)

6. **What laboratory test is usually positive for type II hypersensitivity that causes anemia?**
   Coombs test (usually the direct Coombs test).

7. **What causes type III hypersensitivity? List some classic clinical examples.**
   Type III (immune complex–mediated) hypersensitivity is due to antigen-antibody complexes that are usually deposited in vessels and cause an inflammatory response. Examples include serum sickness, lupus erythematosus, rheumatoid arthritis, polyarteritis nodosa, cryoglobulinemia, and certain types of glomerulonephritis (e.g., from chronic hepatitis).

8. **What causes type IV hypersensitivity? How is it related to tuberculosis testing?**
   Type IV (cell-mediated/delayed) hypersensitivity is due to sensitized T lymphocytes that release inflammatory mediators. The tuberculosis skin test (PPD) exploits this immune system reaction. Other examples include contact dermatitis (especially on contact with

poison ivy, nickel earrings, cosmetics, and medications), chronic transplant rejection, and granulomas (e.g., sarcoidosis).

9. **How do you recognize and treat true anaphylaxis?**
Look for the classic triggers mentioned in Question 2 just before the patient becomes agitated and flushed and develops itching (urticaria), facial swelling (angioedema), and difficulty in breathing. Symptoms tend to develop rapidly and dramatically.

Treat immediately by giving intramuscular epinephrine and securing the airway (laryngeal edema may prevent intubation, in which case perform a cricothyroidotomy if needed). Adjuvant treatments include corticosteroids, which will work slowly to prevent a biphasic reaction. H_1 antihistamines treat the cutaneous reactions and itching but do not treat airway involvement. There is no significant evidence supporting the use of H_2 antihistamines, but they are often given because of a theoretical benefit.

10. **What usually causes hereditary angioedema?**
A deficiency of **C1 esterase inhibitor** (complement) is the usual cause of hereditary angioedema. Patients have diffuse swelling of the lips, eyelids, and possibly the airway that is unrelated to allergen exposure. The disease is autosomal dominant; look for a positive family history. C4 complement levels are low. Acute treatment is the same as for anaphylaxis, except if the diagnosis is known, fresh frozen plasma has C1 esterase inhibitor and can be considered. Recombinant C1 esterase inhibitor products are also available. Androgens are used for long-term treatment because they increase liver production of C1 esterase inhibitor.

11. **What type of testing can identify an allergen if it is not obvious?**
Skin or patch testing.

INFECTIONS

1. **What triad indicates a diagnosis of Wiskott-Aldrich syndrome?**
Wiskott-Aldrich deficiency is an X-linked recessive disorder that affects males. The classic triad consists of eczema, thrombocytopenia (look for bleeding), and recurrent infections (usually respiratory).

2. **How do you recognize Chediak-Higashi syndrome?**
Chediak-Higashi syndrome is usually an autosomal-recessive disorder characterized by giant granules in neutrophils, infections, and often oculocutaneous albinism. It is caused by a defect in microtubule polymerization.

3. **Cover the right-hand column in the following table and specify what each Gram stain most likely represents.**

GRAM STAIN RESULT	MEANING
Blue-purple color	Gram-positive organism
Red color	Gram-negative organism
Gram-positive cocci in chains	Streptococci
Gram-positive cocci in clusters	Staphylococci
Gram-positive cocci in pairs (diplococci)	*Streptococcus pneumoniae*
Gram-negative coccobacilli (small rods)	*Haemophilus* species
Gram-negative diplococci	*Neisseria* species (sexually transmitted disease, septic arthritis, meningitis) or *Moraxella* species (lungs, sinusitis)
Plump gram-negative rod with thick capsule (mucoid appearance)	*Klebsiella* species
Gram-positive rods that form spores	*Clostridium* species, *Bacillus* species
Pseudohyphae	*Candida* species

GRAM STAIN RESULT	MEANING
Acid-fast organisms	*Mycobacterium* (usually M. *tuberculosis*), *Nocardia* species
Gram-positive with sulfur granules	*Actinomyces* species (pelvic inflammatory disease in intrauterine device users; rare cause of neck mass/cervical adenitis)
Silver staining	*Pneumocystis jirovecii* and cat-scratch disease
Positive India ink preparation (thick capsule)	*Cryptococcus neoformans*
Spirochete	*Treponema* species, *Leptospira* species (both seen only on dark-field microscopy), *Borrelia* species (seen on regular light microscopy)

4. Cover the middle and right-hand columns in the following table and specify which organisms are associated with each type of infection and what type of empiric antibiotic should be used while waiting for culture results.

CONDITION	MAIN ORGANISM(S)	EMPIRIC ANTIBIOTICS
Urinary tract infection	*Escherichia coli*	Trimethoprim-sulfamethoxazole, nitrofurantoin, amoxicillin, quinolones
Bronchitis	Virus, *Haemophilus influenzae*, *Moraxella* species	Usually no benefit from antibiotics; may consider macrolides or doxycycline
Pneumonia (classic)	*Streptococcus pneumoniae*, *H. influenzae*	3rd-generation cephalosporin, azithromycin
Pneumonia (atypical)	*Mycoplasma*, *Chlamydia* species	Macrolide antibiotic, doxycycline
Osteomyelitis	*Staphylococcus aureus*, *Salmonella* species	Oxacillin, cefazolin, vancomycin
Cellulitis	Streptococci, staphylococci	Cephalexin, dicloxacillin, trimethoprim-sulfamethoxazole, doxycycline, or clindamycin are often used as first-line agents owing to the emergence of MRSA
Meningitis (neonate)	Group B *Streptococcus*, *E. coli*, *Listeria* species	Ampicillin + aminoglycoside (usually gentamicin); an expanded spectrum 3rd-generation cephalosporin (cefotaxime) should be added if a gram-negative organism is suspected
Meningitis (child/adult)	*S. pneumoniae*, *Neisseria meningitidis**	Cefotaxime or ceftriaxone + vancomycin
Endocarditis (native valve)	Staphylococci, streptococci	Antistaphylococcal penicillin† (or vancomycin if allergic to penicillin) + aminoglycoside
Endocarditis (prosthetic valve)	Numerous different organisms	Vancomycin + gentamicin + cefepime or a carbapenem
Sepsis	Gram-negative organisms, streptococci, staphylococci	3rd-generation penicillin/cephalosporin + aminoglycoside, or imipenem

Continued

CONDITION	MAIN ORGANISM(S)	EMPIRIC ANTIBIOTICS
Septic arthritis‡	*S. aureus*	Vancomycin
	Gram-negative bacilli	Ceftazidime or ceftriaxone
	Gonococci	Ceftriaxone, ciprofloxacin, or spectinomycin

MRSA, Methicillin-resistant *S. aureus*.

H. influenzae is no longer as common a cause of meningitis in children because of widespread vaccination. In a child with no history of immunization, *H. influenzae* is the most likely cause of meningitis.

†Examples: oxacillin, nafcillin.

‡Think of staphylococci if the patient is monogamous or not sexually active. Think of gonorrhea for younger adults who are sexually active.

5. Cover the right-hand columns in the following table and specify the empiric antibiotic of choice for each organism.

ORGANISM*	ANTIBIOTIC	OTHER CHOICES
Streptococcus A or B	Penicillin, cefazolin	Erythromycin
S. pneumoniae	3rd-generation cephalosporin + vancomycin	Fluoroquinolone
Enterococcus	Penicillin or ampicillin + aminoglycoside	Vancomycin + aminoglycoside
Staphylococcus aureus	Antistaphylococcus penicillin (e.g., methicillin)	Vancomycin, trimethoprim-sulfamethoxazole, doxycycline, clindamycin, or linezolid for MRSA
Gonococcus†	Ceftriaxone	Cefixime or high-dose azithromycin followed by test of cure in 1 wk
Meningococcus	Cefotaxime or ceftriaxone	Chloramphenicol or penicillin G if proven to be penicillin susceptible
Haemophilus	2nd- or 3rd-generation cephalosporin	Amoxicillin
Pseudomonas	Antipseudomonal penicillin (ticarcillin, piperacillin) ± beta-lactamase inhibitor (clavulanate, tazobactam)	Ceftazidime, cefepime, aztreonam, imipenem, ciprofloxacin
Bacteroides	Metronidazole	Clindamycin
Mycoplasma	Erythromycin, azithromycin	Doxycycline
Treponema pallidum	Penicillin	Doxycycline
Chlamydia	Doxycycline, azithromycin	Erythromycin, ofloxacin
Lyme disease (*Borrelia* species)	Cefuroxime, doxycycline, amoxicillin	Erythromycin

MRSA, Methicillin-resistant *S. aureus*.

*Always use culture sensitivity to guide therapy once available. Local resistance patterns and institutional standards may vary.

†For genital infections, always treat for presumed *Chlamydia* coinfection using azithromycin or doxycycline.

6. Cover the two right-hand columns in the following table and specify the organism after looking at the scenario associated with it.

SCENARIO	ORGANISM(S)	COMMENTS
Stuck with thorn or gardening	*Sporothrix schenckii*	Treat with itraconazole
Aplastic crisis in sickle cell disease	Parvovirus	B19
Sepsis after splenectomy	*Streptococcus pneumoniae, Haemophilus influenzae, Neisseria meningitis* (encapsulated bacteria)	
Pneumonia in the Southwest (California, Arizona)	*Coccidioides immitis*	Treat with itraconazole or fluconazole, amphotericin B for severe disease
Pneumonia after cave exploring or exposure to bird droppings in Ohio and Mississippi River valleys	*Histoplasma capsulatum*	
Pneumonia after exposure to a parrot or exotic bird	*Chlamydia psittaci*	
Fungus ball/hemoptysis after tuberculosis or cavitary lung disease	*Aspergillus* species	Treat with voriconazole
Pneumonia in a patient with silicosis	Tuberculosis	
Diarrhea after hiking/drinking from a stream	*Giardia lamblia*	Stool cysts; treat with metronidazole
Pregnant woman with cats	*Toxoplasma gondii*	Treat infected pregnant women with spiramycin
B_{12} deficiency and abdominal symptoms	*Diphyllobothrium latum* (intestinal tapeworm)	
Seizures with ring-enhancing brain lesion on CT	*Taenia solium* (cysticercosis) or toxoplasmosis	Treat neurocysticercosis with albendazole or praziquantel, usually with steroids; consider anticonvulsants
Squamous cell bladder cancer in Middle East or Africa	*Schistosoma haematobium*	
Worm infection in children	*Enterobius* species	Positive tape test, perianal itching; treat with mebendazole or albendazole
Fever, muscle pain, eosinophilia, and periorbital edema after eating raw meat	*Trichinella spiralis* (trichinosis)	
Gastroenteritis in young children	Rotavirus, Norwalk virus	
Food poisoning after eating reheated rice	*Bacillus cereus*	Infection is usually self-limited
Food poisoning after eating raw seafood	*Vibrio parahaemolyticus*	

Continued

SCENARIO	ORGANISM(S)	COMMENTS
Diarrhea after travel to Mexico	*Escherichia coli* (Montezuma's revenge)	Treat with ciprofloxacin
Diarrhea after antibiotics	*Clostridium difficile*	Use oral metronidazole or oral vancomycin
Baby paralyzed after eating honey	*C. botulinum*	Toxin blocks acetylcholine release
Genital lesions in children in the absence of sexual abuse or activity	*Molluscum contagiosum*	
Cellulitis after cat/dog bite	*Pasteurella multocida*	Treat high-risk animal bite wounds with prophylactic amoxicillin-clavulanate
Slaughterhouse worker with fever	Brucellosis	
Pneumonia after being in a hotel or near an air conditioner or water tower	*Legionella pneumophila*	Treat with azithromycin or levofloxacin
Burn wound infection with blue-green color	*Pseudomonas* species	*S. aureus* is also a common cause of burn infection, but it lacks blue-green color

7. **How is syphilis diagnosed?**
   Screen for syphilis with an RPR or VDRL test. Confirm a positive test with a fluorescent treponemal antibody absorption (FTA-ABS) or microhemagglutination (MHA-TP) test because false positives occur with the RPR and VDRL tests, classically in patients with lupus erythematosus. Once syphilis is treated, the RPR and VDRL tests become negative, whereas the FTA-ABS and MHA-TP tests often remain positive for life. You also can scrape the base of a genital chancre or condyloma lata and look for spirochetes on dark-field microscopy.

8. **How is syphilis treated?**
   With penicillin. Use doxycycline for penicillin-allergic patients unless they are pregnant or have neurosyphilis (in these cases, desensitization therapy is recommended, and penicillin is still the treatment of choice).

9. **Describe the three stages of syphilis.**
   Primary stage: Look for a painless chancre that resolves on its own within 8 weeks.
   Secondary stage: Roughly 6 weeks to 18 months after infection; look for condyloma lata, a maculopapular rash (classically involves palms and soles of the feet; Fig. 15-1), and lymphadenopathy.
   Tertiary stage: Years after the initial infection (between the secondary and tertiary stages is the latent phase, in which the disease is quiet and asymptomatic). Look for gummas (granulomas in many different organs), neurologic symptoms and signs (e.g., neurosyphilis, Argyll-Robertson pupil, dementia, paresis, tabes dorsalis, Charcot joints), and thoracic aortic aneurysms.

10. **Describe the classic findings for Epstein-Barr virus (EBV) infection (infectious mononucleosis).**
    Look for fatigue, fever, pharyngitis, and cervical lymphadenopathy in a young adult. The signs and symptoms are similar to those for streptococcal pharyngitis, but malaise tends to be prolonged and pronounced in EBV infection. To differentiate from streptococcal pharyngitis, look for the following:
    • Splenomegaly (patients are at increased risk of splenic rupture and should avoid contact sports and heavy lifting)
    • Hepatomegaly

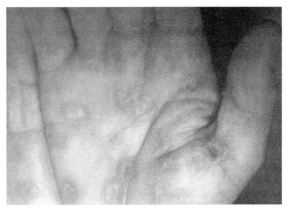

Figure 15-1. Palmar lesions of secondary syphilis. (*From Mandell GL, Bennett JE, Dolin R*. Mandell, Douglas, and Bennett's principles and practice of infectious diseases. *7th ed. Philadelphia: Churchill and Livingstone, 2009.*)

- Atypical lymphocytes (bizarre forms that may resemble leukemia) with lymphocytosis, anemia, or thrombocytopenia
- Positive serology (heterophile antibodies [e.g., monospot test] or specific EBV antibodies (viral capsid antigen, Epstein-Barr nuclear antigens)

11. What is an important differential in the diagnosis of EBV infection?
Acute HIV infection, which can cause a mononucleosis-type syndrome.

12. What is the association between EBV and cancer?
EBV is associated with nasopharyngeal cancer, African Burkitt lymphoma, and posttransplant lymphoproliferative disorder.

13. Describe the classic clinical vignette for Rocky Mountain spotted fever. What causes it? What is the treatment?
Look for history of a tick bite 1 week before the development of a high fever or chills, severe headache, and prostration or severe malaise. A rash appears roughly 4 days later on the palms and wrists and soles and ankles and spreads rapidly to the trunk and face (unique pattern of spread). Patients often look quite ill (e.g., disseminated intravascular coagulation, delirium). The infection is caused by *Rickettsia rickettsii*. Treat with doxycycline; chloramphenicol is a second choice.

14. In what clinical scenario does rabies occur in the United States? Describe the classic physical findings.
Rabies in the United States is due to bites from bats, skunks, raccoons, or foxes; rabies caused by dog bites is extremely rare because of vaccination. The incubation period is usually around 1 to 2 months. The classic findings are hydrophobia (fear of water because of painful swallowing) and central nervous system signs (e.g., paralysis).

15. What should you do after a patient is bitten by an animal?
1. Treat the local wound. Cleanse thoroughly with soap. Do *not* cauterize or suture the wound. Amoxicillin-clavulanate is often given for cellulitis prophylaxis.
2. Observe the animal. If possible, capture and observe the animal for ten days to see if it develops rabies. If a wild animal is caught, it should be killed and the brain tissue examined for rabies.
3. If the wild animal escapes or has rabies, give rabies immunoglobulin and vaccinate the patient. In cases of a dog or cat bite, do *not* give prophylaxis or vaccine unless the animal acted strangely or bit the patient without provocation and rabies is prevalent in the area (rare). Do not give prophylaxis or vaccine for bites from rabbits or small rodents (e.g., rats, mice, squirrels, chipmunks).

16. **What are the two main infections caused by *Streptococcus pyogenes* (group A *Streptococcus*)? What are the common sequelae?**
    S. pyogenes causes pharyngitis and skin infections. Sequelae include rheumatic fever, scarlet fever, and poststreptococcal glomerulonephritis.

17. **Other than pneumonia, what infections does *Streptococcus pneumoniae* commonly cause?**
    Otitis media, meningitis, sinusitis, and spontaneous bacterial peritonitis.

18. **What are the main infections caused by *Staphylococcus aureus*?**
    The list is long. *S. aureus* is a common cause of the following infections:
    - Skin and soft-tissue abscesses (especially in the breast after breastfeeding or in the skin after a furuncle)
    - Endocarditis (especially in drug users)
    - Osteomyelitis (the most common cause, unless sickle cell disease is present)
    - Septic arthritis
    - Food poisoning (via a preformed toxin)
    - Toxic shock syndrome (via a preformed toxin)
    - Scalded skin syndrome (via a preformed toxin; affects younger children who often have impetigo and subsequent desquamation)
    - Impetigo
    - Cellulitis
    - Wound infections
    - Pneumonia (often forms a lung abscess or empyema)
    - Furuncles and carbuncles

19. **What is the treatment of choice for staphylococcal infections on the USMLE?**
    An antistaphylococcal penicillin (e.g., methicillin, dicloxacillin). Use vancomycin, clindamycin, doxycycline, trimethoprim-sulfamethoxazole, or linezolid if the staphylococcal species is known to be methicillin resistant or if methicillin-resistant *S. aureus* (MRSA) is suspected. MRSA is a rapidly growing problem. Most abscesses (regardless of the causative organism) must be treated first with surgical incision and drainage because antibiotics cannot penetrate through the walls of an abscess cavity.

20. **Distinguish between preorbital (preseptal) and orbital cellulitis.**
    The symptoms for both conditions may include swollen eyelids; fever; a history of facial laceration, trauma, insect bite, or sinusitis; and chemosis (edema of the conjunctiva). However, if ophthalmoplegia, proptosis, severe eye pain, or decreased visual acuity is present, the patient has orbital cellulitis. Orbital cellulitis is an ophthalmologic emergency because it may extend into the skull and cause meningitis, venous thromboses, and/or blindness.

21. **What are the common bacterial causes of preorbital and orbital cellulitis? How are they treated?**
    The most common bacteria in both are *Streptococcus pneumoniae*, *Haemophilus influenzae* type B, and *Staphylococcus aureus* or other streptococcal species (in patients with a history of trauma). For both conditions, obtain blood cultures and administer broad-spectrum antibiotics until the culture results are known. A typical regimen for preorbital cellulitis is monotherapy with clindamycin or combination therapy with trimethoprim-sulfamethoxazole plus either amoxicillin or amoxicillin-clavulanic acid or cefpodoxime or cefdinir. A typical regimen for orbital cellulitis is vancomycin plus either ceftriaxone or cefotaxime or ampicillin-sulbactam, or piperacillin-tazobactam. Although preorbital cellulitis may be treated on an outpatient basis with close follow-up, orbital cellulitis requires hospital admission and intravenous antibiotics.

22. **What prophylactic medication should be given to contacts of a patient with *Neisseria meningitidis* infection?**
    Rifampin, ciprofloxacin, or ceftriaxone.

CHAPTER 16

CLINICAL CASE SCENARIOS

CASE 1

History of present illness (HPI): A 60-year-old man with a history of hypertension has right lower leg redness, swelling, and warmth. He states that about 1 week ago he hit his shin while working on his car, which left a small laceration on his skin. Initially it seemed to heal well, but for the past 3 days the skin around the site has become increasingly red, warm, painful, and swollen and is now "the size of a half dollar." He says that he felt like he may have had a fever at home, but did not take his temperature. He denies any other symptoms.

Vital signs: Temperature 98.2° F (36.8° C), pulse 80 beats/min, blood pressure (BP) 140/78 mm Hg, respiratory rate (RR) 16 breaths/min.

Additional history: The patient takes hydrochlorothiazide for hypertension. He occasionally consumes alcohol; he denies smoking and drug use.

1. **What is the differential diagnosis?**
   Cellulitis, erysipelas, fasciitis, thrombophlebitis, stasis dermatitis.

2. **What components of the physical examination do you perform?**
   General appearance, cardiovascular, lungs, skin/extremities.
   Physical examination:
   General: Well-developed, overweight man in no apparent distress.
   Cardiovascular: Within normal limits (WNL).
   Lungs: WNL
   Skin/extremities: 4×4-cm^2 region of poorly demarcated erythema on the anterolateral surface of the right mid-calf with associated warmth and edema. Small 1-cm laceration at the middle of the erythema, healed, without purulence or discharge. No crepitus, no tenderness proximally, no other skin changes. Distal pulses 2+.

3. **What are your initial orders?**
   Complete blood count (CBC), chemistry 8 panel (chem 8), analgesia, antibiotics (e.g., trimethoprim/sulfamethoxazole, cephalexin).
   Advance clock:
   CBC WNL, no leukocytosis. Chem 8 WNL. Patient feels better after analgesia.

4. **What are your follow-up actions?**
   Discharge with a prescription for appropriate antibiotics and analgesics, follow up in 2 to 3 days for wound check.
   Advance clock:
   The patient has been taking antibiotics as prescribed. The erythema has significantly decreased.
   Case ends.
   Critical actions:
   Recognition of cellulitis, understanding of causative organisms (e.g., *Staphylococcus* and *Streptococcus*), administration of appropriate antibiotics, follow up for wound check, consideration of more serious infections.
   Discussion:
   This patient has cellulitis, an infection of the dermis and subcutaneous tissue. Infections of skin and soft tissue range from erysipelas involving the superficial layers of the dermis to cellulitis affecting the dermis and subcutaneous tissue to fasciitis affecting the fascia. The erythema in erysipelas, because of its superficial nature, typically has very well-demarcated borders and is raised; this is typically caused by *Streptococcus* species. Cellulitis has less well-defined margins and varying degrees of erythema and is typically caused by either

Streptococcus or *Staphylococcus aureus*. Fasciitis affects deeper layers and can be life threatening, such as in the case of necrotizing fasciitis, and the presenting symptoms can include even fewer skin signs given its deep nature. However, presenting symptoms for necrotizing fasciitis can also include bulla formation and crepitus; this infection is usually polymicrobial but can be due to *Streptococcus pyogenes* or *Clostridium* species. Differentiating erysipelas, cellulitis, and fasciitis is important in prognosis and in management.

Diagnosis of cellulitis is primarily clinical. Symptoms may include fever and pain in the affected areas. On examination, the affected areas will be warm, erythematous, and tender. The area should be examined for areas of fluctuance that signify abscess formation. Risk factors include skin breakdown (trauma, burns, bites, etc.), poor circulation to the affected area (resulting from diabetes, lymphatic stasis, peripheral vascular disease), and poor immune function (human immunodeficiency virus infection/acquired immune deficiency syndrome [HIV/AIDS], renal or hepatic failure, steroid use).

Simple cellulitis can be treated on an outpatient basis, but patients with more severe involvement or immunocompromised states should be hospitalized for parenteral antibiotic administration. An outpatient regimen in an immunocompetent host should cover *Staphylococcus* if the patient has cellulitis with purulence or evidence of an abscess (and drain the abscess if indicated) and *Streptococcus* for cellulitis without purulence or abscess. Therefore a regimen of trimethoprim-sulfamethoxazole and/or cephalexin would cover *Staphylococcus* (including methicillin-resistant *S. aureus* [MRSA]) and *Streptococcus*, respectively, and would be an appropriate choice.

Diagnosis: Cellulitis

CASE 2

HPI: An 11-day-old previously healthy and ex-full-term infant boy is brought to his pediatrician by his concerned parents because his "skin and eyes look yellow." The parents state that they think that he has been yellow now for about 2 days, but are unsure. They state that he is interacting with them normally, is wetting a normal number of diapers, has normal bowel movements, is breastfeeding exclusively, and is breastfeeding the appropriate number of times (about 10 times a day, 20 minutes per breast each time). No fever, vomiting, cough, runny nose, or other concerns.

Vital signs: Temperature 98.2° F (36.8° C), pulse 120 beats/min, BP 72/40 mm Hg, RR 35 breaths/min.

Additional history: Unremarkable prenatal course. No birth complications. Mother delivered at 39 weeks via normal spontaneous vaginal delivery; no cephalohematoma or bruising during delivery. According to the pediatrician's records, the patient is growing appropriately and is at the 80th percentile for height and weight.

1. **What is the differential diagnosis?**
   Neonatal hyperbilirubinemia: breast milk jaundice, breastfeeding jaundice, physiologic jaundice (but too old), breakdown of blood (e.g., from cephalohematoma), infection, hemolysis, genetic defects, biliary atresia.

2. **What components of the physical examination do you perform?**
   General appearance, skin, cardiovascular, lungs, abdomen, genitalia.
   Physical examination:
   General: Well-developed, well-nourished infant in no distress, latching appropriately onto the mother's breast with good sucking. Cries when examined with good tear production but is easily consoled by parents.
   Skin: Good skin turgor, capillary refill less than 2 seconds. Jaundiced from face to midchest. No signs of skin or soft-tissue infection.
   Cardiovascular: WNL
   Lungs: WNL
   Abdomen: WNL
   Genitalia: Normal uncircumcised boy, testes descended bilaterally.

3. **What are your initial orders?**
   Bilirubin level.
   Advance clock:
   Bilirubin level: 8 mg/dL.

4. What are your follow-up actions?

Counseling on disease process, follow-up bilirubin check.

Advance clock:

The parents are relieved that you reassured them about the jaundice. They return in 1 week and the bilirubin level is 2 mg/dL.

Case ends.

Critical actions:

Recognition of neonatal hyperbilirubinemia, consideration of benign and serious causes of hyperbilirubinemia, recognition of treatment levels when bilirubin is significantly abnormal.

Discussion:

This patient has breast milk jaundice, which is caused by an unknown mechanism in breast milk that leads to increased bilirubin levels, usually in the second week of life. Neonatal jaundice (hyperbilirubinemia) is extremely common: over half of full-term neonates (and more than three quarters of preterm neonates) will have jaundice. Neonatal jaundice is usually benign and does not require treatment. However, jaundice that is present at birth (or within 24 hours), increases rapidly, or occurs in an ill-appearing baby is pathologic and requires a workup to identify the underlying cause (sepsis, hemolysis, congenital infection, etc.). Similarly, very high bilirubin levels can be associated with kernicterus, irreversible brain damage caused by deposition of bilirubin. Very high bilirubin levels (see later discussion) require phototherapy or exchange transfusion. Jaundice can be caused by a number of conditions:

- **Physiologic jaundice:** Caused by immature hepatic conjugation combined with fetal erythrocyte breakdown.
- **Breastfeeding jaundice** (should be called *lack of* breastfeeding jaundice): Caused by inadequate intake of calories and resolves when nutritional intake is adequate.
- **Breast *milk* jaundice:** Breast milk itself can cause increased bilirubin levels through a mechanism that is unclear but may include increased enterohepatic recycling of bilirubin and/or substances in breast milk that block conjugation of bilirubin. In this patient, given that feeding and growth are normal and the level of bilirubin is not dangerous, the mother can continue to breastfeed. In instances in which the bilirubin is high enough to warrant treatment, some physicians recommend stopping breastfeeding and switching to formula briefly.
- **Extravascular blood:** Breakdown of blood products leads to increased bilirubin. If an infant suffers from cephalohematoma or bruising during birth, the blood involved will break down and cause increased bilirubin production.

In infants with more severe hyperbilirubinemia or those who appear ill, other causes such as infection, hemolysis (from ABO compatibility or rhesus factor [Rh] alloimmunization), genetic defects (including conjugation diseases such as Crigler-Najjar syndrome, red blood cell [RBC] defects such as spherocytosis, and inborn errors of metabolism), or obstructed bile flow (such as biliary atresia, etc.) should be investigated. Treatment levels for hyperbilirubinemia depend on the patient's risk factors (e.g., premature, etc.), age in hours, and level of bilirubin (this can be plotted on a nomogram to determine whether phototherapy is indicated). In general, any level greater than 20 mg/dL at any time is abnormal and warrants treatment. Phototherapy converts unconjugated bilirubin into a water-soluble molecule that the kidneys can excrete. Exchange transfusion replaces newborn blood with donor blood, removing bilirubin in the process, and is indicated only for very high bilirubin levels, neurologic symptoms consistent with kernicterus or encephalopathy, or failure of phototherapy.

Diagnosis: Breast milk jaundice

CASE 3

HPI: A 36-year-old woman attends the urgent care center complaining of 1 day of chills, fever, and a cough that produces rust-colored sputum. She states that she has had a runny nose, dry cough, and sore throat for a week but thought she was getting better until today. She denies any hemoptysis, prolonged immobilization, shortness of breath, or other symptoms.

Vital signs: Temperature 98.2° F (38.6° C), pulse 96 beats/min, BP 118/68 mm Hg, RR 18 breaths/min.

Additional history: Previously healthy, no medications except acetaminophen for the fever (last dose 10 hours before arrival). Denies tobacco, drug, or alcohol use. Sexually active with protection with one male partner. Denies travel outside the country, incarceration, recent hospitalization, or close contact with individuals with tuberculosis (TB).

1. What is the differential diagnosis?
   Community-acquired pneumonia, viral upper respiratory tract infection, TB, pulmonary embolism.

2. What components of the physical examination do you perform?
   General appearance; head, eyes, ears, nose, and throat (HEENT); cardiovascular; lungs; abdomen.
   Physical examination:
   General: Well-developed, well-nourished woman in no apparent distress, coughing up rust-colored sputum during examination.
   HEENT: No sinus tenderness, oropharynx WNL.
   Cardiovascular: WNL
   Lungs: Crackles heard in the left lower lobe on auscultation.
   Abdomen: WNL

3. What are your initial orders?
   Chest x-ray (CXR), acetaminophen.
   Advance clock:
   CXR shows an infiltrate that silhouettes the left diaphragm. Temperature 1 hour after acetaminophen administration is 99.7° F (37.6° C) and the heart rate is now 90 beats/min.

4. What are your follow-up actions?
   Single dose of intravenous (IV) ceftriaxone. Discharge with a prescription for a macrolide antibiotic such as azithromycin or a fluoroquinolone that covers atypical organisms, such as levofloxacin, with a follow-up appointment. Counseling on the disease process.
   Advance clock:
   The patient is seen 7 days later for a follow-up appointment: her symptoms have resolved and she is asymptomatic. If the patient is reexamined, there will be no crackles in the left lower lobe of the lung.
   Case ends.
   Critical actions:
   Recognition of pneumonia, appropriate treatment, recognition that the patient does not need to be treated as an inpatient.
   Discussion:
   This patient has community-acquired pneumonia, usually caused by typical pathogens such as *Streptococcus pneumoniae* and *Haemophilus influenzae* or atypical pathogens such as *Legionella*, *Mycoplasma*, and *Chlamydophila pneumoniae* (previously referred to as *Chlamydia pneumoniae*). In the timeframe of an emergency department (ED) or urgent care visit, the type of bacteria causing the pneumonia will not be identified; therefore, antibiotic coverage against all likely agents is appropriate. This is typically done on an inpatient basis with ceftriaxone (for typical bacteria) and azithromycin (for atypical bacteria because some lack a cell wall and therefore beta-lactam antibiotics are ineffective). Outpatient regimens for a young healthy adult are typically a macrolide antibiotic alone (such as azithromycin), doxycycline alone, or a fluoroquinolone that covers atypical organisms, such as levofloxacin or moxifloxacin. Pneumonia associated with a health care setting or pneumonia in those with an underlying lung disease (such as bronchiectasis) typically requires broader coverage because bacteria such as S. *aureus* and *Pseudomonas aeruginosa* are also possible infectious agents.

   Diagnosis of pneumonia is on the basis of history, physical examination, and X-ray imaging. The history typically involves a cough that produces purulent sputum with a fever and possibly shortness of breath. On examination of the lungs, localized crackles in the area of the pneumonia are common. Imaging may show a lobar infiltrate or patchy interstitial infiltrates. The possibility of unusual organisms should be considered by identifying risk factors: (1) Is the patient immunocompromised (e.g., on steroids, risk factors for HIV)? (2) Could the patient have aspirated fluid (risk of *Klebsiella* and polymicrobial anaerobic infections)? (3) Has the patient recently been hospitalized (risk of MRSA or *Pseudomonas*)? (4) Could the patient have TB?

   The most important decision after diagnosing pneumonia is whether the patient can be treated as an outpatient or needs to be admitted to the hospital. Many prediction rules have been developed to help in this decision. One approach is to apply the **CURB-65** criteria, whereby you assign 1 point each for **c**onfusion, **u**rea (blood urea nitrogen [BUN] >19 mg/dL), **R**R >30 breaths/min, **B**P less than 90 mm Hg systolic or 60 mm Hg diastolic, and age older than **65** years. Patients with a score of 0 or 1 can be treated as outpatients, those with a score of 4 or 5 should be admitted, and the decision for those with an intermediate score (2 or 3) should be on a case-by-case basis. The more complicated **PORT** score is also available for use. In this case, the patient appears well, is young, and has no other comorbidities and can be safely treated as an outpatient without the need to draw blood tests. Some guidelines recommend that patients with risk factors for malignancy should have a follow-up CXR 6 weeks later to confirm resolution of the infiltrate. Failure of the infiltrate to resolve requires additional evaluation such as a computed tomography (CT) scan to assess the possibility of an underlying malignancy.

    Diagnosis: Pneumonia

CASE 4

HPI: A 26-year-old woman attends her primary care doctor with right arm weakness and numbness that started gradually the previous day while she was working outside. She states that she could still move the arm, but that it felt much weaker than usual and as if "pins and needles" were sticking into her. She denies any numbness or weakness elsewhere or trauma to her arm. She states that her symptoms have already significantly improved, but she is scared that the condition could be permanent.

Vital signs: Temperature 98.2° F (36.8° C), pulse 76 beats/min, BP 155/78 mm Hg, RR 16 breaths/min.

Additional history: The patient was diagnosed with optic neuritis 6 months ago, but this has since resolved and she essentially has normal vision. There is no other medical history. No medications, allergies, or use of alcohol, drugs, or tobacco.

1. What is the differential diagnosis?

   Transient ischemic attack (TIA), stroke, cervical radiculopathy, peripheral neuropathy, multiple sclerosis (MS), acute disseminated encephalomyelitis, subacute combined degeneration of the spinal cord, HIV-associated neuropathies (e.g., progressive multifocal leukoencephalopathy), vasculitis (e.g., polyarteritis nodosa), neuromyelitis optica.

2. What components of the physical examination do you perform?

   General appearance, HEENT/neck, lungs, cardiovascular, neuro/psych.

   Physical examination:

       General: Well-developed, well-nourished woman in no distress.

       HEENT/neck: On flexion of the neck, the patient says she feels as if "shocks of electricity" are going down her spine.

       Cardiovascular: WNL

       Lungs: WNL

       Neuro/psych Alert and oriented to name, time, place, situation. Cranial nerves II to XII intact. Strength of right arm 4+/5, rest of body 5/5. Minimally diminished sensation to a light touch and pinprick over the right arm.

3. What are your initial orders?

   CBC, chem 8, antinuclear antibody (ANA), erythrocyte sedimentation rate (ESR), vitamin B_{12} level, HIV screening, brain CT, magnetic resonance imaging (MRI) scan of the brain/spine.

   Advance clock:

   CBC, chem 8, ANA, ESR, B_{12}, HIV all negative/WNL.

   Brain CT negative.

   MRI scan of the brain/spine shows multiple demyelinating plaques in various stages throughout the central nervous system (CNS).

4. What are your follow-up actions?

   Counseling on the disease process, lumbar puncture (to look for oligoclonal bands), begin disease-modifying therapy (e.g., interferon-beta, glatiramer) or consult with the neurology department for the same.

   Advance clock:

   Case ends.

Critical actions:
Recognition of MS as a likely cause of the patient's symptoms, investigation of disease, counseling, initiation of appropriate therapy.

Discussion:
This patient has MS, an autoimmune disorder in which CNS neurons become demyelinated. Depending on where the demyelination occurs, patients can have a variety of symptoms; the most common include optic neuritis, sensory or motor changes in the extremities, and ataxia. The demyelination does not occur all at once (but rather over time), so MS is described as involving lesions separated in space (multiple locations within the CNS) and time (multiple episodes). MS can follow one of four general courses: relapsing remitting (most common, characterized by exacerbations and remissions); primary progressive (slowly worsening symptoms without marked exacerbations or remissions); secondary progressive (after an initial relapsing remitting course); and progressive relapsing (least common; progressive but with exacerbations on top of the progression). The cause of MS is unknown, but as for many autoimmune diseases, it is more common in women than in men. It is also more common in younger individuals (age 20 to 40 years).

Diagnosis of MS is on the basis of a history and physical examination leading to clinical suspicion of the disease. After this, studies can further support the diagnosis, such as an MRI scan of the brain/spine showing demyelination in multiple areas, cerebrospinal fluid (CSF) analysis showing oligoclonal bands, and possibly visual or auditory evoked potentials showing subclinical demyelinating disease. Other causes of demyelination should be investigated and ruled out (e.g., HIV, vitamin B_{12} deficiency, other autoimmune conditions). There is no cure for MS. The mainstay of treatment for exacerbations is steroids. For maintenance, glatiramer (structurally similar to myelin basic protein, which MS attacks) is often used, as well as interferon beta.

Diagnosis: MS

CASE 5

HPI: A 40-year-old woman attends her primary care doctor and reports 8 months of progressive weakness, dizziness, and fatigue. She states that whenever she stands up she feels like she is "going to pass out" and finds it hard to even get out of bed in the morning. She states that despite not going outside much because of her weakness, her skin has been getting darker. She has lost 20 lb over the 8-month period and states she does not have much of an appetite, but her husband remarks on how much salt she uses at the dinner table. She affirms that she is too thin and wants to gain her weight and strength back. She denies any syncopal episodes.

Vital signs: Temperature 98.2° F (36.8° C), pulse 60 beats/min, BP 108/60 mm Hg, RR 16 breaths/min.

Additional history: No suicidal ideation, homicidal ideation, or auditory or visual hallucinations. No medical or psychiatric history. Denies use of alcohol, tobacco, or drugs.

1. **What is the differential diagnosis?**
   Chronic adrenal insufficiency (Addison disease), anorexia nervosa, occult malignancy, hemochromatosis, hypothyroidism.

2. **What components of the physical examination do you perform?**
   General appearance, HEENT, cardiovascular, lungs.

   Physical examination:
   General: Thin woman in no apparent distress with generalized hyperpigmentation.
   HEENT: No goiter or palpable thyroid nodules. Buccal mucosal hyperpigmentation. Dry mucous membranes.
   Cardiovascular: WNL
   Lungs: WNL

3. **What are your initial orders?**
   Orthostatic vital signs, electrocardiography (ECG), CBC, chem 8.

   Advance clock:
   Orthostatic vital signs are positive; BP on standing 80/50 mm Hg and pulse 108 beats/min. ECG shows normal sinus rhythm. CBC WNL, chem 8 remarkable for a potassium level of 5.5 mEq/dL, sodium of 134 mEq/dL, and bicarbonate of 20 mmol/L.

4. **What are your follow-up actions?**
Early morning cortisol level. Fluid replacement.
Advance clock:
Early morning cortisol is undetectable.

5. **What are your follow-up actions?**
Start hydrocortisone and fludrocortisone replacement.
Advance clock:
The patient feels much better.
   Case ends.
Critical actions:
Recognition of chronic primary adrenal insufficiency, appropriate workup (e.g., chem panel and cortisol level) and treatment (e.g., steroid replacement).
Discussion:
This patient has chronic primary adrenal insufficiency, also known as Addison disease. The adrenal cortex has three layers, the zona glomerulosa (which makes aldosterone, a mineralocorticoid), the zona fasciculata (which makes cortisol, a glucocorticoid), and the zona reticularis (which makes dehydroepiandrosterone sulfate [DHEAS], an androgen). Aldosterone acts to reclaim sodium and excrete potassium and acid in the distal nephron, so loss of this hormone leads to hypotension and **hyperkalemic metabolic acidosis**. Cortisol also has a role in catecholamine sensitization, and loss of this hormone can lead to resistant hypotension. Loss of the androgenic hormones is less noticeable.

Addison disease is most commonly of autoimmune origin in developed countries, but TB is the most common cause worldwide. Loss of cortisol production causes increased adrenocorticotropic hormone (ACTH) levels; one breakdown product of this is α-melanocyte–stimulating hormone (α-MSH), which leads to characteristic hyperpigmentation, especially in the buccal mucosa, genital area, and areola. Symptoms include fatigue, salt craving, memory impairment, depression, and vague nonspecific symptoms.

Acute adrenal insufficiency can be seen with sepsis, especially infections with *Neisseria meningitidis* causing Waterhouse-Friderichsen syndrome. Iatrogenic causes such as acute cessation of chronic steroid therapy or administration of medications that inhibit cortisol production (e.g., etomidate, ketoconazole) are also precipitating factors.

Screening can be performed via measurement of the early morning cortisol level; a level greater than 20 μg/dL excludes adrenal insufficiency, very low levels (<3 μg/dL) are diagnostic, and intermediate levels require further investigation. An ACTH (cosyntropin) stimulation test can be performed in which baseline cortisol is measured, ACTH is administered, and 30- and 60-minute cortisol levels are measured. Low initial and 30- and 60-minute levels confirm the diagnosis of primary adrenal insufficiency. A low initial level and normal 30- and 60-minute levels indicate pituitary dysfunction, because the pituitary gland is functional (normal ACTH response) but is not secreting enough ACTH, or the hypothalamus is not sending enough corticotropin-releasing hormone (CRH) to the pituitary.

Management involves administration of hydrocortisone and fludrocortisone, with increases in the hydrocortisone dose during illness or before a stressful medical procedure to mimic the body's endogenous cortisol spikes during these times.
Diagnosis: Adrenal insufficiency

CASE 6

HPI: A 12-year-old boy attends the ED complaining of a sore throat and fever for the past 2 days. He denies a cough, runny nose, or sick contacts. He states that he has significant pain on swallowing that is limiting his ability to eat.
Vital signs: Temperature 101.8° F (38.8° C), pulse 94 beats/min, BP 116/70 mm Hg, RR 18 breaths/min.
Additional history: Denies sexual activity. No known drug allergies. Vaccinations up to date.

1. **What is the differential diagnosis?**
Viral pharyngitis, streptococcal pharyngitis, infectious mononucleosis, peritonsillar abscess, retropharyngeal abscess, diphtheria, Lemierre syndrome, gonococcal pharyngitis.

2. **What components of the physical examination do you perform?**
   General appearance, HEENT, cardiovascular, lungs, skin.
   Physical examination:
   General: Mild distress due to throat pain, speaks with a normal voice in full sentences.
   Cardiovascular: WNL
   Lungs: WNL
   HEENT: Tonsillar exudates bilaterally; tender, diffuse, anterior cervical lymphadenopathy; erythematous and inflamed posterior oropharynx; mild petechiae on the palate; uvula midline; no meningismus; and full range of motion of the neck.
   Skin: WNL

3. **What are your initial orders?**
   Acetaminophen or ibuprofen, one dose of intramuscular (IM) benzathine penicillin or a 10-day course of PO penicillin or amoxicillin, PO challenge, dexamethasone.
   Advance clock:
   Patient feels much better, his symptoms have improved.

4. **What are your follow-up actions?**
   Follow up in 1 week.
   Advance clock:
   Case ends.
   Critical actions:
   HEENT examination to rule out peritonsillar abscess or more serious cause of the sore throat; analgesics; recognition that according to the Centor criteria, neither a rapid antigen test nor a throat culture is indicated and that empiric treatment with antibiotics should be started.
   Discussion:
   Streptococcal pharyngitis (so-called strep throat) accounts for approximately 30% of acute pharyngitis in children and is caused by group A beta-hemolytic streptococci (S. pyogenes). Once the diagnosis of acute pharyngitis is established clinically, the Centor criteria can be applied to direct testing and/or treatment, whereby 1 point is given for each of the following: (1) tonsillar exudates, (2) tender anterior cervical lymphadenopathy, (3) fever, and (4) absence of cough. The modified Centor criteria add 1 point for age younger than 15 years and subtract 1 point for age older than 44 years. However, strep throat in children younger than 3 years is very rare.

   A score of 0 or 1 has a positive predictive value (PPV) of 1% to 5% for strep throat, which means that testing should not be undertaken because the likelihood of disease is so low that positive tests are likely to be false positives. Similarly, a score of 4 points has such a high PPV for disease that no testing should be performed and antibiotics should be prescribed; any negative test results are more likely to be false negatives. Therefore, only patients with a score in the intermediate range (2 to 3 points) should be tested using the rapid antigen detection test (RADT); if the result is positive, treatment should be started. If the RADT is negative, a throat culture should be ordered, and if positive, antibiotics should be prescribed.

   Complications of strep throat include suppurative complications such as peritonsillar abscesses, otitis media, retropharyngeal abscess, Lemierre syndrome, and mastoiditis. Nonsuppurative complications such as acute rheumatic fever (can be prevented with antibiotics) and poststreptococcal glomerulonephritis (PSGN; cannot be prevented with antibiotics) can also occur.
   Diagnosis: Streptococcal pharyngitis

CASE 7

HPI: A 22-year-old woman was brought in by her boyfriend 4 hours after she ingested an unknown number of pills from her medicine cabinet. Emergency medical service personnel stated that there were no prescription medications in the cabinet, just aspirin and acetaminophen. The patient states that she feels fine and wants to go home. She denies any nausea, vomiting, abdominal pain, or current suicidal ideation.
Vital signs: Temperature 98.2° F (36.8° C), pulse 80 beats/min, BP 112/64 mm Hg, RR 16 breaths/min.
Additional history: None

1. **What is the differential diagnosis?**
   Overdose of acetaminophen, salicylates, ferrous sulfate, and other medications.

2. **What components of the physical examination do you perform?**

General appearance, cardiovascular, lungs, abdomen, neuro/psych.

Physical examination:

General: No acute distress, no scleral icterus. Pupils equal and round, reactive to light and accommodation (PERRLA). No diaphoresis.

Cardiovascular: WNL

Lungs: WNL

Abdomen: WNL

3. **What are your initial orders?**

Chem 8, CBC, coagulation studies, liver function tests (LFTs), acetaminophen level, salicylate level, ethanol (EtOH) level, urinary toxicology screen, urinary pregnancy test, ECG.

Advance clock:

CBC, chemistry panel, coagulation studies, LFTs, salicylate level, EtOH level, pregnancy test, and ECG are all WNL/negative. Acetaminophen level is 200 μg/L (high). Urine toxicology screen is positive for cannabinoids.

4. **What are your follow-up actions?**

Administration of N-acetylcysteine (NAC), psychiatry consultation for involuntary ("5150") hold and further psychiatric evaluation, admission to a monitored bed for continued NAC therapy and monitoring of LFTs.

Advance clock:

Case ends.

Critical actions:

Recognition of acetaminophen toxicity, appropriate treatment even in the absence of symptoms (because early symptoms are rare), admission for continued therapy.

Discussion:

This patient attended the hospital without symptoms after a suicidal gesture involving ingestion of pills. The lack of symptoms does not rule out such ingestion, because many cases are initially asymptomatic. This patient had a negative laboratory workup except for an elevated acetaminophen level. At 4 hours, the treatment threshold for acetaminophen ingestion is 150 μg/L according to the Rumack-Matthew nomogram, which was surpassed in this patient. In addition, if the amount of acetaminophen ingested is known, acute ingestion of more than 150 mg/kg acetaminophen is also an indication for treatment.

The initial treatment is 150 mg/kg NAC, which helps to inactivate the hepatotoxic metabolic product N-acetyl-p-benzoquinone imine and prevents the complications of acetaminophen overdose. Therapy is then typically continued for 72 hours on an inpatient basis (although shorter regimens are becoming more popular) with a comprehensive psychiatric evaluation. Because the ingestion occurred 4 hours previously in this case, activated charcoal would not be beneficial. For acute ingestion or ingestion of time-release medications for which the ingested substance can bind to charcoal, administration of activated charcoal can be beneficial.

It is important to rule out coingestion of other medication/substances. The patient had a normal ECG and no access to prescription medications, making tricyclic antidepressant (TCA) overdose less likely (the classic three Cs for TCA overdose are cardiotoxicity, convulsions, and coma). The patient's salicylate level was negligible, and salicylate toxicity would be expected to produce a mixed acid-base disorder of respiratory alkalosis (tachypnea from direct stimulation of medullary respiratory centers) and metabolic acidosis (uncoupling of oxidative phosphorylation). A significant dose of opioids should cause symptoms and signs such as respiratory depression and miosis. There is no evidence of a sympathomimetic agent (e.g., cocaine, amphetamine) or cholinergic toxidrome. The lack of metabolic acidosis (normal bicarbonate) makes ingestion of a substance such as methanol or ethylene glycol much less likely.

Diagnosis: Acetaminophen toxicity

CASE 8

HPI: A 40-year-old woman who was previously healthy attends the ED after having had two car accidents in which she had hit parked cars. She states that she did not see them in her peripheral vision and is usually a good driver. She is also concerned because although she typically has regular menstrual cycles, she has not had menses in 3 months. She notes that she has had some bilateral nipple discharge.

Vital signs: Temperature 98.2° F (36.8° C), pulse 76 beats/min, BP 114/64 mm Hg, RR 16 breaths/min.

Additional history: No other medical history. The patient has not been sexually active for more than 2 years.

1. **What is the differential diagnosis?**
   Prolactinoma, pregnancy, primary brain malignancy.

2. **What components of the physical examination do you perform?**
   General appearance, breast, neuro/psych.
   Physical examination:
   General: WNL
   Breast: A small amount of milky discharge can be expressed from each nipple. No masses are palpable.
   Neuro/psych: Bitemporal hemianopsia, otherwise WNL.

3. **What are your initial orders?**
   Prolactin level, brain MRI scan, urinary pregnancy test.
   Advance clock:
   Prolactin level 200 ng/mL (elevated). Pregnancy test negative. Brain MRI scan shows a 12-mm mass in the anterior pituitary gland, with a mass effect on the optic chiasm.

4. **What are your follow-up actions?**
   Begin dopamine agonist therapy (e.g., bromocriptine, cabergoline).
   Consult neurosurgery; no surgical intervention recommended at this time.
   Counsel the patient regarding her disease.
   Advance clock:
   The patient's visual complaints have resolved.
   (If follow-up MRI scan ordered, the mass has shrunk on treatment to 5 mm.)
   Case ends.
   Critical actions:
   Recognition of prolactinoma, ordering of a pregnancy test for a woman of reproductive age with amenorrhea (regardless of reported sexual activity), and initiation of appropriate therapy for prolactinoma (dopamine agonist therapy).
   Discussion:
   This patient has a prolactinoma, a benign tumor of the lactotroph cells in the anterior pituitary gland. This is the most common tumor of the pituitary. Prolactin secretion by a prolactinoma causes downregulation of the release of sex hormones and therefore amenorrhea, infertility, and/or loss of libido can occur. Prolactin stimulates milk production, so affected females often have bilateral nipple discharge.
   As the size of the tumor increases (>10 mm is classified as a macroadenoma versus a smaller microadenoma), there can be mass effect on the optic chiasm, which compresses the crossing fibers from the nasal retina, causing bitemporal hemianopsia. In this patient, loss of these visual fields caused her to accidentally hit the parked cars that were outside her visual field.
   The cornerstone of therapy is dopamine agonists such as bromocriptine and cabergoline. Dopamine exerts negative feedback on the anterior pituitary gland, decreasing prolactin release. This causes the tumor to produce less prolactin and decrease in size; this is why the patient had an improvement in visual symptoms after treatment. The differential diagnosis for hyperprolactinemia includes medication use (e.g., dopamine antagonists), renal failure (from decreased clearance and disordered hypothalamic regulation), and hypothyroidism (because thyrotropin-releasing hormone [TRH] stimulates prolactin release). Surgical therapy is an option, but dopamine agonist therapy is the first-line treatment for most patients.
   Diagnosis: Prolactinoma

CASE 9

HPI: You are called to the inpatient unit because a 10-year-old boy started shaking and became unresponsive; the episode was witnessed by his parents and the nursing staff. The boy was visiting his mother, who is ill. He started shaking 3 minutes ago. He has never had this problem before. The parents deny any trauma or ingestions. The patient was apparently sitting and talking with his mother when he suddenly became unresponsive, his entire body started shaking, and he exhibited urinary incontinence. He is currently still shaking and is unresponsive.

Vital signs: Temperature 98.2° F (36.8° C), pulse 98 beats/min, BP 110/60 mm Hg, RR 22 breaths/min.

Additional history: No medical history, vaccines up to date, no allergies.

1. **What is the differential diagnosis?**
   Seizure secondary to epilepsy, hypoglycemia, hypoxemia, toxin ingestion, infection (meningitis, encephalitis), trauma, mass lesion, bleeding, or electrolyte disturbances (e.g., hyponatremia).

2. **What components of the physical examination do you perform?**
   Defer examination because the patient requires immediate intervention.

3. **What are your initial orders?**
   Cardiac monitoring, pulse oximetry, oxygen, fingerstick blood glucose, lorazepam.
   Advance clock:
   Oxygen saturation 100%, fingerstick glucose 108 mg/dL. After administration of one dose of lorazepam, the seizure stops.

4. **What are your follow-up actions?**
   Transfer to the ED; perform CBC, chem 8, noncontrast head CT scan, physical examination.

5. **What components of the physical examination do you perform?**
   General appearance, HEENT/neck, lungs, cardiovascular, abdomen, neuro/psych.
   Physical examination:
   General: Slowly responds to questions, no shaking activity, breathing on his own.
   HEENT/neck: No meningismus, small superficial laceration to the lateral tongue.
   Cardiovascular: WNL
   Lungs: Tachypnea.
   Abdomen: WNL
   Neuro/psych: Moving all his extremities, alert and oriented to name only, no focal neurologic deficits.
   Advance clock:
   CBC, chem 8, noncontrast head CT scan all WNL.
   Patient returns to baseline, no neurologic deficits, alert and oriented to name, time, place, situation, and conversing normally.

6. **What are your follow-up actions?**
   Counseling on the disease process, neurology consult, electroencephalography (EEG) as an outpatient, MRI scan of the brain as an outpatient, discharge with follow-up appointment.
   Advance clock:
   Case ends.
   Critical actions:
   Recognition of active seizure, immediate supportive care and treatment with benzodiazepine, appropriate workup for seizure.
   Discussion:
   This patient had a generalized tonic-clonic seizure. Seizures are due to uncontrolled firing of neurons in the brain resulting from any number of possible inducing agents (e.g., infections, toxins, trauma). Seizure types include generalized tonic-clonic seizures, simple partial seizures (normal level of consciousness), complex partial seizures (altered level of consciousness), secondarily generalized seizures (start as partial, then become generalized), and absence seizures (characterized by numerous episodes of short seizures with abrupt impairment of consciousness and a blank stare lasting for seconds each time). This patient cannot have had a febrile seizure because he does not have a fever and is also outside the typical age range for febrile seizures (6 months to 6 years). The current definition of SE is a seizure lasting more than 5 minutes or two seizures without a return to baseline between seizures (e.g., the patient is still postictal when the second seizure occurs). SE is a life-threatening condition.
   Treatment for active seizures includes standard supportive care (oxygen, monitoring, airway management if required), followed by benzodiazepines (e.g., lorazepam) as first-line

agents, with other agents such as phenytoin (or the more soluble fosphenytoin), levetirace-tam, or phenobarbital as second-line therapy if the patient does not respond. The blood sugar level should be checked for all patients who have a seizure or are actively seizing, because glucose administration can stop seizures in hypoglycemic patients. A woman of child-bearing age should have a pregnancy test. After the seizure terminates, basic laboratory tests are help-ful in excluding electrolyte abnormalities (e.g., hyponatremia). A head CT scan should be obtained for all patients with first-time seizures (except simple febrile seizures, see Case 44 for details). Outpatient EEG and MRI scanning are indicated for most patients. Counsel patients that 40% of cases will have another seizure.

Diagnosis: Seizure

CASE 10

HPI: A 60-year-old woman attends the ED with chronic constipation, fatigue, memory deficits, and nausea for months. She was referred to the ED by her primary care physician when routine tests for these symptoms showed that her calcium level was elevated. She denies any weight loss, night sweats, or other symptoms.

Vital signs: Temperature 98.6° F (37° C), pulse 96 beats/min, BP 140/90 mm Hg, RR 16 breaths/min.

Additional history: Kidney stones, spine compression fracture, hip fracture with prosthetic hip replacement.

1. What is the differential diagnosis?

   Hypercalcemia due to primary hyperparathyroidism (PHPT) or malignancy. Less likely causes include medications, milk alkali syndrome, hyperthyroidism, immobilization.

2. What components of the physical examination do you perform?

   General appearance, cardiovascular, lungs, abdomen.

   Physical examination:
   General: Comfortable woman with appearance in agreement with stated age, dry mucous membranes.
   Cardiovascular: WNL
   Lungs: WNL
   Abdomen: Mild diffuse tenderness on palpation of the abdomen, no rebound or guarding.

3. What are your initial orders?

   Chem 14, CBC (because the calcium level is known to be elevated already, parathyroid hor-mone [PTH] measurement can be ordered at this point or later), ECG, and albumin (for correct determination of the calcium level) or ionized calcium (not impacted by the albumin level).

   Advance clock:
   Chem 14 remarkable for a calcium level of 13.6 mg/dL (albumin level normal). CBC unremarkable. If an ECG is ordered it shows a normal sinus rhythm with a short QT interval.

4. What are your follow-up actions?

   IV fluid administration, calcitonin, bisphosphonate, PTH level.

   Advance clock:
   PTH result 55 pg/mL (normal 10 to 60 pg/mL).
   Patient feels much better after IV fluid administration.
   If imaging of the parathyroid glands (e.g., sestamibi scan, ultrasound) is ordered, scans will show a solitary parathyroid adenoma.
   Surgery consultation.
   If any other imaging is ordered (e.g., CXR, CT scan), the results will be negative.
   If the PTH-related protein (PTHrP) level is measured, it will be undetectable.
   Case ends.

   Critical actions:
   Recognition of hypercalcemia, treatment with at least IV fluids, recognition that high normal PTH in the setting of high calcium levels is abnormal and confirms the diagnosis of PHPT. Referral for definitive surgical treatment. Initiation of bisphosphonate therapy to reduce the risk of worsening osteoporosis in a patient who already has multiple fractures, presumably because of her underlying condition.

Discussion:

This patient has hypercalcemia, a calcium level greater than 10.5 mg/dL. Although the differential diagnosis for hypercalcemia is broad, over 90% of cases result from one of two conditions: (1) PHPT or (2) malignancy. Abnormal PTH production in PHPT is typically due to a solitary parathyroid adenoma that overproduces PTH (80%), diffuse parathyroid hyperplasia (15%), or, in rare cases, parathyroid carcinoma (5%).

Malignancy can cause hypercalcemia either directly because of bone degradation or via PTHrP. In this case, the PTH level was high for the level of calcium (in the presence of hypercalcemia the PTH level should be less than the lower normal limit because of negative feedback). This confirms the diagnosis of PHPT.

Treatment of hypercalcemia is threefold: (1) IV fluids to reduce calcium levels and improve symptoms, (2) calcitonin to temporarily decrease calcium levels (not a long-term solution because of tachyphylaxis), and (3) bisphosphonate therapy to prevent further bone loss. Further treatment depends on the cause of the patient's hypercalcemia. In PHPT, surgical treatment is first-line therapy. Loop diuretics such as furosemide were previously used as first-line therapy but are now reserved for when urine output is inadequate despite aggressive fluid resuscitation. Sestamibi scans or ultrasound can show whether the parathyroid glands have an adenoma or diffuse hyperplasia. In cases of malignancy, the underlying cancer must be treated.

Diagnosis: Hypercalcemia due to PHPT

CASE 11

HPI: A 72-year-old man attends his primary care physician complaining of red urine for the past 3 months. Initially his urine was just slightly off-colored and brown and the patient thought he was dehydrated, but it has since progressed to a deep red color every time he urinates. The patient denies dysuria, hesitancy, or nocturia. He denies any fevers or chills or weight loss.

Vital signs: Temperature 98.2° F (36.8° C), pulse 76 beats/min, BP 135/78 mm Hg, RR 16 breaths/min.

Additional history: Takes hydrochlorothiazide for hypertension. No other medications and no allergies. Previously smoked for 40 years, 2 packs/day, but quit 3 years ago. Occasional alcohol consumption, no drug use.

1. **What is the differential diagnosis?**

   Hematuria due to bladder cancer, renal cancer, urinary tract infection (UTI), interstitial cystitis, nephrolithiasis, or prostate cancer; nephritic syndrome if urinalysis for hematuria reveals RBC casts.

2. **What components of the physical examination do you perform?**

   General appearance, cardiovascular, lungs, abdomen.

   Physical examination:

   General: Well-developed, well-nourished man in no apparent distress.
   Cardiovascular: WNL
   Lungs: WNL
   Abdomen: Firm mass in the pelvis, otherwise WNL.

3. **What are your initial orders?**

   CBC, chem 8, coagulation profile, urinalysis, urine culture, urine cytology.

   Advance clock:

   CBC normal except hemoglobin (Hb) 11 mg/dL and a mean corpuscular volume (MCV) of 70 fL. Chem 8 and coagulation profile WNL. Urinalysis reveals a high level of blood with too many RBCs to count, no RBC casts, otherwise WNL. Urine culture and cytology pending.

4. **What are your follow-up actions?**

   CT urogram, urology consult for cystoscopy and biopsy.

   Advance clock:

   CT urogram demonstrates a 5-cm bladder mass without evidence of hydronephrosis or metastatic disease. Cystoscopy is performed and demonstrates a bladder mass; biopsy and urine cytology both consistent with transitional cell carcinoma of the bladder. Urine culture negative.

   Case ends.

Critical actions:
Recognition that painless hematuria in an older patient has a high likelihood of malignancy, ordering of appropriate workup, urology referral for cystoscopy and biopsy.

Discussion:
This patient has bladder cancer. Painless gross hematuria is the most common presentation, and almost 100% of patients with bladder cancer will have some amount of microscopic hematuria on urinalysis. Hematuria is often the only symptom, but patients can also have dysuria or frequent urination. A patient may experience urinary retention if the lesion is obstructive. Bladder cancer is more common in men than in women (3:1), older patients (median age is >70 years), and those with a history of smoking. Patients may have multiple tumors in the bladder at the same time because of the field effect, whereby the entire bladder is exposed to urinary carcinogens (e.g., from smoking), so multiple malignant foci can be present simultaneously.

Diagnosis is on the basis of a history of painless hematuria in an appropriately aged patient, followed by urinalysis, urine culture, and urine cytology. A CT urogram can define the anatomy and assess for obstruction and metastatic disease and is recommended for all patients thought to have a malignancy of the urinary system. The gold standard is cystoscopy with biopsy to visualize the lesion and send it for histopathology. Transitional cell carcinoma (urothelial carcinoma) is the most common type of bladder cancer in the United States (almost all cases), followed by the much rarer squamous cell carcinoma and adenocarcinoma. All patients should be assessed for obstruction or severe anemia.

Treatment depends on the depth of invasion and the presence or absence of metastatic disease. Low-grade lesions can be completely resected via transurethral resection of bladder tumor (TURBT), but more advanced disease can require radical cystectomy with or without chemotherapy and possibly radiation if isolated metastases exist. The 5-year survival for localized lesions is good (>75%), but for metastatic disease the prognosis is poor.

Diagnosis: Hematuria due to bladder cancer

CASE 12

HPI: A 50-year-old woman attends the ED complaining of a headache. She says that she was watching television and at 5:13 pm (approximately 1 hour ago) she instantly developed a severe headache over her entire head that caused her to vomit twice. She states that lights now bother her and her neck feels stiff, as if she "slept on it wrong." She denies any history of headaches, except for 1 week ago when she had a similar episode lasting for hours, but that episode was much less severe and she did not seek medical evaluation.

Vital signs: Temperature 98.2° F (36.8° C), pulse 98 beats/min, BP 120/78 mm Hg, RR 18 breaths/min.

Additional history: Occasional alcohol use, no use of drugs or tobacco. No medical or surgical history.

1. **What is the differential diagnosis?**
   Subarachnoid hemorrhage (SAH), migraine, meningitis, hemorrhagic stroke, intracranial hemorrhage, mass lesion, obstructive hydrocephalus.

2. **What components of the physical examination do you perform?**
   General appearance, HEENT/neck, cardiovascular, lungs, neuro/psych.
   Physical examination:
   General: Well-developed, well-nourished woman in moderate distress due to pain.
   HEENT/neck: Meningismus, PERRLA.
   Cardiovascular: WNL
   Lungs: WNL
   Neuro/psych: Normal strength, sensation, reflexes, and tone. Cranial nerves intact.

3. **What are your initial orders?**
   Immediate noncontrast head CT scan. CBC, chem 8, coagulation profile, analgesics (e.g., morphine).
   Advance clock:
   Noncontrast head CT scan: negative for bleeding or a mass effect.
   CBC, chem 8, coagulation profile: WNL
   Patient feels slightly better after analgesia.

4. **What are your follow-up actions?**
Lumbar puncture with a cell count and differential, protein, glucose, Gram stain, culture.
Advance clock:
Lumbar puncture shows more than 100,000 RBCs in all tubes, xanthochromia, otherwise normal.

5. **What are your follow-up actions?**
Neurosurgery consult, admit to the intensive care unit (ICU).
Advance clock:
Case ends.
Critical actions:
Recognition of the possibility of SAH, appropriate diagnostic testing (CT scan and, if negative, a lumbar puncture), admission to the ICU for close monitoring.
Discussion:
This patient has an SAH, which is blood inside the subarachnoid space (where the CSF resides), a life-threatening condition. This is usually due to rupture of a preexisting saccular aneurysm in the circle of Willis but can also be traumatic in origin. The classic presentation is a sudden-onset "thunderclap" headache, which is the worst of the patient's life, with or without loss of consciousness. The blood irritates the meninges, so patients can exhibit neck stiffness, nausea, vomiting, seizures, and an altered level of consciousness. Some patients with SAH have a sentinel bleed days to weeks previously, which this patient exhibited.

Diagnosis is on the basis of a noncontrast CT scan of the head that demonstrates blood inside the subarachnoid space. If positive, the diagnosis is clear and treatment can proceed. If the CT scan is negative, this does not rule out SAH (CT is not sensitive enough) and therefore the patient requires a lumbar puncture for detection of blood in the CSF (or xanthochromia from blood breakdown if the bleed is slightly older). After diagnosis, treatment includes BP management (avoiding hypertension and hypotension), volume management (avoiding hypovolemia), preventing vasospasm with nimodipine (a calcium channel blocker), and preventing seizures with anticonvulsants (typically phenytoin, but anticonvulsants are controversial for SAH). These patients should be admitted to the ICU for close observation for complications such as continued bleeding, vasospasm, hyponatremia, and obstructive hydrocephalus. In cases of aneurysmal SAH, the aneurysm can be coiled or clipped to prevent future episodes of bleeding.
Diagnosis: SAH

CASE 13

HPI: A 22-year-old woman attends the clinic at her university for a rash on her lip. She says that she has had a mild fever (maximum temperature recorded 100.8° F [38.2° C]) and a mild, gradual-onset headache over her bitemporal area without phonophotophobia or neck stiffness for the past 2 days. Today she developed a painful rash on her left lower lip. She denies any history of similar symptoms. She admits that she had protected sex with a man she met at a party last week but says he did not have any rashes that she noticed.
Vital signs: Temperature 99.7° F (37.6° C), pulse 58 beats/min, BP 118/58 mm Hg, RR 16 breaths/min.
Additional history: Twenty lifetime sexual partners, all male, occasional protection. Last menses 3 weeks ago. Moderate alcohol use. No cigarette use, smokes marijuana weekly. No medical problems, medications, allergies, or surgeries.

1. **What is the differential diagnosis?**
Primary herpes simplex virus (HSV) infection, impetigo, herpangina, aphthous stomatitis, herpes zoster, primary syphilis, chancroid, perioral dermatitis.

2. **What components of the physical examination do you perform?**
General appearance, HEENT, cardiovascular, lungs.
Physical examination:
General: Well-developed, well-nourished woman in no apparent distress.
HEENT: Groups of vesicles on an erythematous base at the vermillion border of the left lower lip measuring 8 mm in total. No intraoral lesions. Submandibular and cervical lymphadenopathy. No meningismus.
Cardiovascular: WNL
Lungs: WNL

3. **What are your initial orders?**

Urinary pregnancy test; *Chlamydia*, gonorrhea, HIV screening. Counsel the patient on safe sex techniques, birth control. Optional: HSV polymerase chain reaction (PCR) of lesion.

Advance clock:

Urinary pregnancy test, *Chlamydia*, gonorrhea, HIV negative. HSV PCR of lesion, if ordered, will be positive.

4. **What are your follow-up actions?**

Acyclovir or valacyclovir treatment. Counseling on disease.

Advance clock:

Case ends.

Critical actions:

Recognition of the signs and symptoms of primary HSV infection. Appropriate screening for sexually active young adults, counseling. Treatment of HSV.

Discussion:

This patient has a primary infection with HSV. HSV-1 classically causes oral herpes, whereas HSV-2 classically causes genital herpes, but either one can cause an infection in either location. Outbreaks can be classified as primary or secondary and have different signs and symptoms. The first outbreak (primary) of oral herpes is usually much more severe than subsequent outbreaks and is characterized by mononucleosis-like symptoms such as fever, fatigue, and headache often associated with lymphadenopathy. The rash is vesicular, and a small group of vesicles will manifest itself, usually on the outer edge of the vermillion border. Recurrent outbreaks occur on reactivation of the herpes virus (which is latent in the nerve), are less severe, and often have a prodrome of neuropathic pain and burning before the vesicular lesion (cold sore or fever blister) appears. HSV can also infect the genital region, cause encephalitis (HSV-1 is the most common cause of viral encephalitis), infect the skin via direct contact (herpes gladiatorum), infect skin that is susceptible because of eczema (eczema herpeticum), infect the fingers (herpetic whitlow), or infect the cornea (herpetic keratitis).

The diagnosis is made on a clinical basis because many individuals have asymptomatic infections and antibody tests are of limited use. A viral culture or PCR can be used if the clinical diagnosis is not straightforward. For cases of suspected encephalitis, a lumbar puncture should be performed and sent for HSV PCR. For herpetic keratitis, a fluorescein dye used on the eye will demonstrate dendritic lesions.

Treatment is with acyclovir or valacyclovir for primary infection and to prevent or treat recurrences. Those with a primary HSV infection may never have another outbreak. Patients should be counseled on transmission of HSV and asymptomatic shedding, whereby the virus can still be transmitted even if no lesions are visible. As an aside, the Centers for Disease Control recommends annual screening for *Chlamydia* for all sexually active women younger than 25 years; screening for gonorrhea is indicated for those at risk of infection, and HIV screening should be discussed.

Diagnosis: HSV-1 primary infection

CASE 14

HPI: A 56-year-old man with a medical history of alcoholic cirrhosis is brought to the ED by his wife. He complains of 1 day of gradually worsening, dull abdominal pain. The pain is now moderate and associated with subjective fever. He denies coffee-ground emesis or blood in his stool.

Vital signs: Temperature 100.8° F (38.2° C), pulse 105 beats/min, BP 110/78 mm Hg, RR 12 breaths/min.

Additional history: Diagnosed with alcoholic cirrhosis 2 years previously. No longer drinks alcohol.

1. **What is the differential diagnosis?**

Spontaneous bacterial peritonitis (SBP), secondary bacterial peritonitis, appendicitis, diverticulitis, cholecystitis, pancreatitis, perforated viscus.

2. **What components of the physical examination do you perform?**

General appearance, HEENT, cardiovascular, lungs, abdomen, extremities.

Physical examination:

General: No acute distress.

HEENT: Dry cracked lips, scleral icterus.

Cardiovascular: Tachycardia, otherwise WNL.

Lungs: WNL

Abdomen: Distended with a fluid wave and shifting dullness; soft, moderate tenderness that is diffuse; no rebound or guarding.

Extremities: Pitting edema (score 2+) to the knees.

3. **What are your initial orders?**

Pulse oximetry, BP/cardiac monitor, CBC, chem 8, LFTs, prothrombin time (PT)/ partial thromboplasin time (PTT), lipase/amylase, blood cultures, urinalysis, urine culture, paracentesis (cell count, protein, albumin, glucose, lactate dehydrogenase [LDH], Gram stain, culture), morphine.

Advance clock:

Elevated white blood cell (WBC) count, mild anemia and thrombocytopenia, elevated PT/PTT, low albumin.

Ascitic fluid: More than 250 polymorphonuclear neutrophil (PMN) cells/mL, total protein less than 1 g/dL, glucose greater than 50 g/dL, LDH greater than 225 U/L, Gram stain reveals gram-negative rods.

Other studies: WNL

4. **What are your follow-up actions?**

Ceftriaxone IV, albumin IV, admit to inpatient unit. Vital signs observed every 4 hours, CBC and chem 8 next day. Counseling before discharge.

Advance clock:

Culture is positive for *Escherichia coli* on hospital day 2. Sensitive to ceftriaxone.

WBC count normalizes, vital signs normalize, and the patient's symptoms are greatly improved. Case ends.

Critical actions:

Abdominal examination, paracentesis with ascitic fluid studies, IV antibiotics, admit to inpatient unit.

Discussion:

SBP is a serious medical condition that typically occurs in cirrhotic patients with existing large-volume ascites. The classic presenting symptoms are fever, diffuse abdominal pain/tenderness, and altered mental status. All three of these features may be subtle, however, because cirrhotic patients tend to be hypothermic at baseline and the presence of ascites obscures the physical examination finding of an acute rigid abdomen. Altered mental status may take the form of full delirium or a subtle behavioral change (and can be obscured by baseline hepatic encephalopathy). The most common organisms responsible for SBP are *E. coli*, *Streptococcus*, and *Klebsiella*.

SBP is diagnosed on the basis of an ascites PMN count of greater than 250 cells/mL or a WBC count of greater than 500 cells/mL, especially in the context of a positive Gram stain or culture. A cell count is thus the only ascitic fluid test needed to rule out SBP if clinical suspicion is low. A diagnosis of SBP can only be established, however, in the absence of a secondary cause of peritonitis. To assess for secondary bacterial peritonitis, other ascites studies include ascitic protein, albumin, glucose, LDH, and amylase. Ascites findings that indicate **secondary** peritonitis include protein greater than 1 g/dL, glucose less than 50 mg/dL, and LDH greater than 225 U/L. Elevated amylase or bilirubin in ascitic fluid may indicate pancreatic or biliary causes of peritonitis. If secondary bacterial peritonitis cannot be ruled out, a search for a secondary source must begin. CT imaging can help in evaluating for most pancreatic, biliary, and bowel pathologies. Once a diagnosis of SBP is established, the patient should be treated with a third-generation cephalosporin (ceftriaxone). Albumin IV also decreases the risk of renal failure and mortality. Patients with one episode of SBP are at high risk of recurrence and should be discharged on a prophylactic antibiotic regimen such as norfloxacin or ciprofloxacin.

Diagnosis: SBP

CASE 15

HPI: A 36-year-old woman attends the ED after noticing swelling and pain in her left leg. She does not recall any trauma to the leg. She noticed that the leg was painful and tender this morning when she tried to walk. She has had no fevers, chills, chest pain, cough, or shortness of breath. She was recently on a flight from Australia to New York.

Vital signs: Temperature 98.6° F (37.0° C), pulse 78 beats/min, BP 110/78 mm Hg, RR 15 breaths/min.

Additional history: The patient takes an oral contraceptive. No other medical history or medications. No use of drugs, tobacco, or alcohol.

1. **What is the differential diagnosis?**
   Deep venous thrombosis (DVT), superficial thrombophlebitis, cellulitis, muscle strain, fracture, venous insufficiency.

2. **What components of the physical examination do you perform?**
   General appearance, HEENT, cardiovascular, lungs, abdomen, extremities.
   Physical examination:
   General: No acute distress.
   HEENT: WNL
   Cardiovascular: WNL
   Lungs: WNL
   Abdomen: WNL
   Extremities: Swelling and erythema of left calf compared to right. Tenderness along the posterior calf with a deep palpable cord. Peripheral pulses 2+.

3. **What are your initial orders?**
   Pulse oximetry, ultrasound of the leg, CBC, chem 8, PT/PTT.
   Advance clock:
   Ultrasound reveals a noncompressible popliteal vein consistent with venous thrombosis. All other studies WNL.

4. **What are your follow-up actions?**
   Low-molecular-weight heparin (LMWH; subcutaneous [SC] enoxaparin), warfarin PO, follow up in 3 days to check PT/international normalized ratio (INR), discontinue oral contraceptive pill (OCP), counseling.
   Advance clock:
   Case ends.
   Critical actions:
   Examination of the extremities, ultrasound of the leg, discontinuation of OCP, anticoagulation therapy (e.g., LMWH and warfarin).
   Discussion:
   This patient has unilateral swelling of the leg with risk factors for DVT (OCP use and recent travel). The physical examination in this case is suggestive of DVT and further diagnostic testing is warranted. In patients with low risk of DVT, a single negative D-dimer result may be sufficient to rule out thrombosis. In this intermediate-risk patient (based on history and physical findings), the workup should proceed directly to ultrasound because a negative D-dimer result is insufficient to rule out DVT. Most cases of DVT can be treated on an outpatient basis with anticoagulation therapy. This typically consists of warfarin and LMWH bridging (usually enoxaparin). The initial laboratory screening tests can identify those at risk of anticoagulation complications. Patients should be scheduled for follow up in 2 to 3 days to check the PT/INR and adjust the warfarin dosage. When applicable, OCPs should be discontinued and patients should be counseled about alternative contraceptive methods. In first-time provoked (known risk factors such as OCP use) cases of DVT, anticoagulation therapy is continued for 3 to 6 months and screening for hypercoagulability is generally not warranted. In patients with unprovoked or recurrent DVT, a hypercoagulable workup is performed that includes testing for protein C, protein S, antithrombin III, factor V Leiden, antiphospholipid antibodies, and prothrombin G20210A gene mutation. These tests are usually ordered at follow-up because some are influenced by oral anticoagulation use and the clotting event itself. The evaluation and treatment of DVT are primarily to prevent the complications of venous thromboembolism, including pulmonary embolism (discussed separately). Any patient with DVT should be evaluated for signs and symptoms related to pulmonary embolism (chest pain, shortness of breath, hypoxia).
   Diagnosis: DVT

CASE 16

HPI: A 4-year-old boy is brought to the ED by his parents, who are concerned about their child's fever. They state that they have taken his temperature for the past 6 days and it was always greater than 100.4° F (38° C) and did not seem to resolve on acetaminophen or ibuprofen administration. The patient denies a cough, runny nose, urinary problems, or sore throat. The parents state that he has had red eyes for the past 2 days but that they do not hurt, and on the first day of illness he had a rash on his chest that felt rough but has since resolved.

Vital signs: Temperature 101.5° F (38.6° C), pulse 120 beats/min, BP 110/80 mm Hg, RR 20 breaths/min.

Additional history: No medical history, no hospitalizations, all vaccines up to date.

1. **What is the differential diagnosis?**
   Kawasaki disease, viral exanthem, conjunctivitis (e.g., adenovirus), infectious mononucleosis.

2. **What components of the physical examination do you perform?**
   General appearance, HEENT, skin, cardiovascular, lungs, abdomen.
   Physical examination:
   General: Well-developed, well-nourished boy in no acute distress.
   HEENT: Bilateral conjunctivitis with perilimbic sparing, no exudates. Tongue has diffuse inflamed red papillae. Anterior cervical adenopathy bilaterally, largest 2 cm.
   Skin: No rashes.
   Cardiovascular: WNL
   Lungs: WNL
   Abdomen: WNL

3. **What are your initial orders?**
   Admit to the inpatient unit, aspirin, IV immunoglobulin (IVIG), transthoracic echocardiogram (TTE).
   Advance clock:
   The patient's fever resolves with treatment. TTE shows no evidence of coronary artery aneurysm.

4. **What are your follow-up actions?**
   Discharge with follow-up for serial TTE and recheck.
   Advance clock:
   Case ends.
   Critical actions:
   Recognition of Kawasaki disease as a clinical diagnosis; initiation of treatment.
   Discussion:
   This patient has Kawasaki disease, an acute vasculitis of childhood primarily involving the coronary arteries. The diagnosis is on a clinical basis, but for incomplete Kawasaki disease (previously called atypical), laboratory findings support the diagnosis (see below). Untreated patients are at much higher risk (20% to 25%) of coronary artery aneurysms than treated patients (4%), so prompt recognition is essential.
   The clinical diagnosis of Kawasaki disease can be remembered by the **CRASH and burn** mnemonic. The burn refers to the 5 days of fever, and **CRASH** is a mnemonic for **c**onjunctivitis (nonexudative bilateral, perilimbic sparing), **r**ash (anything but petechiae), **a**denopathy (cervical), **s**trawberry tongue or other oral mucous membrane changes, and **h**ands and feet (erythema, edema, desquamation). At least **four** of the **CRASH** mnemonic findings must be present, as well as fever for 5 days. If two or three CRASH findings are present, then there are laboratory criteria to support the diagnosis of incomplete Kawasaki disease (hypoalbuminemia, anemia, alanine aminotransferase [ALT] elevation, thrombocytosis, leukocytosis, urinary WBCs).
   Treatment is with IVIG and acute high-dose aspirin administration, followed by low-dose aspirin for a longer period of time (6 to 8 weeks). TTE should be performed on initial diagnosis and at 2 weeks and 2 months to rule out interval development of coronary artery aneurysms.
   Diagnosis: Kawasaki disease

CASE 17

HPI: A 35-year-old woman attends the ED with intense, intermittent right flank pain for the past 2 days. During this time she has also noticed that her urine has taken on a darker appearance. She states that when she has the pain she cannot seem to get comfortable; the pain is alleviated somewhat by ibuprofen. She denies any history of similar symptoms. No fevers, cough, dysuria, nausea, vomiting, or trauma.

Vital signs: Temperature 98.2° F (36.8° C), pulse 64 beats/min, BP 115/68 mm Hg, RR 16 breaths/min.

Additional history: No use of drugs, alcohol, or tobacco. No medical history.

1. **What is the differential diagnosis?**
   Nephrolithiasis, pyelonephritis, right lower-lobe pneumonia, musculoskeletal pain, abdominal aortic aneurysm (AAA), cholecystitis.

2. **What components of the physical examination do you perform?**
   General, cardiovascular, lungs, abdominal, back.
   Physical examination:
   General: Well-developed and well-nourished woman in moderate distress due to pain, writhing uncomfortably on the gurney.
   Cardiovascular: WNL
   Lungs: WNL
   Abdomen: WNL
   Back: Significant right-sided flank pain. No overlying skin changes or evidence of trauma.

3. **What are your initial orders?**
   CBC, chem 8, urinalysis, urinary pregnancy test, nonsteroidal antiinflammatory drug (NSAID; e.g., ketorolac, ibuprofen), opioid analgesic (e.g., morphine).
   Advance clock:
   CBC and chem 8 WNL. Urinalysis blood 3+ with more than 182 RBCs per high-power field (hpf), otherwise WNL. Urinary pregnancy test negative. Patient feels much better after pain medication.

4. **What are your follow-up actions?**
   Noncontrast CT scan of the abdomen/pelvis.
   Advance clock:
   CT scan shows 3-mm kidney stone at the right ureterovesicular junction (UVJ) with mild hydronephrosis.

5. **What are your follow-up actions?**
   Prescription for ibuprofen, an opioid, and tamsulosin. Follow up after 1 week. Counsel the patient on the disease process and advise her to strain her urine.
   Advance clock:
   Patient returns stating she passed the stone and her pain has resolved; she was unable to catch the stone.
   Case ends.
   Critical actions:
   Recognition of nephrolithiasis, appropriate treatment and follow-up.
   Discussion:
   This patient has urolithiasis (a kidney stone) in the urogenital tract. Kidney stones typically cause severe intermittent (colicky) pain due to intermittent spasm of an irritated ureter. The three most common locations of stones are the ureteropelvic junction (where the renal pelvis joins the ureter), the pelvic brim (where the stone can get caught as the ureter passes over the iliac arteries), and the UVJ (where the ureters enter the bladder). The likelihood of stone passage is related to the size and location of the stone. Stones smaller than 5 mm usually pass, whereas stones larger than 10 mm almost never pass spontaneously. The most common stone is a calcium oxalate stone, but other stones can also occur. Struvite stones can occur when patients have infections from urea-splitting organisms such as *Proteus* because the free ammonia from the split urea makes up part of the struvite stone; these stones can completely fill the renal pelvis and are referred to as staghorn calculi.

Diagnosis is via history and physical examination. For patients who have a kidney stone without a prior history of stones, a CT scan is typically performed to evaluate the size and location of the stone. Complications include obstructing stones (which block urinary flow from the kidney and are associated with hydronephrosis), infected stones (which can prevent infected urine from passing), and renal failure if obstruction persists for too long. Management is with a combination of NSAIDs and opioids (the NSAIDs help prevent prostaglandin-mediated ureter pain), as well as tamsulosin, which is an alpha-antagonist that helps dilate the smooth muscle in the urogenital tract to facilitate stone passage. Patients with uncomplicated nephrolithiasis can be managed as outpatients with urologic follow-up if the stone is unlikely to be passed on its own. Urgent urologic consultation and/or admission are indicated for concurrent infection with hydronephrosis, renal failure, uncontrollable pain, or inability to tolerate oral intake. In older patients with symptoms consistent with nephrolithiasis, an AAA must always be considered.

Diagnosis: Nephrolithiasis

CASE 18

HPI: A 26-year-old man is brought to the ED by his friends because he "wasn't making sense" when he talked and was becoming less responsive. The friends say that he takes insulin, but ran out a little less than a week ago and has not been able to get a refill. They deny any ingestion or any other complaints from the patient.

Vital signs: Temperature 98.2° F (36.8° C), pulse 120 beats/min, BP 100/70 mm Hg, RR 28 breaths/min.

Additional history: Unknown.

1. **What is the differential diagnosis?**
   Altered mental status: **AEIOU TIPS** mnemonic: **a**cidosis; **e**lectrolytes, **e**ncephalopathy, **e**ndocrine (e.g., diabetic ketoacidosis [DKA]); **i**nsulin causing hypoglycemia; **o**piates or overdose; **u**remia; **t**rauma, **t**emperature, **t**oxemia; **i**nfections; **p**ulmonary embolism or **p**sychogenic; **s**pace-occupying lesions, **s**trokes, **s**hock, **s**eizure.

2. **What components of the physical examination do you perform?**
   General appearance, cardiovascular, lungs, neuro/psych.
   Physical examination:
   General: Obtunded but able to be aroused, breathing rapidly and deeply.
   Cardiovascular: Tachycardic but no murmurs, rubs, or gallops.
   Lungs: WNL
   Neuro/psych: Able to say name on stimulation, knows year. No obvious focal neurologic deficits but limited examination secondary to obtundation.

3. **What are your initial orders?**
   CBC, chem 8, serum ketones, urinalysis, ECG, venous blood gas, portable CXR, IV fluids.
   Advance clock:
   CBC shows leukocytosis of 16×10^3 cells/mL with a left shift but no bandemia; otherwise normal. Chem 8 remarkable for sodium 130 mEq/L, potassium 4.8 mEq/L, bicarbonate 10 mEq/L (anion gap 26 mEq/L), normal creatinine, and glucose 500 mg/dL; otherwise normal. Serum ketones elevated. Urinalysis reveals a high ketone level, high specific gravity, and a high glucose level; otherwise negative. ECG sinus tachycardia at 125 beats/min. Venous blood gas pH 7.05. Portable CXR negative. After IV fluids, the heart rate decreases to 110 beats/min.

4. **What are your follow-up actions?**
   Begin regular insulin IV drip, continue high rate of IV fluid administration with potassium supplementation, admit to the ICU.
   Advance clock:
   Case ends.
   Critical actions:
   Recognition of DKA as the cause of the patient's altered mental status; fluid resuscitation, waiting for potassium value before starting insulin.
   Discussion:
   This patient has DKA secondary to running out of insulin. Lack of insulin causes increased gluconeogenesis and lipolysis, leading to ketosis and acidosis. These factors, paired with

an inability to import glucose into cells, lead to significant hyperglycemia. After diagnosis, fluid resuscitation should be initiated because osmotic diuresis arising from hyperglycemia typically causes profound hypovolemia. In children, however, there is controversy about whether aggressive fluid resuscitation causes cerebral edema. Insulin therapy should not be initiated until a potassium level is obtained: patients experience whole-body potassium depletion but often have normal or high potassium values because of acidosis. If potassium is low (<3.3 mEq/L), insulin should not be administered until potassium is replete. If the potassium is normal, potassium can be added to IV fluids; if high (>5.5 mEq/L), no potassium should be added. The dose of insulin is 0.1 U/kg/hr via a regular insulin IV drip; an initial bolus of 0.1 U/kg is controversial and probably unnecessary. Sodium is classically low because hyperglycemia causes water to shift into the intravascular space, where it dilutes sodium. The correction is 1.6 mEq/L added for every 100 mg/dL by which glucose exceeds 100 mg/dL.

Although missing insulin doses are a common precipitant for DKA, there should be a high index of suspicion for alternative causes. Infection is a common inducing factor, as are myocardial infarction (MI) and substance ingestion. Alcoholic ketoacidosis should also be included in the differential diagnosis. Close monitoring of electrolytes and glucose is required, and once glucose falls below 250 mg/dL, glucose should be added to the IV fluids. The insulin drip can be stopped when the acidosis and ketosis resolve, and the patient can be transitioned to SC insulin. Admission to a monitored bed or ICU is usually warranted for initial management.

Diagnosis: DKA

CASE 19

HPI: An 84-year-old man is brought to his primary care physician by his family because of concerns about increased forgetfulness. The family states that for the past 5 to 6 years he has progressively worsened in his ability to remember things. Initially, he needed help with his finances and taxes but otherwise was able to live independently and carry out his daily activities. However, over the past year or so he has been getting lost when he goes out driving or walking, and has been forgetting to do things like turn off the stove and forgetting the names of family members. The patient denies being forgetful and says that he never gets lost. The family and the patient deny any abrupt decline in function, changes in medication, or new exposures. The patient does not have any difficulty in walking, sleeping, or eating, and has no weakness.

Vital signs: Temperature 98.2° F (36.8° C), pulse 66 beats/min, BP 135/78 mm Hg, RR 16 breaths/min.

Additional history: History only significant for hyperlipidemia, for which he takes atorvastatin. No other medical problems or allergies. No use of drugs, alcohol, or tobacco.

1. **What is the differential diagnosis?**
   Dementia: Alzheimer (most likely), vascular, frontotemporal, Lewy body. Other causes: hypothyroidism, vitamin B_{12} deficiency, calcium derangement, depression, medication effects.

2. **What components of the physical examination do you perform?**
   General appearance, lungs, cardiovascular, neuro/psych.
   Physical examination:
   General: Well-developed, well-nourished man in no apparent distress.
   Cardiovascular: WNL
   Lungs: WNL
   Neuro/psych: Cranial nerves II through XII intact. Strength, sensation, reflexes, and gait all WNL. Alert and oriented to name only. Remembers 0/3 objects at 5 minutes. Cannot subtract serial 7s from 100, and cannot spell WORLD backwards. Can name a pen, but not a watch. Can follow one-step commands, but not more complicated commands.

3. **What are your initial orders?**
   CBC, chem 8, ESR, vitamin B_{12}, thyroid function tests, noncontrast head CT scan.
   Advance clock:
   All the studies ordered are WNL.

4. **What are your follow-up actions?**
   Counseling on the disease process and the need to stop driving, social work consult, consider starting medication such as donepezil.
   Advance clock:
   Case ends.
   Critical actions:
   Recognition of dementia, basic evaluation to rule out reversible causes, counseling on disease process and prognosis.
   Discussion:
   This patient has dementia, a chronic and often irreversible global decline in cognitive function. Dementia has many subtypes, including Alzheimer disease (most common), vascular dementia, frontotemporal dementia, and Lewy body dementia, among others. It is important to rule out a reversible cause of dementia and its mimics (e.g., hypothyroidism, pseudodementia caused by depression, medication effects in older individuals leading to cognitive impairment), as well as delirium (change in level of consciousness with acute or subacute onset, often caused by a medical problem and usually reversible if identified).
   Diagnosis is on the basis of history and physical examination and a ruling out of reversible causes. A mental status examination should be performed in all patients to evaluate their cognitive function. Basic laboratory tests such as CBC, serum chemistry (to rule out electrolyte/metabolic disturbances and uremia), vitamin B_{12} level (evaluate for subacute combined degeneration of the spinal cord), and thyroid tests (evaluate for hypothyroidism) should be performed, and a CT scan is often ordered to rule out hydrocephalus and other lesions. Depending on the history, additional tests may be required (e.g., evaluation for neurosyphilis, HIV, autoimmune disease, carotid ultrasound if vascular dementia is being considered, LFTs if hepatic encephalopathy is considered, ESR if screening for occult inflammatory states or malignancy). Treatment is mainly supportive because current medications (e.g., donepezil, memantine) have limited efficacy. Ensuring a safe home environment, counseling patients and their caregivers/family on the disease course, and appropriate follow-up to track disease progression are required.
   Diagnosis: Dementia

CASE 20

HPI: An 18-month-old boy is brought to the ED with abdominal pain for the past 24 hours. The mother states that he appears well and is acting normally but then periodically starts to cry and brings his legs to his chest and vomits. During these episodes he says "Ow" and points to his abdomen. He has also been eating less and making fewer wet diapers during this time. The mother denies any changes in bowel movements.

Vital signs: Temperature 99.7 ° F (37.6° C), pulse 110 beats/min, BP 100/70 mm Hg, RR 30 breaths/min.

Additional history: All vaccinations up to date. Delivered at full term. No previous surgeries.

1. **What is the differential diagnosis?**
   Intussusception, incarcerated hernia, adhesions (if patient had history of surgery), constipation (if change in bowel movements), volvulus, testicular torsion.

2. **What components of the physical examination do you perform?**
   General appearance, cardiovascular, lungs, abdomen, genitalia.
   Physical examination:
   General: Well-appearing infant who occasionally has fits of crying and appears to be in moderate distress due to pain.
   Cardiovascular: WNL
   Lungs: WNL
   Abdomen: Soft, nondistended, tender to palpation during episodes of pain, sausage-like mass in the right abdomen.
   Genitalia: Testes descended bilaterally and nontender.

3. **What are your initial orders?**
   Ultrasound of abdomen, optional KUB, urinalysis.
   Advance clock:
   Ultrasound demonstrates the target sign, suggestive of intussusception.

4. **What are your follow-up actions?**
   Air/barium enema, surgical consult, admission to inpatient unit, counseling.
   Advance clock:
   Case ends.
   Critical actions:
   Recognition of intussusception as the cause of the abdominal pain, ordering appropriate workup, appropriate disposition. Checking the testes in male patients with abdominal pain because testicular torsion has a bimodal peak and can occur in both adolescence and early infancy.
   Discussion:
   This patient has ileocolic intussusception, whereby one part of the bowel (the intussusceptum) invaginates into a distal adjoining part of the bowel (the intussuscipiens). This typically occurs in patients between 3 months and 2 years of age but can also occur in older individuals with a lead point that drags the proximal bowel into the distal bowel. Examples are polyps, lymphoid hyperplasia from infections or lymphoma, a Meckel diverticulum, and submucosal hematomas seen in Henoch-Schönlein purpura.
   The classic presentation of intussusception involves the triad of intermittent colicky abdominal pain, vomiting, and a stool resembling red currant jelly, which is a late finding due to intestinal necrosis. The patient may draw the legs up during the pain, and the vomiting due to the intestinal obstruction may be bilious. On examination there may be a sausage-like mass that can be palpated. Diagnosis is made on the basis of ultrasound showing a target sign, but plain X-rays can also be beneficial.
   An air (or barium) enema is both diagnostic and therapeutic because the intussusception is often reduced by the enema (90% of cases). Management also includes fluid resuscitation if needed, antibiotics if there is evidence of peritonitis due to perforation, and a surgical consult and admission to the hospital regardless of whether or not the intussusception is reduced by the enema, because the early recurrence risk is highest within the first 24 hours.
   Diagnosis: Intussusception

CASE 21

HPI: A 66-year old man attends the clinic complaining of several weeks of decreased energy. He feels so fatigued that he can barely get out of bed. When he does move he feels short of breath. He has found several large bruises over his body as a result of minor trauma. He cut himself while preparing dinner last week and the bleeding did not stop for an abnormally long time.
Vital signs: Temperature 99.3° F (37.4° C), pulse 92 beats/min, BP 110/76 mm Hg, RR 18 breaths/min.
Additional history: No medical history. No use of drugs, tobacco, or alcohol.

1. **What is the differential diagnosis?**
   Anemia, thrombocytopenia, leukemia, congestive heart failure (CHF), pneumonia, viral infection, depression.

2. **What components of the physical examination do you perform?**
   General appearance, skin, lymph nodes, HEENT, cardiovascular, lungs, abdomen, extremities.
   Physical examination:
   General: No acute distress.
   Skin/lymph nodes: Two 5×5-cm² ecchymoses over lateral thigh and arm.
   HEENT: Conjunctival pallor.
   Cardiovascular: WNL
   Lungs: WNL
   Abdomen: WNL
   Extremities: WNL

3. **What are your initial orders?**
   Pulse oximetry, CBC with differential, peripheral smear, chem 8, PT/PTT, CXR.
   Advance clock:
   CBC reveals 72,000 WBCs/mL with a high percentage of blasts, Hb 9.1 mg/dL, MCV 92 fL, platelets 82,000 cells/μL. Peripheral smear notable for presence of Auer rods. Other studies WNL.

4. What are your follow-up actions?
Uric acid, LDH, LFTs, oncology consult, bone marrow biopsy.
Advance clock:
Case ends.
Critical actions:
CBC, hematology-oncology consult.
Discussion:
This patient has vague symptoms of fatigue and shortness of breath. Although this indicates a broad differential, the signs and symptoms of easy bruising indicate the possibility of a hematologic issue. CBC is an excellent screening test for hematologic issues, and the peripheral smear can offer more specific information. A thorough physical examination and CXR can exclude some other causes in the differential. The presence of hyperleukocytosis (>50,000 WBCs/mL), anemia, and thrombocytopenia points to a hematologic malignancy. The presence of blasts is suggestive of leukemia, and the presence of Auer rods is highly suggestive of acute myelogenous leukemia (AML). Once leukemia is suspected, a hematologist-oncologist should be consulted. The hematologist-oncologist will perform a bone marrow biopsy to confirm the diagnosis.

Urgent considerations in management include the exclusion of complications such as tumor lysis syndrome, leukostasis, and infection. Tumor lysis syndrome is evidenced by very high levels of uric acid, LDH, potassium, and phosphorous. It causes renal, cardiac, and neurologic complications. Treatment involves IV hydration, correction of electrolyte abnormalities, and administration of uric-acid–lowering agents such as allopurinol. Leukostasis may occur because of the high viscosity of the blood, particularly when the WBC count exceeds 100,000 cells/mL. This may cause renal, neurologic, and pulmonary symptoms. The treatment is aggressive hydration and a hematology consult for initiation of leukapheresis and chemotherapy. Patients with leukemia may be febrile secondary to the disease process or to bacterial infection. It is often difficult to distinguish the cause, so cultures should be sent and empiric antibiotic therapy should be initiated in patients with leukemia and fever.
Diagnosis: AML

CASE 22

HPI: A 53-year-old woman attends the ED complaining of 2 days of fatigue and 1 day of mild confusion. Her daughter says she is normally in excellent health but has had difficulty getting out of bed over the past several days. She has felt feverish, but no temperature was recorded at home. Her daughter also noted a few small purple specks on her mother's skin. Today her mother seemed very confused so her daughter brought her to the ED.
Vital signs: Temperature 100.6° F (38.1° C), pulse 92 beats/min, BP 120/76 mm Hg, RR 18 breaths/min.
Additional history: No medical history. No use of drugs, tobacco, or alcohol.

1. What is the differential diagnosis?
Anemia, thrombocytopenia, leukemia, immune thrombocytopenic purpura (ITP), stroke, thrombotic thrombocytopenic purpura (TTP), vasculitis, infection (including pneumonia, UTI, meningitis, influenza), disseminated intravascular coagulation (DIC).

2. What components of the physical examination do you perform?
General appearance, skin, lymph nodes, HEENT, cardiovascular, lungs, abdomen, extremities, neuro/psych.
Physical examination:
General: No acute distress.
Skin: Few scattered petechiae.
Lymph nodes: WNL
HEENT: Conjunctival pallor.
Cardiovascular: WNL
Lungs: WNL
Abdomen: WNL
Extremities: WNL
Neuro/psych: Alert and oriented to person and place but not time, no focal neurologic deficits, neck supple.

3. **What are your initial orders?**
   Pulse oximetry, CBC with differential, peripheral smear, chem 14, PT/PTT, CXR, urinalysis.
   Advance clock:
   CBC reveals platelets 25,000 cells/μL, Hb 7.0 mg/dL. Peripheral smear notable for presence of schistocytes. Mildly elevated BUN, creatinine, and bilirubin. Urinalysis blood 2+. Other studies WNL.

4. **What are your follow-up actions?**
   Reticulocyte count, haptoglobin, LDH, hematology consult for plasma exchange, corticosteroids (e.g., prednisone), fresh frozen plasma (FFP) transfusion, admit to ICU.
   Advance clock:
   Case ends.
   Critical actions:
   CBC, hematology-oncology consult, admission, avoid transfusion of platelets.
   Discussion:
   TTP is recognized clinically by a pentad described by the mnemonic **FAT RN: f**ever, **a**nemia (microangiopathic hemolytic anemia [MAHA]), **t**hrombocytopenia, **r**enal failure, and **n**eurologic deficits. The condition is caused by a deficiency of the protease ADAMTS13, usually due to autoantibodies. Under normal conditions, ADAMTS13 cleaves von Willebrand factor (vWF) multimers into smaller parts. ADAMTS13 deficiency causes vWF to agglutinate platelets in small vessels. As platelets clump in the small vessels, they create a shearing force on passing RBCs that causes MAHA (characterized by anemia, schistocytes, and elevated bilirubin). Occlusion of the microvasculature also causes renal failure and neurologic signs (e.g., coma, confusion, seizures). The complete pentad is present in only 50% of cases, however, so the presence of MAHA and thrombocytopenia should trigger a hematology consult. The diagnosis may not be suspected until routine laboratory tests for evaluation of the presenting complaint have been completed. CBC will reveal thrombocytopenia and anemia. A chemistry panel may reveal renal insufficiency. A peripheral smear will reveal schistocytes. LDH, bilirubin, and reticulocytes will all be elevated. Unlike DIC, the PT/PTT/INR will be normal because these parameters are not affected in TTP.
   Treatment of TTP is initiated in consultation with a hematologist. The treatment of choice is plasmapheresis, which removes the patient's autoantibodies and ultralarge vWF. Then dysfunctional ADAMTS13 is replaced with functional ADAMTS13 in FFP. Plasmapheresis is rarely available immediately, so temporizing measures should be undertaken. These include corticosteroid administration to address the autoimmune component and FFP transfusion to replace dysfunctional ADAMTS13. Despite often profound thrombocytopenia, platelets should not be transfused. Additional platelets will also become occluded in small vessels, worsening the microangiopathic process.
   Although hemolytic uremic syndrome (HUS) and TTP appear similar clinically, they are caused by different mechanisms and ADAMTS13 is not implicated in HUS. HUS is more likely to occur in children, to be accompanied by diarrhea, and to have more profound kidney injury. Classically, HUS is caused by *E. coli* O157:H7. TTP is more likely to have neurologic sequelae.
   Diagnosis: TTP

CASE 23

HPI: A 19-year-old man is brought to the ED by ambulance after becoming confused in his dormitory. He was complaining of a headache and fever before he became confused. Two other students in the same dormitory have recently been hospitalized for similar symptoms.

Vital signs: Temperature 102.2° F (39° C), pulse 130 beats/min, BP 90/62 mm Hg, RR 20 breaths/min.

Additional history: No medical history, no use of drugs, alcohol, or tobacco.

1. **What is the differential diagnosis?**
   Meningitis, encephalitis, sepsis, intracranial hemorrhage, brain abscess, hemolytic uremic syndrome, TTP, Rocky Mountain spotted fever, other rickettsial disease.

2. **What components of the physical examination do you perform?**
   General appearance, HEENT, cardiovascular, lungs, abdomen, skin, neuro/psych.

Physical examination:
General: Lethargic, not answering questions appropriately, alert and oriented to name only.
HEENT: Withdraws when light is shined in eyes. Neck stiff to movement, positive Brudzinski sign.
Cardiovascular: Tachycardic.
Lungs: WNL
Abdomen: WNL
Skin: Diffuse, scattered petechiae, nonblanching.
Neuro/psych: Difficult to assess given mental status, but moving all extremities. Positive Kernig sign.

3. **What are your initial orders?**
Head CT scan, ceftriaxone 2 g IV, vancomycin 1 g IV, with or without dexamethasone before antibiotics, CBC, chem 8, coagulation studies, IV fluids, antipyretics.
Advance clock:
Head CT scan normal. CBC remarkable for WBC count of 26,000 cells/mL with 20% bands. Chem 8 unremarkable. Coagulation studies unremarkable. After IV fluid administration, the patient's BP has improved to 118/70.

4. **What are your follow-up actions?**
Lumbar puncture with CSF cell count, glucose, protein, Gram stain, culture.
Advance clock:
Lumbar puncture demonstrates opening pressure of 35 cm H_2O (elevated), 2400 WBCs/mL (95% neutrophils), protein 500 mg/dL, glucose 20 mg/dL. Gram stain shows numerous gram-negative diplococci.

5. **What are your follow-up actions?**
Admit to the ICU, prophylaxis of close contacts, counseling.
Critical actions:
Recognition of meningitis, ordering a CT scan before a lumbar puncture in a patient with altered mental status. Ordering appropriate antibiotics. Ordering a lumbar puncture and CSF studies.
Discussion:
This patient has meningococcal meningitis caused by *Neisseria meningitidis*, an encapsulated, aerobic, gram-negative diplococcus that classically occurs in crowded living situations such as military camps and dormitories. *N. meningitidis* causes a spectrum of disease that ranges from occult bacteremia to meningococcal meningitis to septicemia and adrenal hemorrhage (called Waterhouse-Friderichsen syndrome). Although meningitis of any cause typically leads to fever, headache, and eventually neck stiffness and confusion, only meningococci cause petechial lesions. This is because *N. meningitidis* releases blebs of endotoxin into the bloodstream that lodge in capillaries and cause inflammatory reactions that break down the capillary bed and lead to small petechial hemorrhages.
   The treatment of meningitis in adults involves recognition, early administration of dexamethasone (as discussed later) and appropriate antibiotics, and a CT scan if the patient has focal neurologic deficits, altered mental status, a recent seizure, a known CNS lesion, immunocompromised state, age older than 60 years, or papilledema. If the CT scan does not show evidence of increased intracranial pressure, it is safe to perform a lumbar puncture. It has been shown that dexamethasone improves outcomes in pneumococcal meningitis but not necessarily in other forms of meningitis, and it must be given before antibiotics to be effective. A lumbar puncture in a patient with bacterial meningitis classically shows elevated opening pressure, a high WBC count with neutrophil predominance, high protein, and low glucose. In this case the patient demonstrated all of these signs and the Gram stain showed *N. meningitidis*, confirming the diagnosis. Because of his hypotension, admission to the ICU for close monitoring in case of adverse effects such as adrenal hemorrhage is warranted.
   The other possible causes of bacterial meningitis in this age group include *Streptococcus pneumoniae* and, albeit much less likely, *Listeria monocytogenes*. Ceftriaxone provides excellent coverage for both *N. meningitidis* and *S. pneumoniae*, and vancomycin can be added to ensure coverage for any resistant *S. pneumoniae* species. Ampicillin can be added for coverage of *L. monocytogenes* in susceptible patients (immunocompromised, older, pregnant, or very

young patients). All close contacts should be given prophylaxis with either rifampin (600 mg PO every 12 hours for 2 days) or ciprofloxacin (500 mg PO, single dose) to prevent the development of meningitis.

Diagnosis: Meningitis

CASE 24

HPI: A 70-year-old man attends his primary care physician because yesterday he suddenly felt part of his face and his right arm go numb and limp while eating dinner. His wife states that his face looked asymmetric and he was unable to speak or move his right arm. She thinks those symptoms lasted about 20 minutes but then completely resolved. She wanted to go to the ED last night but he refused because his symptoms resolved. He denies any history of similar symptoms and currently "feels OK."

Vital signs: Temperature 98.2° F (36.8° C), pulse 80 beats/min, BP 160/98 mm Hg, RR 16 breaths/min.

Additional history: Has a history of type 2 diabetes, hypertension, and dyslipidemia. Takes metformin, glipizide, hydrochlorothiazide, amlodipine, and simvastatin. No allergies. Occasional alcohol use, no tobacco or drugs.

1. **What is the differential diagnosis?**
   TIA, hypoglycemia, complicated migraine, seizure with Todd paralysis, demyelinating diseases.

2. **What components of the physical examination do you perform?**
   General appearance, lungs, cardiovascular, neuro/psych.
   Physical examination:
   General: Overweight man in no apparent distress.
   Cardiovascular: WNL
   Lungs: WNL
   Neuro/psych: Cranial nerves II through XII intact. Strength 5/5 and symmetric over all extremities. Normal sensation, reflexes 2+ throughout, downgoing Babinski response bilaterally. No ataxia, no dysdiadochokinesia, normal gait.

3. **What are your initial orders?**
   CBC, chem 8, coagulation profile, fingerstick blood glucose, ECG, noncontrast head CT scan.
   Advance clock:
   CBC, chem 8, coagulation profile, fingerstick glucose, ECG WNL.
   Noncontrast head CT scan unremarkable.

4. **What are your follow-up actions?**
   Admit to inpatient unit, aspirin, neurology consult. Order TTE, MRI scan, carotid ultrasound, fasting lipid panel. Counseling on disease process.
   Advance clock:
   TTE, MRI, and carotid ultrasound negative. Fasting lipid panel WNL.
   Case ends.
   Critical actions:
   Recognition of TIA in a high-risk patient, checking blood glucose, obtaining a head CT scan before starting antiplatelet therapy, admission for high-risk TIA and neurologic consult. Inpatient workup of TIA including TTE, MRI, carotid ultrasound, and fasting lipid panel.
   Discussion:
   This patient has had a TIA, which is "a transient episode of neurologic dysfunction caused by focal brain, spinal cord, or retinal ischemia, *without* acute infarction" according to the American Stroke Association (previously it was defined as resolving within 24 hours). If acute infarction has occurred, the patient would instead be diagnosed with a stroke. Although this patient's symptoms have completely resolved, the risk of a subsequent stroke is high; the highest risk of a subsequent stroke is in the first week after a TIA, and 17% of patients will have a stroke within the first 3 months after their TIA. Predisposing factors include hypertension, diabetes, dyslipidemia, and atrial fibrillation (AF).

   Diagnosis is according to history and physical examination demonstrating a neurologic deficit that follows a vascular distribution; therefore, knowledge of the basic vascular distribution

Table 16-1. ABCD2 Score and Prediction of Stroke Risk After Transient Ischemic Attack

SCORE	AGE	BLOOD PRESSURE	CLINICAL FEATURES	SYMPTOM DURATION	DIABETES
0	<60 yr	Normal	Other	<10 min	No
1	≥60 yr	≥140/90 mm Hg	Speech disturbance, no weakness	10-59 min	Yes
2			Unilateral weakness	≥60 min	

of the brain is important. Blood glucose should be checked in all such patients because hypoglycemia can mimic stroke symptoms. An immediate head CT scan should be obtained for any patient suspected of having had a stroke or TIA to rule out hemorrhage because antiplatelet agents are contraindicated in such patients. Treatment (if not contraindicated) involves antiplatelet agents, such as aspirin, and control of the patient's risk factors. The ABCD2 score assigns the risk of having a subsequent stroke after TIA (Table 16-1). For example, a score of 0 or 1 corresponds to a risk of stroke in the next 2 days of nearly 0%, whereas a score of 6 or 7 indicates an 8% chance of stroke in the next 2 days. There is controversy, but any patient with a score of 4 or higher should be admitted for observation and urgent TIA workup. Other patients can be worked up on an outpatient basis if they have an expedient neurologic evaluation (including MRI, TTE, carotid ultrasound, and fasting lipid panel).

Diagnosis: TIA

CASE 25

HPI: A 42-year-old man attends his primary care physician because of dizziness. He says that this morning he rolled over in bed and all of a sudden "the whole room was spinning" and he vomited once. The entire episode was severe and lasted for about 5 seconds before resolving. Since then, whenever he turns to the right the symptoms are reproduced and he feels nauseated. Symptoms never last for more than 30 seconds, and when he continues to turn right, the symptoms get less and less severe each time. He denies any trauma, numbness, weakness, changes in hearing, recent or current illness, or other symptoms. As long as he sits still, he says he feels fine.

Vital signs: Temperature 98.2° F (36.8° C), pulse 76 beats/min, BP 126/68 mm Hg, RR 16 breaths/min.

Additional history: No medical history. Has smoked 1 pack of cigarettes per day for 10 years, occasional alcohol consumption, no drug use. No surgeries or allergies.

1. **What is the differential diagnosis?**
   Vertigo, either central or peripheral (but most likely peripheral).
   • Central vertigo: Cerebellar or brainstem infarction or bleeding, tumors such as acoustic neuroma, demyelinating disease such as MS.
   • Peripheral vertigo: Benign positional paroxysmal vertigo (BPPV), labyrinthitis, vestibular neuronitis, Ménière disease, perilymphatic fistula, herpes zoster oticus, otosclerosis, cholesteatoma.

2. **What components of the physical examination do you perform?**
   General appearance, HEENT/neck, lungs, cardiovascular, neuro/psych.
   Physical examination:
   General: Well-developed, well-appearing male in no distress when sitting still, but severe distress when moving head to the right.
   HEENT/neck: Neck with full range of motion, no carotid bruit, bilateral ear canals and tympanic membranes normal.
   Cardiovascular: WNL
   Lungs: WNL
   Neuro/psych: Cranial nerves II through XII intact, strength 5/5 in bilateral upper and lower extremities, reflexes 2+ throughout, normal sensation throughout, PERRLA without nystagmus. When the patient is rapidly laid down with his head tilted 45 degrees to the right, he develops nystagmus and his symptoms are reproduced.

3. What are your initial orders?
   Epley maneuver, fingerstick glucose.
   Advance clock:
   Fingerstick glucose 105 mg/dL.
   Epley maneuver performed; patient states he no longer has symptoms.

4. What are your follow-up actions?
   Disease counseling, meclizine prescription, follow up after 1 week.
   Advance clock:
   Patient states that he had occasional episodes of symptoms soon after the visit but they have since resolved.
   Case ends.
   Critical actions:
   Recognition of vertigo, consideration of central versus peripheral causes.
   Discussion:
   This patient has vertigo, a perception of abnormal movement (usually a sensation that the room is spinning). Any patient who complains of dizziness must further describe what they mean, because "dizziness" can mean lightheadedness (presyncope), imbalance (ataxia), or vertigo. For a patient with vertiginous symptoms, it should be determined whether the vertigo is likely to be central or peripheral.

   Causes of central vertigo include lesions in the brainstem or cerebellum (e.g., infarction, bleeding, tumors [e.g., vestibular schwannoma, also known as an acoustic neuroma], demyelination [e.g., MS], or toxins) and are typically more serious. Peripheral vertigo can be caused by lesions in the inner ear or vestibular system, including BPPV (caused by otolith displacement from the normal position in the utricle into one of the semicircular canals), labyrinthitis (inflammation of the vestibular organs, usually due to a virus), and vestibular neuronitis (inflammation of the vestibular nerve, also usually caused by a virus) or Ménière disease (increased volume of endolymph in semicircular canals, characterized by vertigo, hearing loss, feeling of ear fullness, and tinnitus). There are also rarer causes of peripheral vertigo such as perilymphatic fistulas, herpes zoster oticus (Ramsay Hunt syndrome), otosclerosis, and cholesteatomas, which are not covered here.

   The general characteristics that can help in differentiating central from peripheral vertigo are listed in Table 16-2.

   In this case, the patient has symptoms and an examination consistent with peripheral vertigo, specifically BPPV, and has a positive Dix-Hallpike test. The otoliths can be repositioned using the Epley maneuver, but medications often have to be prescribed to ameliorate symptoms until recovery (1 to 2 weeks). First-line treatment is with an anticholinergic medication such as meclizine or scopolamine, with possible addition of a benzodiazepine such as diazepam if needed. Antiemetic agents can also be added for symptom control. In general, patients with peripheral vertigo can be discharged home. Patients with central vertigo will need urgent imaging (CT or MRI scan), a neurologic consult, and admission to the hospital.

   Diagnosis: Vertigo due to BPPV

Table 16-2. Differentiation of Central Vertigo from Peripheral Vertigo

	PERIPHERAL	CENTRAL
Onset	Sudden	Sudden or slow
Severity	Intense	Less intense, ill defined
Pattern	Paroxysmal, intermittent	Persistent
Worse with motion	Yes	Sometimes
Nausea	Often	Rarer
Fatigue of symptoms on movement	Yes	No
Other neurologic findings	No	Often

CASE 26

HPI: An 8-year-old boy attends his pediatrician because his mother thinks his urine "has looked funny" for the past 2 days. The boy says he feels tired all the time since the condition started and thinks his body "seems puffy" as well. He has never had similar symptoms before and otherwise feels okay. His mother accompanies him on the visit and is concerned that this is some type of reaction to the antibiotic he received 2 weeks ago for a sore throat (finished a 10-day course a few days ago). The patient denies any joint pain, rashes, nausea, vomiting, dysuria, or shortness of breath.

Vital signs: Temperature 98.2° F (36.8° C), pulse 80 beats/min, BP 130/90 mm Hg, RR 16 breaths/ min.

Additional history: Culture-positive group A streptococcal pharyngitis 2 weeks ago, treated with penicillin twice daily for 10 days. No other medical history. No other medications or allergies.

1. **What is the differential diagnosis?**
   Glomerular disease, probably nephritic syndrome: PSGN, rapidly progressive glomerulone-phritis, immunoglobulin A (IgA) nephropathy (Berger disease), HUS, lupus nephritis.
   Nonglomerular hematuria: interstitial cystitis, UTI.

2. **What components of the physical examination do you perform?**
   General appearance, cardiovascular, lungs, abdomen.
   Physical examination:
   General: Well-developed, well-nourished boy in no apparent distress. Mildly edematous,
     especially in the periorbital area.
   Cardiovascular: WNL
   Lungs: WNL
   Abdomen: Mild tenderness over bilateral flanks.

3. **What are your initial orders?**
   CBC, chem 8, coagulation profile, urinalysis (with microscopy).
   Advance clock:
   CBC, chem 8, coagulation profile all WNL.
   Urinalysis demonstrates a high level of blood with numerous RBC casts, moderate protein;
   otherwise WNL.

4. **What are your follow-up actions?**
   Antistreptolysin O (ASO) titer, anti-DNAse B titer, serum C3 and C4 levels, nephrology consult. Follow-up appointment for rechecking of laboratory tests. Counseling.
   Advance clock:
   ASO and anti-DNAse B titers strongly positive. Serum C3 and C4 undetectable.
   Nephrology has no recommendations at this time; supportive care only.
   Patient follow-up in 3 days and repeat laboratory tests are all WNL, hematuria is decreasing,
   patient states that he feels better.
   Case ends.
   Critical actions:
   Recognition of nephritic syndrome, consideration of PSGN as the likely cause,
   supportive care.
   Discussion:
   This patient has PSGN, an immunologic response after an infection with group A beta-hemolytic streptococcal (GAS) infection. In children and young adults, PSGN can follow either a skin infection (e.g., impetigo) or an infection of the pharynx (e.g., streptococcal pharyngitis, strep throat). Young children (under 7) are most commonly affected. Unfortunately, treatment of the initial infection with antibiotics does not prevent this immunologic complication. There are other forms of postinfectious glomerulonephritis; IgA nephropathy (Berger disease) classically occurs after a viral infection of the upper respiratory tract. IgA nephropathy has a faster onset (1 to 2 days, often called *synpharyngitic* because the nephropa-thy occurs with the infection) than PSGN (weeks). PSGN is a nephritic syndrome and therefore there will be RBC casts in the urine and some proteinuria.
   Diagnosis of PSGN is on the basis of a history suggestive of recent infection (as well as lab-oratory testing to confirm recent GAS infection with ASO and anti-DNAse B titers) and evi-dence of a nephritic syndrome. Urine microscopy will demonstrate RBC casts and moderate

proteinuria. If complement levels (e.g., C3, C4) are ordered, they will be low, but these are not specific to PSGN. A renal biopsy is not required in stable patients for whom the diagnosis is clear, but patients who rapidly deteriorate or have an unclear diagnosis may require a biopsy to exclude other treatable causes. Treatment is primarily supportive, guided in conjunction with a nephrologist, and may include antihypertensive medication and/or diuresis. Any underlying infection should be treated (although antibiotics do not seem to prevent PSGN, patients with PSGN and an active GAS infection do better with early antibiotic treatment).

Diagnosis: PSGN

CASE 27

HPI: A 21-year-old man with known sickle cell disease attends the ED with severe aches and pains in his ribs and both legs. The pain started while he was playing soccer outside earlier today with friends. He describes the pain as an ache of 10/10 in intensity consistent with multiple prior exacerbations of his condition. He has these exacerbations approximately twice a year. He usually takes oral hydromorphone at home to help with mild to moderate pain, but he ran out of his home medication. He denies fevers or vomiting.

Vital signs: Temperature 97.7° F (36.5° C), pulse 112 beats/min, BP 122/84 mm Hg, RR 18 breaths/min.

Additional history: Takes hydroxyurea. No other medical history. No use of tobacco, alcohol, or drugs.

1. **What is the differential diagnosis?**
   Sickle cell pain crisis, acute chest syndrome, muscle strain.

2. **What components of the physical examination do you perform?**
   General appearance, HEENT, cardiovascular, lungs, abdomen, extremities.
   Physical examination:
   General: Moderate distress secondary to pain.
   HEENT: Dry mucous membranes, conjunctival pallor, mild scleral icterus.
   Cardiovascular: Tachycardic.
   Lungs: WNL
   Abdomen: WNL
   Extremities: WNL

3. **What are your initial orders?**
   Pulse oximetry, normal saline IV, analgesia (hydromorphone) IV, CBC, CXR, reticulocyte count.
   Advance clock:
   The patient's pain is well controlled, heart rate normalizes. O_2 saturation 100% on room air. Hb 9 g/dL; other studies WNL.

4. **What are your follow-up actions?**
   Discharge home with hydromorphone PO and follow up after 1 week. Counseling.
   Advance clock:
   Case ends.
   Critical actions:
   Recognition of sickle cell pain crisis, aggressive analgesia, consideration of other complications of sickle cell disease.
   Discussion:
   Sickle cell anemia is a genetic condition caused by homozygosity for the atypical Hb molecule HbS. This form of Hb is prone to polymerization under conditions of stress and causes erythrocytes to form a sickle shape that can lead to vasoocclusive events. Acute painful episodes are the most common manifestation of vasoocclusive events. They may be triggered by exertion, hypoxia, or dehydration, but often there is no recognizable underlying trigger. The mainstay of management for acute painful episodes is aggressive analgesia, often requiring IV opioids. Correction of reversible causes should be addressed. This patient appears dehydrated after playing soccer and will benefit from hydration. Correction of hypoxia, when present, is also warranted. It is also important to consider other sickle cell crises. Patients with chest pain, cough, or fever should be evaluated for acute chest syndrome using CXR. The presence of acute chest

syndrome warrants hospital admission and antibiotics (because it cannot be clinically distinguished from pneumonia). Patients with neurologic symptoms should be evaluated for stroke. Hb measurement can help in screening for hemolytic and aplastic crises when compared to baseline data. Hydroxyurea increases the presence of HbF in the circulation, which decreases the frequency of vasoocclusive events and the need for transfusions but is not helpful in the acute setting. Hydroxyurea is indicated for patients with more than two vasoocclusive events per year and those with other severe complications (e.g., acute chest syndrome).

Diagnosis: Sickle cell pain crisis

CASE 28

HPI: A 40-year-old woman with a history of hypertension complains of chronic fatigue that started months ago and has not abated. She admits not sleeping well and not being able to stay focused on her job because of her fatigue. She also states she has gained 20 lb during this time and complains of dry scaly skin. She feels that she is losing more hair than normal but attributes this to the stress of her inability to sleep.

Vital signs: Temperature 98.2° F (36.8° C), pulse 60 beats/min, BP 110/78 mm Hg, RR 16 breaths/min.

Additional history: Takes amlodipine for hypertension. Denies suicidal ideations, homicidal ideations, or auditory or visual hallucinations.

1. **What is the differential diagnosis?**
   Hypothyroidism (caused by Hashimoto thyroiditis, iodine deficiency, de Quervain thyroiditis, Reidel thyroiditis), chronic fatigue syndrome, depression, anemia.

2. **What components of the physical examination do you perform?**
   General appearance, HEENT, cardiovascular, lungs, abdomen, neuro/psych.
   Physical examination:
   General: Well-developed woman, no pallor, no apparent distress.
   HEENT: Slightly enlarged thyroid, nontender, no nodules.
   Cardiovascular: WNL except for bilateral nonpitting edema of the extremities.
   Lungs: WNL
   Abdomen: WNL
   Neuro/psych: Normal strength and sensation; reflexes abnormal because of prolonged relaxation phase.

3. **What are your initial orders?**
   CBC, chem 8, thyroid-stimulating hormone (TSH) (free T_4, T_3, can order once TSH result comes back).
   Advance clock:
   CBC and chem 8 WNL, no anemia. TSH markedly elevated and free T_4 nearly undetectable.

4. **What are your follow-up actions?**
   Levothyroxine PO, follow-up appointment.
   Advance clock:
   Patient's symptoms significantly improved, feels much better.
   Case ends.
   Critical actions:
   Recognition of hypothyroidism and differential diagnosis that includes depression and anemia. Appropriate workup and treatment.
   Discussion:
   This patient has hypothyroidism, which is underproduction of thyroid hormone. The most common cause is Hashimoto thyroiditis, an autoimmune disease affecting the thyroid gland. Unlike Graves disease, in which autoantibodies stimulate the TSH receptor, in Hashimoto thyroiditis, antibodies block the TSH receptor and thyroid peroxidase (TPO) and elicit T-cell attack of the thyroid gland. Other causes of hypothyroidism include iodine deficiency (incredibly rare in industrialized countries), thyroiditis syndromes, hypothalamic/pituitary causes, and drug-related causes, but all of these are much rarer than Hashimoto thyroiditis.
   Symptoms of hypothyroidism are consistent with generalized slowing of the metabolism (because thyroid hormone is the main metabolic regulator). These symptoms include dry,

rough skin; brittle nails; myxedema because of decreased turnover of glycosaminoglycans; cold intolerance because of a decrease in body heat production; fatigue; constipation; and weight gain. Patients can also experience myopathy characterized by proximal muscle weakness, myalgias, elevated creatine kinase (CK) levels, and stiffness; a decreased relaxation phase may also be apparent during reflex responses.

Diagnosis is via laboratory testing, which reveals elevated TSH and depressed free T_4. Treatment is with levothyroxine (synthetic T_4). Myxedema coma is a life-threatening complication of untreated hypothyroidism for which the symptoms are hypothermia, altered mental status, and hypotension; it is treated with high-dose thyroid hormone.

Diagnosis: Hypothyroidism

CASE 29

HPI: A 40-year-old man attends his primary care physician complaining of progressive weakness in his legs and arms for the past year. He denies any changes in sensation. His weakness has worsened to the point that he cannot perform his normal daily activities and can no longer work. His symptoms are similar all day and do not seem to get better or worse with continued use of his muscles. He has also noticed that his tongue wiggles continuously.

Vital signs: Temperature 98.6° F (37° C), pulse 80 beats/min, BP 118/60 mm Hg, RR 16 breaths/min.

Additional history: None. Previously healthy, no medications. Works as a day laborer, denies exposure to any chemicals.

1. **What is the differential diagnosis?**
   Amyotrophic lateral sclerosis (ALS; Lou Gehrig disease), tick paralysis, MS, spinal muscular atrophy, myasthenia gravis (MG), Lambert-Eaton myasthenic syndrome.

2. **What components of the physical examination do you perform?**
   General appearance, lungs, neuro/psych.
   Physical examination:
   General: Comfortable, speaking in full sentences.
   Lungs: Slightly shallow breaths; no cyanosis, wheezes, crackles, or rhonchi.
   Neuro/psych: Diffuse atrophy of all muscle groups, visible fasciculations of the tongue and the thigh and arm. Normal sensation to light tough, pinprick, and vibration. Hyperreflexia of the upper extremities and hyporeflexia of the lower extremities. Abnormal Babinski sign on the right foot but normal on the left. Cranial nerves intact.

3. **What are your initial orders?**
   Neurology consult, pulmonary function tests, admit to a monitored bed, electromyography (EMG)/nerve condition studies (optional), MRI scan of the brain/spinal cord (optional).
   Advance clock:
   EMG/nerve conduction studies show evidence of both upper and lower motor neuron disease.
   Pulmonary function tests show low risk of respiratory compromise.
   If an MRI scan of the brain and spinal cord is ordered, the results are normal.

4. **What are your follow-up actions?**
   Start riluzole therapy, counsel the patient on the disease, physical therapy.
   Advance clock:
   Case ends.
   Critical actions:
   Recognition of both upper and lower motor neuron disease as characteristics of ALS, prompt neurology consult, pulmonary function tests to ensure the patient is not at risk of respiratory compromise.
   Discussion:
   This patient has ALS, a progressive, incurable, and ultimately fatal disease affecting both upper and lower motor neurons in the brain, brainstem, and spinal cord. Although some cases of ALS are genetic (associated with superoxide dismutase mutations), most are sporadic and onset typically occurs between the ages of 40 and 70 years. Other motor neuron diseases and autoimmune diseases are initially in the differential diagnosis. Patients with spinal muscular atrophy should have only lower motor neuron signs; patients with MS would not have a normal MRI

scan and would be unlikely to have such an abrupt and diffuse onset; those with MG should have symptoms that worsen on repeated muscle use; and those with Lambert-Eaton myasthenic syndrome should have symptoms that improve on repeated muscle use.

Treatment of ALS is mostly supportive, aided by physical, occupational, and speech therapy. There is one medication approved for use, riluzole, which lengthens survival by slowing disease progression, but the survival benefit is measured in months, not years. Patients will eventually need to decide if they want more aggressive measures, such as a feeding tube and ventilator, as their disease progresses further.

Diagnosis: ALS

CASE 30

HPI: A 28-year-old woman attends the outpatient clinic complaining of increased fatigue and occasional blurry vision. She states that she works as a receptionist and for the past 2 months has noticed that by the end of the day she is extremely tired and "can barely keep her eyes open" and the screen becomes more blurry. If she takes a break she can go back to work, but the symptoms then start again. She states she is getting enough sleep, does not use caffeine or drink alcohol, and overall feels well other than this complaint. She says her diet is good but she has moved to eating softer foods recently because she is so tired that even chewing can be difficult. She denies any history of similar symptoms and any numbness or tingling.

Vital signs: Temperature 98.2° F (36.8° C), pulse 76 beats/min, BP 120/70 mm Hg, RR 16 breaths/min.

Additional history: No medical history, no medications, no allergies.

1. **What is the differential diagnosis?**
   Myasthenia gravis (MG), botulism, Lambert-Eaton myasthenic syndrome, cholinergic crisis/ toxicity, depression.

2. **What components of the physical examination do you perform?**
   General appearance, lungs, cardiovascular, neuro/psych.
   Physical examination:
   General: Well-developed, well-nourished woman in no apparent distress.
   Cardiovascular: WNL
   Lungs: WNL
   Neuro/psych: Strength initially 5/5 but on repetitive testing becomes weaker and weaker to 3/5. PERRLA, extraocular movements intact, but during a sustained gaze to one side the patient develops diplopia in about 30 seconds. Sensation intact, reflexes 2+ throughout, cranial nerves II through XII intact but motor cranial nerves fatigue on test repetition.

3. **What are your initial orders?**
   EMG; can also consider Tensilon (edrophonium) test.
   Advance clock:
   EMG demonstrates decreasing amplitude of muscle contraction on repetitive muscle stimulation, relieved by rest.
   Tensilon (edrophonium) test performed; when edrophonium is injected the patient shows a marked improvement in symptoms.

4. **What are your follow-up actions?**
   Rheumatology consult, start acetylcholine esterase inhibitor (e.g., pyridostigmine) treatment, counseling on the disease process. Follow-up appointment.
   Advance clock:
   Patient states she has good symptom control with the new medication.
   Case ends.
   Critical actions:
   Recognition of the classic presentation of MG, ordering basic diagnostic tests (mostly a clinical diagnosis), starting medication for symptom control.
   Discussion:
   This patient has MG, an autoimmune disorder in which autoantibodies attack and block acetylcholine receptors at the neuromuscular junction. This leads to generalized muscle weakness, including the eye muscles (diplopia, ptosis), that is worse on repetitive movement.

This worsening on repetitive movement is unlike Lambert-Eaton myasthenic syndrome (anti–calcium channel antibodies), which gets *better* on repetitive movement because of an increase in calcium release with each movement. Myasthenic crisis is a potentially life-threatening condition in which there is an acute increase in weakness; if the weakness involves the respiratory muscles, respiratory failure can occur.

Diagnosis of MG is on the basis of history and physical examination but can be supported by laboratory testing (such as acetylcholine receptor autoantibody screens [AChR-Ab] and antibodies against muscle-specific receptor tyrosine kinase [anti-MuSK]), EMG showing decreased amplitude of contraction with repetitive stimulation, and the rarely used Tensilon (edrophonium) test, in which improvement after administration of an acetylcholine esterase inhibitor is diagnostic of MG. All patients with MG should be investigated for the presence of a thymoma; thymomas are common in MG and improvements in symptoms can occur if the thymoma is removed.

Treatment involves three different approaches: (1) symptom control, (2) immunosuppression, and (3) surgical removal of any thymoma. Symptom control with pyridostigmine is common; by increasing the amount of acetylcholine in the neuromuscular junction, patients will have increased strength. Immunosuppression with prednisone or other immunosuppressants helps to decrease autoantibody production. Lastly, thymectomy should be considered.

A myasthenic crisis can be treated with plasmapheresis to remove autoantibodies from the blood or with IVIG. In myasthenic crisis, the patient's respiratory status must be closely monitored (e.g., forced vital capacity and/or negative inspiratory force) to watch for any deterioration.

Diagnosis: MG

CASE 31

HPI: An 18-month-old boy is brought to the ED because of "high-pitched sounds" on breathing in for the past 2 hours. His parents state that the patient has had a fever, runny nose, and cough for 2 days. The parents deny any possibility of foreign body ingestion.

Vital signs: Temperature 101.5° F (38.6° C), pulse 130 beats/min, BP 96/60 mm Hg, RR 40 breaths/min.

Additional history: Ex-full term, no complications, no hospitalizations, no medical history, medications, or allergies. Vaccinations are up to date.

1. **What is the differential diagnosis?**
   Stridor due to laryngotracheobronchitis (croup), foreign body, epiglottitis, bacterial tracheitis, laryngomalacia, subglottic stenosis, or retropharyngeal abscess.

2. **What components of the physical examination do you perform?**
   General appearance, HEENT, cardiovascular, lungs.
   Physical examination:
      General: Well-developed, well-nourished infant in moderate respiratory distress. A barking cough is present.
      HEENT: No foreign body visualized on inspection of the oropharynx. Clear rhinorrhea. Moist mucous membranes.
      Cardiovascular: Tachycardic, regular.
      Lungs: Tachypneic. Diffuse symmetric inspiratory stridor at rest with some expiratory wheezes. Using subcostal and intercostal accessory muscles.

3. **What are your initial orders?**
   Racemic epinephrine via nebulizer, dexamethasone. Antipyretics. CXR optional. Cool mist optional.
   Advance clock:
   After administration of racemic epinephrine and dexamethasone, the patient no longer exhibits stridor and is breathing comfortably without accessory muscle use. If a CXR is ordered, it will show a steeple sign in the upper airway.

4. **What are your follow-up actions?**
   Observe for 4 hours; if stridor returns before then, admit to the hospital; if not, discharge with return precautions.

Advance clock:
Case ends.
Critical actions:
Recognition of croup as a common cause of stridor, administration of racemic epinephrine and dexamethasone, observation for an appropriate amount of time before disposition.
Discussion:
This patient has laryngotracheobronchitis (croup) caused by parainfluenza virus or other viruses. Croup typically occurs between 6 months and 3 years of age and causes (as the name implies) predominantly upper airway obstruction that leads to stridor. The classic cough associated with croup resembles a seal barking. Croup lasts for 3 to 5 days but the second or third night is when the most intense symptoms typically occur, as in this case. There is another condition called spasmodic croup that is noninfectious and affects those with a history of upper airway disease and/or reactive airway disease.

Diagnosis of croup is primarily on a clinical basis. Foreign body aspiration must be ruled out because a foreign body in the upper airway can cause stridor. In this case, the viral symptoms, barking cough, and lack of aspiration history make this situation less likely. Epiglottitis is a particularly dangerous cause of stridor, as is bacterial tracheitis; patients with these conditions typically appear much more ill. Findings on CXR in epiglottitis typically include the thumbprint sign, whereby the enlarged epiglottis looks like a thumb-sized mark on the lateral view.

Management of croup of any severity includes dexamethasone administration to decrease airway inflammation. Severe croup, in which patients have stridor at rest, should be treated with racemic epinephrine via a nebulizer, which decreases swelling and inflammation with effects lasting approximately 2 hours. This is why patients must be observed for 4 hours, even if they appear well immediately after treatment, to watch for the return of symptoms after the epinephrine wears off (dexamethasone takes hours to have an effect but is long lasting). Cool mist has been used in croup for decades, but there is no evidence that it provides benefit; however, there is little harm in cool mist administration, so this strategy is optional.

Diagnosis: Croup

CASE 32

HPI: A 60-year-old man with a history of small cell lung cancer complains of headache, nausea, weakness, generalized fatigue, and muscle cramps for the past 3 days. He states that the symptoms all occurred progressively and there was no inducing event. He denies any vomiting, fever, chills, visual changes, or significant changes in weight.
Vital signs: Temperature 98.2° F (36.8° C), pulse 92 beats/min, BP 150/80 mm Hg, RR 16 breaths/min.
Additional history: Localized small cell lung cancer diagnosed 1 year ago without evidence of metastatic disease; 50 pack-year smoking history (quit after diagnosis). The patient denies alcohol or drug use. No recent chemotherapy or radiotherapy.

1. What is the differential diagnosis?
   Metastases to brain, paraneoplastic syndrome such as syndrome of inappropriate antidiuretic hormone (SIADH) causing hyponatremia, malnutrition from cachexia, other electrolyte imbalances, hyperglcemia or hypoglycemia, chemotherapy side effects, tumor lysis syndrome.

2. What components of the physical examination do you perform?
   General appearance, cardiovascular, lungs, neuro/psych.
   Physical examination:
   General: Mildly cachectic male, sleeping but can be aroused and converses appropriately.
   Cardiovascular: WNL, no jugular venous distention (JVD), no pitting edema.
   Lungs: Dullness on percussion and decreased breath sounds in the right upper lobe.
   Neuro/psych: Strength 4/5 diffusely, sensation intact, gait normal, cranial nerves II through XII intact, no papilledema, visual fields full, PERRLA, reflexes normal.

3. What are your initial orders?
   Noncontrast head CT scan, fingerstick blood glucose, oxygen saturation, CBC, chem 8.

Advance clock:
Head CT scan shows no evidence of bleeding, metastatic disease, or midline shift. Finger-stick blood glucose 115 mg/dL. Oxygen saturation 97% on room air. CBC WNL. Chem 8 significant for sodium 120 mEq/L, all other electrolytes WNL. If a uric acid level is ordered to evaluate for tumor lysis syndrome, it is normal.

4. **What are your follow-up actions?**

Serum osmolality (will be low), urine osmolality (will be inappropriately high), urine electrolytes (urine sodium will be high), admit to a ward bed, fluid restriction, start IV saline with correction no faster than 0.5 mEq/L, serial sodium checks.

Advance clock:
Case ends.

Critical actions:
Checking glucose and oxygen saturation for altered patient, head CT scan in a patient with headache and malignancy, recognition of SIADH as a common paraneoplastic syndrome for small cell lung cancer, admission and appropriate treatment of hyponatremia.

Discussion:
This patient has hyponatremia, which is a sodium level of less than 135 mEq/L. However, the sodium value should first be corrected for hyperglycemia, if present. This is because glucose is an osmotic agent that draws water into the vasculature, causing relative dilution of sodium. Therefore, for each 100 mg/dL by which the glucose level exceeds 100 mg/dL, 1.6 mEq/L must be added to the sodium value; for instance, if the glucose level is 500 mg/dL (400 mg/dL higher than normal), the sodium value should be increased by 1.6 mEq/L × 4 = 6.4 mEq/L.

There are many causes of hyponatremia; the condition is usually classified as hypovolemic, euvolemic, or hypervolemic hyponatremia, each with different causes. Hypovolemic hyponatremia is usually due to extrarenal fluid losses via diarrhea, third spacing of fluids, poor intake, and increased insensible losses. Hypovolemic hyponatremia can also be due to renal losses caused by diuretic usage, cerebral salt wasting, and mineralocorticoid deficiency. Euvolemic hyponatremia (what this patient has) is typically due to SIADH but in rare cases can be due to primary polydipsia, in which the patient drinks gallons of water a day. Hypervolemic hyponatremia can be caused by hypervolemic states such as CHF, cirrhosis, nephrotic syndrome, and renal failure.

The first step in the workup is measurement of plasma and urine osmolality and assessment of volume status during a physical examination. This patient is euvolemic and has low plasma osmolality but high urine osmolality. The body should completely shut off ADH production to dilute the urine as much as possible to correct low plasma osmolality. In this case, the kidneys are inappropriately concentrating the urine, exacerbating the problem. This is known as SIADH. This patient has a history of small cell lung cancer, which can secrete ADH. Treatment involves fluid restriction and slow correction of the sodium level to normal using saline, salt tablets, or a vasopressin antagonist (e.g., vaptan drugs such as conivaptan and tolvaptan). Rapid correction can lead to central pontine myelinolysis, an irreversible and potentially fatal condition.

Diagnosis: Hyponatremia

CASE 33

HPI: A 23-year-old woman attends your clinic because of jitteriness and weight loss. She states that she feels her heart racing intermittently and she sweats easily; she wears much less clothing than her friends for this reason. She has also lost 10 lb unintentionally in the past 3 months, although she states that her appetite has decreased. She denies any caffeine or stimulant use, any history of similar symptoms, and any significant life stressors.

Vital signs: Temperature 98.2° F (36.8° C), pulse 90 beats/min, BP 120/70 mm Hg, RR 16 breaths/min.

Additional history: Works as a cashier. No medical history and no medications. No recent infections.

1. **What is the differential diagnosis?**

Hyperthyroidism (Graves disease, toxic multinodular goiter, toxic adenoma, de Quervain thyroiditis, Hashitoxicosis, exogenous thyroid hormone use), anxiety disorder, panic disorder, pheochromocytoma, stimulant abuse.

2. **What components of the physical examination do you perform?**
   General appearance, HEENT, cardiovascular, lungs.
   Physical examination:
   General: Well-developed woman in no apparent distress.
   HEENT: Mild goiter noted, palpation of the thyroid gland reveals no tenderness and no discrete nodules. Lid lag is noted.
   Cardiovascular: Rate 96 beats/min and regular, holosystolic murmur throughout the precordium.
   Lungs: WNL

3. **What are your initial orders?**
   ECG, TSH (optional free T_4 and T_3, but should be ordered if TSH is abnormal if not ordered now).
   Advance clock:
   ECG shows normal sinus rhythm, rate 96 beats/min. TSH undetectable, free T_4 and T_3 elevated. (If TSH were normal, consider urine metanephrines for pheochromocytoma and a urine toxicology screen for evidence of stimulant abuse.)

4. **What are your follow-up actions?**
   Counsel the patient on disease, propranolol for symptomatic relief, methimazole or propylthiouracil to decrease thyroid hormone production, appointment to reassess symptoms. Consider measurement of anti-TPO antibodies, ordering a thyroid uptake scan, or endocrinology referral for radioactive iodine ablation.
   Advance clock:
   Case ends.
   Critical actions:
   Recognition of the symptoms of hyperthyroidism, appropriate diagnostic testing (e.g., at least TSH), treatment (symptom control with propranolol, blockade of thyroid hormone production with propylthiouracil or methimazole).
   Discussion:
   This patient has hyperthyroidism, characterized by increased thyroid hormone levels in the setting of decreased TSH levels. Graves disease is the most common cause of hyperthyroidism in children and young adults; it is an autoimmune disease characterized by stimulatory antibodies that bind to TSH receptors, causing increased thyroid hormone production. Toxic multinodular goiter (TMG) is the most common cause of hyperthyroidism in older individuals. Graves disease stimulates fibroblasts and causes lymphocytic infiltration in the periorbital space, so patients can have exophthalmos, a finding specific to this disease. The most common cause of hypothyroidism is Hashimoto thyroiditis (also an autoimmune disease), and early in its course, inflammation in the thyroid can cause thyroid hormone to leak out, leading to transient hyperthyroidism (Hashitoxicosis). Painful (and rarer) causes of hyperthyroidism include de Quervain thyroiditis (a postviral thyroiditis) and postpartum thyroiditis.
   Diagnosis of hyperthyroidism is on the basis of increased T_3 or free T_4 levels (not total T_4) and decreased TSH. If the cause of the hyperthyroidism is in question, a radioiodine uptake scan can be performed. In Graves disease, diffuse overproduction of thyroid hormone leads to diffuse radioiodine uptake. In TMG, there are multiple nodules of uptake. In exogenous thyroid ingestion and thyroiditis, there is little uptake because the thyroid gland is not stimulated to produce thyroid hormone. Treatment is aimed at reducing symptoms from high sympathetic tone (e.g., a nonselective beta-blocker such as propranolol), reducing TPO enzyme activity to decrease hormone production (with methimazole or propylthiouracil), and possibly administering radioactive iodine to ablate the thyroid gland and destroy it permanently.
   Diagnosis: Hyperthyroidism

CASE 34

HPI: A 5-year-old girl is brought to the pediatrician by her father. Her parents have noticed that her gums have been bleeding a small amount when they brush her teeth. They have also noticed that small purple dots have appeared on her ankles. She has been acting normally and does not appear to be bothered by the skin changes. She has always been a healthy child although she occasionally suffers from viral respiratory infections. She had symptoms of an upper respiratory tract infection approximately 2 weeks ago.

Vital signs: Temperature 98.2° F (36.8° C), pulse 80 beats/min, BP 100/70 mm Hg, RR 20 breaths/min.

Additional history: No other medical history. Vaccinations up to date.

1. **What is the differential diagnosis?**
   Immune/idiopathic thrombocytopenic purpura (ITP), HUS, TTP, drug-induced thrombocytopenia, leukemia.

2. **What components of the physical examination do you perform?**
   General appearance, HEENT, skin/lymph nodes, cardiovascular, lungs, abdomen, neuro/psych.
   Physical examination:
   General: No acute distress.
   HEENT: WNL
   Skin/lymph nodes: Scattered bilateral petechiae over the lower extremities, no lymphadenopathy.
   Cardiovascular: WNL
   Lungs: WNL
   Abdomen: WNL, no splenomegaly.
   Neuro/psych: WNL

3. **What are your initial orders?**
   CBC, peripheral smear, chem 14, PT/PTT.
   Advance clock:
   Platelets 28,000 cells/mL, other studies WNL

4. **What are your follow-up orders?**
   Prednisolone PO, repeat CBC in 5 days, follow up in 5 days and 2 weeks.
   Advance clock:
   After 2 weeks the patient's platelet count has normalized and her symptoms have resolved.
   Critical actions:
   Skin examination, lymph node examination, abdominal examination, CBC, peripheral smear, consideration of steroid therapy.
   Discussion:
   ITP is a condition characterized by platelet counts of less than 100,000 cells/mL and symptoms of thrombocytopenia (petechiae, bruising, bleeding). The condition can range from mild asymptomatic thrombocytopenia to severe life-threatening hemorrhage, including intracranial hemorrhage. In children, ITP is most common between the ages of 2 and 5 years. It tends to be acute in onset and resolves spontaneously or with steroid administration. ITP is often preceded by a viral infection during the previous month. In adults, ITP tends to be more indolent. It occurs over a long period of time and is more refractory to treatment. A careful history and physical examination can reveal suspicion of thrombocytopenia, and a CBC can quickly provide a platelet count. Once a diagnosis of thrombocytopenia is established, other causes should be evaluated. A normal peripheral smear helps to rule out TTP. In patients at risk, infectious causes should be evaluated, including HIV and *Helicobacter pylori*. The size of the spleen should be evaluated using at least a physical examination, and any suspicion of splenomegaly warrants advanced imaging. Any precipitating agents should be stopped if possible; common offenders are antihistamines, proton pump inhibitors, and sulfa drugs. Children with mild manifestations can usually be monitored as outpatients and do not need treatment. Moderate cases can be treated with steroids alone. Severe cases require steroids, IVIG, platelet transfusion, and a hematology consult. Refractory cases may benefit from splenectomy. A bone marrow biopsy is indicated in patients who are refractory to treatment and those in whom malignancy is a possibility (e.g., lymphadenopathy, weight loss, atypical cells on smear).
   Diagnosis: ITP

CASE 35

HPI: A 9-year-old girl is brought to an urgent care clinic because of redness and swelling around her right eye for the past day that is worsening. There is no discharge from the eye according to her mother, and she states that the child is using her eye normally otherwise. The patient states that she has 6/10 pain over the skin around the eye but no pain in the eye itself. She recently had sinusitis, which has since resolved. The patient denies neck stiffness, pain on eye movements, and visual changes.

Vital signs: Temperature 98.2° F (36.8° C), pulse 80 beats/min, BP 110/60 mm Hg, RR 16 breaths/min.

Additional history: Immunizations up to date.

1. **What is the differential diagnosis?**
    Periorbital (preseptal) cellulitis, orbital cellulitis, conjunctivitis, dacryoadenitis, dacryocystitis, hordeolum, chalazion.

2. **What components of the physical examination do you perform?**
    General appearance, HEENT.
    Physical examination:
    General: Well-developed, well-nourished girl in no apparent distress.
    HEENT: Right eye has significant periorbital swelling, warmth, and erythema encircling the skin around the entire eye and upper and lower eyelids. No conjunctival injection. No proptosis. PERRLA. Extraocular movements intact. Visual acuity 20/20 in both eyes.

3. **What are your initial orders?**
    Antibiotics (e.g., oral amoxicillin-clavulanate for 10 days), analgesia. Discharge home with follow-up appointment in 24 to 48 hours for recheck. Counseling on periorbital cellulitis.
    Advance clock:
    The patient has been taking antibiotics as prescribed and the erythema has significantly receded.

4. **What are your follow-up actions?**
    Follow-up appointment in 7 to 10 days to ensure complete resolution.
    Advance clock:
    Case ends.
    Critical actions:
    Recognition of periorbital cellulitis, consideration of other causes of redness around the eye, ruling out orbital cellulitis according to the history and physical examination.
    Discussion:
    This patient has periorbital (also known as preseptal) cellulitis, which is a bacterial cellulitis involving the area of the orbits and limited to tissues anterior to the orbital septum. Periorbital cellulitis is typically caused by spread from the paranasal sinuses and therefore infection is most commonly due to organisms involved in sinusitis (*Streptococcus* species, *H. influenzae*, anaerobes, and *S. aureus*). The infection causes warmth, swelling, and erythema of the eyelid and skin around the orbit. Periorbital cellulitis must be distinguished from the emergent condition orbital cellulitis. Orbital cellulitis has more severe symptoms and may involve proptosis, decreased or painful extraocular motility, ocular pain, and visual changes. Whereas periorbital cellulitis can often be treated with antibiotics (such as amoxicillin-clavulanate) on an outpatient basis with close follow-up, orbital cellulitis is an emergency and requires admission to the hospital for parenteral antibiotics and a CT scan of the orbits to rule out retroorbital air or abscess formation.
    There should always be close follow-up of patients with periorbital cellulitis because complications can occur. Periorbital cellulitis can progress to orbital cellulitis. The veins that drain the periorbital area lead into the cavernous sinus; the infection can predispose patients to cavernous sinus thrombosis. The close proximity of the paranasal sinuses to the CSF also means that meningitis is a possible complication. Patients with orbital cellulitis can have retroorbital involvement, including air or abscesses.
    Diagnosis: Periorbital cellulitis

CASE 36

HPI: A 38-year-old woman with recent diagnoses of hypertension and diabetes attends her primary care doctor for follow-up. She says that she had numerous symptoms in the time around her diagnoses, including fatigue, insomnia, and inability to concentrate. She also says she is embarrassed to say that she is gaining weight around her abdomen and is developing stretch marks and that she has recently had to shave her facial hair, although she has never had this problem before. She is concerned about these changes in her body because she was previously healthy, exercised frequently, and never had any complaints.

Vital signs: Temperature 98.2° F (36.8° C), pulse 90 beats/min, BP 160/90 mm Hg, RR 16 breaths/min.

Additional history: Diagnosed with hypertension and diabetes 2 months ago. Takes hydrochlorothiazide, amlodipine, metformin, and glipizide. No allergies. No surgeries. No use of alcohol, tobacco, or drugs. Not sexually active, menses previously regular every 4 weeks but currently irregular for the past 4 or 5 months.

1. **What is the differential diagnosis?**
   Hypercortisolism: excess exogenous glucocorticoid, ACTH-dependent endogenous glucocorticoid production (e.g., pituitary adenoma, ectopic ACTH production), ACTH-independent endogenous glucocorticoid production (e.g., adrenal tumor).
   Depression, polycystic ovarian syndrome, metabolic syndrome.

2. **What components of the physical examination do you perform?**
   General appearance, HEENT, cardiovascular, lungs, abdomen, extremities, neuro/psych.
   Physical examination:
   General: Overweight woman in no apparent distress.
   HEENT: Presence of a dorsocervical fat pad, moon facies, acne, mild hirsutism.
   Cardiovascular: WNL
   Lungs: WNL
   Abdomen: Centripetal obesity with purple-red striae.
   Extremities: Decreased muscle mass over extremities, peripheral edema 1+.
   Neuro/psych: 4/5 strength in proximal muscle groups diffusely, otherwise 5/5 strength.
   Neurologic signs otherwise WNL. Psychologic signs WNL.

3. **What are your initial orders?**
   CBC, chem 8, CK, urinalysis, urinary pregnancy test, hypercortisolism screening (24-hour urinary free cortisol or salivary cortisol or dexamethasone suppression test).
   Advance clock:
   CBC WNL. Chem 8 demonstrates blood glucose 240 mg/dL and potassium 3 mEq/L but otherwise WNL. CK WNL. Urinalysis WNL and urinary pregnancy test negative. Marked elevation of 24-hour urinary free cortisol. Salivary cortisol markedly elevated. Dexamethasone suppression test shows no suppression at a low dose but suppression at a high dose.

4. **What are your follow-up actions?**
   ACTH level.
   Advance clock:
   ACTH level markedly elevated.

5. **What are your follow-up actions?**
   Brain CT/MRI scan.
   Advance clock:
   CT or MRI scan of the brain shows a pituitary mass.

6. **What are your follow-up actions?**
   Neurosurgery consult, transsphenoidal surgery to remove the mass.
   Advance clock:
   The pituitary mass is removed. The patient sees you in 6 months and now has no symptoms.
   Case ends.
   Critical actions:
   Recognition of hypercortisolism as a likely cause of the patient's symptoms, testing for hypercortisolism, determination of the cause of the hypercortisolism, and initiation of appropriate treatment.
   Discussion:
   This patient has hypercortisolism (Cushing syndrome) caused by an ACTH-secreting pituitary adenoma (Cushing disease). Hypercortisolism can be caused by a number of factors,

ranging from exogenous intake of glucocorticoids (e.g., prolonged steroid use), excess stimulation of glucocorticoid release (e.g., pituitary tumor secreting ACTH, ectopic ACTH-secreting tumor, or corticotropin-releasing hormone [CRH]–producing tumor), or a tumor of the zona fasciculata of the adrenal glands that directly produces glucocorticoids. Knowledge of the physiology of glucocorticoid release will help in understanding the diagnosis and treatment. In brief, the hypothalamus secretes CRH, leading to ACTH release by the anterior pituitary gland. This ACTH then acts on the zona fasciculata of the adrenal gland to promote secretion of glucocorticoids, which then exert negative feedback on the hypothalamus and pituitary gland to decrease CRH and ACTH production, respectively. This ensures tight control of glucocorticoid production.

Diagnosis is on the basis of history and a physical examination showing classic central obesity, a buffalo hump (fat on the back of the neck), moon facies (rounded face), acne, hirsutism, and hemorrhagic purple-red striae. Basic laboratory tests may reveal hyperglycemia arising from the diabetogenic effect of glucocorticoids in increasing insulin resistance, and vital signs may demonstrate hypertension because glucocorticoids in high doses have mineralocorticoid-like effects (act like aldosterone). Diagnosis of hypercortisolism involves first determining that hypercortisolism exists, usually by measurement of urinary free cortisol or late-night salivary cortisol. A dexamethasone suppression test can be performed to assess if the hypercortisolism decreases when dexamethasone (a steroid) is administered; this should cause ACTH suppression via negative feedback. In the case of an ACTH-secreting pituitary tumor, high-dose dexamethasone will suppress production. However, if the ACTH is being secreted by another ectopic source (e.g., small cell carcinoma of the lung) or the tumor was not ACTH-dependent to begin with (e.g., tumor in the adrenal gland that directly secretes cortisol), no negative feedback will occur. An ACTH level can also help in differentiating between an adrenal tumor (low ACTH because of negative feedback) and an ACTH-dependent tumor. Treatment depends on the cause: if exogenous steroid use is the cause, tapering of the steroid regimen is warranted. If the cause is endogenous (e.g., a tumor), surgery is the therapy of choice.

Diagnosis: Hypercortisolism from Cushing disease

CASE 37

HPI: A 50-year-old woman attends the clinic because of heavy vaginal bleeding and fatigue. Until 1 year ago she had regular menses every month that lasted for 5 days with a normal flow. She now has irregular menses that last as long as 14 days. She has a very heavy flow and occasional passage of clots. Recently she has also been feeling fatigued. She has never lost consciousness, although at times she does have a vague dizzy sensation. She has no personal or family history of bleeding disorders.

Vital signs: Temperature 99.1° F (37.3° C), pulse 88 beats/min, BP 112/77 mm Hg, RR 18 breaths/min.

Additional history: No medical history. No use of drugs, tobacco, or alcohol.

1. What is the differential diagnosis?

   Vaginal bleeding due to dysfunctional uterine bleeding (DUB), fibroids, endometrial carcinoma, endometrial polyp, cervical lesion, bleeding disorder.

2. What components of the physical examination do you perform?

   General appearance, lymph nodes, HEENT, cardiovascular, lungs, abdomen, extremities, genitalia.

   Physical examination:
   General: No acute distress.
   Lymph nodes: WNL
   HEENT: Conjunctival pallor.
   Cardiovascular: WNL
   Lungs: WNL
   Abdomen: WNL
   Extremities: WNL
   Genitalia: Scant blood visualized in the vaginal vault. No cervical lesions.

3. **What are your initial orders?**
   CBC with differential, PT/PTT, TSH, pelvic ultrasound, Papanicolaou (Pap) smear, urinary pregnancy test, endometrial biopsy.
   Advance clock:
   CBC reveals Hb 10.1 mg/dL, MCV 69 fL. Other studies WNL.

4. **What are your follow-up actions?**
   Ferrous sulfate PO, medroxyprogesterone IM (Depo-Provera), follow up in 2 months.
   Advance clock:
   Case ends.
   Critical actions:
   Genitalia examination, CBC, Pap smear, endometrial biopsy, hormonal treatment of DUB.
   Discussion:
   This patient has heavy/irregular bleeding (menometrorrhagia). She is in the perimenopausal period, and in this setting DUB due to anovulatory cycles is the most common cause. Anovulatory DUB arises from the unopposed effect of estrogen on the endometrium. Without ovulation, the corpus luteum is not able to secrete progesterone to stabilize the endometrial lining. The lining thus builds up and sheds in an irregular pattern with a heavy flow. Although DUB is the most common cause of perimenopausal bleeding, DUB is a diagnosis of exclusion and other causes of vaginal bleeding should be investigated. A Pap smear can evaluate the cervical pathology and pelvic ultrasound can assess for structural problems such as uterine fibroids and endometrial polyps. Endometrial biopsy is indicated in women older than 35 years with abnormal vaginal bleeding to assess for endometrial carcinoma. For any patient with concerning bleeding, a CBC should be performed to assess Hb and platelet levels. Transfusion may be indicated in some patients with symptomatic anemia, but ferrous sulfate is often sufficient to replenish iron stores. Although many hormonal methods can be used to treat DUB, in the perimenopausal period, medroxyprogesterone IM (Depo-Provera) is often used to address the underlying hormonal imbalance. Nondrug therapies are also available for patients with contraindications to hormonal treatment or refractory symptoms despite hormonal treatment. Endometrial ablation and hysterectomy provide definitive management of DUB.
   Diagnosis: DUB

CASE 38

HPI: An 85-year-old woman with a history of hypertension is brought to the ED by ambulance after she fell at her assisted living facility. Caregivers saw the patient slip and fall while getting out of the bath this morning. Initially she complained of a mild headache, but did not lose consciousness. According to the caregivers she has become progressively more confused over the past 6 hours. They deny any possibility of syncope or seizure as a cause of the fall. The caregivers say she normally knows her name and the date and can carry on a conversation, but now does not make sense when she talks.

Vital signs: Temperature 98.2° F (36.8° C), pulse 80 beats/min, BP 145/80 mm Hg, RR 16 breaths/min.

Additional history: No use of alcohol, tobacco, or drugs. Medical history only significant for hypertension controlled with hydrochlorothiazide. No history of dementia.

1. **What is the differential diagnosis?**
   Blunt head trauma causing epidural hematoma, subdural hematoma, SAH, intraparenchymal hemorrhage, traumatic brain injury, diffuse axonal injury.
   Altered mental status arising from another cause: infection/sepsis, stroke/TIA, opioid overdose, alcohol overdose, acute renal failure, electrolyte derangement, calcium derangement, hypoglycemia, MI.

2. **What components of the physical examination do you perform?**
   General appearance, skin, HEENT/neck, lungs, cardiovascular, abdomen, extremities, neuro/psych.
   Physical examination:
   General: Confused and disoriented.

HEENT/neck: 5-cm hematoma over the right frontal bone, no evidence of a depressed skull fracture. No posterior auricular hematoma, no hemotympanum. Pupils are 6 mm and reactive bilaterally.

Lungs: WNL

Cardiovascular: WNL

Abdomen: WNL

Extremities: WNL

Neuro/psych: Alert and oriented to name only. Opens eyes spontaneously, localizes pain but does not obey simple commands. Speaks in sentences but the sentences do not make sense (Glasgow Coma Scale 4-5-4).

3. **What are your initial orders?**

IV fluids, oxygen, pulse oximetry, cardiac monitor. Fingerstick blood glucose. CBC, chem 8, coagulation profile. Immediate noncontrast head CT scan. ECG. Consider troponin, CXR, urinalysis/culture.

Advance clock:

Pulse oximetry 100% O_2 saturation on nonrebreather mask. Fingerstick blood glucose 160 mg/dL. Other laboratory tests WNL.

Noncontrast head CT scan reveals a right-sided concave density consistent with subdural hematoma. No evidence of midline shift.

4. **What are your follow-up actions?**

Neurosurgery consult. Admit to ICU.

Advance clock:

Case ends.

Critical actions:

Recognition and evaluation of altered mental status, stabilization of the patient, evaluation of intracranial pathology in a patient with head trauma, neurosurgery consult.

Discussion:

This patient has an acute subdural hematoma, a life-threatening neurosurgical emergency. It most commonly occurs as a result of injury to the bridging veins in the skull that penetrate the dura, leading to bleeding in the potential space between the dura and the arachnoid (because the bleeding is under the dura, it is a *sub*dural hematoma). In patients with atrophic brains (e.g., older individuals, alcoholic patients), the causative trauma can be minor. As the bleed expands, the patient is at risk of herniation and death.

Diagnosis is on the basis of a noncontrast CT scan of the brain showing a sickle-shaped (concave) bleed that can cross suture lines (unlike epidural hematomas). Management is first supportive (airway, breathing, circulation) with reversal of anticoagulation if the patient is taking an anticoagulant. Seizure prophylaxis is typically given as well. Treatment includes admission to an ICU and possible neurosurgical intervention, depending on the extent of the bleeding and the patient's symptoms.

Diagnosis: Subdural hematoma

CASE 39

HPI: A 62-year-old man attends the ED complaining of weakness for the past few days. He has a history of diabetes and oliguric end-stage renal disease on hemodialysis, but he admits that he has missed the past two dialysis sessions because of his hectic work schedule. When asked to elaborate on his weakness, he states "I don't know, I just can't walk as far as normal, and I feel like my whole body isn't as strong as it usually is."

Vital signs: Temperature 98.2° F (36.8° C), pulse 54 beats/min, BP 166/94 mm Hg, RR 16 breaths/min.

Additional history: Occasional alcohol use.

1. **What is the differential diagnosis?**

Hyperkalemia, fluid overload, hyperglycemia, other electrolyte derangements (e.g., hypercalcemia), CHF, uremia, anemia.

2. **What components of the physical examination do you perform?**

General appearance, cardiovascular, lungs, abdomen, neuro/psych.

Physical examination:
General: Comfortable.
Cardiovascular: WNL
Lungs: WNL
Abdomen: WNL
Neuro/psych: 4+/5 strength in all extremities, symmetric.

3. **What are your initial orders?**
ECG, chem 14, CBC, CXR, brain natriuretic peptide (BNP), troponin, LFTs.
Advance clock:
ECG shows sinus bradycardia with diffuse peaked T waves, a PR interval of 0.24 seconds, and a QRS duration of 0.16 seconds.
Chem 14 remarkable for potassium 7.4 mEq/L, BUN 80 mg/dL, creatinine 12 mg/dL.
CBC remarkable for Hb 11.2 mg/dL.
CXR shows mild cephalization of the pulmonary vasculature, no pulmonary edema or effusions, no cardiomegaly.

4. **What are your follow-up actions?**
Calcium chloride, insulin and glucose, sodium bicarbonate, albuterol, furosemide, sodium polystyrene sulfonate (Kayexalate), urgent nephrology consult for hemodialysis, admit to inpatient unit.
Advance clock:
Case ends.
Critical actions:
Recognition of hyperkalemia, rapid intervention, nephrology consult for definitive treatment (dialysis).
Discussion:
This patient has potentially life-threatening hyperkalemia as a result of missing dialysis sessions. Normally, individuals take in more potassium than they need and the excess is excreted by the kidneys. However, patients with renal failure are prone to accumulation of excess potassium and the development of hyperkalemia. The presenting symptoms for hyperkalemia can be generalized weakness or malaise, palpitations because of cardiac arrhythmia, or cardiac arrest. A potassium level greater than 5 mEq/L is generally considered hyperkalemia. The differential diagnosis for generalized weakness in a renal failure patient should also include fluid overload from a decreased glomerular filtration rate, as well as anemia due to decreased erythropoietin production.
    Causes of hyperkalemia fall into three categories: (1) decreased elimination of potassium (renal insufficiency, medications such as angiotensin-converting enzyme [ACE] inhibitors, conditions with decreased aldosterone such as adrenal insufficiency); (2) increased potassium release from cells (rhabdomyolysis, blood transfusions, acidosis); and (3) excessive potassium intake (rare). These must be distinguished clinically from a laboratory error caused by RBC hemolysis during blood draw from the patient, leading to spuriously elevated potassium levels.
    Treatment of hyperkalemia involves three targets: (1) temporary stabilization of the myocardium to prevent arrhythmias using calcium chloride or calcium gluconate; (2) a temporary shift in intracellular potassium using agents such as insulin (IV, not SC, and with glucose administration to prevent hypoglycemia), bicarbonate, and albuterol; and (3) elimination of potassium from the body, which can be accomplished via the urine with loop diuretics (furosemide), via the stool with ion exchange resins (sodium polystyrene sulfonate [Kayexalate]), and via the blood with dialysis. It should be emphasized that (1) and (2) are merely temporizing measures: the myocardial stabilizing activity of calcium lasts for just 30 minutes and the activity of agents that shift potassium intracellularly typically last for a few hours. In all cases of hyperkalemia, the underlying cause should be determined and corrected if possible.
    Diagnosis: Hyperkalemia

CASE 40

HPI: A 10-day-old infant boy is brought to the ED because of poor feeding, vomiting, fever, and abdominal distention for 1 day. The parents state that he was born at 35 weeks of gestation and the mother had preeclampsia, but the hospital stay was uncomplicated and they were released from the hospital just 3 days previously, after the infant's feeding was monitored.

Vital signs: Temperature 102.2° F (39° C), pulse 160 beats/min, BP 64/40 mm Hg, RR 60 breaths/min.
Additional history: None. Received birth vaccinations. Breastfed only.

1. **What is the differential diagnosis?**
   Necrotizing enterocolitis (NEC), malrotation/midgut volvulus, strangulated hernia.

2. **What components of the physical examination do you perform?**
   General appearance, cardiovascular, lungs, abdomen.
   Physical examination:
   General: Lethargic, ill-appearing neonate, unresponsive but breathing.
   Cardiovascular: Tachycardic, weak and thready pulses, no murmur.
   Lungs: Tachypneic, but lungs clear on auscultation; using accessory muscles.
   Abdomen: Distended, diffusely tender to palpation, absent bowel sounds.

3. **What are your initial orders?**
   IV fluid bolus of normal saline, nothing by mouth (NPO), nasogastric/orogastric tube, blood cultures, CBC, chem 14, broad-spectrum antibiotics (e.g., ampicillin, gentamycin, metronidazole), fingerstick blood glucose, abdominal x-ray.
   Advance clock:
   After fluid resuscitation the patient's BP is 90/60 mm Hg and the heart rate is 140 beats/min.
   An abdominal x-ray shows pneumatosis intestinalis, and dilated loops of bowel.
   Blood glucose is normal.
   CBC demonstrates leukocytosis with a left shift.

4. **What are your follow-up actions?**
   Surgery consult. Admit to ICU.
   Advance clock:
   Case ends.
   Critical actions:
   Recognition of vital sign abnormalities in the neonate, resuscitation. Recognition of NEC as a possible cause of the abdominal pain, ordering an appropriate workup, appropriate disposition.
   Discussion:
   NEC is the most common neonatal GI emergency, with high morbidity and mortality. NEC is caused by bowel ischemia, which causes translocation of bacteria through the bowel wall. Risk factors are prematurity and any cause of a low-flow state to the bowel, including congenital heart disease, maternal cocaine use, maternal preeclampsia, and hypotension. NEC presentation to the ED is uncommon because it classically occurs in more premature or otherwise ill neonates who would have reasons to remain in hospital. In term babies, NEC typically occurs within the first week of life, and within weeks 2 to 3 of life in premature babies.
       The presenting symptoms for NEC are abdominal distention, fever, irritability, and possibly peritoneal signs, with progression to shock. Plain abdominal x-rays are often sufficient to make the diagnosis and classically show (1) pneumatosis intestinalis, (2) free portal vein air, and/or (3) dilated loops of bowel.
       Management includes NPO, nasogastric or orogastric tube placement, fluid resuscitation, blood cultures, broad-spectrum antibiotics, glucose testing, abdominal x-ray, and ICU admission. In this case the neonate was hypotensive (systolic BP should be a **minimum** of 70 + [2 × age in years] up to the age of 10 years and 90 mm Hg thereafter) and needed fluid resuscitation. Poor glycogen stores in neonates necessitate blood sugar checks for ill-appearing patients.
       Diagnosis: NEC

CASE 41

HPI: A 27-year-old man attends the clinic complaining of 1 week of fever and malaise. He states that he has been feeling "hot" all week and has had frequent shaking chills. He has also noticed some pink patches on his skin that are painful to touch. He has never had any similar symptoms. He denies a cough, shortness of breath, other skin changes, sick contacts, or recent travel history.
Vital signs: Temperature 100.8° F (38.2° C), pulse 90 beats/min, BP 125/78 mm Hg, RR 16 breaths/min.

Additional history: No medical history. Uses IV heroin two or three times per week, smokes marijuana, drinks occasional alcohol, and smokes one pack of cigarettes daily. Not currently sexually active.

1. **What is the differential diagnosis?**
   Bacteremia, endocarditis, autoimmune disease, malignancy.

2. **What components of the physical examination do you perform?**
   General appearance, HEENT, cardiovascular, lungs, extremities.
   Physical examination:
   General: Mildly disheveled male in no apparent distress.
   HEENT: Fundoscopy shows small retinal hemorrhages with pale white centers, no papilledema, otherwise WNL.
   Cardiovascular: IV/VI holosystolic murmur at the left lower sternal border, otherwise WNL.
   Lungs: Occasional crackles throughout the lung fields bilaterally.
   Extremities: Multiple tender erythematous nodules on the hands and feet. Splinter hemorrhages seen on the nail beds of the hands and feet bilaterally.

3. **What are your initial orders?**
   CBC, chem 8, blood cultures, rapid HIV test, CXR, antipyretics (e.g., acetaminophen).
   Advance clock:
   CBC remarkable for leukocytosis of 17,000 cells/mL with neutrophil predominance. Chem 8 WNL. Blood cultures pending. Rapid HIV test negative. CXR shows evidence of septic pulmonary emboli in both lung fields.

4. **What are your follow-up actions?**
   Admit to monitored bed. Echocardiogram. Infectious disease consult.
   Advance clock:
   Echocardiogram shows large vegetation on the tricuspid valve. Blood cultures grow methicillin-sensitive S. aureus.

5. **What are your follow-up actions?**
   Start oxacillin administration via a peripherally inserted central catheter line for 4 to 6 weeks.
   Advance clock:
   Case ends.
   Critical actions:
   Recognition of infective endocarditis (IE), admission, ordering of appropriate workup, initiation of appropriate treatment.
   Discussion:
   This patient has IE, an infection of the endocardium of the heart, typically on the valvular surfaces. The most common causes are S. aureus (especially for acute presentations) and Viridans group Streptococcus species (for subacute presentations). In this individual with a history of IV drug use, S. aureus is the most likely agent. IE should be suspected in patients with fever and a heart murmur. Classic examination findings in IE include Roth spots (retinal emboli causing hemorrhages, often with white or pale centers); splinter hemorrhages in the nailbed; Janeway lesions; which are nontender purple macular lesions; and Osler nodes, which are similar to Janeway lesions but are raised and painful (remember Osler – Ow!).
   The diagnosis of IE is made according to the Duke criteria whereby (1) two major criteria or (2) one major and three minor criteria or (3) five minor criteria are met. The two major criteria are:
   1. Positive blood cultures for organisms causing endocarditis (e.g., Viridans group streptococci, S. aureus, and HACEK species*).
   2. Evidence of endocardial involvement (e.g., a positive echocardiogram showing a vegetation or new valvular regurgitation).

---

*HACEK is a mnemonic for slow-growing gram-negative bacteria that are difficult to culture but rarely can cause endocarditis. They include *Haemophilus*, *Actinobacillus*, *Cardiobacterium*, *Eikenella*, and *Kingella* species.

The minor criteria are conditions that are also common to many other diseases and therefore are not as specific for endocarditis. They are:

1. Fever.
2. Predisposition (e.g., IV drug use, damaged heart valve).
3. Vascular phenomena (e.g., emboli, Janeway lesions).
4. Immunologic phenomena (e.g., Osler nodes, Roth spots).
5. Positive blood cultures that do not meet major criteria. Typically, multiple sets of blood cultures will need to be obtained before antimicrobial treatment is started to ensure adequate isolation of the causative organism.

Treatment is with long-term parenteral antibiotics (4 to 6 weeks). An infectious disease consult should be sought to ensure appropriate antimicrobial coverage. Abscess formation, hemodynamic instability, and decompensation are all indications for surgical management. The most common two complications are CHF from valvular dysfunction and embolization (through the pulmonary circulation [lungs] for tricuspid vegetations or the systemic circulation [e.g., brain, kidneys] for mitral and aortic vegetations). The disposition for all patients with suspected or confirmed endocarditis is admission.

Diagnosis: IE

CASE 42

HPI: A 36-year-old woman attends her regular doctor 48 hours after receiving a tuberculin skin test (TST) as a condition of her new employment as a nurse at a nursing home. Since the skin test was placed on her right forearm she has noticed the development of a large bump in the area. She has worked at other nursing homes in the past and her TST was always negative. She denies any cough, fevers, chills, night sweats, weight loss, or other symptoms.

Vital signs: Temperature 98.2° F (36.8° C), pulse 76 beats/min, BP 115/68 mm Hg, RR 16 breaths/min.

Additional history: No medical history. Occasional alcohol use, denies smoking or use of other drugs. Sexually active with one male partner. Born in Mexico and has received the bacillus Calmette-Guérin (BCG) vaccine.

1. What is the differential diagnosis?
   TB, latent versus active.

2. What components of the physical examination do you perform?
   General appearance, cardiovascular, lungs, extremities.
   Physical examination:
   General: Well-developed, well-nourished woman in no apparent distress.
   Cardiovascular: WNL
   Lungs: WNL
   Extremities: 11-mm induration over the volar aspect of the right forearm.

3. What are your initial orders?
   CXR, CBC, chem 7, LFTs.
   Advance clock:
   CXR negative. CBC, chem 7, and LFTs all WNL.

4. What are your follow-up actions?
   Begin isoniazid and pyridoxine treatment for 9 months. Counsel patient on disease. Consider periodic LFTs to monitor for isoniazid-induced hepatitis.
   Advance clock:
   Case ends.
   Critical actions:
   Recognition of what classifies a positive TST in each risk group, understanding the difference between latent and active TB, appropriate treatment.
   Discussion:
   This patient has latent TB, a contagious bacterial infection due to *Mycobacterium tuberculosis*. TB has a wide spectrum of disease, ranging from latent (asymptomatic) TB to primary or reactivated pulmonary TB to disseminated TB. An asymptomatic individual with a newly

positive TST and no evidence of active disease has latent TB; treatment for these patients involves 9 months of isoniazid therapy. Active TB is characterized by clinical symptoms such as chronic cough, hemoptysis, fever, night sweats, and weight loss, as well as a positive TST. Patients with active TB are treated with four drugs (isoniazid, rifampin, pyrazinamide, and ethambutol) for 2 months and then two drugs (isoniazid and rifampin) for a further 4 months over a total treatment time of 6 months. This can be remembered by the "4-for-2 and 2-for-4" mnemonic (4 drugs for 2 months, 2 drugs for 4 months). Extrapulmonary TB is typically treated in the same way as active TB, except a longer course is used for spinal involvement (Pott disease) and TB meningitis. All patients on isoniazid should receive pyridoxine (vitamin B_6) because isoniazid can cause pyridoxine deficiency and subsequently lead to neuropathy and seizures.

Multidrug-resistant (MDR) TB is becoming more common and is resistant to isoniazid and rifampin, requiring other agents such as fluoroquinolones. However, an even more resistant strain called extensively drug-resistant (XDR) TB is emerging and is resistant to many of these second-line drugs as well. Patients with HIV have a 10% per year risk of reactivation of latent TB; this is in contrast to immunocompetent individuals, who have a 10% lifetime risk of reactivation.

A positive TST is defined differently for different risk groups, but the measurement (in millimeters) is always based on induration (not erythema). Whether or not the patient has received the BCG vaccine should not impact management:

- 5 mm or greater for high-risk patients, including HIV-positive individuals, immunosuppressed individuals, patients with a CXR consistent with TB, and individuals who have had recent contact with someone known to have active TB.
- 10 mm or greater for intermediate-risk patients, including immigrants from a high-prevalence country, IV drug users, residents or employees of a high-risk setting (e.g., jail, homeless shelter, nursing home, hospital), and individuals with a high-risk comorbid condition (e.g., diabetes, chronic kidney disease).
- 15 mm or greater for low-risk patients who have no risk factors for TB.

The patient in this case falls into the category for which the TST is positive at 10 mm because she is a health care worker in a high-risk environment. Therefore, she should be treated. She did not have evidence of active TB and therefore has latent TB.

Diagnosis: Latent TB

CASE 43

HPI: A 6-week-old infant boy is brought to the ED because he is "throwing up everything he eats" according to his parents. For the past few days, his condition has worsened to the point that he was vomiting 100% of his meals. Initially the patient would want to feed immediately afterward, but recently has been less interactive with his mother. The mother describes the vomitus as "the same color as the formula" with no blood.

Vital signs: Temperature 98.2° F (36.8° C), pulse 170 beats/min, BP 60/40 mm Hg, RR 50 breaths/min.

Additional history: Ex-full term, no complications.

1. **What is the differential diagnosis?**
   Pyloric stenosis, malrotation with midgut volvulus, duodenal atresia, gastroesophageal reflux disease (GERD), antral web or atresia, adrenal insufficiency, inborn error of metabolism, improper feeding practices.

2. **What components of the physical examination do you perform?**
   General appearance, cardiovascular, lungs, abdomen, skin, extremities.
   Physical examination:
   General: Lethargic infant, responding poorly to stimuli but breathing on his own.
   Cardiovascular: Tachycardic for age, holosystolic murmur throughout the precordium.
   Lungs: Tachypneic but lungs clear on auscultation.
   Abdomen: Soft, nontender, nondistended, small olive-like structure palpated superiorly and to the right of the umbilicus.
   Skin: No rash.
   Extremities: Delayed capillary refill.

3. **What are your initial orders?**
IV normal saline bolus, blood glucose test, CBC, chem 8, abdominal ultrasound when stable.
Advance clock:
After a bolus of normal saline the patient's heart rate is 140 beats/min and BP is 80/55 mm Hg. He is now interacting with his mother. Blood glucose 30 mg/dL. CBC remarkable for hemoconcentration. Chem 8 remarkable for potassium 3 mEq/L, bicarbonate 30 mEq/L, chloride 80 mEq/L, normal renal function. Abdominal ultrasound shows a hypertrophied pylorus.

4. **What are your follow-up actions?**
IV 10% dextrose, maintenance fluids 5% dextrose in quarter-strength normal saline with KCl 20 mEq/L, NPO, surgery consult, admit.
Advance clock:
Case ends.
Critical actions:
Recognition of pyloric stenosis as the cause of vomiting, consideration of other life-threatening causes, correction of metabolic abnormalities, patient stabilization, admission and surgical consult.
Discussion:
This patient has pyloric stenosis caused by hypertrophy of the gastric pylorus leading to obstruction. This classically occurs early in life, between the ages of 2 and 8 weeks. The vomiting is always nonbilious because bile is introduced in the duodenum, but the blockage is proximal to this. As the hypertrophy progresses, the patient vomits more frequently and forcefully (projectile vomiting), which often leads to dehydration and lethargy.

Findings are typically hypochloremic and hypokalemic metabolic acidosis arising from both vomiting of HCl and K^+ from the stomach and upregulation of the renin-angiotensin-aldosterone system. An olive-type mass can sometimes be palpated over the area of the pylorus, as in this case. Definitive diagnosis is via ultrasound, which will demonstrate a thick wall (>3 mm) and a long length (>16 mm) for the pylorus.

Management is with fluid resuscitation, if required, and correction of metabolic abnormalities (electrolyte derangements, hypoglycemia because of poor glycemic stores). Surgical pyloromyotomy is definitive but not emergent because the patient will stabilize once resuscitated.
Diagnosis: Pyloric stenosis

CASE 44

HPI: A 4-year-old, previously healthy boy is brought to the ED by his parents after he had a single 30-second episode of "shaking of his whole body." He was unresponsive during this episode and was briefly confused afterward but has since returned to normal.
Vital signs: Temperature 102.2° F (39° C), pulse 120 beats/min, BP 100/64 mm Hg, RR 24 breaths/min.
Additional history: Patient has had a runny nose, cough, and fever for the past 3 days. No history of ingestions, headache, or vision changes.

1. **What is the differential diagnosis?**
Seizure secondary to febrile illness, meningitis, intracranial hemorrhage, toxic ingestion, intracranial mass.

2. **What components of the physical examination do you perform?**
General appearance, HEENT, cardiovascular, lungs, neuro/psych.
Physical examination:
General: Well-developed, well-nourished boy in no distress, nontoxic, smiling.
HEENT: No evidence of trauma, neck supple without meningeal signs. Mild posterior oropharynx erythema and cobblestoning. Small tongue laceration. Rhinorrhea. Tympanic membranes normal.
Cardiovascular: WNL
Lungs: WNL
Neuro/psych: Appropriate for developmental age. Normal strength, sensation, and reflexes. Cranial nerves II through XII intact. No focal neurologic deficits.

3. **What are your initial orders?**
   Fingerstick glucose test, acetaminophen PO.
   Advance clock:
   Glucose 110 mg/dL, repeat temperature check 99.7° F (37.6° C).

4. **What are your follow-up actions?**
   Counsel the parents on simple febrile seizures.
   Follow up with primary doctor.
   Advance clock:
   Case ends.
   Critical actions:
   Recognition of simple febrile seizure, ruling out of more serious etiologies (e.g., meningitis) according to the history and physical examination, not pursuing an aggressive workup for simple febrile seizure.
   Discussion:
   This patient had a simple febrile seizure. A simple febrile seizure occurs in patients aged 3 months to 6 years with a temperature of 100.4° F (38° C) or greater and must meet **all** of the following criteria: (1) generalized tonic-clonic seizure, (2) less than 15 minutes in duration, (3) only occurs once in a 24-hour period, and (4) no focal features. Any exceptions to these four criteria will classify the condition as a complex febrile seizure, which may require a more thorough workup.
      The differential diagnosis for a patient who otherwise meets all the criteria for a simple febrile seizure includes any febrile illness (usually viral) but can also include more serious causes such as meningitis, intracranial hemorrhage, toxic ingestion, and intracranial mass. These other causes should be ruled out on the basis of the history and physical examination alone. In this case, the child currently appears well and nontoxic, does not have meningeal signs, has no abnormalities on neurologic examination, and has an examination consistent with an alternative diagnosis (viral upper respiratory tract infection). Therefore, the patient and his parents can be reassured that this condition is common (up to 5% of the population), does not significantly increase the risk of long-term seizure disorder, is not harmful, and does not require antiepileptic medications.
      Diagnosis: Simple febrile seizure

CASE 45

HPI: A 70-year-old woman attends your clinic for follow-up of thoracic back pain that has persisted for the past 3 weeks. She denies any similar history of pain. She denies any antecedent trauma or numbness or weakness in her body. She states that her back pain still occurs with activity and describes it as knifelike and nonradiating. She has also noticed that her posture has changed; she stoops forward from her upper back since the pain began.
Vital signs: Temperature 98.2° F (36.8° C), pulse 76 beats/min, BP 130/68 mm Hg, RR 16 breaths/min.
Additional history: 20–pack-year smoking history, quit 30 years ago. Hypertension controlled with amlodipine.

1. **What is the differential diagnosis?**
   Vertebral compression fracture secondary to osteoporosis, malignancy (pathologic fracture, especially lung cancer in this former smoker), hyperparathyroidism, Cushing syndrome or steroid use, Paget disease of bone.

2. **What components of the physical examination do you perform?**
   General appearance, back, neuro/psych.
   Physical examination:
      General: Well-developed female in no apparent distress.
      Back: Significant kyphosis with a dowager hump, mild tenderness to palpation over the midthoracic vertebrae, no paraspinal tenderness.
      Neuro/psych: Normal strength, sensation, and reflexes in all extremities. Cranial nerves II through XII intact.

3. **What are your initial orders?**
   CBC, chem 8, thoracic spine x-ray, acetaminophen or other analgesia.

Advance clock:
CBC and chem 8 normal, no evidence of hypercalcemia. Thoracic spine x-ray shows wedge fractures of T6 and T7 vertebrae and generalized decreased bone density with degenerative joint disease.

4. **What are your follow-up actions?**
   Dual-energy x-ray absorptiometry (DXA) scan, counseling on osteoporosis.
   Advance clock:
   DXA scan shows osteoporosis with a T score of −3.0. The patient's pain has improved with acetaminophen.

5. **What are your follow-up actions?**
   Vitamin D (can order a vitamin D level before supplementation), calcium, consider bisphosphonates.
   Advance clock:
   Case ends.
   Critical actions:
   Recognition of osteoporosis, appropriate workup and treatment.
   Discussion:
   This patient has osteoporosis, which is decreased bone density characterized by a DXA T value of −2.5 or lower (−1 to −2.5 is osteopenia). This value is the number of standard deviations by which the patient's density differs from a normal peak bone density. A DXA scan should be performed for women older than 65 years, men older than 70 years, and individuals older than 50 years with a fracture. Those with risk factors for osteoporosis (e.g., chronic glucocorticoid use) should be screened at an earlier age.
   Treatment of osteoporosis includes lifestyle modifications (e.g., smoking cessation, increased weight-bearing exercise), nutrition (e.g., vitamin D and calcium supplementation), and pharmacologic therapy (e.g., bisphosphonates, PTH analogues such as teriparatide).
   In a patient without prior trauma, underlying malignancy must remain in the differential diagnosis, particularly for older patients and for this patient, who is a former smoker. Remember the mnemonic "BLT with a kosher pickle" for malignancies that commonly metastasize to bone: **b**reast, **l**ung, **t**hyroid, **k**idney, and **p**rostate. Also remember multiple myeloma as a possible cause of bone pain that is commonly missed in the initial evaluation of a patient.
   Diagnosis: Osteoporosis

CASE 46

HPI: A 28-year-old man attends the ED complaining of bilateral lower extremity weakness for 4 days. He states that his symptoms began gradually, with his feet tripping as he walked up stairs, but they have now progressed and he finds it difficult to walk on flat ground. He denies any trauma or travel history.

Vital signs: Temperature 98.2° F (36.8° C), pulse 76 beats/min, BP 155/78 mm Hg, RR 16 breaths/min.

Additional history: Occasional marijuana use. Had diarrhea that was occasionally bloody 2 weeks ago, but this has since completely resolved.

1. **What is the differential diagnosis?**
   Guillain-Barré syndrome (GBS), transverse myelitis, spinal cord compression, tick paralysis, vitamin B_{12} deficiency resulting in subacute combined degeneration of the spinal cord (Lichtheim disease).

2. **What components of the physical examination do you perform?**
   General appearance, cardiovascular, lungs, neuro/psych.
   Physical examination:
   General: Comfortable, no distress, speaking in full sentences.
   Cardiovascular: WNL
   Lungs: Unlabored breathing.
   Neuro/psych: Strength in bilateral upper extremities 5/5, strength in hips 4/5, strength in knees 3/5, strength in ankles 3/5. No patellar or Achilles reflexes. Mild decreased sensation to pinprick in bilateral lower extremities. Cranial nerves intact.

3. **What are your initial orders?**

Chem 14, CBC, bedside pulmonary function tests, lumbar puncture (CSF cell count with differential, protein, glucose, Gram stain and culture), vitamin B_{12} level.

Advance clock:

Chem 14 and CBC unremarkable. Bedside pulmonary function tests WNL. Lumbar puncture shows high protein but normal cell count and no organisms on Gram stain. Vitamin B_{12} level normal.

4. **What are your follow-up actions?**

Neurology consultation, plasmapheresis or IVIG, admit to inpatient unit.

Advance clock:

Case ends.

Critical actions:

Recognition of GBS, appropriate diagnostic testing including lumbar puncture, assessment of pulmonary function to predict early respiratory compromise, admission to a monitored bed.

Discussion:

This patient has GBS, an autoimmune disease affecting the Schwann cells of the peripheral nervous system and characterized by ascending paralysis with areflexia and sensory changes. GBS classically follows an infection, especially with *Campylobacter jejuni*, as in this patient, but it can also occur without a known prior infection. GBS is also rarely (1 in 1,000,000) associated with influenza vaccination.

There are different GBS subtypes. The most important variant is Miller Fisher syndrome, which has *descending* paralysis, affects the cranial nerves, and is associated with positive anti-GQ1b antibodies. Although at times severe enough to require intubation, GBS commonly resolves completely in most patients. The hallmark diagnostic finding in GBS is albumino-cytologic dissociation in the CSF, meaning that there is a high protein level without a corresponding increase in cell count.

The treatment for GBS is plasmapheresis to remove autoantibodies or IVIG to neutralize them. Supportive care with pulmonary function tests and close monitoring is also a cornerstone of therapy to ensure that the patient does not develop respiratory compromise.

Diagnosis: GBS

CASE 47

HPI: A 26-year-old, previously-healthy woman attends the ED complaining of fever and right-sided back pain for the past 3 days. She states that the pain started approximately 1 week ago with a burning sensation during urination but has now progressed to significant pain in her back. She denies any history of similar symptoms. She states that she has had mild nausea but no vomiting.

Vital signs: Temperature 101.1° F (38.4° C), pulse 120 beats/min, BP 110/68 mm Hg, RR 18 breaths/min.

Additional history: 1-week history of dysuria and urinary urgency and frequency. Denies hematuria. Denies IV drug use. Denies sexual activity.

1. **What is the differential diagnosis?**

Pyelonephritis (with or without perinephric abscess), lower UTI (e.g., cystitis), urethritis (e.g., gonococcal or nongonococcal), pelvic inflammatory disease (PID), nephrolithiasis, pregnancy (including ectopic pregnancy).

2. **What components of the physical examination do you perform?**

General appearance, cardiovascular, abdomen, back, genitalia.

Physical examination:

General: Uncomfortable female sitting up in bed, mild distress.

Cardiovascular: WNL

Abdomen: Tenderness to palpation in the suprapubic area without rebound or guarding.

Back: Costovertebral angle tenderness on the right side.

Genitalia: No urethral prolapse, no vaginal discharge. No vaginal, cervical, or vulvar lesions. No cervical motion tenderness.

3. **What are your initial orders?**

   Urinalysis with microscopy, urine culture, CBC, chem 8, urinary pregnancy test, analgesia/antipyretics/antiemetics (e.g., morphine and ondansetron), IV fluids. (Consider gonococcal and *Chlamydia* testing.)

   Advance clock:

   Urinalysis with microscopy significant for positive leukocyte esterase and nitrites, 50 WBCs/hpf, 5 RBCs/hpf, no squamous epithelial cells. Urinary pregnancy test negative.

   CBC significant for leukocytosis of 16,000 cells/mL with 95% neutrophils. Other studies WNL.

   Patient feels much better after analgesics, antipyretics, and antiemetics.

   After IV fluids, her heart rate is 80 beats/min.

   If gonococcal/*Chlamydia* testing is ordered, it will be negative.

4. **What are your follow-up actions?**

   Appropriate antibiotics for pyelonephritis (e.g., fluoroquinolone such as ciprofloxacin for 10 to 14 days). Appropriate analgesics and antiemetics (e.g., hydrocodone/acetaminophen, ondansetron). Counseling. Discharge with close follow-up.

   Advance clock:

   Case ends.

   Critical actions:

   Diagnosis of acute pyelonephritis, assessment of pregnancy status, appropriate analgesia and supportive care, antibiotics appropriate for treatment of acute pyelonephritis.

   Discussion:

   This patient has a UTI that initially started as cystitis, an ascending bacterial infection of the bladder. It then ascended further to the kidneys, causing pyelonephritis. By far the most common cause of UTIs is *E. coli*, followed by *Staphylococcus saprophyticus*. Whereas cystitis typically does not cause fever, pyelonephritis often leads to fever because bacteria can now reach the bloodstream. UTIs can be divided into complicated and uncomplicated. Uncomplicated UTI **only** occurs in otherwise healthy women with a normal urinary tract who are not pregnant. Therefore any patient who does not meet these criteria has, by definition, a complicated UTI (e.g., all males, all pregnant women, all diabetic patients).

   Diagnosis of a UTI is based on history, physical examination, and results of urinalysis with microscopy. A positive nitrite test on urinalysis is the most specific indicator of a UTI (e.g., a positive result in the right clinical context virtually guarantees a UTI) but is not sensitive because only some bacteria (including *E. coli*) have the ability to reduce nitrate to nitrite and the reaction is slow. Leukocyte esterase is a more sensitive (e.g., more likely to be positive in the presence of a UTI) but less specific indicator. In a sample with few or no squamous cells (indicating a sample not contaminated by the perineum or vagina), a high WBC count (>5 cells/hpf) supports diagnosis of a UTI.

   Whereas uncomplicated simple cystitis usually does not require a urine culture, complicated cases or any case of pyelonephritis will benefit from a urine culture in case treatment fails and the bacterial type and antibiotic sensitivity need to be known. Blood cultures in pyelonephritis are controversial but are probably diagnostically redundant because a good urine sample will grow the causative organism nearly 100% of the time, whereas blood cultures are positive much less frequently. In sexually active patients with symptoms of urethritis (e.g., dysuria, frequency), *Chlamydia* or gonorrhea should be considered.

   If a patient with uncomplicated pyelonephritis can take PO medication, has adequate pain control, and has appropriate follow-up, she can be treated as an outpatient with a 10- to 14-day course of a fluoroquinolone such as ciprofloxacin or levofloxacin; folate inhibitors such as trimethoprim/sulfamethoxazole are second-line agents because of resistance patterns.

   Diagnosis: Pyelonephritis

CASE 48

HPI: A 12-year-old girl attends the ED complaining of a severe, nonproductive cough for the past 5 days. She says that the cough comes in forceful spurts and she needs to catch her breath afterward. She has vomited twice today because of the coughing. She says that a week or two ago her condition started with mild fever, a runny nose, and a normal cough, but her parents did not take her to see the doctor because they thought it was a common cold.

Vital signs: Temperature 98.2° F (36.8° C), pulse 76 beats/min, BP 115/68 mm Hg, RR 16 breaths/min.

Additional history: No medical history.

1. **What is the differential diagnosis?**

   Pertussis, cough-variant asthma, viral upper respiratory tract infection, pneumonia, mononucleosis, TB, foreign body aspiration.

   For older patients, consider other causes of chronic cough: GERD, postnasal drip, ACE-associated cough.

2. **What components of the physical examination do you perform?**

   General appearance, HEENT, cardiovascular, lungs.

   Physical examination:

   General: Well-developed, well-nourished girl, occasionally coughing in forceful paroxysms and inhaling forcefully afterward.

   HEENT: WNL

   Cardiovascular: WNL

   Lungs: WNL

3. **What are your initial orders?**

   CXR optional. Pertussis PCR. Azithromycin for patient and close contacts.

   Advance clock:

   Pertussis PCR positive for *Bordatella pertussis*.

4. **What are your follow-up actions?**

   Counseling on disease process.

   Advance clock:

   Case ends.

   Critical actions:

   Recognition of pertussis, azithromycin to reduce the infectivity of patient and close contacts.

   Discussion:

   Pertussis (whooping cough) is a bacterial infection with droplet transmission caused by *B. pertussis*, a gram-negative rod bacterium. There are classically three stages of pertussis: (1) the catarrhal stage, characterized by typical upper respiratory tract symptoms such as rhinorrhea and cough; followed by (2) the paroxysmal stage, with the classic cough in paroxysms followed by an inspiratory whoop and posttussive emesis; and finally (3) the convalescent stage, during which a chronic cough develops that lasts for weeks. Unfortunately, very young individuals do not have the classic symptoms and can have apnea as the presenting symptom.

   Diagnosis is mostly on a clinical basis, but the recommended diagnostic test is a pertussis PCR of a nasopharyngeal swab. Culture on Bordet-Gengou medium can also be performed. If a CBC is ordered, it may show severe leukocytosis because of a stimulating factor made by the bacteria (called a leukemoid reaction because the high WBC count is similar to that seen in acute leukemia). Treatment is with azithromycin (or erythromycin), which reduces infectivity but does not significantly impact symptom duration or severity unless started very early in the course of the illness. Close contacts should be treated as well, regardless of immunization status.

   Diagnosis: Pertussis

CASE 49

HPI: A 65-year-old man attends the ED complaining of right knee pain and swelling for the past day that prevent him from being able to walk without extreme pain. The symptoms are associated with fever and malaise. He denies any trauma or a history of similar symptoms.

Vital signs: Temperature 101.8° F (38.8° C), pulse 100 beats/min, BP 155/78 mm Hg, RR 16 breaths/min.

Additional history: History of hypertension and diabetes, moderately controlled. One sexual partner, monogamous. Occasional alcohol consumption, no use of tobacco or drugs.

1. **What is the differential diagnosis?**
   Monoarticular arthritis: septic arthritis, gout, pseudogout, trauma, osteoarthritis, psoriatic arthritis. (If patient were a child, transient synovitis would be included in the differential.)

2. **What components of the physical examination do you perform?**
   General appearance, cardiovascular, lungs, extremities.
   Physical examination:
   General: Well-developed, well-nourished man in mild distress due to pain.
   Cardiovascular: WNL
   Lungs: WNL
   Extremities: Right knee joint swollen with evidence of large effusion. Markedly diminished range of motion because of pain. Distal sensation, motion, and pulses intact. Further examination of the knee limited because of pain. Skin intact, no evidence of skin infection or breakdown.

3. **What are your initial orders?**
   CBC, chem 8, x-ray series of the right knee, ESR, C-reactive protein (CRP), arthrocentesis of right knee (with Gram stain, culture, cell count with differential, crystal analysis), analgesics.
   Advance clock:
   CBC remarkable for leukocytosis of 17,000 cells/mL with neutrophil predominance. Chem 8 unremarkable. ESR 80 mm/h and CRP 10 mg/dL (both elevated). X-ray series of the right knee remarkable for joint effusion; otherwise no evidence of fracture, dislocation, or osteomyelitis. Arthrocentesis of the right knee produces purulent liquid for which a Gram stain shows gram-positive cocci in clusters and a cell count of 120,000 WBCs/μL with a neutrophil predominance, culture pending.

4. **What are your follow-up actions?**
   IV vancomycin, admit for antibiotic therapy, serial aspiration. Orthopedic surgery consult for arthrotomy or arthrocentesis.
   Advance clock:
   Case ends.
   Critical actions:
   Recognition of septic arthritis, early aspiration and diagnosis, IV antibiotics, and admission.
   Discussion:
   This patient has septic arthritis, which is infection of a joint space. Most often, septic arthritis is monoarticular, involves a painful and swollen joint, and may have systemic symptoms such as fever. The causes is usually *S. aureus* (such as in this case); in patients with gonococcal arthritis (which can be monoarticular or oligoarticular), the causative agent is *Neisseria gonorrhoeae*. Septic arthritis should be considered in any patient with acute monoarticular arthritis, although the differential includes gout, pseudogout, trauma, osteoarthritis, psoriatic arthritis, and transient synovitis (in children; previously called toxic synovitis). Transient synovitis is a common condition in children aged 3 to 10 years (peak incidence 5 to 6 years) and differs from septic arthritis in that there will typically be no fever, the child will be able to bear weight, and the ESR and WBC count will not be as elevated as in septic arthritis (and if joint aspiration is performed there will be no evidence of infection). Transient synovitis is self-limiting and will resolve with supportive measures (decreased activity, NSAIDs).
   Definitive diagnosis of septic arthritis is on the basis of joint aspiration. The most important test is a bacterial culture, but if enough fluid is aspirated, a Gram stain, cell count with differential, and crystal analysis should be performed. A cell count greater than 50,000 cells/μL, a positive Gram stain, or a positive culture requires immediate treatment. The initial antibiotic choice depends on what the likely organism is and the patient's age, but definitive management is via needle aspiration and/or surgical drainage of the joint. Studies have shown that for most joints (not the hip and not for joints with prostheses in them), serial needle aspiration is as effective as surgical drainage of the joint. All patients with septic arthritis should be admitted for parenteral antibiotic therapy and definitive management.
   Diagnosis: Septic arthritis

CASE 50

HPI: An 80-year-old man attends the ED because of sudden-onset weakness and numbness of the left arm and left lower face that started 90 minutes ago. He was watching television when the symptoms suddenly started, and they have not improved at all since onset. He says that it feels like the left side of his mouth is not moving when he speaks and that he cannot move his left arm at all, but can still walk. He denies any history of similar symptoms and at baseline takes care of himself and lives with his wife. He denies any recent falls or trauma.

Vital signs: Temperature 98.2° F (36.8° C), pulse 76 beats/min, BP 160/90 mm Hg, RR 16 breaths/min.

Additional history: Has hypertension controlled with amlodipine. No other medical problems, medications, or allergies. No alcohol, tobacco, or drug use.

1. What is the differential diagnosis?
   Acute stroke (ischemic vs. hemorrhagic), TIA, hypoglycemia, seizure with Todd paralysis.

2. What components of the physical examination do you perform?
   General appearance, lungs, cardiovascular, neuro/psych.
   Physical examination:
   General: Well-developed, well-nourished man in no apparent distress.
   Cardiovascular: WNL
   Lungs: WNL
   Neuro/psych: Cranial nerves II through XII intact except the left lower face has 1/5 strength; left upper face normal. Strength 5/5 and symmetric over all extremities except for the left arm, which has 1/5 strength. Decreased sensation to light touch and pinprick over the left arm. No ataxia, no dysdiadochokinesia, normal gait.

3. What are your initial orders?
   CBC, chem 8, coagulation profile, fingerstick blood glucose, immediate noncontrast head CT scan.
   Advance clock:
   CBC, chem 8, coagulation profile, fingerstick blood glucose WNL.
   Noncontrast head CT scan unremarkable, no evidence of intracranial hemorrhage.

4. What are your follow-up actions?
   Neurology consult. NPO. Head of bed at least 30 degrees. Thrombolytic agents (e.g., tissue plasminogen activator [tPA]). Admit to ICU for close monitoring after thrombolytic administration. Counseling on disease process.
   Advance clock:
   Patient admitted to ICU after thrombolytic administration.
   Patient's weakness resolves and he returns to baseline.
   Case ends.
   Critical actions:
   Recognition of acute stroke; ruling out hypoglycemia and hemorrhagic stroke by fingerstick glucose and head CT scan, respectively; and thrombolytic administration for patients who are within the time window and do not have contraindications.
   Discussion:
   This patient had an ischemic stroke, an infarction of an area of brain due to interruption of arterial blood flow. Strokes can be either ischemic (85%) or hemorrhagic (15%). It is important to determine which type of stroke has occurred (with a head CT scan) because their management differs greatly. Strokes are sudden-onset neurologic deficits that follow a vascular distribution, so it is important to understand the vascular distribution of the brain. Strokes are the third leading cause of death in adults in the United States and often occur in older individuals with risk factors for atherosclerosis (hypertension, diabetes, dyslipidemia, tobacco use) and/or emboli (AF).
   Diagnosis is on the basis of history and physical examination. Blood glucose should be measured in all patients suspected of having a stroke because hypoglycemia can mimic stroke symptoms. An immediate noncontrast head CT scan should be performed. Early in the course of an *ischemic* stroke, a head CT scan will often be normal or show subtle changes. However, the CT scan is important to exclude a hemorrhagic stroke. If a diagnosis of stroke is made, the next step is to find out for exactly how long the symptoms have been present.

Thrombolytic agents are recommended for patients who do not have contraindications and attend within 3 hours of symptom onset (and some patients within 4.5 hours, but this is less likely to be tested). Treatment of ischemic stroke also includes permissive hypertension, whereby BP of up to 220/120 mm Hg should be allowed initially (although the maximum acceptable BP is lower than that in patients who are to receive thrombolytics), because acute BP lowering can increase the infarct size and extent. All patients should have an emergent neurology consult, especially if thrombolytic agents are considered. All patients should be admitted to a monitored bed; if thrombolytic agents are administered, ICU admission should be strongly considered because these patients have a 6% risk of intracranial hemorrhage.

Diagnosis: Ischemic stroke

CASE 51

HPI: A 45-year-old man attends his primary care physician because he was at a health fair last week and was told his blood sugar was 300 mg/dL. He was not sure if the result was accurate because he says that he does not have any problems. He denies any polyuria or polydipsia, changes in vision, weight changes, or other symptoms. He read online that you should not eat before you get your blood sugar checked so he has not eaten today.

Vital signs: Temperature 98.2° F (36.8° C), pulse 76 beats/min, BP 120/70 mm Hg, RR 16 breaths/min.

Additional history: Body mass index 30 (obese). Patient works as a receptionist and does not exercise. No medical history, no medications, no allergies. Occasional alcohol consumption, no use of tobacco or drugs.

1. **What is the differential diagnosis?**
   Hyperglycemia due to diabetes, medication effect (but patient not on medications), other endocrine disorders (e.g., hypercortisolism, hypothyroidism).

2. **What components of the physical examination do you perform?**
   General appearance, HEENT, cardiovascular, lungs, neuro/psych.
   Physical examination:
   General: Obese male in no apparent distress.
   HEENT: Fundoscopic examination shows mild nonproliferative diabetic retinopathy.
   Cardiovascular: WNL
   Lungs: WNL
   Neuro/psych: Sensation intact to pinprick, light touch, and two-point discrimination in all extremities. Proprioception in distal extremities intact. Rest of neurologic examination WNL.

3. **What are your initial orders?**
   Fingerstick blood glucose, Hb A_{1C}, CBC, chem 8, urinalysis, fasting lipid panel.
   Advance clock:
   Fingerstick blood glucose (fasting): 200 mg/dL.
   HbA1c: 7.9%.
   CBC WNL; chem 8 glucose 200 mg/dL, otherwise WNL; low-density lipoprotein (LDL) 65 mg/dL.
   Urinalysis: Moderate glucose, trace protein, otherwise WNL.

4. **What are your follow-up actions?**
   Counsel patient on disease process, lifestyle modification, exercise. Initiate metformin therapy. Measure urinary microalbumin. Refer for retinal photography. Follow-up appointment in 2 to 3 months.
   Advance clock:
   Patient returns for visit. States that he has not had medication side effects and has lost 20 lb since changing his diet and starting to exercise. Fingerstick glucose (fasting) 120 mg/dL. Urinary microalbumin negative. Retinal photography shows mild nonproliferative diabetic retinopathy.
   Case ends.
   Critical actions:
   Recognition of hyperglycemia, knowing diagnostic criteria, initiation of treatment for (likely) type 2 diabetes mellitus (T2DM).

Discussion:
This patient has T2DM, a chronic disorder characterized by insulin resistance and dysfunction of the insulin-producing beta-cells in the islets of Langerhans in the endocrine pancreas. Individuals most at risk include those with a positive family history, obesity, a sedentary lifestyle, and increasing age. Hyperosmolar hyperglycemic state (HHS) is an acute complication of T2DM in which severe hyperglycemia occurs without significant ketosis because there is enough insulin to prevent fatty acid breakdown and ketone production. Another acute complication is diabetic ketoacidosis (DKA), which can occur in T2DM when beta-cells have failed over time, leading to a marked insulin deficiency and thus hyperglycemia and ketosis. Chronic complications include retinopathy, nephropathy, neuropathy, and accelerated atherosclerosis (leading to increased rates of stroke and MIs, as well as peripheral vascular disease and impotence).

Diagnosis is on the basis of any two of the following criteria: Hb A$_{1C}$ of 6.5% or greater, fasting glucose of 126 mg/dL or greater, and/or random plasma glucose of 200 mg/dL or greater *with symptoms of hyperglycemia*. A 2-hour glucose tolerance test (75 g) with a result of 200 mg/dL or greater can also be applied as a criterion, but this is rarely used outside of pregnancy. Results should be confirmed by a second test unless the results are unequivocal (e.g., fasting glucose of 250 mg/dL certainly represents diabetes). After diagnosis, patient testing should include Hb A$_{1C}$, basic laboratory tests, urinary albumin to assess for nephropathy, a fasting lipid profile to assess for concomitant dyslipidemia, referral for retinal photography to assess for retinopathy, counseling on the disease process, and instructions to check their feet daily for foot ulcers (because sensation is diminished with diabetic neuropathy). Treatment always includes lifestyle modifications (patient education, dietary modification, and exercise) with an Hb A$_{1C}$ goal of less than 7.0% in most patients. The first-line medication is metformin to increase insulin sensitivity and decrease hepatic gluconeogenesis, as long as there are no contraindications (e.g., renal failure). Second-line agents include oral drugs such as a sulfonylurea (e.g., glipizide), a glucagon-like peptide-1 (GLP-1) receptor agonist, or insulin. Insulin is now being recommended earlier in the management of diabetes, especially for patients with marked hyperglycemia. Management of comorbidities is also important. Patients with dyslipidemia should be started on a statin with an LDL goal of less than 100 mg/dL (<70 mg/dL for concomitant cardiovascular disease). BP should be controlled with a systolic goal of less than 140/80 mm Hg. An ACE inhibitor or angiotensin receptor blocker (ARB) is the first-line therapy for patients with diabetes and either hypertension or albuminuria. Aspirin therapy should be initiated in patients with increased cardiovascular risk (most men >50 years and women >60 years who have at least one major cardiovascular risk factor).

Diagnosis: Uncontrolled T2DM

CASE 52

HPI: A 29-year-old man attends the ED with an altered mental status. He was brought in by his friend, who says that he was walking home with the patient when they were both assaulted about 1 hour ago. The patient was hit on the right side of his head with a baseball bat and was unconscious for 1 minute, but then felt normal. He did not want to go to the hospital and wanted to "sleep it off." However, before they got home the patient became less responsive and could no longer walk, so his friend called 911. The friend does not think the patient has any other medical problems or injuries.

Vital signs: Temperature 98.2° F (36.8° C), pulse 50 beats/min, BP 175/98 mm Hg, RR 14 breaths/min.

Additional history: Unknown. Patient's friend denies any alcohol or drug use before the assault.

1. **What is the differential diagnosis?**
   Blunt head trauma causing epidural hematoma, subdural hematoma, SAH, intraparenchymal hemorrhage, traumatic brain injury/diffuse axonal injury.
   Altered mental status from another cause: opioid overdose, alcohol overdose.

2. **What components of the physical examination do you perform?**
   General appearance, skin, HEENT/neck, lungs, cardiovascular, abdomen, extremities, neuro/psych.

Physical examination:
General: Lethargic, responds to painful stimuli but not voice. Obvious trauma to the right temporal area of his head. Breathing irregularly.
HEENT/neck: Depression of the skull over the right temporal bone without any laceration. No posterior auricular hematoma, no hemotympanum. Pupils are 6 mm and reactive bilaterally.
Lungs: Irregular respirations but lungs clear bilaterally on auscultation.
Cardiovascular: Bradycardic, otherwise WNL.
Abdomen: WNL
Extremities: WNL
Neuro/psych: Opens eyes to verbal stimuli, localizes pain but does not follow commands, and utters inappropriate words (Glasgow Coma Scale 3-5-3). Moving all extremities equally.

3. **What are your initial orders?**
   IV fluids, oxygen, pulse oximetry, cardiac monitor. Fingerstick blood glucose. Ethanol level. CBC, chem 8, coagulation profile. Immediate noncontrast head CT scan.
   Advance clock:
   Pulse oximetry: 100% O_2 saturation on nonrebreather mask.
   Fingerstick blood glucose: 160 mg/dL.
   CBC, chem 8, coagulation profile WNL.
   Noncontrast head CT scan: Right-sided biconvex density consistent with acute epidural hematoma. Midline shift of 5 mm. Depressed skull fracture of right temporal bone.
   Ethanol level: 0 mg/dL.

4. **What are your follow-up actions?**
   Neurosurgery consult, admit to the ICU.
   Advance clock:
   Case ends.
   Critical actions:
   Recognition of altered mental status, patient stabilization, evaluation for intracranial pathology in a patient with head trauma, neurosurgery consult.
   Discussion:
   This patient has an epidural hematoma, a life-threatening neurosurgical emergency. The condition most commonly occurs as a result of injury to the middle meningeal artery during trauma, leading to bleeding in the potential space between the dura and the skull (above the dura, and hence *epi*dural, vs. a venous *sub*dural hematoma with bleeding below the dura). The classic presentation is a patient who has suffered significant head trauma (often with loss of consciousness) followed by an asymptomatic lucid period during which the patient is bleeding but has not developed symptoms. As the bleed progresses, the patient will exhibit a rapid deterioration in consciousness and potentially brain herniation and death. This patient has Cushing triad, a combination of bradycardia, hypertension, and irregular breathing, which indicates increased intracranial pressure and should raise the level of suspicion for an intracranial bleed.
   Diagnosis is on the basis of a noncontrast CT scan of the brain showing a lens-shaped bleed that does not cross suture lines (because the dura adheres to the skull at the suture lines, the blood cannot cross). Treatment includes stabilizing the patient (airway, breathing, circulation), correcting any underlying coagulopathy, reducing intracranial pressure if signs of herniation are present, and an emergent neurosurgical consult for craniotomy. Seizure prophylaxis is also commonly given to such patients.
   Diagnosis: Epidural hematoma

CASE 53

HPI: A 30-year-old man attends the ED with a headache and lightheadedness that began after he woke up this morning. The headache is described as affecting "the whole head" and is a dull pain that is nonradiating. No visual changes, fever or chills, weakness or numbness. The lightheadedness has been occurring all day, is not positional, and is not associated with vertigo or unsteadiness. The patients reports that he lives with his girlfriend and his brother, both of whom are in the ED with the same symptoms.

Vital signs: Temperature 98.2° F (36.8° C), pulse 80 beats/min, BP 125/78 mm Hg, RR 16 breaths/min.

Additional history: No medical history. Denies use of alcohol, tobacco, or drugs.

1. **What is the differential diagnosis?**
   Carbon monoxide (CO) poisoning, cyanide poisoning, headache (migraine, tension, etc.) sedative overdose, hypoxemia, meningitis, viral syndrome.

2. **What components of the physical examination do you perform?**
   General appearance, cardiovascular, lungs, neuro/psych.
   Physical examination:
   General: No apparent distress.
   Cardiovascular: No cyanosis, WNL.
   Lungs: WNL
   Neuro/psych: Cranial nerves II through XII intact; motion, sensation, and reflexes normal. No focal neurologic deficits.

3. **What are your initial orders?**
   Pulse oximetry, arterial blood gas, CBC, chem 8, ECG.
   Advance clock:
   Pulse oximetry reveals 100% O_2 saturation on room air, arterial blood gas normal except for a CO level of 20%. CBC, chem 8, ECG all WNL.

4. **What are your follow-up actions?**
   Oxygen via nonrebreather mask (100%), admit for observation.
   Advance clock:
   Case ends.
   Critical actions:
   Recognition of CO toxicity as a cause of headache and dizziness, especially in multiple patients in the same building. Treatment with 100% oxygen.
   Discussion:
   This patient has CO poisoning. CO is produced when there is incomplete combustion of fuel, such as by gas-powered heaters, barbecues, or any fire. CO binds avidly to Hb and therefore prevents oxygen from binding. Although the oxygen-carrying capacity is diminished, the oxygen saturation as measured by normal pulse oximetry will be normal because pulse oximetry cannot distinguish between the waveforms of CO bound to Hb and oxygen bound to Hb. Symptoms are classically flulike symptoms, headaches, and dizziness. Diagnosis of CO poisoning is on the basis of blood gas analysis demonstrating elevated levels of CO in the blood.
   Treatment is via high-flow oxygen (e.g., a nonrebreather mask) because the half-life of CO is about 4 to 6 hours on room air but decreases to 1 hour on 100% oxygen (and even lower with hyperbaric oxygen therapy). Indications for hyperbaric treatment are controversial but include neurologic deficits, pregnancy, and cardiovascular compromise.
   Diagnosis: CO poisoning

CASE 54

HPI: A 67-year-old woman attends the ED with shortness of breath. The patient has noticed 1 week of gradually worsening dyspnea. She is now unable to walk at all without becoming short of breath. She has never smoked cigarettes and has no history of asthma.

Vital signs: Temperature 98.8° F (37.1° C), pulse 115 beats/min, BP 90/70 mm Hg, RR 30 breaths/min.

Additional history: Metastatic breast cancer.

1. **What is the differential diagnosis?**
   Pulmonary embolism, CHF, pericardial effusion, pneumothorax, pulmonary metastatic disease, malignant pleural effusion.

2. **What components of the physical examination do you perform?**
   General appearance, HEENT, cardiovascular, lungs, abdomen, extremities.

Physical examination:
General: Tachypneic.
HEENT: WNL
Cardiovascular: Elevated jugular venous pressure (JVP), tachycardia, muffled heart sounds.
Lungs: Tachypnea but otherwise WNL.
Abdomen: WNL
Extremities: WNL

3. **What are your initial orders?**
Pulse oximetry, BP/cardiac monitoring, CBC, chem 8, coagulation panel, blood typing and screening, troponin every 8 hours, arterial blood gas, ECG, CXR, TTE, IV fluids.
Advance clock:
ECG: Low voltage throughout, alternation of QRS amplitude between beats.
CXR: Enlarged cardiac silhouette.
TEE: Pericardial effusion with tamponade physiology.
All other studies WNL
Patient update: The patient's dyspnea worsens and she becomes obtunded.

4. **What are your follow-up actions?**
Pericardiocentesis (the patient's symptoms improve and vital signs normalize).
Cardiothoracic surgery consult. Admit to the ICU; morning ECG, CXR, CBC, chem 8. Counseling.
Advance clock:
Case ends.
Critical actions:
Cardiac and pulmonary examination, ECG, echocardiogram, pericardiocentesis.
Discussion:
This patient has a pericardial effusion with tamponade physiology, probably secondary to her metastatic breast cancer. Other causes of pericardial effusion include aortic dissection, radiation, trauma, and pericarditis. The patient's chief complaint of shortness of breath has a broad differential, but the physical examination strongly suggests pericardial effusion. Furthermore, the triad of JVD, muffled heart sounds, and hypotension is consistent with tamponade. As soon as tamponade is suspected, the patient should be given a large bolus of IV fluids as a temporizing measure. IV fluids can increase the preload and cardiac output. CXR may reveal an enlarged cardiac silhouette and ECG may reveal electrical alternans. The diagnosis of pericardial effusion should be confirmed with an echocardiogram, and an unstable patient should be treated promptly with pericardiocentesis. A cardiothoracic surgery consult should be requested to consider definitive management with a pericardial window. This intervention is probably necessary in this patient because malignant effusions tend to recur.
Diagnosis: Pericardial effusion

CASE 55

HPI: A 50-year-old woman attends the clinic complaining of burning epigastric abdominal pain that radiates to the throat. It is worse when she lies flat and improves when she is upright for a prolonged period. It has been occurring daily for several months and is worse after large meals. She reports occasional difficulty in swallowing foods such as steak and bread. She says that these foods sometimes feel stuck in her throat. She denies weight loss, odynophagia, and early satiety. She has never noticed blood in her stool.
Vital signs: Temperature 98.8° F (37.1° C), pulse 72 beats/min, BP 115/75 mm Hg, RR: 16 breaths/min.
Additional history: No medical history. No use of tobacco, alcohol, or drugs.

1. **What is the differential diagnosis?**
GERD, esophageal malignancy, achalasia, peptic ulcer disease, coronary artery disease (CAD).

2. **What components of the physical examination do you perform?**
General appearance, skin, lymph nodes, HEENT, cardiovascular, lungs, abdomen, rectal, extremities, neuro/psych.

Physical examination:
General: No acute distress.
Skin/lymph nodes/HEENT: WNL
Cardiovascular: WNL
Lungs: WNL
Abdomen: WNL
Genitalia/rectal: Brown-colored stool, no palpable masses.
Extremities: WNL
Neuro/psych: WNL

3. **What are your initial orders?**
Counseling (including diet), omeprazole PO, upper GI tract endoscopy, follow up at clinic in 1 month.
Advance clock:
Endoscopy: WNL
Patient returns to clinic and symptoms have greatly improved.
Case ends.
Critical actions:
Abdominal examination, upper GI tract endoscopy, proton pump inhibitor (PPI) or H₂-blocker.
Discussion:
This patient has classic GERD symptoms and a physical examination that is nonconcerning. All patients with GERD should receive dietary counseling and advice on elevating the head of the bed. Calcium carbonate can be used as needed for occasional symptom relief, but the fact that this patient has daily symptoms indicates the need for an H₂-blocker or a PPI. Either would be a reasonable starting agent in this case. However, if the H₂-blocker does not relieve her symptoms, a change to a PPI would be indicated. CAD should at least be in the differential for any patient with GERD symptoms, especially women, who may exhibit atypical cardiac symptoms. On the basis of her history, this patient has a very low risk of CAD. However, ordering an ECG would be unlikely to lose points in the exam. To avoid missing a serious diagnosis, all patients with GERD symptoms should be assessed for red-flag signs (weight loss, dysphagia, odynophagia, GI bleeding, and early satiety). This patient's mild dysphagia is reason enough to perform upper GI tract endoscopy to assess for Barrett esophagus and dysplasia. If Barrett esophagus with low-grade dysplasia is present, surveillance endoscopy should initially be performed every 6 months. High-grade dysplasia is treated with esophagectomy or endoscopic ablative therapies. The selection of the modality is beyond the scope of this case.
   Diagnosis: GERD

CASE 56

HPI: A 28-year-old woman attends the ED with acute-onset shortness of breath and a sharp chest pain that is worse when she takes a deep breath. She has had no fever, but does report a mild, nonproductive cough. She takes no medications except for an OCP.
Vital signs: Temperature 99.9° F (37.7° C), pulse 103 beats/min, BP 130/80 mm Hg, RR 31 breaths/min.
Additional history: No tobacco, alcohol, or drug use. Car accident 2 months previously that resulted in a fractured tibia.

1. **What is the differential diagnosis?**
Pneumonia, pneumothorax, pulmonary embolism, asthma, costochondritis, pericarditis.

2. **What components of the physical examination do you perform?**
General appearance, HEENT, cardiovascular, lungs, abdomen, extremities.
General: Increased work of breathing.
HEENT: WNL
Cardiovascular: Tachycardic.
Lungs: Tachypneic, breath sounds normal.
Abdomen: WNL
Extremities: WNL

3. **What are your initial orders?**
   Pulse oximetry/oxygen, BP/cardiac monitor, CXR, CBC, chem 8, PT/PTT, arterial blood gas, troponin, urinary pregnancy test.
   Advance clock:
   O_2 saturation: 90% on room air, arterial blood gas shows hypoxia.
   Laboratory and radiologic studies: WNL

4. **What are your follow-up actions?**
   Chest CT-angiogram, lower extremity ultrasound.
   Advance clock:
   Chest CT-angiogram chest: Pulmonary embolism on the left.
   Lower extremity ultrasound: Common femoral vein DVT.

5. **What are your follow-up actions?**
   Stop the OCP (okay to start nonhormonal birth control); start enoxaparin and warfarin. Admit to ward. Can stop enoxaparin and discharge home when warfarin is therapeutic, the patient is stable on room air, and her pain is controlled. Follow up after 1 week. Counseling.
   Case ends.
   Critical actions:
   Pulmonary examination, extremity examination, pulse oximetry and/or oxygen, CT-angiogram, warfarin plus LMWH such as enoxaparin (or other appropriate anticoagulation agent).
   Discussion:
   This patient's history alone raises concerns for pulmonary embolism and she should be evaluated using a reliable imaging method. CT-angiography has largely taken the place of ventilation-perfusion scans. A D-dimer test alone would be insufficient to confirm or rule out pulmonary embolism in this high-probability pretest setting. Once the diagnosis is established, appropriate anticoagulation therapy should be initiated (usually warfarin with LMWH). Thrombolytic therapy with tPA is indicated in hemodynamically unstable patients. A hypercoagulability workup is unlikely to award any extra points in the setting of acute/provoked DVT, but it is not likely that points would be deducted. This patient's therapy should be continued for a minimum of 3 months because she has had a provoked first episode. Patients with recurrent pulmonary embolism or persistent risk factors may require lifelong anticoagulation therapy.
   Diagnosis: Pulmonary embolism

CASE 57

HPI: A 51-year-old man arrives by ambulance complaining of three episodes of passage of bright red blood from the rectum. He has no abdominal pain and denies nausea and vomiting. He has previously had a few episodes of a maroon-colored stool, but has never passed frank blood. He denies recent weight loss.
Vital signs: Temperature 98.2° F (36.8° C), pulse 92 beats/min, BP 120/75 mm Hg, RR 15 breaths/min.
Additional history: No medical or surgical history.

1. **What is the differential diagnosis?**
   Lower GI tract bleed: Arteriovenous malformation, bleeding hemorrhoids, bleeding diverticulosis, colon cancer, angiodysplasia, anal fissure.
   Brisk upper GI tract bleed: Peptic ulcer disease, varices.

2. **What components of the physical examination do you perform?**
   General appearance, HEENT, cardiovascular, lungs, abdomen, rectal.
   Physical examination:
   General: Mild pallor.
   HEENT: WNL
   Cardiovascular: WNL
   Lungs: WNL
   Abdomen: WNL
   Rectal: Bright red blood in the rectal vault.

3. **What are your initial orders?**
   Pulse oximetry, cardiac/BP monitor, CBC, chem 8, LFTs, PT/PTT, blood type and cross-match, IV normal saline, NPO, GI consult, colonoscopy, admit to inpatient unit.
   Advance clock:
   Hb 10.2 mg/dL.
   Colonoscopy reveals bleeding diverticulosis. Hemostasis is achieved with intervention.
   All other studies WNL.

4. **What are your follow-up actions?**
   CBC every 4 hours (can decrease frequency if stable). Counseling before discharge (including dietary counseling), follow up in 1 week.
   Advance clock:
   Case ends.
   Critical actions:
   Abdominal examination, rectal examination, IV fluids, GI consult, colonoscopy.
   Discussion:
   This patient has a lower GI tract bleed, anatomically defined as bleeding distal to the ligament of Treitz. The vast majority of lower GI tract bleeds localize to the colon, and the small intestine is a rare source of bleeding. Presenting symptoms for slow lower GI tract bleeds may be microcytic anemia with occult blood. Bright red blood passed through the rectum corresponds to a high degree of suspicion for a lower GI tract source; however, brisk upper GI tract bleeds may also cause frankly bloody stools. In the United States, diverticular bleeding is the most common cause of lower GI tract bleeding. Diverticula tend to occur around the vasa recta, where the penetrating blood vessels create local areas of weakness. The associated vasa recta are then protected only by the overlying mucosa and are at risk of bleeding.
   The first step in assessing an acute GI bleed is to stabilize the patient. This patient's stable vital signs indicate that he does not need aggressive resuscitation or transfusion, but he should be monitored closely. Transfusion strategies vary widely but almost always include transfusion for Hb of less than 7 mg/dL or hemodynamic instability. Although most lower GI tract bleeds resolve spontaneously, they should be evaluated with colonoscopy for diagnostic and therapeutic purposes. Treatment strategies for actively bleeding sites include mechanical clips, injection of epinephrine, and bipolar coagulation. Upper GI tract endoscopy would be indicated if colonoscopy were negative to evaluate for a brisk upper GI tract bleed. Once bleeding is controlled, the patient can be monitored and eventually discharged home with counseling and close follow-up.
   Diagnosis: Bleeding diverticulosis

CASE 58

HPI: A 42-year-old man is brought by ambulance to the ED. He was observed sitting at a bus stop when he suddenly slumped over, fell to the ground, and had total body convulsions. These convulsions stopped spontaneously and he was brought directly to the ED.
Vital signs: Temperature 98.6° F (37.0° C), pulse 110 beats/min, BP 145/90 mm Hg, RR 19 breaths/min.
Additional history: Patient is unable to provide additional history.

1. **What is the differential diagnosis?**
   Hypoglycemic seizure, underlying primary generalized epilepsy, alcohol withdrawal, convulsive syncope, psychogenic nonepileptic seizure.

2. **What components of the physical examination do you perform?**
   General appearance, HEENT, cardiovascular, lungs. abdomen, neuro/psych.
   Physical examination:
   General: Disheveled appearance, smells of alcohol.
   HEENT: Soft-tissue swelling of the scalp over the parietal region.
   Cardiovascular: Tachycardic.
   Lungs: WNL
   Abdomen: WNL
   Neuro/psych: Postictal, alert and oriented to person and place but not time, follows commands, eyes open, tremor of hands and tongue, no focal neurologic deficits.

3. **What are your initial orders?**
   Random glucose test, pulse oximetry, IV normal saline, BP/cardiac monitor, IV diazepam, CBC, chem 8, urine toxicology, noncontrast head CT scan.
   Advance clock:
   Hb 10.2 mg/dL, MCV 107 fL, other studies WNL.
   Tremor improves, heart rate 90 beats/min.

4. **What are your follow-up actions?**
   Multivitamin, thiamine, folate, admit to inpatient unit, vital signs every 4 hours, continuous pulse oximetry, CBC and chem 8 in the morning, social work consult, addiction unit consult, counseling (including alcohol cessation).
   Advance clock:
   Case ends.
   Critical actions:
   Glucose level, benzodiazepine (e.g., diazepam, chlordiazepoxide), counseling, thiamine.
   Discussion:
   An undifferentiated patient with acute seizures should trigger a broad initial workup, especially because the medical history is often limited. Rapid assessment for hypoglycemia, traumatic brain injury, and pregnancy (in females) can help to narrow the differential and guide management. Presenting symptoms for alcohol withdrawal can include agitation, visual hallucinations, delirium tremens (delirium with unstable vital signs), and seizures. The mainstay of alcohol withdrawal treatment is benzodiazepines. Mild withdrawal can be treated on an outpatient basis; however, patients with first-time seizures, delirium tremens, or symptoms requiring large doses of benzodiazepines should be admitted to the hospital. It is prudent to give thiamine before administering any glucose because of the theoretical concern of precipitating thiamine depletion and Wernicke encephalopathy. Many clinicians also provide folic acid and a multivitamin. Counseling on alcohol cessation should be given to all patients.
   Diagnosis: Alcohol withdrawal

CASE 59

HPI: A 36-year-old woman attends the clinic complaining of several months of joint pain. She has noticed pain in her hands, wrists, elbows, and knees bilaterally that seems to move from joint to joint. During this time she has had an increasing feeling of fatigue and finds it difficult to get out of bed some days. She has also noticed a rash that appears over her face when her symptoms are at their worst. Her symptoms seem to worsen when she is exposed to the sun.
Vital signs: Temperature 99.3° F (37.4° C), pulse 85 beats/min, BP 120/74 mm Hg, RR 18 breaths/min.
Additional history: No medical history. No use of tobacco, drugs, or alcohol. No medications.

1. **What is the differential diagnosis?**
   Systemic lupus erythematosus (SLE), rheumatoid arthritis (RA), Lyme disease, fibromyalgia, osteoarthritis (OA), depression.

2. **What components of the physical examination do you perform?**
   General appearance, skin, lymph nodes, HEENT, cardiovascular, lungs, abdomen, genitalia, rectal, extremities, neuro/psych.
   Physical examination:
   General: No acute distress.
   Skin/lymph nodes/HEENT: Erythematous rash over the cheeks sparing the nasolabial folds. Painless oral ulcerations.
   Cardiovascular: WNL
   Lungs: WNL
   Abdomen: WNL
   Genitalia/rectal: WNL
   Extremities: Tenderness to palpation over the hand, wrist, and elbow joints. Mild effusion in the knees bilaterally.
   Neuro/psych: WNL

3. **What are your initial orders?**
   Pulse oximetry, CBC, chem 14, PT/PTT, ESR, CRP, ANA, complement screen, urinalysis, rheumatoid factor (RF), x-ray of affected joints, ibuprofen PO (or other NSAID).
   Advance clock:
   ESR/CRP elevated, ANA positive, C3/C4 low, other studies WNL. Minimal symptom improvement with NSAIDs.

4. **What are your follow-up actions?**
   Anti-dsDNA (positive), rheumatology consult, prednisone PO, hydroxychloroquine PO, counseling, physical therapy, occupational therapy, follow up in 4 weeks.
   Advance clock:
   Case ends.
   Critical actions:
   Extremities examination, analgesia (NSAID), ANA test, rheumatology consult.
   Discussion:
   The diagnosis of SLE is based on at least four of 11 criteria remembered by the mnemonic **SOAP BRAIN MD**: **s**erositis, **o**ral ulcerations, **a**rthritis, **p**hotosensitivity, **b**lood disorders, **r**enal involvement, **A**NA positive, **i**mmunologic abnormalities, **n**eurologic disease, **m**alar rash, **d**iscoid rash.

   This patient has a migratory symmetric polyarthritis with malar rash, photosensitivity, and oral ulcers. This collection of signs and symptoms should trigger a workup for a rheumatologic condition. ANA is a fairly sensitive test in screening for SLE, and anti-dsDNA is highly specific. ESR, CRP, and complement levels are nonspecific markers for inflammation but may suggest an autoimmune process. Once the diagnosis of SLE is suspected, consultation with a rheumatologist is warranted. Other tests such as antiphospholipid, anti-SSA/SSB, antihistone, anti-Smith, and antiribonucleoprotein antibodies may be ordered; however, for testing purposes a rheumatology consult will be sufficient. Most patients will benefit from NSAIDs for analgesia (if renal function is normal).

   Hydroxychloroquine is an immunomodulatory agent that is first-line therapy for symptom management and prevention of lupus flares. When symptoms are not controlled with NSAIDs and hydroxychloroquine alone, corticosteroids can provide a significant improvement. Given their side-effect profile, they should be used at the lowest effective dose for the shortest possible duration. Patients should be regularly monitored by a rheumatologist for symptom control, progression of disease, and systemic complications. A nephrology consult may be indicated for patients with renal involvement. Patients on long-term corticosteroids should be monitored for associated complications.
   Diagnosis: SLE

CASE 60

HPI: A 45-year-old woman attends the ED. She has had 24 hours of gradually worsening abdominal pain in the right upper quadrant. She has had seven episodes of vomiting and feels like she has a fever.
Vital signs: Temperature 100.8° F (38.2° C), pulse 105 beats/min, BP 156/98 mm Hg, RR 14 breaths/min.
Additional history: Hyperlipidemia, on atorvastatin. No other medical history.

1. **What is the differential diagnosis?**
   Acute cholecystitis, cholangitis, pancreatitis, symptomatic cholelithiasis.

2. **What components of the physical examination do you perform?**
   General appearance, HEENT, cardiovascular, lungs, abdomen.
   Physical examination:
   General: Moderate distress secondary to pain.
   HEENT: Dry cracked lips.
   Cardiovascular: Tachycardia, otherwise WNL.
   Lungs: WNL
   Abdomen: Obese abdomen; soft, severe tenderness to right upper quadrant with voluntary guarding; positive Murphy sign, no rebound.

3. **What are your initial orders?**
   Pulse oximetry, BP/cardiac monitor, urinary pregnancy test, urinalysis, urine culture, CBC, chem 8, LFTs, lipase/amylase, blood cultures, gallbladder ultrasound, IV normal saline, morphine, ondansetron, acetaminophen.
   Advance clock:
   WBC: Elevated with left shift.
   Gallbladder ultrasound: Gallstones, thickened gallbladder wall, pericholecystic fluid, normal common bile duct, positive sonographic Murphy sign. Other studies WNL.
   The patient's symptoms are moderately improved.

4. **What are your follow-up actions?**
   PT/PTT, blood type and screen, NPO, IV antibiotics (ceftriaxone and metronidazole), surgery consult, laparoscopic cholecystectomy, admit to inpatient unit. Check vital signs every 4 hours, CBC and chem 8 next day. Counseling before discharge.
   Advance clock:
   Case ends.
   Critical actions:
   Gallbladder ultrasound, IV fluids, morphine, ondansetron, antibiotics, laparoscopic cholecystectomy.
   Discussion:
   Acute-onset abdominal pain in the right upper quadrant should warrant evaluation for hepatobiliary pathology including cholecystitis, cholangitis, and pancreatitis. Acute pancreatitis can be excluded if a lipase test is normal. The classic presentation of cholangitis is the Charcot triad: fever, right upper quadrant abdominal pain, and jaundice. Cholecystitis can be diagnosed according to the combination of historical features, physical examination, laboratory values, and ultrasound.
       Acute cholecystitis is an inflammatory process of the gallbladder usually secondary to stasis arising from a stone lodged in the cystic duct. Acalculous cholecystitis may occur in critically ill patients. Once the diagnosis is established, patients should be given IV fluid and NPO. *E. coli* is the most common bacterial source, but gram-positive, gram-negative, anaerobic, and aerobic organisms are all possible causes. Broad-spectrum antibiotics such as ceftriaxone and metronidazole are therefore indicated. Early cholecystectomy is generally the preferred approach because prompt surgical intervention decreases hospital readmission rates and mortality. Ascending cholangitis is treated with IV fluids, endoscopic retrograde cholangiopancreatography, admission, and metronidazole/cefepime (or other broad-spectrum combination for gram-negative, gram-positive, and anaerobic bacteria). If the patient had symptomatic cholelithiasis without cholecystitis, the treatment would include control of symptoms (analgesia and antiemetics) and elective surgery.
       Diagnosis: Acute cholecystitis

CASE 61

HPI: An 18-year-old woman attends the ED. She has had 12 hours of gradually worsening abdominal pain in the right lower quadrant. She has vomited many times and has been unable to eat or drink anything since the pain started. She has never had similar pain before this event.
Vital signs: Temperature 101.3° F (38.5° C), pulse 115 beats/min, BP 118/78 mm Hg, RR 23 breaths/min.
Additional history: Sexually active with one male partner. No other medical history.

1. **What is the differential diagnosis?**
   Acute appendicitis, PID, tuboovarian abscess, ectopic pregnancy, ovarian torsion.

2. **What components of the physical examination do you perform?**
   General appearance, HEENT, cardiovascular, lungs, abdomen, genitalia.
   Physical examination:
   General: Moderate distress secondary to pain.
   HEENT: WNL
   Cardiovascular: Tachycardia, otherwise WNL.

Lungs: Tachypnea, otherwise WNL.

Abdomen: Soft, severe tenderness to right lower quadrant with voluntary guarding, no rebound.

Genitalia: No cervical motion tenderness or discharge. No adnexal tenderness.

3. **What are your initial orders?**

Pulse oximetry, cardiac/BP monitoring, urinary pregnancy test, urinalysis, urine culture, CBC, chem 8, LFTs, lipase/amylase, blood cultures, wet mount, gonorrhea/*Chlamydia*, ultrasound of the abdomen/pelvis, IV normal saline, morphine, ondansetron, acetaminophen.

Advance clock:

WBC count elevated with left shift.

Ultrasound: Noncompressible, dilated appendix. Periappendiceal fluid collection. No pelvic pathology.

Other studies WNL.

The patient feels a moderate improvement in her pain and is no longer nauseated.

4. **What are your follow-up actions?**

Coagulation panel, blood type and screen, NPO, IV antibiotics (cefoxitin), surgery consult, appendectomy, admit to inpatient unit, monitor vital signs every 4 hours, CBC and chem 8 next day. Counseling before discharge.

Advance clock:

Case ends.

Critical actions:

Abdominal examination, pelvic examination, IV fluids, antibiotics, appendectomy.

Discussion:

Appendicitis is caused by appendiceal obstruction and subsequent inflammation. In adults this is usually caused by a fecalith, whereas in children it is usually caused by lymphoid hyperplasia from a preceding viral illness. This patient's history and physical examination are classic for appendicitis; however, in women of reproductive age, pregnancy must be excluded and ovarian/pelvic pathology must be considered. A thorough history and physical examination by an experienced clinician may be adequate to diagnose appendicitis in the context of a classic presentation. Advanced imaging is necessary, however, in equivocal cases. In this patient, ultrasound has the benefit of assessing the pelvic organs and can diagnose appendicitis mimics such as tuboovarian abscesses and ovarian torsion. Although ultrasound is specific for appendicitis, it is insensitive, especially in overweight patients. A CT scan is both sensitive and specific but is not as good at evaluating for pelvic pathology. A CT scan also has the disadvantage of radiation exposure. MRI scanning is both sensitive and specific but its availability is limited.

Once a diagnosis of appendicitis is made, the patient should proceed to surgery as soon as possible for an urgent appendectomy. IV fluids are indicated for all septic patients. Antibiotics should be given preoperatively to cover aerobic and anaerobic gram-negative organisms. For simple appendicitis, cefoxitin or ampicillin-sulbactam is often used. Symptom control should also be achieved with IV analgesia and antiemetics (e.g., morphine and ondansetron).

In cases of a contained perforated appendix, patients are often treated with a period of bowel rest and IV antibiotics (e.g., ceftriaxone and metronidazole). They may require percutaneous drainage of infected material and/or delayed appendectomy. Patients with a noncontained perforation are often quite ill with an acute abdomen on physical examination. They require immediate surgical management.

Diagnosis: Acute appendicitis

CASE 62

HPI: A 68-year-old man is brought by ambulance to the ED. Over the past several days he has been gradually getting more short of breath. Previously he could walk a block without feeling winded, but now he feels out of breath while sitting.

Vital signs: Temperature 97.7° F (36.5° C), pulse 110 beats/min, BP 195/98 mm Hg, RR: 35 breaths/min.

Additional history: Hypertension, high cholesterol, previous MI. On hydrochlorothiazide and simvastatin.

1. **What is the differential diagnosis?**
   CHF exacerbation, chronic obstructive pulmonary disease (COPD) exacerbation, pneumonia, pulmonary embolism, pneumothorax.

2. **What components of the physical examination do you perform?**
   General appearance, HEENT, cardiovascular, lungs, abdomen, extremities.
   Physical examination:
   General: Sitting upright in bed, increased work of breathing.
   HEENT: WNL
   Cardiovascular: JVP 10 cm, tachycardia with a regular rhythm, loud S3, displaced point of maximal impulse.
   Lungs: Crackles in bilateral lower and middle lung fields.
   Abdomen: WNL
   Extremities: Bilateral pitting edema 2+ to the knees.

3. **What are your initial orders?**
   Pulse oximetry, BP/cardiac monitor, CBC, chem 8, ECG, troponin, CXR, BNP, furosemide IV, nitroglycerin.
   Advance clock:
   O_2 saturation: 94% on room air.
   ECG: Sinus tachycardia, Q waves in leads II, III, aV_F.
   CXR: Cephalization, alveolar edema, perihilar fullness, and septal lines.
   BNP: 2543 pg/mL
   The patient is still mildly short of breath but feels better.

4. **What are your follow-up actions?**
   Admit to inpatient unit, continuous monitoring, DVT prophylaxis, cardiology consult. Check vital signs every 4 hours, low-sodium diet, troponin every 8 hours. CBC and chem 8 in morning, TTE (reveals left ventricular ejection fraction [EF] of 40%). Aspirin, ACE inhibitor (lisinopril PO), beta-blocker on discharge, counseling (including medication compliance, nutrition), cardiac rehabilitation, follow up in 1 week.
   Advance clock:
   Case ends.
   Critical actions:
   Furosemide, TTE (or measure of left ventricular function), ACE inhibitor, beta-blocker, aspirin, counseling on diet and medication.
   Discussion:
   This patient has newly diagnosed acute decompensated heart failure. The immediate symptoms can be treated by reducing cardiac preload with nitroglycerin and furosemide. Newly diagnosed CHF warrants initiation of aspirin therapy and an ACE inhibitor. EF should be measured, usually via TTE. A beta-blocker, usually carvedilol, should be initiated for EF of 40% or less (but this patient requires a beta-blocker regardless of EF because of his history of MI). Counseling should be part of every case but is particularly important in CHF. An implantable cardiac defibrillator is indicated for prevention of sudden cardiac death in patients with EF of less than 35% despite optimal medical therapy or history of a serious dysrhythmia (ventricular fibrillation/tachycardia) and/or cardiac arrest.
   The initial treatment strategy for acute decompensated heart failure can be remembered by the mnemonic **UNLOAD ME**: **u**pright position, **n**itroglycerin, **l**evophed (if in cardiogenic shock), **o**xygen with noninvasive positive-pressure ventilation (NIPPV), **A**CE inhibitors, **d**iuresis (furosemide), **m**echanical ventilation (if NIPPV does not work), and **e**lectricity (if dysrhythmia is the cause of the decompensation). Just as important as the treatment is consideration of why the patient had new CHF or an exacerbation; consider medication/dietary noncompliance, ischemia, dysrhythmia, new valvular disease, and anemia.
   Diagnosis: Acute decompensated CHF

CASE 63

HPI: A 42-year-old man attends the ED with chest pain. The patient has noticed 1 day of gradually worsening retrosternal chest pain. It has been constant, sharp, and worse when breathing deeply or lying flat.

Vital signs: Temperature 100.0° F (37.8° C), pulse 88 beats/min, BP 110/75 mm Hg, RR 14 breaths/min.
Additional history: 10–pack-year smoker. Drinks three beers a week.

1. **What is the differential diagnosis?**
   Acute coronary syndrome (ACS), pulmonary embolism, pericarditis (with or without myocarditis), pneumothorax.

2. **What components of the physical examination do you perform?**
   General appearance, HEENT, cardiovascular, lungs, abdomen, extremities.
   Physical examination:
      General: Nothing abnormal detected.
      HEENT: WNL
      Cardiovascular: Regular rate and rhythm. Normal S1, S2. High-pitched rub.
      Lungs: WNL
      Abdomen: WNL
      Extremities: WNL

3. **What are your initial orders?**
   Pulse oximetry, BP/cardiac monitoring, CBC, chem 8, PT/PTT, ECG, troponin every 8 hours, CXR, ESR, CRP.
   Advance clock:
   ECG: ST-segment elevations diffusely across all leads. PR segment depression.
   ESR and CRP elevated.
   Other studies WNL.

4. **What are your follow-up actions?**
   Administer ibuprofen, omeprazole. Admit to inpatient unit, check vital signs every 4 hours, TTE. Counseling (including diet and smoking cessation). Discharge home with outpatient follow-up after negative cardiac biomarkers on three occasions and TTE without evidence of large pericardial effusion or tamponade.
   Advance clock:
   Case ends.
   Critical actions:
   Cardiovascular exam, ECG, ibuprofen (or other NSAID).
   Discussion:
   This patient's history and physical examination are suggestive of pericarditis. ECG with diffuse ST-segment elevations and PR depression confirms this diagnosis. The treatment of choice for pericarditis is an NSAID such as ibuprofen. A PPI is also used for GI protection given the large dose of NSAIDs necessary. Colchicine therapy can be started initially but is often reserved for refractory or recurrent cases. Although not always necessary, an echocardiogram can rule out a large or complex pericardial effusion that may necessitate pericardiocentesis. Anticoagulation therapy should be avoided given the possibility of bleeding into a pericardial effusion. An afebrile immunocompetent patient without a large pericardial effusion can usually be safely discharged home. In the USMLE, however, a more conservative approach is rarely penalized. Thus admission with three sets of troponin measurements to rule out ACS and perimyocarditis (in which the inflammation extends into the myocardium) is a reasonable disposition.
   Diagnosis: Pericarditis

CASE 64

HPI: A 65-year-old woman attends the ED with shortness of breath and a cough productive of thick sputum. The symptoms were gradual in onset. She has smoked 1 pack of cigarettes daily for 50 years. About twice yearly she has episodes such as this one that require her to go to the ED.
Vital signs: Temperature 100.0° F (37.8° C), pulse 90 beats/min, BP 135/85 mm Hg, RR 29 breaths/min.
Additional history: No other medical history. No alcohol or drug use.

1. **What is the differential diagnosis?**
   COPD exacerbation, pneumonia, CHF exacerbation, pulmonary embolism, ACS.

2. **What components of the physical examination do you perform?**
   General appearance, HEENT, cardiovascular, lungs, abdomen.
   Physical examination:
   General: Moderately increased work of breathing.
   HEENT: WNL
   Cardiovascular: WNL
   Lungs: Tachypneic, diffuse wheezing, hyperresonance, coarse crackles.
   Abdomen: WNL

3. **What are your initial orders?**
   Pulse oximetry, BP/cardiac monitor, CXR, albuterol, ipratropium.
   Advance clock:
   O_2 saturation: 94% on room air.
   The patient's symptoms are improved. CXR reveals a flattened diaphragm and hyperlucent lung fields.

4. **What are your follow-up actions?**
   Repeat pulmonary examination (decreased wheezing, improved air movement, no increased work of breathing). Steroids (prednisone), antibiotics (azithromycin), counseling (including smoking cessation), follow up in 1 week.
   Advance clock:
   Case ends.
   Critical actions:
   Lung examination, albuterol, ipratropium, steroids, smoking cessation counseling.
   Discussion:
   This patient's acute episode of shortness of breath with a cough and a significant smoking history is consistent with COPD, especially given the history of several prior exacerbations. COPD is characterized by airway inflammation with partially reversible bronchospasm (chronic bronchitis) and pulmonary parenchymal destruction (emphysema). This patient is having an acute COPD exacerbation that is responsive to initial medical management. Treatment for COPD exacerbation includes inhaled albuterol/ipratropium (to address bronchospasm) and a steroid taper (to address inflammation). Because the patient has dyspnea, increased sputum production, and sputum purulence, she is a good candidate for antibiotic therapy. Azithromycin is a common outpatient choice, although more intensive gram-positive coverage with a second- or third-generation cephalosporin in addition to a macrolide is also appropriate. Because the patient greatly improved on albuterol and ipratropium, she is a good candidate for discharge and close follow-up. If the case continued, you could consider pulmonary function tests, pneumococcal vaccine, and influenza vaccine. Long-term management of poorly controlled symptoms may also include long-acting bronchodilators (a beta-agonist such as salmeterol or an anticholinergic agent such as tiotropium), inhaled corticosteroids, supplemental oxygen (if chronic hypoxia is present), and pulmonary rehabilitation.
   Diagnosis: COPD exacerbation

CASE 65

HPI: A 76-year-old man is brought by ambulance to the ED because of chest pain and back pain. Thirty minutes before arrival he was watching television when he experienced 9/10 tearing retrosternal chest pain that radiated to his back. The pain has been constant ever since.
Vital signs: Temperature 98.6° F (37.0° C), pulse 110 beats/min, BP 195/65 mm Hg, RR 20 breaths/min.
Additional history: Hypertension, ran out of medications.

1. **What is the differential diagnosis?**
   Aortic dissection, ACS, hypertensive emergency, pulmonary embolism, pneumothorax, pericarditis.

2. **What components of the physical examination do you perform?**
   General appearance, HEENT, cardiovascular, lungs.
   Physical examination:
   General: Visible discomfort from chest pain.
   HEENT: WNL
   Cardiovascular: Tachycardia.
   Lungs: WNL

3. **What are your initial orders?**
   Pulse oximetry, BP/cardiac monitoring, CBC, chem 8, coagulation panel, ECG, troponin, D-dimer, blood type and screen, CXR, morphine. When stable, chest CT with contrast (or TEE).
   Advance clock:
   CXR: Widened mediastinum.
   CT scan: Ascending aortic dissection.
   Follow-up: The patient's symptoms are improved. BP 135/70 mm Hg.

4. **What are your follow-up actions?**
   Esmolol drip IV, surgery consult, surgical repair of aortic dissection, admit to ICU, continuous monitoring, check vital signs every 2 hours, additional BP control if needed, CBC, chem 8 in the morning, counseling.
   Advance clock:
   Case ends.
   Critical actions:
   Cardiovascular examination, TEE or chest CT scan, esmolol or labetalol, morphine, surgical consult.
   Discussion:
   This patient has a history and physical examination suggestive of aortic dissection. Classically, pain from aortic dissection is sharp or tearing in quality, may radiate to the back, and may be associated with unequal pulses (or unequal BPs). To confirm the diagnosis, you should obtain a CT scan (if the patient is stable) or TEE if the patient is unstable. The presence of an ascending aortic dissection (type A) is a surgical emergency. You should stabilize the patient with IV beta-blockers and immediately ask for a thoracic surgery consult. An esmolol drip (or other beta-blocker) is the medication of choice to control BP and heart rate with a systolic BP goal of 100 to 120 mm Hg and a heart rate of 60 beats/min or lower. If the patient requires further antihypertensive therapy after high-dose beta-blockers, nitroprusside or nicardipine administration can be initiated. It is important not to start those medications first, however, because reflex tachycardia from the afterload reduction can increase wall stress and make the dissection worse.
   Unlike BP reduction strategies in most situations, systolic BP can and should be reduced to 100 to 120 mm Hg regardless of the initial BP (recall that in most cases of elevated BP, the mean arterial pressure should not be reduced acutely by more than 25% because of the risk of decreased cerebral perfusion). Aortic dissection can be complicated by cardiac tamponade (if the dissection extends into the pericardium), MI (if the dissection extends into the coronary arteries, usually the right coronary artery), aortic regurgitation, stroke (carotid artery extension), or limb ischemia.
   Morphine should be given because the patient is in pain. If this were a dissection of the descending aorta (type B), then medical management with BP control would be warranted. Uncomplicated descending dissections are not surgical emergencies, but surgical or endovascular repair should be considered.
   Diagnosis: Aortic dissection

CASE 66

HPI: A 23-year-old woman attends the clinic complaining of heavy vaginal bleeding. She has had irregular periods over the past 10 months, many of which were heavier than usual or lasted longer than usual. She occasionally has intermenstrual bleeding. She takes no medications. She is sexually active with one partner and uses condoms. She does not desire immediate fertility.

Vital signs: Temperature 97.2° F (36.2° C), pulse 92 beats/min, BP 135/78 mm Hg, RR 17 breaths/min.

Additional history: No medical history. No use of tobacco, drugs, or alcohol.

1. **What is the differential diagnosis?**
   DUB, polycystic ovary syndrome (PCOS), endometriosis, uterine fibroid, endometrial polyp, pregnancy (with possible pathology such as threatened abortion).

2. **What components of the physical examination do you perform?**
   General appearance, skin, lymph nodes, HEENT, cardiovascular, lungs, abdomen, genitalia, extremities, neuro/psych.
   Physical examination:
   General: No acute distress.
   Skin: Acne.
   HEENT: Mild hirsutism.
   Lymph nodes: WNL
   Cardiovascular: WNL
   Lungs: WNL
   Abdomen: Obese abdomen, soft, nontender.
   Genitalia: WNL
   Extremities/neuro/psych: WNL

3. **What are your initial orders?**
   Pulse oximetry, urinary pregnancy test, CBC, chem 8, PT/PTT, serum testosterone, DHEAS, luteinizing hormone (LH), follicle-stimulating hormone (FSH), TSH, 17-hydroxyprogesterone, prolactin, fasting lipid panel, Hb A_{1C}, pelvic ultrasound.
   Advance clock:
   Urinary pregnancy test negative, testosterone elevated, elevated LH/FSH ratio, ultrasound reveals polycystic ovaries. Other studies WNL.

4. **What are your follow-up actions?**
   Counseling (including diet, weight loss, exercise), OCP, follow up in 8 weeks.
   Advance clock:
   The patient's symptoms are greatly improved.
   Critical actions:
   Assessment of hyperandrogenism (physical examination and/or serum testosterone), OCP (if patient does not desire fertility), counseling (including weight loss).
   Discussion:
   PCOS is diagnosed according to the presence of two of the three Rotterdam criteria: (1) oligo/anovulation, (2) hyperandrogenism, and (3) polycystic ovaries. Oligoanovulation manifests as irregular menses. Hyperandrogenism may manifest as hirsutism, acne, virilization, or deepening of the voice. A serum testosterone level can confirm the presence of hyperandrogenism. Polycystic ovaries are diagnosed using ultrasound.
      The patient should be evaluated for other causes of oligomenorrhea such as prolactinoma and hypothyroidism. Recall that elevated prolactin downregulates gonadotropin-releasing hormone, causing amenorrhea. Furthermore, hypothyroidism causes increased TRH, which stimulates prolactin release, in turn causing amenorrhea. Checking TSH and prolactin levels can screen for these conditions. Checking DHEAS assesses whether an androgen-secreting tumor is the cause of hirsutism. You should also consider diagnosing and treating common comorbidities of PCOS by checking a lipid panel and Hb A_{1C}.
      Treatment for all patients with PCOS begins with weight loss to attempt to restore normal ovulation and menstruation. For those who do not desire immediate fertility, OCPs can regulate menstruation and reduce hirsutism. An antiandrogen (spironolactone) can be added for persistent hirsutism. Metformin should be added for patients with T2DM.
      In patients with PCOS who desire fertility, consultation with a gynecologist is recommended. Treatment includes weight loss, clomiphene (induces ovulation), and metformin.
   Diagnosis: PCOS

CASE 67

HPI: A 55-year-old male attends the ER with rapid-onset severe pain in his right knee that started 4 hours ago. The pain is now so severe that he can barely put weight on the knee. The patient also noted some swelling and stiffness of the joint over the past several days. He denies fever, trauma, or recent infection.

Vital signs: Temperature 99.1° F (37.3° C), pulse 90 beats/min, BP 135/75 mm Hg, RR 14 breaths/min.

Additional history: Takes hydrochlorothiazide for hypertension. No use of tobacco or drugs. Drinks three glasses of wine daily.

1. **What is the differential diagnosis?**

   Septic arthritis, gout, pseudogout, hemarthrosis, OA, meniscal tear.

2. **What components of the physical examination do you perform?**

   General appearance, skin, HEENT, cardiovascular, lungs, abdomen, extremities, neuro/psych.

   Physical examination:

   General: No acute distress.
   Skin/HEENT: WNL
   Cardiovascular: WNL
   Lungs: WNL
   Abdomen: WNL
   Extremities: Moderate swelling of the right knee. Decreased range of motion and inability to bear weight secondary to pain.
   Neuro/psych: WNL

3. **What are your initial orders?**

   Knee x-ray, knee arthrocentesis (with Gram stain, culture, cell count with differential, crystal analysis), CBC, chem 8, PT/PTT.

   Advance clock:

   Knee arthrocentesis: 23,000 WBCs/mL, needle-shaped negatively birefringent crystals, Gram stain negative. Other studies WNL.

4. **What are your follow-up actions?**

   Naproxen (the patient's symptoms greatly improve), discontinue hydrochlorothiazide, counseling (including diet and alcohol cessation), follow up in 2 weeks, uric acid level at follow-up.

   Advance clock:

   Case ends.

   Critical actions:

   Extremity examination, arthrocentesis, NSAID, discontinue hydrochlorothiazide.

   Discussion:

   This patient has acute monoarticular arthritis. Septic arthritis should be assumed until proven otherwise, and arthrocentesis should not be delayed. The presence of needle-shaped negatively birefringent crystals is diagnostic of gout. Synovial WBCs may be elevated to a count that can range from 1000 to 50,000 cells/mL in inflammatory conditions, whereas WBC counts greater than 50,000 cells/mL are suggestive of septic arthritis.

   Gout is caused by an inflammatory response to monosodium urate crystals in the joint space. Ninety percent of cases involve in the first metatarsophalangeal joint, but any joint may be affected. NSAIDs are the first-line treatment modality for acute episodes of gout. Oral colchicine and steroids are second- and third-line agents, respectively, but are often avoided because of their side-effect profiles. They can be used in patients who cannot tolerate NSAIDs or who have insufficient relief of symptoms. Thiazide diuretics should be discontinued because they decrease the renal clearance of uric acid. Patients should also be counseled on dietary triggers. A uric acid level can be checked 2 weeks after the episode (because it may be falsely low during the acute event). Patients with elevated uric acid and repeated attacks may take a urate-lowering drug such as allopurinol. Allopurinol therapy should not be started, however, during an acute flare.

   Diagnosis: Gout

CASE 68

HPI: A 29-year-old woman attends the clinic complaining of 5 weeks of diarrhea and mild cramping pain in her lower abdomen. She has been passing around four loose stools per day that are streaked with blood and mucus. She has not been out of the country or camping recently and has no sick contacts.

Vital signs: Temperature 98.2° F (36.8° C), pulse 82 beats/min, BP 125/75 mm Hg, RR 17 breaths/min.

Additional history: No medical history. No use of tobacco, alcohol, or drugs.

1. **What is the differential diagnosis?**
   Infectious colitis, ulcerative colitis, Crohn disease, celiac disease, diverticulitis, giardiasis, amoebiasis.

2. **What components of the physical examination do you perform?**
   General appearance, skin, lymph nodes, HEENT, cardiovascular, lungs, abdomen, rectal, extremities, neuro/psych.
   Physical examination:
   General: No acute distress.
   Skin/lymph nodes/HEENT: WNL
   Cardiovascular: WNL
   Lungs: WNL
   Abdomen: Mild tenderness of the left lower quadrant.
   Rectal: Blood and stool in the rectal vault.
   Extremities: WNL
   Neuro/psych: WNL

3. **What are your initial orders?**
   Pulse oximetry, CBC, chem 8, LFTs, lipase, urinary pregnancy test, stool culture, stool WBC count, stool ova and parasites, ESR, CRP, colonoscopy.
   Advance clock:
   Hb 10.9 mg/dL, fecal WBCs present, mildly elevated ESR and CRP, all other laboratory tests WNL.
   Colonoscopy with rectal biopsy: Continuous inflammation of the rectum with friability. Biopsy consistent with ulcerative colitis.

4. **What are your follow-up actions?**
   Mesalamine suppository, counseling, follow up in 2 weeks.
   Advance clock:
   The patient's symptoms are greatly improved.
   Case ends.
   Critical actions:
   Abdominal examination, colonoscopy, 5-aminosalicylic acid (5-ASA) agent (mesalamine).
   Discussion:
   This patient has bloody diarrhea and cramping abdominal pain consistent with colitis. Radiation colitis can be ruled out by history, but infectious colitis should be worked up with stool studies. ESR and CRP help determine severity of disease, and a pregnancy test is always a good idea in a woman of reproductive age. A colonoscopy is the best way to differentiate between the other causes of colitis. In this case it is consistent with ulcerative colitis. Initial therapy consists of mesalamine suppositories (or enema if inflammation extends beyond the rectum). Persistent symptoms can be treated with topical steroids (e.g., hydrocortisone) or oral mesalamine. Systemic steroids are indicated if the patient is having a severe flare (more than five stools daily, severe pain, fever, tachycardia, or ESR >30 mm/hour). The evaluation and treatment of mild Crohn disease are very similar, although oral rather than rectal 5-ASA agents are preferred and the oral corticosteroid budesonide is considered a first-line agent.
   Diagnosis: Ulcerative colitis

CASE 69

HPI: A 19-year-old woman (gravida 1 para 0) at 38+0 weeks of gestation attends the ED complaining of intermittent blurry vision and a frontal headache that has not responded to acetaminophen. The headache has been present for 4 hours and is gradually worsening. The pregnancy has been uncomplicated to this point, and the patient has had regular prenatal care. She denies abdominal pain, contractions, loss of fluids, or vaginal bleeding. She takes a prenatal vitamin, but otherwise takes no medications.

Vital signs: Temperature 97.9° F (36.6° C), pulse 91 beats/min, BP 165/100 mm Hg, RR 19 breaths/min.

Additional history: No medical history. No use of tobacco, drugs, or alcohol.

1. **What is the differential diagnosis?**

   Pregnancy-induced hypertension (gestational hypertension), chronic hypertension, pre-eclampsia, HELLP syndrome (**h**emolysis, **e**levated **l**iver enzymes, **l**ow **p**latelets, and right upper quadrant or epigastric **p**ain).

2. **What components of the physical examination do you perform?**

   General appearance, skin/HEENT, cardiovascular, lungs, abdomen, genitalia, extremities, neuro/psych.

   Physical examination:
   General: No acute distress.
   Skin/HEENT: WNL
   Cardiovascular: WNL
   Lungs: WNL
   Abdomen: Fundal height 38 cm, nontender.
   Genitalia: Cervix soft and dilated to 4 cm, 60% effaced, fetal station −1. No pooling of
     fluids. Cephalic presentation.
   Extremities: Edema 1+ in lower extremities.
   Neuro/psych: WNL

3. **What are your initial orders?**

   Pulse oximetry, BP/cardiac monitor, CBC, chem 8, PT/PTT, LFTs, uric acid, LDH, blood type and screen, urinalysis, 24-hour urinary protein, urine output, fetal ultrasound, fetal monitor, magnesium sulfate IV, labetalol IV, obstetrics consult.

   Advance clock:
   O_2 saturation: 100% on room air.
   Repeat vital signs: BP 128/80 mm Hg.
   Blood type O positive, urinalysis protein 2+, laboratory tests otherwise WNL.
   Symptoms are greatly improved.

4. **What are your follow-up actions?**

   Admit to inpatient unit, induction of labor (oxytocin or misoprostol), counseling.

   Advance clock:
   Case ends.

   Critical actions:
   Genital examination, neurologic exam, urinalysis, urine output monitoring, fetal monitoring, magnesium IV, obstetrics consult.

   Discussion:
   Any gravid woman with symptoms suggestive of preeclampsia (headache, blurry vision, right upper quadrant pain, oliguria, edema) should be promptly evaluated for hypertension, protein-uria, thrombocytopenia, elevated liver enzymes, and hemolysis (LDH/uric acid). Preeclampsia is defined by BP greater than 140/90 mm Hg with proteinuria. BP greater than 160/110 or the presence of symptoms is sufficient for the diagnosis of severe preeclampsia. Treatment includes seizure prophylaxis using magnesium and BP control with labetalol or hydralazine. Once the patient is stabilized, the only definitive treatment is delivery. Because this patient is full term and has a favorable cervix, induction of labor is a reasonable approach; however, prolonged inductions should be avoided, and cesarean section is indicated if the baby cannot be delivered within a reasonable period of time. Induction can be achieved with oxytocin or misoprostol; however, on an exam, credit will be given if you simply consult obstetrics. Antenatal corticosteroids are indicated for gestational ages greater than 34 weeks. Blood type should be determined for all gravid women, and Rho(D) immune globulin (RhoGAM) should be administered within 72 hours of delivery if the mother is rhesus (Rh)-negative.

   Diagnosis: Preeclampsia

CASE 70

HPI: A 72-year-old man attends the clinic with leg pain. He describes an ache in both calves that occurs after walking two city blocks. If he rests the pain goes away, but further activity brings the pain back. His legs become uncomfortable when he props them up and are relieved by dangling them over the edge of the bed. He denies numbness or weakness. He has a 50-pack-year smoking history and continues to smoke. He does not exercise and has a sedentary lifestyle.

Vital signs: Temperature 97.9° F (36.6° C), pulse 72 beats/min, BP 120/78 mm Hg, RR 16 breaths/min.

Additional history: No alcohol or drug use. History of hypertension, well controlled on hydrochlorothiazide.

1. **What is the differential diagnosis?**
   Peripheral arterial disease (PAD), spinal stenosis, peripheral neuropathy, venous insufficiency, Raynaud phenomenon.

2. **What components of the physical examination do you perform?**
   General appearance, HEENT, cardiovascular, lungs, abdomen, extremities.
   Physical examination:
   General: No acute distress.
   HEENT: WNL
   Cardiovascular: WNL
   Lungs: WNL
   Abdomen: WNL
   Extremities: Hair loss and shiny skin over bilateral lower extremities. Thick toenails. Faint dorsalis pedis and posterior tibial pulses. Lower-extremity pallor with passive leg raise. Sensation and strength intact. No ulcerations.

3. **What are your initial orders?**
   Pulse oximetry, ankle-brachial index (ABI), Hb A_{1C}, fasting lipid panel, ECG, vascular surgery consult.
   Advance clock:
   ABI 0.8, elevated LDL, all other studies WNL.

4. **What are your follow-up actions?**
   Aspirin PO, statin PO, counseling (including smoking cessation and exercise), follow up in 1 month.
   Advance clock:
   Case ends.
   Critical actions:
   Extremity examination, ABI, lipid profile, aspirin, counseling.
   Discussion:
   This patient has bilateral lower extremity aching provoked by exercise and relieved by rest. This is the classic presentation of claudication, which represents exercise-induced limb ischemia due to atherosclerotic disease. PAD is a manifestation of atherosclerotic disease that is usually present throughout the vascular system. Claudication is the peripheral equivalent of angina from CAD. Risk factors include age, tobacco use, diabetes mellitus (DM), hypertension, and hyperlipidemia.
   Physical examination often reveals shiny, hairless skin over the lower legs with decreased pulses and brittle nails. ABI is the systolic BP in the leg divided by the systolic BP in the arm. It provides information on the presence and severity of disease (normal is >0.9). ABI can also be used to track progression of disease. It should be interpreted with care, however, in patients with calcified vessels, as occurs in DM. Calcified vessels are less compressible and may result in falsely high ankle systolic BP, leading to false negative ABIs. All patients should be assessed for critical limb ischemia, which manifests as the five Ps (pain at rest, pulselessness, palor, paresthesia, paralysis, and poikilothermia [cold]). A cold, pulseless foot is an emergency that requires initiation of anticoagulation therapy (heparin drip) and an emergent vascular surgery consult.
   Treatment for ABI begins with risk factor modification to prevent progression of disease. Smoking cessation and an exercise regimen can improve symptoms and prevent progression of disease. Assessment for and control of BP, hyperlipidemia, and diabetes are also important in disease management. Aspirin reduces disease progression and the risk of stroke and MI, which often occur together in vasculopathic patients. Clopidogrel (in place of aspirin), pentoxifylline, and cilostazol may also be considered for patients with PAD. New-onset PAD warrants a consultation with a vascular specialist to identify any need for procedural revascularization including stenting or bypass grafting.
   Diagnosis: PAD

CASE 71

HPI: A 29-year-old woman (gravida 1 para 0) at 9 weeks of gestation attends the clinic complaining of intractable nausea and vomiting. She has been vomiting four or five times daily for the past 10 days. Today she has been unable to drink or eat anything without immediately vomiting. She has lost 4 kg in weight since her last visit. The pregnancy has been uncomplicated up to this point. She takes no medications other than a prenatal vitamin. She denies fever, chills, constipation, diarrhea, and abdominal pain.

Vital signs: Temperature 98.4° F (36.9° C), pulse 111 beats/min, BP 120/80 mm Hg, RR 17 breaths/min.

Additional history: No medical history. No tobacco, drugs, or alcohol use.

1. What is the differential diagnosis?

   Hyperemesis gravidarum, viral gastroenteritis, pyelonephritis, cholecystitis, appendicitis, hepatitis.

2. What components of the physical examination do you perform?

   General appearance, skin, lymph nodes, HEENT, cardiovascular, lungs, abdomen, genitalia, extremities, neuro/psych.

   Physical examination:

   General: Mild distress due to nausea. Dry mucous membranes.
   Skin/lymph nodes/HEENT: WNL
   Cardiovascular: Tachycardic, regular rhythm.
   Lungs: WNL
   Abdomen: WNL
   Genitalia: WNL
   Extremities: WNL
   Neuro/psych: WNL

3. What are your initial orders?

   Pulse oximetry, CBC, chem 8, orthostatic vital signs, fetal ultrasound, urinalysis, ondansetron IV, normal saline IV.

   Advance clock:

   Urinalysis ketones 2+, otherwise studies WNL.
   The patient's symptoms have mildly improved, but she is still unable to tolerate fluids without emesis.

4. What are your follow-up actions?

   Admit to ward, pyridoxine, doxylamine, ondansetron, repeat chem 8 and urinalysis, counseling.

   Advance clock:

   Urinalysis WNL with no ketones.
   The patient's symptoms have greatly improved. She is able to tolerate a full diet.
   Case ends.

   Critical actions:

   Abdominal examination, IV fluids, antiemetics.

   Discussion:

   Nausea and vomiting are common symptoms during pregnancy, although other intraabdominal processes should also be considered in the differential diagnosis. When pregnancy-induced vomiting causes dehydration, weight loss, or ketonuria, it is on the severe side and is termed *hyperemesis gravidarum*. Diagnostic criteria for hyperemesis gravidarum include weight loss of greater than 5% of the prepregnancy weight and prolonged severe nausea and vomiting, after ruling out other causes. It is thought to be caused by the emetogenic properties of human chorionic gonadotropin (hCG) and other hormonal changes in pregnancy. It normally starts at 4 weeks of gestation and resolves by 20 weeks. Evaluation should include orthostatic vital signs, chem 8, and urinalysis to assess ketonuria. Treatment of all nausea and vomiting in pregnancy begins with IV fluids as needed. Mild symptoms can be treated with dietary changes alone. Pyridoxine with doxylamine is considered first-line therapy for mild to moderate symptoms. Persistent symptoms are usually treated with ondansetron. Other agents considered safe in pregnancy include diphenhydramine, prochlorperazine, and metoclopramide. Patients are stable for discharge home when any ketonuria resolves, they can tolerate PO, and their symptoms are controlled without IV medications.

   Diagnosis: Hyperemesis gravidarum

CASE 72

HPI: A 19-year-old woman attends the ED complaining of 2 days of abdominal pain in the right lower quadrant. The pain was gradual in onset and associated with one episode of vomiting. She has had a moderate amount of green vaginal discharge. The patient came to the ED today because she thought she had a fever.

Vital signs: Temperature 102.6° F (39.2° C), pulse 115 beats/min, BP 122/80 mm Hg, RR 14 breaths/min.

Additional history: Sexually active with one male partner. No tobacco, alcohol, or drug use.

1. What is the differential diagnosis?

   Acute appendicitis, ectopic pregnancy, PID, septic abortion, pyelonephritis, ovarian torsion, ruptured ovarian cyst.

2. What components of the physical examination do you perform?

   General appearance, skin, lymph nodes, HEENT, cardiovascular, lungs, abdomen, genitalia, extremities, neuro/psych.

   Physical examination:
   General: Moderate distress secondary to pain.
   Skin/lymph nodes/HEENT: WNL
   Cardiovascular: Tachycardia.
   Lungs: WNL
   Abdomen: Soft, moderate tenderness in the right lower quadrant without guarding or rebound.
   Genitalia: Right adnexal tenderness, positive cervical motion tenderness, moderate mucopurulent discharge from the cervical os.

3. What are your initial orders?

   Pulse oximetry, cardiac/BP monitor, urinary pregnancy test, urinalysis, urine culture, CBC, chem 8, LFTs, lipase, amylase, blood cultures, wet mount, *Gonococcus*, *Chlamydia*, abdomen/pelvis ultrasound, IV fluids, cefoxitin IV, doxycycline PO, morphine, ondansetron, acetaminophen.

   Advance clock:
   WBC: 14.0 x10³/μL
   Urinary pregnancy test: Negative.
   Gonococcus antigen: Positive.
   Ultrasound: Thickening of fallopian tube. No tuboovarian abscess.
   The patient feels mild improvement, but remains in significant pain. She continues to be nauseated.
   Temperature 101.1° F (38.4° C), pulse 101 beats/min, BP 130/82 mm Hg, RR 13 breaths/min.

4. What are your follow-up actions?

   Admit to inpatient unit, check vital signs every 4 hours, HIV antibody test, rapid plasma reagin (RPR). CBC and chem 8 next day. Counseling (including safe sex and partner treatment). Discharge home when vital signs are normalized, symptoms have improved, and the patient is tolerating food.

   Advance clock:
   Case ends.

   Critical actions:
   CBC, abdominal examination, pelvic examination, IV fluids, testing for sexually transmitted illnesses, antibiotics for gonorrhea and *Chlamydia*.

   Discussion:
   PID is an ascending infection that spreads from the lower genital tract to involve the uterus, fallopian tubes, ovaries, and/or peritoneum. It typically begins with the sexually transmitted organisms *N. gonorrhoeae* and *Chlamydia trachomatis*, although PID is a polymicrobial process and must be treated as such. The differential for lower abdominal pain and pelvic pain is broad in female patients. We can substantially limit our differential immediately by ruling out pregnancy. PID is a clinical diagnosis that is suggested by the physical examination (adnexal tenderness, cervical motion tenderness, mucopurulent cervical discharge). Diagnostic tests can support the diagnosis, especially if they detect gonorrhea or *Chlamydia*. Ultrasound can provide further evidence of PID while assessing for other conditions in the differential

diagnosis (appendicitis, ovarian cyst, ovarian torsion). Ultrasound can also evaluate potential complications such as tuboovarian abscess.

Because the patient is septic with significant symptoms, she meets admission criteria and will need IV antibiotics that cover *N. gonorrhoeae* and *C. trachomatis*. IV cefoxitin with PO doxycycline is a common inpatient regimen that provides coverage for gram-negative enteric organisms, streptococci, and anaerobes. Outpatients are more commonly treated with a single dose of IM ceftriaxone and a course of PO doxycycline. Patients should also be tested for other sexually transmitted infections, and their sexual partners should be treated.

Diagnosis: PID

CASE 73

HPI: A 47-year-old man attends the clinic complaining of decreased energy. For the past 6 weeks he has felt like he lacks his normal amount of energy. He has been waking early in the morning and having trouble getting back to sleep. He believes that this has affected his concentration and caused him to perform poorly at work. He feels sad most days. He denies hallucinations, delusions, past manic episodes, suicidal ideation, and homicidal ideation. He has not recently experienced the death of a loved one.

Vital signs: Temperature 98.2° F (36.8° C), pulse 65 beats/min, BP 115/75 mm Hg, RR 17 breaths/min.

Additional history: No medical history. No tobacco, alcohol, or drug use.

1. What is the differential diagnosis?

   Major depressive disorder, dysthymia, adjustment disorder, bipolar disorder, hypothyroidism, anemia, substance abuse disorder.

2. What components of the physical examination do you perform?

   General appearance, skin, lymph nodes, HEENT, cardiovascular, lungs, abdomen, extremities, neuro/psych.

   Physical examination:
   General: No acute distress.
   Skin/lymph nodes/HEENT: WNL
   Cardiovascular: WNL
   Lungs: WNL
   Abdomen: WNL
   Extremities: WNL
   Neuro/psych: Depressed mood/affect. No focal neurologic deficits.

3. What are your initial orders?

   CBC, TSH, citalopram, no-suicide contract, follow up in 2 weeks, therapy, counseling.
   Advance clock:
   Studies WNL.
   The patient's symptoms are improved.
   Advance clock:
   Case ends.
   Critical actions:
   Thorough physical examination, CBC, TSH, antidepressant (selective serotonin reuptake inhibitor [SSRI] or serotonin-norepinephrine reuptake inhibitor [SNRI]), follow up.
   Discussion:
   This patient has depressed mood/affect, guilt, sleep disturbance, low energy, and poor concentration. These symptoms have caused functional impairment and lasted for longer than 2 weeks. *The Diagnostic and Statistical Manual of Mental Disorders*, fifth edition (DSM V), did not change the criteria for major depressive disorder; the diagnosis remains depressed mood for more than 2 weeks that is a change in baseline and causes impaired function and specific symptoms. The specific symptoms are at least five of the following eight, which can be remembered by the mnemonic **SIG E CAPS**: (1) **s**leep changes, (2) **i**nterest loss (anhedonia), (3) **g**uilt, (4) **e**nergy decrease, (5) **c**ognition/concentration reduction, (6) **a**ppetite decrease, (7) **p**sychomotor changes (agitation or lethargy), and (8) **s**uicide/death preoccupation. The symptoms are not due to loss of a loved one (grief reaction) or a substance (substance-induced mood disorder). This fits the diagnostic criteria for depression. Laboratory

studies can rule out nonpsychological causes of these symptoms, including anemia and hypothyroidism. Treatment can begin with psychotherapy, counseling, and an SSRI or SNRI. Symptoms may not improve for 4 to 6 weeks despite appropriate therapy. It is important to schedule regular follow-up to reassess for suicidal thinking.

Diagnosis: Depression

CASE 74

HPI: A 45-year-old woman attends the clinic complaining of several months of gradually worsening joint pain and stiffness. The pain mostly affects the small joints of her hands and has recently included her wrists as well. Both the right and left sides are affected equally. The patient finds the pain and stiffness worse in the morning. Her symptoms are somewhat improved by activity. She notes occasional swelling of the affected joints. She has not had any rash or fever.

Vital signs: Temperature 99.0° F (37.2° C), pulse 79 beats/min, BP 115/75 mm Hg, RR 16 breaths/min.

Additional history: No medical history. No tobacco, alcohol, or drug use.

1. **What is the differential diagnosis?**

   Rheumatoid arthritis (RA), osteoarthritis (OA), psoriatic arthritis, systemic lupus erythematosus (SLE), fibromyalgia, gout, Lyme disease.

2. **What components of the physical examination do you perform?**

   General appearance, skin, lymph nodes, HEENT, cardiovascular, lungs, abdomen, extremities, neuro/psych.

   Physical examination:
   General: No acute distress.
   Skin/lymph nodes/HEENT: WNL
   Cardiovascular: WNL
   Lungs: WNL
   Abdomen: WNL
   Extremities: Tenderness to palpation over interphalangeal, metacarpophalangeal (MCP), and wrist joints, with moderate swelling and effusion present. Subcutaneous nodules over MCP joints. No visible bony deformities. Decreased range of motion in wrists bilaterally.
   Neuro/psych: WNL

3. **What are your initial orders?**

   Pulse oximetry, CBC, chem 14, ESR, CRP, RF, cyclic citrullinated peptide antibody (anti-CCP), x-ray of affected joints, ibuprofen (or other NSAID), synovial fluid analysis (cell count, crystals, bacterial culture).

   Advance clock:
   CBC mild anemia, ESR and CRP elevated. RF strongly positive, anti-CCP positive. Other studies WNL.

4. **What are your follow-up actions?**

   Rheumatology consult, counseling, methotrexate or other disease-modifying antirheumatic drug (DMARD), physical therapy, occupational therapy, exercise, follow up in 4 weeks.

   Advance clock:
   The patient's symptoms have improved.
   Case ends.

   Critical actions:
   Extremities examination, analgesia (NSAIDs or acetaminophen), methotrexate (or other DMARD).

   Discussion:
   This patient has gradual onset of symmetric joint pain, morning stiffness, and inflammation suggestive of RA. RA usually involves smaller joints, especially of the hands and feet. Wrists, elbows, shoulders, knees, and hips may also be affected. Involvement of the distal interphalangeal joints is more suggestive of OA. The presence of effusions and rheumatoid nodules in this patient are highly suggestive of RA and should trigger a laboratory assessment for this

condition. There is no test that is both sensitive and specific for RA, but several laboratory tests can suggest the disease. Anti-CCP is the most specific test at greater than 90%, but it is not sensitive. RF is 70% sensitive and 85% specific. Other nonspecific findings include increased ESR and CRP and the presence of microcytic anemia. Synovial fluid may reveal mild inflammation and may be useful in distinguishing from septic arthritis and gout when these are in the differential diagnosis. X-rays may reveal osteopenia, joint space narrowing, and deformities consistent with RA.

Barring contraindications, most patients with undifferentiated arthritis will benefit from therapy with NSAIDs. Once a diagnosis of RA has been established, initiation of DMARD therapy will not only improve symptoms but will also prevent progression of disease. Methotrexate is the most frequently used DMARD, but leflunomide, sulfasalazine, and hydroxychloroquine also have efficacy. In acute flares, a brief course of corticosteroids may be indicated. Patients with severe or refractory disease should be evaluated for treatment with a biologic agent such as etarnecept (TNF-alpha antagonist). Patients on biologic agents are at higher risk of infectious complications. Counseling, physical therapy, and occupational therapy all play a role in disease management as well.

Diagnosis: RA

CASE 75

HPI: A 23-year-old woman (gravida 1 para 0) at 36 weeks of gestation attends the ED complaining of vaginal bleeding. The bleeding started approximately 6 hours ago and has included passage of clots. She does not think that her water has broken, but she has been experiencing frequent contractions. She admits using cocaine several times during the pregnancy, including earlier today. She takes no medications other than a prenatal vitamin.

Vital signs: Temperature 98.8° F (37.1° C), pulse 90 beats/min, BP 118/74 mm Hg, RR 19 breaths/min.

Additional history: No medical history. Smokes two packs of cigarettes per week. Uses cocaine twice per month. No alcohol.

1. **What is the differential diagnosis?**
   Placental abruption, placenta previa, preterm labor.

2. **What components of the physical examination do you perform?**
   General appearance, skin, lymph nodes, HEENT, cardiovascular, lungs, abdomen, genitalia, extremities, neuro/psych.
   Physical examination:
   General: No acute distress.
   Skin/lymph nodes/HEENT: WNL
   Cardiovascular: WNL
   Lungs: WNL
   Abdomen: Fundal height 34 cm; fundus is mildly tender and feels firm.
   Genitalia: Scant blood at the vaginal introitus.
   Extremities: WNL
   Neuro/psych: WNL

3. **What are your initial orders?**
   Pulse oximetry, CBC, chem 8, PT/PTT, blood type and screen, urine toxicology, fetal ultrasound, fetal monitoring.
   Advance clock:
   Blood type O positive, Hb 11.3 mg/dL, ultrasound reveals placental abruption, fetal monitoring reveals late decelerations. Other studies WNL except urine toxicology, which is positive for cocaine.

4. **What are your follow-up actions?**
   Obstetric consult, cesarean section, child protection services, social work consult, counseling (including drug and tobacco counseling).
   Advance clock:
   Case ends.

Critical actions:
Fetal ultrasound, fetal monitoring, CBC, blood type and screen, toxicology screen, obstetrics consult, social work consult, counseling.

Discussion:
In an examination setting, third-trimester vaginal bleeding can usually be identified as placenta previa or placental abruption. Placenta previa is abnormal implantation of the placenta in the lower uterine segment. The classical presentation is **painless vaginal bleeding** with or without contractions. Placental abruption is abnormal separation of the placenta before delivery. The classical presentation is **painful vaginal bleeding** with contractions.

In both instances, patients should undergo a thorough physical examination. If placenta previa is suspected, speculum and digital examinations are contraindicated because they can cause hemorrhage. Laboratory tests should assess hemoglobin/hematocrit, PT/PTT, and alloimmunization (Rh) status. RhoGAM should be given if fetal-maternal hemorrhage has occurred and the mother is Rh-negative. Fetal ultrasound is very reliable in diagnosing placenta previa, although it is not sensitive enough to rule out placental abruption.

Continuous fetal monitoring can assess fetal distress or stability. In placental abruption, a fetus at less than 34 weeks of gestation can be delivered vaginally if stable or via cesarean section if unstable. In this patient, late decelerations indicate fetal distress so emergent cesarean section is indicated. Placental abruption can cause DIC, so coagulation parameters should be monitored.

Diagnosis: Placental abruption

CASE 76

HPI: A 70-year-old woman attends the ED with a headache. The headache was gradual in onset and is located in the right temporal region. It has continued to worsen over the last 12 hours and seems to worsen when the patient tries to eat. She has never had a previous headache like this. She denies fevers or neck stiffness, but reports muscle aches at her shoulders and hips. She has had no visual changes or recent trauma.

Vital signs: Temperature 98.0° F (36.7° C), pulse 71 beats/min, BP 118/75 mm Hg, RR 16 breaths/min.

Additional history: No medical history. No tobacco, drugs, or alcohol use. No recent psychosocial stressors.

1. **What is the differential diagnosis?**
   Temporal arteritis, intracerebral hemorrhage, neoplasm, tension headache, migraine.

2. **What components of the physical examination do you perform?**
   General appearance, skin, lymph nodes, HEENT, cardiovascular, lungs, abdomen, genitalia, extremities, neuro/psych.
   Physical examination:
   General: No acute distress.
   Skin/lymph nodes/HEENT: Tenderness over the right temporal artery.
   Cardiovascular: WNL
   Lungs: WNL
   Abdomen: WNL
   Genitalia: WNL
   Extremities: Tenderness over shoulders and hips.
   Neuro/psych: WNL

3. **What are your initial orders?**
   Pulse oximetry, CBC, chem 8, ESR, CRP, noncontrast head CT scan.
   Advance clock:
   ESR 110 mm/h, CRP 10 mg/dL, other studies WNL.

4. **What are your follow-up actions?**
   Prednisone, admit to ward, temporal artery biopsy (reveals temporal arteritis), rheumatology consult, repeat ESR, counseling.
   Advance clock:
   Symptoms greatly improved.
   Case ends.

Critical actions:
HEENT/neurologic exam, ESR and/or CRP, immediate prednisone, temporal artery biopsy.
Discussion:
New onset of headaches in the elderly should prompt a thorough evaluation for underlying pathology. This patient's historical features of new-onset temporal headache with jaw claudication are suggestive of temporal arteritis (giant cell arteritis). The presence of temporal artery tenderness further suggests the diagnosis, especially in the setting of elevated ESR/CRP. For individuals younger than 50 years, temporal arteritis essentially never occurs; the mean age at diagnosis is 70 years. The patient's history of proximal muscle pain also indicates she may have polymyalgia rheumatica, which frequently coexists with temporal arteritis (approximately 50% of patients with temporal arteritis also have or develop polymyalgia rheumatica). Temporal artery biopsy is indicated for formal diagnosis, but treatment with corticosteroids should not be delayed because biopsy results are not significantly altered if biopsy is performed within 1 to 2 weeks of starting therapy. If treatment is delayed, spread to the ophthalmic artery can cause irreversible vision loss. Serial ESR measurement can track the response to treatment. Any visual symptoms warrant consultation with an ophthalmologist.
   Diagnosis: Temporal arteritis (giant cell arteritis)

CASE 77

HPI: A 29-year-old woman attends the ED because of epigastric abdominal pain that radiates to her back. The pain was gradual in onset but has been constant and severe for 8 hours. The patient has had nausea and vomiting, but denies fever or diarrhea.
Vital signs: Temperature 99.0° F (37.2° C), pulse 105 beats/min, BP 135/85 mm Hg, RR 16 breaths/min.
Additional history: No medical history. No use of tobacco, alcohol, or drugs.

1. What is the differential diagnosis?
   Peptic ulcer disease, cholecystitis, pancreatitis, esophageal spasm, AAA.

2. What components of the physical examination do you perform?
   General appearance, HEENT, cardiovascular, lungs, abdomen, rectal.
   Physical examination:
      General: Moderate distress due to pain, dry mucous membranes.
      HEENT: WNL
      Cardiovascular: Mild tachycardia.
      Lungs: WNL
      Abdomen: Tenderness to epigastric palpation without rebound or guarding.
      Rectal: WNL

3. What are your initial orders?
   Pulse oximetry, cardiac/BP monitor, CBC, chem 14, lipase, urinalysis, urinary pregnancy test, morphine, ondansetron, IV normal saline, NPO.
   Advance clock:
   Lipase 1129 U/L, all other laboratory tests WNL.
   Pain moderately improved.

4. What are your follow-up actions?
   Abdominal ultrasound, fasting lipid panel (reveals extremely elevated triglycerides), LDH, lactate, CT scan of the abdomen/pelvis with contrast. Admit to ward. Gemfibrozil PO, morning CBC/chem 14. Advance diet as tolerated, follow up in 1 week. Counseling
      Advance clock:
   Case ends.
   Critical actions:
   Abdominal examination, lipase, fasting lipid panel, abdominal ultrasound, IV fluids.
   Discussion:
   This patient has epigastric abdominal pain radiating to the back. A focused physical examination and laboratory assessment for intraabdominal pathology reveal a lipase level that is diagnostic of pancreatitis (three times the upper normal limit). All patients with pancreatitis

should receive IV fluids, pain control, and antiemetics. They should initially be NPO (although there is increasing evidence that early feeding, when tolerated, is safe). Glucose and electrolytes (especially calcium) should be closely monitored. A diagnosis of pancreatitis should trigger evaluation of the cause. In the United States, gallstones, alcohol, medications, and triglycerides are the most common identifiable causes. Alcohol and medications can be ruled out by history. Gallstones should be evaluated using ultrasound, and triglycerides can be identified with lipid panel measurement. As triglyceride levels increase above 500 mg/dL there is a progressive risk of pancreatitis. Gemfibrozil is the agent of choice in this situation because it effectively lowers triglyceride levels. In this case, an LDH test was ordered to calculate a Ranson score for prognosis. A CT scan is not always necessary but can be used in cases of diagnostic uncertainty, suspected complications, or lack of clinical improvement. Patients may be safely discharged home when pain is controlled, vital signs and electrolytes are normalized, and they are tolerating food. Patients with gallstone pancreatitis should have cholecystectomy with common bile duct exploration during the same hospitalization if they are surgical candidates. Patients with necrotizing pancreatitis are often treated with prophylactic antibiotics to prevent superinfection.

Diagnosis: Pancreatitis

CASE 78

HPI: A 71-year-old man attends the ED with 10/10 intensity periumbilical abdominal pain. One hour before his arrival he was walking to the kitchen when he had sudden onset of abdominal pain radiating to his back. The patient felt dizzy at that time and had to lie down. The pain has been constant since then.

Vital signs: Temperature 98.8° F (37.1° C), pulse 110 beats/min, BP 100/75 mm Hg, RR 20 breaths/min.

Additional history: 25–pack-year smoker, hypertension on hydrochlorothiazide, hyperlipidemia on simvastatin.

1. **What is the differential diagnosis?**
   Abdominal aortic aneurysm (AAA), ACS, pancreatitis, small bowel obstruction (SBO).

2. **What components of the physical examination do you perform?**
   General appearance, HEENT, cardiovascular, lungs, abdomen, extremities, rectal.
   Physical examination:
   General: Diaphoretic. Visible discomfort from pain.
   HEENT: WNL
   Cardiovascular: Tachycardia.
   Lungs: WNL
   Abdomen: Palpable pulsatile abdominal mass.
   Extremities: WNL
   Rectal: WNL

3. **What are your initial orders?**
   Pulse oximetry, BP/cardiac monitoring, CBC, chem 8, LFTs, lipase, coagulation panel, urinalysis, troponin, ECG, blood type and crossmatch, CXR, abdominal ultrasound.
   Advance clock:
   Ultrasound: 7-cm AAA.
   All other studies WNL

4. **What are your follow-up actions?**
   Surgical consult, surgical repair of AAA.
   Admit to ICU; check vital signs every 2 hours, CBC every 4 hours, chem 8 in the morning.
   Counseling: activity, diet, smoking cessation.
   Advance clock:
   Case ends.
   Critical actions:
   Abdominal examination, surgical consult, surgical repair of AAA.
   Discussion:
   This patient has a ruptured AAA. The chief complaint and physical examination should prompt you to stabilize the patient and order a rapid imaging modality such as ultrasound

or a CT scan to assess for an aneurysm. IV fluids and blood products can be used to treat hypotension, although there is evidence that the BP should be kept relatively low as long as the patient is stable to prevent further bleeding. An immediate surgical consult and repair are required. The patient should be admitted to the ICU after the surgery. A number of other routine tests can (and should) be ordered, but you should not wait for the results before proceeding with emergent surgical management.

An AAA is an abdominal aortic diameter of greater than 3 cm. Surgical or endovascular repair is generally indicated for any symptomatic aneurysm, an aneurysm larger than 5 cm, or a rapidly enlarging aneurysm. Smaller AAAs can be monitored with serial ultrasound or CT scans. One-time screening is recommended for men of 65 to 75 years of age who have ever smoked. Most AAAs are caused by atherosclerosis but some are caused by connective tissue disorders such as Marfan syndrome and Ehlers-Danlos syndrome. The most common modifiable risk factors are cigarette smoking and hypertension. The mortality rate for ruptured AAAs is very high and the condition should always be considered in any older patient with abdominal pain, back pain, hypotension, or syncope. A ruptured AAA can be mistaken for renal colic in older patients, but a new-onset kidney stone in an older patient without a history of this complaint is uncommon; hematuria can even be the presenting symptom for ruptured AAAs.

Diagnosis: AAA

CASE 79

HPI: A 76-year-old man attends the ED with palpitations. He says he has been having palpitations on and off for a week. Recently he has felt his heart racing extremely fast and has been feeling increasingly weak and short of breath. The patient denies chest pain, fever, and loss of consciousness. He has never had similar symptoms before.

Vital signs: Temperature 98.2° F (36.8° C), pulse 155 beats/min, BP 115/80 mm Hg, RR 17 breaths/min.

Additional history: History of hypertension on hydrochlorothiazide. No drug, tobacco, or alcohol use.

1. What is the differential diagnosis?
   Stable tachycardia: AF, atrial flutter, supraventricular tachycardia (SVT), sinus tachycardia, stable ventricular tachycardia.

2. What components of the physical examination do you perform?
   General appearance, HEENT, cardiovascular, lungs, abdomen, extremities.
   Physical examination:
   General: Mild distress due to palpitations.
   HEENT: WNL
   Cardiovascular: Tachycardic, irregularly irregular rhythm.
   Lungs: WNL
   Abdomen: WNL
   Extremities: WNL

3. What are your initial orders?
   Pulse oximetry, cardiac/BP monitor, ECG, CBC, chem 8, troponin, TSH, CXR.
   Advance clock:
   ECG reveals irregularly irregular narrow complex tachycardia without P-waves.
   Other studies WNL.

4. What are your follow-up actions?
   Atrioventricular (AV) nodal blocking agent (metoprolol), warfarin, admit patient to ward, morning ECG, CBC, chem 8, PT/PTT, TTE, counseling.
   Advance clock:
   TTE reveals dilated right atrium without valvular pathology.
   Heart rate 98 beats/min, patient's symptoms greatly improved.
   Case ends.
   Critical actions:
   Cardiac examination, ECG, rate-controlling agent, anticoagulation therapy.

Discussion:
The patient has AF with rapid ventricular response (RVR). Any patient with hemodynamic instability and AF with RVR should undergo immediate synchronized cardioversion. Patients who have been in AF for less than 48 hours can also undergo cardioversion with low risk of thromboembolism.

Because this patient is stable and has been in AF for longer than 48 hours, he is not a good candidate for cardioversion. His symptoms are probably due to his RVR, and because he does not have underlying causes of tachycardia (e.g., GI bleed, sepsis, CHF), he will benefit from rate control with an AV nodal blocking agent (usually metoprolol or diltiazem).

The major long-term risk associated with AF is thromboembolic disease. This can manifest as stroke, mesenteric ischemia, or limb ischemia. The **CHADS$_2$** score can be used to calculate the long-term risk of stroke. One point is assigned for the presence of **C**HF, **h**ypertension, **a**ge older than 75 years, and **d**iabetes. Two points are assigned if a prior stroke has occurred. Patients with a score of 0 or 1 may take aspirin for stroke prevention, whereas patients with two or more risk factors qualify for anticoagulation therapy (usually with warfarin). This patient has two risk factors (age and hypertension) so he qualifies for anticoagulation therapy. Another management option in this case would involve TEE followed by synchronized cardioversion if no cardiac thrombus is present.

Secondary causes of AF such as electrolyte abnormalities, hyperthyroidism, and structural cardiac problems such as atrial enlargement should be investigated for all new diagnoses of AF. Long-term rate control (to keep the heart rate at <110 beats/min) is beneficial and should be targeted.

Diagnosis: AF with RVR

CASE 80

HPI: A 23-year-old woman attends the clinic because it has been 6 weeks since her last menstrual period. She usually has periods regularly every 28 days that last for 4 days with a moderate flow. She had menarche at 13 years of age and has never been pregnant. The patient is sexually active with one male partner and intermittently uses condoms. She has no history of sexually transmitted infection. She has never had a Pap smear.

Vital signs: Temperature 98.2° F (36.8° C), pulse 77 beats/min, BP 108/70 mm Hg, RR 14 breaths/min.

Additional history: No medical history. Drinks three beers daily. No tobacco or drug use.

1. **What is the differential diagnosis?**
   Amenorrhea due to pregnancy, PCOS, hypothyroidism, hypothalamic amenorrhea, pituitary adenoma, premature ovarian failure.

2. **What components of the physical examination do you perform?**
   General appearance, skin, lymph nodes, HEENT, cardiovascular, lungs, abdomen, genitalia, extremities, neuro/psych.
   Physical examination:
   General: No acute distress.
   Skin/lymph nodes/HEENT: WNL
   Cardiovascular: WNL
   Lungs: WNL
   Abdomen: WNL
   Genitalia: WNL
   Extremities: WNL
   Neuro/psych: WNL

3. **What are your initial orders?**
   Urinary pregnancy test.
   Advance clock:
   Urinary pregnancy test positive. The patient states that this is a desired pregnancy.

4. **What are your follow-up actions?**
   CBC, blood type and screen, Pap smear, RPR, *Chlamydia/gonococcus* screening, hepatitis B surface antigen, HIV antibody test, rubella serology, varicella antibody, TSH, purified protein derivative, Hb A$_{1C}$, urinalysis, urine culture, fetal ultrasound, folic acid PO, obstetrics/gynecology consult, counseling (including alcohol cessation), follow up in 4 weeks.

Advance clock:
Ultrasound reveals intrauterine pregnancy, dating consistent with last menstrual period.
   Case ends.
Critical actions:
Pregnancy test, counseling.
Discussion:
Although the differential for amenorrhea is broad, you should always consider pregnancy first. A thorough physical examination is indicated for amenorrhea, although it rarely can establish the cause on its own. Urine and serum tests for beta-hCG are extremely sensitive and specific for pregnancy. Once you have determined the patient has a desired pregnancy, early prenatal care is important. Establishing dates is most accurate by counting from the first day of the last menstrual period (if known). If this date is not known, an ultrasound can estimate the gestational age.

   Although various guidelines and practitioners have slightly different recommendations, a conservative approach to laboratory testing includes CBC, blood type and screen, urinalysis, urine culture, rubella status, hepatitis B, HIV, syphilis, gonorrhea, *Chlamydia*, Pap smear, TSH, and HbA$_{1C}$. Folic acid supplementation is indicated, although ideally it should have been started before the pregnancy occurred. Thorough counseling is indicated for all patients. Routine follow-up is usually scheduled every 4 weeks for the first 28 weeks, every 2 weeks from 28 to 36 weeks, and weekly after 36 weeks.
   Diagnosis: Uncomplicated pregnancy

CASE 81

HPI: A 27-year-old man attends the ED with acute onset of chest pain and shortness of breath. Twenty minutes ago he was watching television when he noticed sudden onset of shortness of breath. His chest pain is severe and worsens every time he inhales deeply.
Vital signs: Temperature 97.7° F (36.5° C), pulse 125 beats/min, BP 92/60 mm Hg, RR 32 breaths/min.
Additional history: No medical history. An 8–pack-year smoking history.

1. **What is the differential diagnosis?**
   Pulmonary embolism, pericarditis, pneumothorax (tension), aortic dissection.

2. **What components of the physical examination do you perform?**
   General appearance, cardiovascular, lungs.
   Physical examination:
      General: Severe respiratory distress, pale.
      Cardiovascular: Tachycardic, weak peripheral pulses.
      Lungs: Trachea is deviated. No breath sounds on the right side, right side hyperresonance
         on percussion.

3. **What are your initial orders?**
   Needle thoracostomy, pulse oximetry, oxygen, normal saline, BP/cardiac monitor.
   Advance clock:
   A rush of air is heard after needle placement, the patient's symptoms greatly improve, and his breathing normalizes.
   O$_2$ saturation 100%, repeat vital signs WNL.

4. **What are your follow-up actions?**
   Chest tube, CXR, morphine, ECG, CBC, chem 8, admit to inpatient unit, surgery consult, repeat CXR in morning, counseling.
   Advance clock:
   Repeat CXR with resolved pneumothorax. Chest tube to water seal shows no air leak. Laboratory tests WNL.
      Case ends.
   Critical actions:
   Lung examination, immediate needle thoracostomy, chest tube, CXR after chest tube placement.
   Discussion:
   The patient's history of acute onset of pleuritic chest pain and shortness of breath should alert you to a likely pneumothorax. A simple pneumothorax is a nonexpanding collection of

air between the visceral and parietal pleura without respiratory or hemodynamic instability. A tension pneumothorax is an expanding pneumothorax with respiratory or hemodynamic compromise. Tension pneumothorax usually leads to some of the following signs: unilateral absence of breath sounds, deviated trachea, hyperresonance on percussion, distended neck veins, hypoxia, and hypotension. This patient has a primary spontaneous tension pneumothorax. Timing is extremely important in this case. As soon as the absent breath sounds are noted, the patient should be treated immediately with needle thoracostomy. There should be no delay for laboratory analysis, imaging, or a complete physical examination. Once the patient has been stabilized, a chest tube should be placed and a CXR should be ordered to confirm placement. A surgical consult is also appropriate. If the case continues, admit the patient for monitoring and maintain the chest tube until the pneumothorax has resolved and the chest tube to water seal has no air leak.

Diagnosis: Tension pneumothorax

CASE 82

HPI: A 59-year-old male attends the clinic complaining of gradual-onset right knee pain over the past 7 months. The pain is an ache that is usually present, but worsens on exercise. The patient has had mild stiffness of the joint over the previous months. He denies fever, weight loss, or trauma.

Vital signs: Temperature 98.6° F (37.0° C), pulse 75 beats/min, BP 125/73 mm Hg, RR 14 breaths/min.

Additional history: No medical history. No use of tobacco, alcohol, or drugs.

1. **What is the differential diagnosis?**
   OA, ligamentous injury, meniscal tear, RA, gouty arthritis.

2. **What components of the physical examination do you perform?**
   General appearance, skin, HEENT, cardiovascular, lungs, abdomen, genitalia, extremities, neuro/psych.
   Physical examination:
   General: No acute distress.
   Skin/HEENT: WNL
   Cardiovascular: WNL
   Lungs: WNL
   Abdomen: WNL
   Genitalia: WNL
   Extremities: Antalgic gait. Decreased range of motion with crepitus in the right knee. No
       joint line tenderness. Negative anterior drawer, posterior drawer, and Lachman tests.
   Neuro/psych: WNL

3. **What are your initial orders?**
   Knee x-ray.
   Advance clock:
   X-ray reveals joint space narrowing with osteophytes, subchondral sclerosis, and subchondral cysts. Other studies WNL.

4. **What are your follow-up actions?**
   Acetaminophen, physical therapy, NSAIDs, counseling.
   Advance clock:
   The patient's symptoms are greatly improved.
       Case ends.
   Critical actions:
   Extremity examination, acetaminophen and/or NSAID.
   Discussion:
   This patient has monoarticular arthritis consistent with OA according to his history and physical examination. Plain x-ray films also reveal the four classic radiographic findings for OA: (1) joint space narrowing, (2) osteophytes, (3) subchondral sclerosis, and (4) subchondral cysts. Although every monoarticular arthritis should be considered a septic joint until proven otherwise, the patient's chronic course makes this extremely unlikely. Furthermore the presentation

is so classic for OA that the need for further workup with rheumatologic studies and advanced imaging is not necessary. A trial with acetaminophen with or without NSAIDs is the best first step. Physical therapy is also helpful in strengthening the relevant muscles and improving flexibility. If the patient's symptoms were not controlled with these basic modalities, an MRI scan may be indicated to evaluate for ligamentous or meniscal injury of the knee. Other treatment modalities include weight loss, intraarticular glucocorticoids, narcotics (short course), and glucosamine (although there is no strong evidence that glucosamine is beneficial). For persistent pain, referral to an orthopedist and evaluation for total knee arthroplasty are indicated.

Diagnosis: OA

CASE 83

HPI: A 52-year-old man arrives at the ED complaining of severe abdominal pain in the left lower quadrant for 10 hours. He has had two episodes like this in the past, but they were not as painful and he chose not to seek medical attention. He denies nausea, vomiting, diarrhea, or blood in his stool.

Vital signs: Temperature 101.3° F (38.5° C), pulse 95 beats/min, BP 125/80 mm Hg, RR 14 breaths/min.

Additional history: No medical history. No use of tobacco, alcohol, or drugs.

1. **What is the differential diagnosis?**
   Diverticulitis, acute appendicitis, GI malignancy, inflammatory bowel disease (IBD), UTI, prostatitis.

2. **What components of the physical examination do you perform?**
   General appearance, HEENT, cardiovascular, lungs, abdomen, rectal.
   Physical examination:
   General: No acute distress.
   HEENT: WNL
   Cardiovascular: WNL
   Lungs: WNL
   Abdomen: Severe tenderness over left lower quadrant. No rebound or guarding.
   Rectal: WNL

3. **What are your initial orders?**
   Pulse oximetry, cardiac/BP monitor, CBC, chem 8, LFTs, lipase, urinalysis, morphine, acetaminophen.
   Advance clock:
   O_2 saturation 100%.
   WBC x 10^3/μL count 12.2, all other tests WNL.
   Pain and fever improved, but the patient continues to have moderate pain in the left lower quadrant.

4. **What are your follow-up actions?**
   CT scan of the abdomen/pelvis (reveals diverticulitis without phlegmon, stricture, or obstruction). Start metronidazole PO and ciprofloxacin PO for 10 days. Counseling before discharge (including dietary counseling), follow up in 1 week. Colonoscopy at 6 weeks.
   Advance clock:
   Case ends.
   Critical actions:
   Abdominal examination, ciprofloxacin/metronidazole (or other appropriate antibiotics), follow-up colonoscopy.
   Discussion:
   This patient has left lower quadrant pain suggestive of acute abdominal pathology including diverticulitis. It is reasonable to order a set of laboratory tests and treat his pain and fever first, but because he has severe tenderness without a known diagnosis of diverticulosis, a CT scan of the abdomen/pelvis is important to evaluate for other pathology. The CT scan reveals diverticulitis without complications (phlegmon, stricture, obstruction), the patient's pain is well controlled, and he does not have a high fever. Because these conditions are met, oral

antibiotics and discharge home are appropriate. If he had a high fever, complications revealed by the CT scan, severe pain, or other concerning features, inpatient admission with IV antibiotics (ceftriaxone/metronidazole) would be more appropriate. A phlegmon requires interventional radiology or surgical drainage. A stricture or obstruction requires a surgical consult.

After an episode of diverticulitis is treated, all patients need colon cancer screening with colonoscopy because carcinoma of the colon with perforation can mimic diverticulitis clinically and on CT scans. Colonoscopy should be avoided during active diverticulitis because of the increased risk of perforation. A nonurgent surgical consultation is appropriate for recurrent cases of diverticulitis.

Diagnosis: Diverticulitis

CASE 84

HPI: A 43-year-old-man with a medical history of schizophrenia is brought to the ED by ambulance. He is accompanied by his caregiver, who explains that this morning the patient was found in bed unresponsive and sweating. When she tried to rouse him she noticed he felt "stiff as a board." His symptoms of schizophrenia had been under moderate control after his physician recently doubled his dose of haloperidol. Before presentation, the patient was interactive and ambulatory. His prior auditory hallucinations had resolved.

Vital signs: Temperature 104.2° F (40.1° C), pulse 115 beats/min, BP 164/94 mm Hg, RR 24 breaths/min.

Additional history: No other medical history or medications. No use of drugs, tobacco, or alcohol.

1. **What is the differential diagnosis?**
   Neuroleptic malignant syndrome, meningitis, encephalitis, sepsis, catatonic schizophrenia, malignant hyperthermia, serotonin syndrome, dystonic reaction.

2. **What components of the physical examination do you perform?**
   General appearance, HEENT, cardiovascular, lungs, abdomen, extremities, neuro/psych.
   Physical examination:
      General: Ill-appearing man, diaphoretic, tremulous. Protecting his airway without increased work of breathing.
      HEENT: WNL
      Cardiovascular: Tachycardic, otherwise WNL.
      Lungs: Tachypneic.
      Abdomen: WNL
      Extremities: Lead pipe rigidity of all extremities.
      Neuro/psych: Eyes open, nonresponsive to questioning, moves extremities in response to pain.

3. **What are your initial orders?**
   Pulse oximetry, CBC, chem 14, serum CK, urinalysis, CXR, CSF studies (protein, glucose, cell count, Gram stain and culture), discontinue haloperidol, acetaminophen, normal saline IV, bromocriptine, dantrolene.
   Advance clock:
   Laboratory tests reveal CK 3670 U/L. Urinalysis positive for myoglobin. All other studies WNL.

4. **What are your follow-up actions?**
   Serial laboratory tests: CK, chem 14, CBC.
   Admit to ICU.
   Advance clock:
   Case ends.
   Critical actions:
   Neurologic examination, discontinuation of haloperidol, supportive measures (cooling and IV fluids), ICU admission, consideration of bromocriptine/dantrolene.
   Discussion:
   Neuroleptic malignant syndrome is a rare emergent condition caused by the use of dopamine antagonists (usually antipsychotic agents). Dopamine antagonism at the hypothalamus causes

autonomic dysfunction, hyperthermia, lead pipe rigidity, and altered mental status. Any patient on antipsychotic medication may be affected. Higher risk is associated with high-potency drugs, high dosage, or rapid escalation of dosing of antidopaminergic medications.

The differential diagnosis is broad for any patient with fever and altered mental status. Meningitis should be considered and generally should be evaluated using a lumbar puncture. Other infectious causes should be evaluated via urinalysis and CXR. Other toxic causes should be investigated where indicated (e.g., serotonin syndrome, malignant hyperthermia [inhaled anesthetics/succinylcholine], alcohol withdrawal). Treatment for neuroleptic malignant syndrome is primarily supportive, with airway protection, IV fluids, cooling measures, and assessment for rhabdomyolysis. In cases of severe muscle rigidity, treatment is started with bromocriptine (dopamine agonist) and dantrolene (skeletal muscle relaxant).

Diagnosis: Neuroleptic malignant syndrome

CASE 85

HPI: A 52-year-old white woman attends her primary care doctor for a BP check. She has had no recent medical issues, but her BP has been elevated the last two times she was in the office. It has remained elevated despite dietary changes and increased exercise.

Vital signs: Temperature ° F (36.5° C), pulse 78 beats/min, BP 158/98 mm Hg, RR 16 breaths/min.

Additional history: No medical history. Smokes one pack of cigarettes daily.

1. What is the differential diagnosis?
   Essential hypertension, hyperthyroidism, renal artery stenosis, pheochromocytoma.

2. What components of the physical examination do you perform?
   General appearance, skin, lymph nodes, HEENT, lungs, cardiovascular, abdomen, extremities, neuro/psych.
   Physical examination:
   General: No acute distress.
   Skin/lymph nodes/HEENT: WNL
   Cardiovascular: WNL
   Lungs: WNL
   Abdomen: WNL
   Extremities: WNL
   Neuro/psych: WNL

3. What are your initial orders?
   CBC, chem 8, ECG, lipid panel, urinalysis, first-line antihypertensive agent (i.e., thiazide diuretic for most patients), follow up in 1 month, counseling (diet, exercise, smoking cessation).
   Advance clock:
   Repeat BP 152/92 mm Hg. All studies WNL.

4. What are your follow-up actions?
   Add a second antihypertensive agent (e.g., lisinopril, losartan, atenolol, felodipine), follow up in 1 month.
   Advance clock:
   Repeat BP 120/80 mm Hg, no new symptoms.
   Case ends.
   Critical actions:
   First-line antihypertensive agent, add a second agent if BP not controlled; provide counseling, schedule follow-up.
   Discussion:
   Stage 1 hypertension is defined as BP 140-159/90-99 mm Hg measured on more than one occasion. Stage 2 hypertension is defined as BP 160/100 mm Hg or greater. To diagnose hypertension, BP should be measured twice on each of two separate office visits. Stage 1 hypertension can be managed initially with a trial of diet modification and exercise. In patients with stage 2 hypertension or comorbidities (e.g., diabetes or renal disease), early pharmacologic management is preferred.

Because this patient has no comorbidities, a thiazide diuretic (hydrochlorothiazide) is a good first choice. The patient's BP is still not controlled at the follow-up visit, so a second agent such as an ACE inhibitor, ARB, beta-blocker, or calcium channel blocker should be added. If the patient had attended with stage 2 hypertension (BP >160/100 mm Hg), two agents could be started simultaneously. See Chapter 4 for more detail.

Diagnosis: Chronic hypertension

CASE 86

HPI: A 56-year-old man attends the ED because of five episodes of coffee ground emesis over the past 8 hours. He has had two episodes like this in the past 12 months, but never so severe. The patient has also noted a black, tarry quality to his stool. He began to feel weak and dizzy so he called 911.

Vital signs: Temperature 98.6° F (37.0° C), pulse 119 beats/min, BP 115/75 mm Hg, RR 16 breaths/min.

Additional history: Never sought medical care previously. Drinks 1 pt of vodka daily. No NSAID use.

1. **What is the differential diagnosis?**
   Bleeding varices, bleeding peptic ulcer, gastric cancer, erosive gastritis, Mallory-Weiss tear.

2. **What components of the physical examination do you perform?**
   General appearance, HEENT, cardiovascular, lungs, abdomen, rectal.
   Physical examination:
   General: Pale, temporal wasting, scleral icterus.
   HEENT: WNL
   Cardiovascular: Tachycardic.
   Lungs: WNL
   Abdomen: Soft, nontender, moderate distention with shifting dullness and positive fluid wave.
   Rectal: Melena.

3. **What are your initial orders?**
   Pulse oximetry, cardiac/BP monitor, CBC, chem 8, LFTs, PT/PTT, blood type and crossmatch, lipase/amylase, IV normal saline, IV pantoprazole, ceftriaxone, octreotide, ondansetron, NPO.
   Advance clock:
   Hb 6.0 mg/dL, INR 1.3.
   Reassess: The patient's vital signs have normalized and symptoms improved.

4. **What are your follow-up actions?**
   RBC transfusion, gastroenterology consult, upper GI tract endoscopy, admit to ICU, CBC every 4 hours, abdominal ultrasound. Decrease CBC frequency when stabilized and discontinue ceftriaxone and octreotide. Transition to oral PPI. Counseling before discharge, including alcohol cessation. Follow up in 1 week.
   Advance clock:
   Case ends.
   Critical actions:
   Abdominal examination, IV fluids, upper GI tract endoscopy, pantoprazole, octreotide, ceftriaxone, counseling.
   Discussion:
   This patient has an upper GI tract bleed. After a focused physical examination, resuscitation should begin given the patient's tachycardia. IV fluids and blood products should be given as needed until his vital signs improve. A PPI drip should be started for all upper GI tract bleeds. Given the patient's stigmata for liver disease (temporal wasting, scleral icterus, shifting dullness and fluid wave), variceal bleeding is a likely source. Octreotide is indicated for variceal bleeds for splanchnic vasoconstriction. Ceftriaxone should be given to all patients with cirrhosis and an upper GI tract bleed. Upper GI tract endoscopy with variceal ligation is the definitive management and should not be delayed. If the case continues, you can admit the patient to the ICU, monitor for improvement, deescalate care, image for cirrhosis, and schedule close follow-up. When the patient is stable, he should be given counseling, including alcohol cessation.
   Diagnosis: Upper GI tract bleed

CASE 87

HPI: A 31-year-old woman attends the clinic complaining of watery diarrhea for the past 14 days. She complains of approximately four loose, foul-smelling stools daily. The patient has mild cramping abdominal pain, but denies blood or mucus in her stool. She has had no fever or vomiting. She returned from a business trip to South America 2 weeks ago.

Vital signs: Temperature 97.7° F (36.5° C), pulse 90 beats/min, BP 122/82 mm Hg, RR 17 breaths/min.

Additional history: No medical history. No tobacco, alcohol, or drug use.

1. What is the differential diagnosis?

   Giardiasis, amoebiasis, traveler's diarrhea, foodborne illness, intestinal parasitism, *Clostridium difficile*.

2. What components of the physical examination do you perform?

   General appearance, skin, lymph nodes, HEENT, cardiovascular, lungs, abdomen, genitalia, rectal, extremities, neuro/psych.

   Physical examination:
   General: No acute distress.
   Skin/lymph nodes/HEENT: WNL
   Cardiovascular: WNL
   Lungs: WNL
   Abdomen: Hyperactive bowel sounds; no tenderness, rebound, or guarding.
   Genitalia/rectal: WNL
   Extremities: WNL
   Neuro/psych: WNL

3. What are your initial orders?

   Pulse oximetry, fecal WBCs, stool ova and parasites, stool culture, stool *Giardia* antigen, C. *difficile* toxin, counseling (including oral hydration).

   Advance clock:
   Giardia antigen positive, stool ova and parasites positive for *Giardia*, other laboratory tests WNL.

4. What are your follow-up actions?

   Metronidazole PO, counseling, oral hydration, follow up in 2 weeks.

   Advance clock:
   Case ends.

   Critical actions:
   Abdominal examination, stool ova and parasites, metronidazole, counseling.

   Discussion:
   This patient has diarrhea after travelling abroad. Infectious sources should be at the top of your differential diagnosis. Most cases of diarrhea are due to viral illness. Viral gastroenteritis is usually self-limited and does not necessitate any laboratory evaluation. In this case, the prolonged time course and associated cramping indicate a possible parasitic cause and should trigger a laboratory evaluation with stool studies. This patient's studies are positive for *Giardia*, which can be treated with metronidazole. A similar case presentation may appear for many patients with infectious diarrhea. The physical examination and laboratory evaluation are all the same. If this patient happened to be positive for *Entamoeba histolytica*, the treatment would be the same (metronidazole). If the case were consistent with enterotoxigenic *E. coli* (2 to 4 days of profuse watery diarrhea while travelling), the patient could be treated with ciprofloxacin. If it were most consistent with a viral cause, the patient could be treated with oral hydration alone.

   Diagnosis: Acute diarrhea due to giardiasis

CASE 88

HPI: A 25-year-old woman attends the ED with severe abdominal pain in the left lower quadrant and scant vaginal bleeding that has progressively worsened over the past 5 hours. She has never had similar symptoms before. She denies fevers, vomiting, and diarrhea.

Vital signs: Temperature 98.2° F (36.8° C), pulse 110 beats/min, BP 100/70 mm Hg, RR 18 breaths/min.

Additional history: No medical history, sexually active with one male partner.

1. What is the differential diagnosis?

   PID, ectopic pregnancy, fibroids, endometriosis, appendicitis, diverticulitis, ovarian torsion, ovarian cyst.

2. What components of the physical examination do you perform?

   General appearance, skin, HEENT, cardiovascular, lungs, abdomen, genitalia.

   Physical examination:

   General: Moderate distress secondary to pain.

   Skin/HEENT: WNL

   Cardiovascular: Tachycardic.

   Lungs: WNL

   Abdomen: Tenderness over left lower quadrant.

   Genitalia: Scant blood from closed os, tenderness over left adnexa.

3. What are your initial orders?

   Pulse oximetry, BP/cardiac monitor, urinary pregnancy test, IV fluids, CBC, chem 8, PT/PTT, blood type and screen.

   Advance clock:

   Pulse 120 beats/min, BP 90/60 mm Hg.

   Positive urinary pregnancy test, Hemoglobin 10.1 mg/dL, blood type O negative.

4. What are your follow-up actions?

   Serum beta-hCG (4200 mIU/mL), pelvic ultrasound (free pelvic and peritoneal fluid, empty uterus). Gynecology consult, RhoGAM, laparoscopy (left salpingectomy performed), admit to inpatient unit, continuous monitoring, CBC every 4 hours, counseling.

   Advance clock:

   Case ends.

   Critical actions:

   Abdominal/genitalia examination, beta-hCG, pelvic ultrasound, blood type and screen, RhoGAM, laparoscopy.

   Discussion:

   This Rh-negative woman has a ruptured ectopic pregnancy. The differential diagnosis is initially broad; however, early assessment for pregnancy greatly narrows the possibilities. After initial stabilization, you should quickly confirm the pregnancy is ectopic. Occasionally the ectopic pregnancy itself can be visualized on ultrasound, but this is unnecessary for diagnosis. An empty uterus with a beta-hCG level above the discriminatory zone (usually 2000 mIU/mL) corresponds to a high degree of suspicion for an ectopic pregnancy, and an urgent obstetrics/gynecology consult is required. Because this patient has unstable vital signs and free peritoneal fluid according to ultrasound, the ectopic pregnancy has probably already ruptured and will require laparoscopy. Stable patients with small, unruptured ectopic pregnancies may qualify for methotrexate therapy. Because this patient is Rh-negative, she should be treated with RhoGAM to prevent alloimmunization. Of note, RhoGAM is given to Rh-negative women at 28 weeks and during episodes of fetal-maternal hemorrhage.

   Diagnosis: Ruptured ectopic pregnancy

CASE 89

HPI: A 76-year-old man attends the clinic with a chief complaint of fatigue. He has been increasingly tired over the past 5 months and recently felt as if he could barely walk outside to collect his mail. He denies fever, shortness of breath, and chest pain. He has noticed a slight maroon color to his stool recently.

Vital signs: Temperature 97.7° F (36.5° C), pulse 90 beats/min, BP 120/85 mm Hg, RR 19 breaths/min.

Additional history: No medical history. No tobacco, drugs, or alcohol use.

1. What is the differential diagnosis?

   Lower GI tract bleeding due to colorectal cancer, angiodysplasia, diverticulosis, arteriovenous (AV) malformation, hemorrhoids.

   Upper GI tract bleeding due to peptic ulcer disease, gastritis, varices, malignancy.

2. **What components of the physical examination do you perform?**
General appearance, skin, lymph nodes, HEENT, cardiovascular, lungs, abdomen, genitalia, rectal, extremities, neuro/psych.
Physical examination:
General: No acute distress.
Skin/lymph nodes/HEENT: WNL
Cardiovascular: WNL
Lungs: WNL
Abdomen: WNL
Genitalia/rectal: Maroon-colored stool, no palpable masses.
Extremities: WNL
Neuro/psych: WNL

3. **What are your initial orders?**
Pulse oximetry, CBC, chem 8, PT/PTT, LFTs, fecal occult blood test.
Advance clock:
Hb 9.0 mg/dL, MCV 65 fL, heme-positive stool, laboratory tests otherwise WNL.

4. **What are your follow-up actions?**
Ferritin, total iron-binding capacity (TIBC), serum iron, gastroenterology consult for colonoscopy.
Advance clock:
Ferritin is low, TIBC is high, serum iron is low. Colonoscopy reveals adenocarcinoma in the ascending colon.

5. **What are your follow-up actions?**
Surgical consult, carcinoembryonic antigen (CEA), CXR (no evidence of metastases). CT scan of the abdomen/pelvis with contrast reveals a large mass in the ascending colon without evidence of local invasion or distant metastases
Advance clock:
Case ends.
Critical actions:
Abdominal/rectal examination, hemoglobin, colonoscopy, surgical consult.
Discussion:
This patient has an ambiguous chief complaint of fatigue, but the historical component of maroon-colored stools indicates that anemia arising from a GI bleed is the likely cause. His microcytic anemia and heme-positive stool provide further evidence. His iron studies indicate that his microcytic anemia is secondary to iron deficiency. Colonoscopy is the best way to confirm the source because this is probably a lower GI tract bleed. On colonoscopy, a biopsy should be obtained for any suspicious lesions.
In this case, adenocarcinoma of the ascending colon was diagnosed on colonoscopy. Adenocarcinomas account for 98% of colorectal cancer cases. They arise from adenomatous polyps that can be detected on screening colonoscopy. Recall that right-sided colon cancers tend to bleed and left-sided colon cancers tend to obstruct. When malignancy is detected, a surgical consult should be requested because resection is the only possibility of a cure. If the case continues, a CT scan and CXR are helpful in assessing for local invasion and metastases. Colon cancer tends to metastasize to the liver and lungs. CEA testing may be ordered to establish a preoperative baseline.
Diagnosis: Microcytic anemia secondary to colon cancer

CASE 90

HPI: A 32-year-old man attends the clinic because of 4 months of diarrhea and abdominal pain. He reports waxing and waning of mild lower abdominal cramps that are relieved by defecation. He passes up to five loose stools per day that are occasionally streaked with mucus. The symptoms are worse during the day and seem to disappear at night. There is no blood in his stool, and he denies weight loss, fever, nausea, or vomiting. He has not had any recent travel or dietary changes.
Vital signs: Temperature 97.9° F (36.3° C), pulse 82 beats/min, BP 135/85 mm Hg, RR 17 breaths/min.
Additional history: No medical history. No use of tobacco, alcohol, or drugs.

1. **What is the differential diagnosis?**
   Lactose intolerance, infectious diarrhea, Crohn disease, ulcerative colitis, irritable bowel syndrome (IBS), microscopic colitis, celiac disease.

2. **What components of the physical examination do you perform?**
   General appearance, skin, lymph nodes, HEENT, cardiovascular, lungs, abdomen, genitalia, rectal, extremities, neuro/psych.
   Physical examination:
   General: No acute distress.
   Skin/lymph nodes/HEENT: WNL
   Cardiovascular: WNL
   Lungs: WNL
   Abdomen: WNL
   Genitalia/rectal: WNL
   Extremities: WNL
   Neuro/psych: WNL

3. **What are your initial orders?**
   Pulse oximetry, CBC, chem 8, LFTs, lipase, TSH, stool culture, stool WBCs, stool ova and parasites, *Giardia* antibody, transglutaminase antibody.
   Advance clock:
   All studies WNL.

4. **What are your follow-up actions?**
   Counseling (high-fiber diet, lactose-free diet, avoid caffeine), colonoscopy, follow up in 4 weeks.
   Advance clock:
   Colonoscopy WNL. The patient's symptoms are improved.
      Case ends.
   Critical actions:
   Abdominal examination, counseling.
   Discussion:
   This patient has abdominal pain and diarrhea that are consistent with IBS. He meets the Rome III criteria of (1) a change in stool frequency, (2) a change in stool appearance, and (3) abdominal pain relieved by defecation. The history and physical examination lack red flags such as weight loss, hematochezia, nocturnal symptoms, and worsening symptomatology. Laboratory studies also lack red flags such as anemia and electrolyte disturbances. A physical examination, reassurance, and counseling are the most important aspects of this case. Limited diagnostic studies can evaluate for anemia, hyperthyroidism, *Giardia*, infectious diarrhea, and celiac disease. A colonoscopy is warranted for any concerning signs/symptoms and to evaluate for the possibility of IBD. However, other invasive studies should be avoided. If the diarrhea is not improved by counseling alone, a trial of loperamide may be indicated. Persistent symptoms may warrant trial of a TCA (amitriptyline) or antispasmodic agent (dicyclomine). Persistent symptoms despite conservative therapies may warrant referral to a gastroenterologist for further evaluation.
      Diagnosis: IBS

CASE 91

HPI: A 25-year-old man attends the ED because of palpitations of 1 hour in duration. They occurred suddenly when he was watching TV. He says his heart feels as if it is racing extremely fast. The patient has never had similar symptoms before. He denies chest pain or shortness of breath. He has had no loss of consciousness.
Vital signs: Temperature 98.6° F (37.0° C), pulse 205 beats/min, BP 110/80 mm Hg, RR 17 breaths/min.
Additional history: No medical history. No use of drugs, tobacco, or alcohol.

1. **What is the differential diagnosis?**
   Stable tachycardia: AV nodal reentrant tachycardia, AV reciprocating tachycardia, atrial flutter, AF, multifocal atrial tachycardia, ventricular tachycardia, sinus tachycardia.

2. **What components of the physical examination do you perform?**
   General appearance, HEENT, cardiovascular, lungs, extremities.
   Physical examination:
   General: Mild distress due to palpitations.
   HEENT: WNL
   Cardiovascular: Tachycardia, regular rhythm.
   Lungs: WNL
   Extremities: WNL

3. **What are your initial orders?**
   Pulse oximetry, cardiac/BP monitor, ECG, vagal maneuvers.
   Advance clock:
   ECG reveals regular narrow-complex tachycardia without P-waves with a ventricular rate of 205 beats/min.
   Vagal maneuvers have no effect.

4. **What are your follow-up actions?**
   Adenosine IV (the patient's heart rate normalizes). CBC, chem 8, serum magnesium, repeat ECG. Cardiology consult. Counseling. Follow up in 2 days.
   Advance clock:
   Repeat ECG shows normal sinus rhythm without evidence of preexcitation.
   Case ends.
   Critical actions:
   Cardiac examination, ECG, vagal maneuvers, adenosine, synchronized cardioversion if the patient becomes unstable, counseling.
   Discussion:
   Technically, SVT refers to any tachycardia that originates above the bundle of His (although it most commonly refers to AV nodal reentrant tachycardia [AVNRT]). AVNRT usually occurs spontaneously, although it may be triggered by stimulants, exercise, or alcohol. The most common presenting symptom is palpitations. Other symptoms such as chest pain and loss of consciousness represent unstable tachycardia and warrant a more aggressive approach. Because the patient is stable, vagal maneuvers such as the Valsalva maneuver can be attempted. If these fail, adenosine should be used to attempt to convert the heart to a sinus rhythm. Adenosine administration can be repeated three times. Adenosine is successful in inducing cardioversion in most cases. If it fails, however, an AV nodal blocking agent can be used such as a nondihydropyridine calcium channel blocker (diltiazem) or a beta-blocker (metoprolol).
       If at any point the patient becomes unstable (chest pain, hypotension, loss of consciousness), adenosine administration may be tried, but you should proceed quickly to synchronized cardioversion. A repeat ECG after the episode has resolved can screen for underlying dysrhythmias such as the preexcitation seen in Wolff-Parkinson-White syndrome. Patients with a single episode of well-tolerated AVNRT may not require any further treatment. Diltiazem and metoprolol are usually first-line agents for chronic suppressive therapy. In patients with poorly tolerated SVT, definitive management with catheter ablation should be considered. These decisions should be made in conjunction with a cardiologist. Patients with uncomplicated AVNRT without significant comorbidities may be discharged home with close cardiology follow-up. Poorly tolerated AVNRT or the presence of significant comorbidities probably warrants admission for monitoring.
       Diagnosis: SVT

CASE 92

HPI: A 46-year-old man attends the clinic complaining of 1 week of back pain. He had been lifting boxes when he felt acute onset of right lower backache. The pain has been persistent ever since. He denies numbness, weakness, fever, urinary retention, and fecal incontinence.

Vital signs: Temperature 97.2° F (36.2° C), pulse 75 beats/min, BP 108/70 mm Hg, RR 16 breaths/min.

Additional history: No medical history. No drug or alcohol use. Smokes one pack of cigarettes daily.

1. What is the differential diagnosis?
   Muscle strain, sciatica, lumbar radiculopathy, fracture, herniated disc, neoplasm, paraspinal abscess.

2. What components of the physical examination do you perform?
   General appearance, skin, lymph nodes, HEENT, cardiovascular, lungs, abdomen, rectal, extremities, neuro/psych.
   General: No acute distress.
   Skin/lymph nodes/HEENT: WNL
   Cardiovascular: WNL
   Lungs: WNL
   Abdomen: WNL
   Rectal: WNL
   Extremities: Tenderness to palpation over the right paraspinal muscles. Decreased range of motion at hips secondary to pain.
   Neuro/psych: WNL

3. What are your initial orders?
   Counseling (including smoking cessation), ibuprofen, follow up in 1 month.
   Advance clock:
   The patient's symptoms have greatly improved.
   Case ends.
   Critical actions:
   Extremities/neurologic examination, analgesia (NSAIDs, acetaminophen, or short course of narcotics).
   Discussion:
   This patient has acute onset of lower back pain consistent with muscle strain. His history and physical examination lack red flags such as IV drug use, trauma, malignancy, neurologic signs and symptoms, weight loss, or symptoms lasting for longer than 4 weeks. These red flags are reasons to order imaging such as an x-ray or a CT or MRI scan. In this low-risk setting, pursuit of advanced imaging may lead to deduction of points from your score. Analgesia is important in this case. Because the patient has not tried any medications, it is appropriate to start with an NSAID or acetaminophen. A short course of a narcotic (hydrocodone) or muscle relaxant (baclofen) could be added as a second agent for incomplete relief of symptoms. If this case revealed cord compression, cauda equina syndrome, or a significant neurologic deficit, then advanced imaging and an emergent neurosurgical consult would be indicated.
   Diagnosis: Muscle strain

CASE 93

HPI: A 25-year-old woman attends the clinic 4 months after she was assaulted and robbed at knifepoint. Although she suffered no significant physical trauma, she reports she has had difficulty concentrating since the event. When she tries to go to sleep, the experience seems to play over repeatedly in her head. She has even stopped leaving her house at night for fear the event might occur again. She denies suicidal or homicidal ideation. She has experienced no audio or visual hallucinations.

Vital signs: Temperature 97.7° F (36.5° C), pulse 75 beats/min, BP 125/70 mm Hg, RR 17 breaths/min.

Additional history: No medical history. No tobacco, alcohol, or drug use.

1. What is the differential diagnosis?
   Posttraumatic stress disorder (PTSD), major depressive disorder, adjustment disorder, generalized anxiety disorder.

2. What components of the physical examination do you perform?
   General appearance, skin, lymph nodes, HEENT, cardiovascular, lungs, abdomen, extremities, neuro/psych.
   General: No acute distress.
   Skin/lymph nodes/HEENT: WNL
   Cardiovascular: WNL

Lungs: WNL
Abdomen: WNL
Extremities: WNL
Neuro/psych: No focal neurologic deficits. Normal mood and affect.

3. **What are your initial orders?**
Psychiatry consult, follow up in 2 weeks, therapy, counseling, SSRI.
Advance clock:
The patient's symptoms are improved.
   Case ends.
Critical actions:
Neurologic/psychologic examination, therapy, counseling, SSRI.
Discussion:
This patient attends the clinic after a traumatic event with difficulty in concentrating, intrusive thoughts, and avoidance behaviors that interfere with her functioning. Because these symptoms have lasted for longer than 1 month, the patient meets criteria for PTSD. Other symptoms of PTSD include hyperarousal and emotional numbing. Similar symptoms lasting for less than 4 weeks do not meet the criteria for PTSD and instead fall under the diagnosis of acute stress disorder. Inciting events include any major trauma that was experienced personally or witnessed. Events include acts of war, terrorism, physical assault, sexual assault, and serious accidents. The lifetime prevalence of PTSD is higher in women (10%) than men (5%). Risk factors include preexisting psychiatric disorders including anxiety, depression, and substance abuse. The evaluation for PTSD can be limited to a history and physical examination, with laboratory testing only needed if suspicion is raised for underlying pathology. Treatment includes counseling and therapy by a mental health specialist. SSRIs are first-line pharmacotherapy. The patient should be followed up regularly as an outpatient to assess for improvement.
   Diagnosis: PTSD

CASE 94

HPI: A 57-year-old man is brought by ambulance to the ED because of chest pain and shortness of breath. Thirty minutes before his arrival he was mowing the lawn when he noticed retrosternal chest pressure that radiated to his left arm. His pain was 8/10 and improved minimally with rest. When the pain did not resolve he called 911.
Vital signs: Temperature 98.2° F (36.8° C), pulse 76 beats/min, BP 155/78 mm Hg, RR 16 breaths/min.
Additional history: 15–pack-year smoker, hyperlipidemia on atorvastatin.

1. **What is the differential diagnosis?**
ACS, aortic dissection, pulmonary embolism, pneumothorax.

2. **What components of the physical examination do you perform?**
General appearance, HEENT, cardiovascular, lungs, abdomen.
Physical examination:
   General: Diaphoretic. Visible discomfort because of chest pain.
   HEENT: WNL
   Cardiovascular: WNL
   Lungs: WNL
   Abdomen: WNL

3. **What are your initial orders?**
Pulse oximetry, BP/cardiac monitor, aspirin, sublingual nitroglycerin, morphine, CBC, chem 8, ECG/troponin every 8 hours, CXR.
Advance clock:
ECG reveals ST elevation in leads V_2 through V_6 and ST depression in leads II, III, and aV_F. Troponin/CK-MB elevated. Other studies WNL.

4. **What are your follow-up actions?**
Immediate cardiology consult, cardiac catheterization, admit to ICU.

Anticoagulation therapy (e.g., enoxaparin), antiplatelet agent (e.g., clopidogrel), beta-blocker (e.g., metoprolol), ACE inhibitor (e.g., lisinopril), statin (e.g., simvastatin), TTE, troponin/ECG every 8 hours, lipid panel, TSH, CBC, chem 8 in the morning, counseling (including smoking cessation).

Advance clock:
Case ends.

Critical actions:
Aspirin, nitroglycerin, and ECG early. Immediate cardiology consult and cardiac catheterization after ECG result. Anticoagulation therapy, ACE inhibitor, beta-blocker, and antiplatelet agent.

Discussion:
This patient is having an acute ST-elevation MI (STEMI). The history alone should trigger an immediate workup for ACS. An immediate ECG should be ordered, and prompt treatment with aspirin should not be delayed. Standard laboratory tests can also be ordered as long as they do not interfere with the evaluation and treatment of the patient. Nitroglycerin is given for relief of chest pain unless (1) right ventricular infarction is suspected, (2) hypotension or bradycardia is present, or (3) a phosphodiesterase inhibitor (e.g., sildenafil) was used in the previous 24 to 48 hours. As soon as the ECG reveals a STEMI, you should consult cardiology and order cardiac catheterization. Note that even though you have not yet received the results of many laboratory tests, you should proceed to cardiac catheterization (i.e., do not advance the clock before you order cardiac catheterization). The other laboratory results will become available later. If the case does not end after catheterization, continue inpatient ICU management of the STEMI including anticoagulation therapy (enoxaparin), an antiplatelet agent (clopidogrel), a beta-blocker (metoprolol), an ACE inhibitor (lisinopril), a statin, echocardiography, laboratory monitoring, risk factor modification, and counseling.

   Diagnosis: STEMI

CASE 95

HPI: A 23-year-old woman at 11 weeks of gestation (gravida 1 para 0) attends the clinic complaining of vaginal bleeding. The bleeding started approximately 6 hours previously and has included passage of clots and mild abdominal cramping. The pregnancy has been uncomplicated up to this point. The patient takes no medications other than a prenatal vitamin supplement.

Vital signs: Temperature 98.6° F (37.0° C), pulse 81 beats/min, BP 115/80 mm Hg, RR 15 breaths/min.

Additional history: No past medical history. No use of tobacco, drugs, or alcohol. No fertility treatment was used to achieve this pregnancy.

1. **What is the differential diagnosis?**
   Threatened abortion, inevitable abortion, incomplete abortion, complete abortion, missed abortion, septic abortion.

2. **What components of the physical examination do you perform?**
   General appearance, skin, lymph nodes, HEENT, cardiovascular, lungs, abdomen, genitalia, extremities, neuro/psych.
   Physical examination:
      General appearance: No acute distress.
      Skin/lymph nodes/HEENT: WNL
      Cardiovascular: WNL
      Lungs: WNL
      Abdomen: WNL
      Genitalia: Scant blood pooling from open os.
      Extremities: WNL
      Neuro/psych: WNL

3. **What are your initial orders?**
   Pulse oximetry, CBC, blood type and screen, fetal ultrasound.
   Advance clock:
   Blood type O negative; ultrasound reveals an intrauterine pregnancy with no fetal cardiac activity. Other studies WNL.

4. What are your follow-up actions?

Counseling, RhoGAM, misoprostol, follow up after 1 week.

Advance clock:

Case ends.

Critical actions:

Pelvic examination, fetal ultrasound, blood type and screen, RhoGAM.

Discussion:

The most immediate concern for first-trimester vaginal bleeding is to evaluate for ectopic pregnancy. An intrauterine pregnancy visualized on ultrasound is usually sufficient to rule out ectopic pregnancy (the exception being in the setting of fertility treatment, for which heterotopic pregnancies are more common). First-trimester vaginal bleeding is categorized as threatened abortion (os closed); inevitable abortion (os open); incomplete abortion (partial passage of products of conception); complete abortion (complete passage of products of conception); missed abortion (fetal demise without passage of products of conception); or septic abortion (infection during any abortion).

Threatened abortion is managed expectantly and there is no definitive evidence that any medication or behavioral change prevents miscarriage. Inevitable abortion, incomplete abortion, and missed abortion can be managed expectantly, medically (misoprostol), or surgically (dilation and curettage/evacuation). The particular approach is largely based on patient preference. Septic abortion should be managed by stabilizing the patient, obtaining cultures, and initiating broad-spectrum antibiotic therapy (e.g., clindamycin IV and gentamycin IV). Blood type should be determined for all gravid women, and RhoGAM should be administered to Rh-negative women at about 28 weeks of pregnancy or for any antenatal events that are likely to cause fetal-maternal hemorrhage (e.g., procedures such as amniocentesis, spontaneous or therapeutic abortions, abdominal trauma).

Diagnosis: Inevitable abortion

CASE 96

HPI: A 7-year-old boy attends the ED with shortness of breath and wheezing that has gradually worsened over the previous 5 hours. He has never had similar symptoms before. He has had no fever, cough, or sick contacts. His vaccinations are up to date.

Vital signs: Temperature 98.1° F (36.7° C), pulse 85 beats/min, BP 110/80 mm Hg, RR 24 breaths/min.

Additional history: Medical history of eczema and allergic rhinitis.

1. What is the differential diagnosis?

Foreign body aspiration, pneumonia, asthma, bronchitis.

2. What components of the physical examination do you perform?

General appearance, HEENT, cardiovascular, lungs, abdomen.

General: Mild increased work of breathing.

HEENT: WNL

Cardiovascular: WNL

Lungs: Tachypnea, diffuse wheezing in bilateral lung fields, subcostal retractions, increased expiratory phase.

Abdomen: WNL

3. What are your initial orders?

Pulse oximetry, BP/cardiac monitor, albuterol inhaled, ipratropium inhaled, prednisone PO, CXR, peak flow.

Advance clock:

The patient's symptoms are greatly improved.

CXR: No infiltrate; mildly hyperexpanded lungs.

4. What are your follow-up actions?

Repeat the pulmonary examination (decreased wheezing, improved air movement, no increased work of breathing). Monitor vital signs. Discharge home with albuterol inhaler, steroid taper, counseling, follow up after 1 week.

Advance clock:
Case ends.
Critical actions:
Lung examination/reexamination, pulse oximetry and/or oxygen measurement, albuterol, steroids, counseling.
Discussion:
The patient's atopic history (eczema and allergic rhinitis), physical examination, CXR findings, and response to treatment are all consistent with an acute episode of asthma. Asthma is characterized by recurrent and reversible obstruction of the airways caused by inflammation and bronchospasm. The presenting symptoms are wheezing, chest tightness, and shortness of breath. Severe exacerbations are characterized by respiratory distress with tachypnea, increased work of breathing, and use of accessory muscles. It is important to identify and address common triggers when possible. These include respiratory infections, exercise, environmental allergies, and gastric reflux. Initial management of acute asthma exacerbations includes oxygen as needed, along with inhaled albuterol (beta$_2$-agonist) and ipratropium (anticholinergic). These inhaled medications are fast acting and address reversible bronchospasm. Steroids are indicated for incomplete response to inhaled medications and are almost always indicated in exacerbations requiring a trip to the ED. Steroids address the inflammatory component of asthma. CXRs are generally unnecessary for recurrent asthma exacerbations, but CXR is indicated in this situation to rule out other causes because this is the first episode for this patient. Antibiotics are only given if bacterial infection is suspected or present. If the patient does not significantly improve, continuous nebulizers should be given and IV magnesium can be tried to further address bronchospasm. Admission is indicated for refractory symptoms, hypoxia, and respiratory distress. Patients with hypoxic or hypercapnic respiratory failure despite aggressive management will require endotracheal intubation in addition to continued treatments. Mechanical ventilation can be dangerous in these situations, however, given the tendency for air trapping. This can lead to complications from barotrauma and volutrauma. Patients with mild to moderate exacerbations with sustained and significant improvement can be discharged home with follow-up. If the case continues to the outpatient setting, the patient may eventually need to start inhaled corticosteroids for frequent exacerbations.
   Diagnosis: Asthma

INDEX

A

ABCDEs
  of moles, 140
  of trauma, 18
Abdomen, acute condition of, 92
Abdominal aortic aneurysm (AAA), 80,
  339–340
Abdominal trauma
  blunt, management of, 109
  penetrating, management of, 110
Abetalipoproteinemia, 216, 219f
Abnormal reflex, 3
ABO blood group incompatibility, 194–195
Abortion, 198
Abruptio placentae, 200
Abscess, 148
  breast, 175
Accelerated rejection, of transplanted kidney,
  170
Acetaminophen
  for hemophilia with arthritis, 125
  overdose of, 102
  toxicity of, 260–261
Achalasia, 89
Achlorhydria, 92
Acid-base disorders, 172–173
Acid burns, 153
Acidosis, serum, on potassium and calcium
  levels, 172
Acne, 139
  treatment options for, 139
Activated partial thromboplastin time
  (APTT), 227
Acute bowel infarction, 74
Acute lymphocytic leukemia (ALL), 229t,
  230
Acute myelogenous leukemia (AML), 229t,
  276–277
  diagnosis of, 230
  differential diagnosis of, 276
  follow-up actions for, 277
  initial orders for, 276
  physical examination for, 276
  risk and symptoms of, 230
  treatment of, 230, 277
Acute rejection, of transplanted kidney, 170

Acute tubular necrosis, intrarenal failure and,
  168
Acute urinary retention, symptoms and
  management of, 236
Acute withdrawal syndrome, 120
Acyclovir, 151
  for HSV-1 primary infection, 268
ADAMTS13 deficiency, 278
Addison disease, 162, 259
  in shock, 65
Adenomyosis, 177
Adenosine deaminase deficiency, 239
Adhesions, in small bowel obstruction, 96
Adjustment disorder, 114
Admission rate bias, 18
Adnexal mass, 178
Adolescence
  causes of death in, 5
  normal development in, 4–5
Adrenal disorders, 160–162
Adrenal insufficiency, 258–259
Adrenal tumors, 160
Adrenocorticotropic hormone (ACTH), 259
Adrenogenital syndrome, 162
Adult respiratory distress syndrome (ARDS),
  51
Adulthood
  normal development in, 6–8
  vaccines in, 6, 6t
Adults
  cerebellar findings in, 36
  meningitis in, 247t–248t
  neck mass in, 88
Age
  dementia and, 9
  milestones of, 1, 1t
  pattern of development and, 1
  rapidly growing segment of population, 9
Aging
  female sexual function changes and, 9
  hearing and vision changes and, 9
  male sexual function changes and, 9
Airway, breathing *versus*, in trauma protocol,
  18
Airway obstruction, 60
Akathisia, definition of, 113

Page numbers followed by *f* refer to figures, by *b* to boxes, and by *t* to tables.

Albuterol/ipratropium, for COPD exacerbation, 325
Alcohol
abuse, epidemiology of, 119
accidental or intentional death and, 120
as cause of cirrhosis and esophageal varices, 99
chronic intake of, disease and conditions caused by, 119
effects on pregnancy, 209
Alcohol withdrawal, 318–319
differential diagnosis of, 318
follow-up actions for, 319
initial orders for, 319
physical examination for, 318
stages of, 120
treatment of, 120, 319
Alcoholism
treatment of, 120
vitamin, mineral, and electrolyte deficiencies in, 105
Alkali burns, 153
Alkaline phosphatase
elevated levels of, 99
in Paget disease, 130
Alkalosis, serum, on potassium and calcium levels, 172
Allergen, skin/patch testing for identification of, 246
Allergic rhinitis, 51
Allopurinol, as maintenance therapy for gout, 124
Alpha-1-antitrypsin deficiency, and COPD, 47–48
Alpha-blocker, for bladder obstruction, 166
Alpha-fetoprotein (AFP)
in liver cancer, 101
in pregnant patient, 193
Alpha-methyldopa, for hypertension, 68
5-Alpha-reductase inhibitor, for bladder obstruction, 166
Alpha$_1$-antitrypsin (AAT), deficiency of, diagnosis of, 100
Alzheimer dementia, 24
Ambiguous genitalia, 162
Amenorrhea, 180
American Cancer Society, cancer screening guidelines of, 7, 7t–8t
Aminoaciduria, kidney stones and, 171
Aminoglycosides
causing myasthenia gravis, 26
plus loop diuretic, effect of, 21t
renal failure and, 168
Amniotic fluid pulmonary embolism, 206
Amniotomy, 202
Amphetamine, intoxication, symptoms of, 121
Ampicillin, for neonatal sepsis, 213
Amrinone, for shock, 66

Amylase, elevation of, 103
Amyotrophic lateral sclerosis (ALS), 25, 286–287
Anal atresia, 107t
Analysis of variance (ANOVA), 15
Anaphylaxis, 245–246
Androgen insensitivity syndrome, 180–181
Anemia, 215–223
autoimmune, laboratory test for, 225
blood loss and, 215
causes of, 226
of chronic disease, 223
chronic liver disease and, 226
definition of, 215
diagnostic test for, 215–216, 221
hemolysis and, 222
lead poisoning causing, 225
medications for, 215
patient history of, 215
reticulocyte count for, 221
screening for, 3
symptoms and sign of, 215
transfusion and hemoglobin level for, 226
in United States, 222
Anencephaly, 198
Anergy, 240
Anesthesia, in obstetric patients, 190
Angina
stable, 73
unstable, 73
variant, 73
Angioedema, hereditary, 246
Angiography, in GI bleed, 92
Angiosarcoma, 101
Angiotensin-converting enzyme inhibitor (ACEI), for hypertension, 67, 67t–68t
Angiotensin receptor blocker (ARB), for hypertension, 67, 67t–68t
Anorexia, 117
Anterior cruciate ligament (ACL), tears, 131
Anterior fontanelle, closing of, 4
Antibiotics
for COPD exacerbation, 48
long-term parenteral, for infective endocarditis, 301
prophylaxis, for bacterial meningitis, 37
Antibody screen, of pregnant patient, 193
Anticentromere antibody test, 244
Anticholinergic crisis, toxidromes associated with, 19
Anticholinergic medication, for vertigo, 282
Anticipatory guidance, items frequently tested using, 2
Anticoagulant, lupus, clotting and, 84
Anticonvulsants, 34
Anti-DNase antibody, elevated, 52
Antidote, 21, 21t

Antiemetic agents, for vertigo, 282
Antihistamines
    for allergic rhinitis, 51–52
    for anaphylactic shock, 65
Antimitochondrial antibodies, in primary
        biliary cirrhosis, 99
Antinuclear antibody (ANA) test, 244
Antipsychotics
    atypical, side effects of, 122
    classes of, 113t
    extrapyramidal side effects of, 113
    parkinsonism and, 122
    prolactin levels and, 122
    for schizophrenia, 112
Anti-Smith antibody test, 244
Antisocial personality disorder, 119
    conduct disorder and, 118
Antistreptolysin O (ASO), elevated, 52
Antitopoisomerase antibody test, 244
Anxiety disorders, 113–114
Aorta
    coarctation of, 69
    regurgitation in, 81–82
    rupture of, 80
    stenosis of, 81–82
Aortic dissection, 325–326
    chest pain and, 71
    differential diagnosis of, 325
    follow-up actions for, 326
    initial orders for, 326
    physical examination for, 326
APGAR score, 204, 205t
Aplastic anemia, diagnosis of, 226
Appendicitis, 96
    acute, 321–322
Applied biostatistics, 12–18
Aripiprazole, side effects of, 122
Aromatase inhibitors, breast cancer
        and, 186
Arrest disorder, 204
Arrhythmias, 75
Arterial disorders, 242–243
Arthritis
    causes of, 124, 124t
    in Jones criteria for rheumatic fever
        diagnosis, 125
Asbestos, exposure to, 50
Asbestosis, 50
Ascites, in liver failure, 100
Aspergillus species, 249t–250t
Aspirin
    monitoring of, 233
    myocardial infarction and, 74
    nasal polyps and, 245
    pregnancy and, 198
    reversing the effects of, 233
    for STEMI, 72, 74
    strokes and, 29

Asthma, 48, 356–357
    differential diagnosis of, 356
    follow-up actions for, 356
    hyperventilation and normal carbon dioxide
        (CO_2) level in, 49
    initial orders for, 356
    and intubation, 49
    and long-acting beta-agonists (LABAs), 48
    physical examination for, 356
    symptoms of, 357
Atelectasis, 51
Atherosclerosis, 158
Athlete's foot. *see* Tinea pedis
Atrial fibrillation (AF), 76f, 76t, 79, 80t
    with rapid ventricular response (RVR),
        340–341
        differential diagnosis of, 340
        follow-up actions for, 340
        initial orders for, 340
        physical examination for, 340
        secondary causes of, 341
Atrial flutter, 76f–77f, 76t
Atrial septal defect, 85t–86t, 86
Attention-deficit hyperactivity disorder
        (ADHD), 118
Attributable risk, 13, 13t
Autism spectrum disorder, 118
Autoimmune disorder, systemic signs of
        inflammation and, 126
Autosomal dominant polycystic kidney disease
        (ADPKD), 169
Autosomal recessive polycystic kidney disease
        (ARPKD), 169
Avascular necrosis, risk factors and diagnosis
        of, 125
Avoidant personality disorder, 119
Azithromycin (or erythromycin), for pertussis,
        308

B
B-cell lymphoma, CNS, 229t
Babesiosis, 217
Bacillus cereus, 249t–250t
Bacteria, in preorbital/orbital cellulitis, 252
Bacteriuria, asymptomatic, 174
    during pregnancy, 198
Bacteroides, 248t
Baldness, pathologic causes of, 139
Bamboo spine, radiographs of ankylosing
        spondylitis, 126
Barbiturate, intoxication, symptoms and signs
        of, 121
Barium swallow, in achalasia, 89
Barrett esophagus, esophageal cancer
        and, 90
Basal cell cancer, 141, 142f
    develops metastases, 141

Basophilia, 229
Beck Depression Inventory, 111t
Beck triad, 65, 87
Becker muscular dystrophy, 128
Behavioral/emotional disorders, 111–123
Behavioral therapy, for simple phobias, 113
Behçet syndrome, in Step 3 examination, 244
Benign prostatic hyperplasia (BPH)
    postrenal failure and, 168
    symptoms and sequelae of, 236
    treatment of, 236
Benzodiazepines
    for alcohol withdrawal, 319
    intoxication, symptoms and signs of, 121
    for seizure, 263–264
Berger syndrome, 167
Beta-blockers
    in diabetic patients, 160
    for hypertension, 67t–68t
    side effects of, 87
Bile duct obstruction, common, causes
        of, 98
Biliary atresia, jaundice and, 208
Biliary cirrhosis, primary, diagnosis of, 99
Biliary tract obstruction
    signs and symptoms of, 98
    types of, 98
Bilirubin, jaundice and, 208
Biofeedback, for simple phobias, 113
Biophysical profile, 198
Bipolar disorder
    definition and classic symptoms
        of, 115
    treatment of, 115
Bipolar II disorder, definition of, 115
Birth control, forms of, 183
Birth control pills
    for endometriosis, 176–177
    smoking and, 184
Bite cells, with Heinz bodies, 217f
Bitemporal hemianopsia, 39
Bladder cancer
    clinical vignette for, 166
    urinalysis for, 8
Bladder obstruction, 166
Bleeding
    fetal, 200
    platelet-type, causes of, 228
    third-trimester, 191–192, 199
Bleeding disorders, 223–228
Bleeding diverticulosis, 317–318
Bleeding time (BT), 227, 233
Blindness, 42
    with strabismus, 44
Blood, disorders of, 215–233
Blood components, reactions to, 228
Blood dyscrasias, 229
Blood products, use of, indications for, 228

Blood transfusion reaction
    management for, 228
    risks of, 228
    signs and symptoms of, 228
Blood type, of pregnant patient, 193
Blood urea nitrogen (BUN) level, during
        pregnancy, 189
Bloody show, 199
Body dysmorphic disorder, 117
Boerhaave tears, 90
Bone cyst, unicameral, 129, 129f
Bone tumor, metastatic, 129
Borderline personality disorder, 119
Borrelia burgdorferi, as causative bacterium of
        Lyme disease, 131
Borrelia species, 248t
Bouchard nodes, 124
Bowel contrast, for GI perforation, 90
Bowen disease, 141
Brain, cancers metastasize to, 36
Brain atrophy, aging and, 9
Brain tumor
    headache secondary to, 32
    presentations of, 36
    treatment of, 36
Brainstem damage, hyponatremia and, 172
Breast, diseases and disorders of, 175–176
Breast cancer, 176, 185
    in men, 234
    oral contraceptive pills and, 184
Breast-conserving surgery, efficacy of, 186
Breastfeeding, 205
    jaundice, 208, 255
Breast mass, causes of, 175, 185
Breathing, airway *versus*, in trauma protocol,
        18
Broad ligament, diseases and disorders of,
        177–178
Bronchiolitis, 59
Bronchitis, 247t–248t
Bronze diabetes, 99–100
Brucellosis, 249t–250t
Bruton agammaglobulinemia, 239
Buerger disease, 47
Bulimia, definition and classic findings for, 117
Bulla, 135t
Bullous pemphigoid, 138, 138f
"Bunch of grapes," in vagina, 179
Burkitt lymphoma, 229t
Burns
    causes of, 152
    severity classified, 153

C

C1 esterase inhibitor, 246
Café-au-lait macules, 144
    multiple, 145f

Caffeine, withdrawal, symptoms of, 122
Calcium channel blocker (CCB),
    hypertension, 67, 67t–68t
Calories, 9
Cancer
  associated with alcohol intake, 120
  in children and young adults, 231
  diseases risk for, 243
  Epstein-Barr virus (EBV) infection-
    associated, 251
  metastasize to brain, 36
  Paget disease and, 130
  screening of, 7, 7t–8t
Candidal infection, vaginitis and, 179
Candidiasis, 146
  chronic mucocutaneous, 239
  treatment of, 147
Capillary hemangiomas, 144
Caput succedaneum, 211
Carbamazepine, side effects of, 122
Carbon monoxide (CO) poisoning, 313–314
Carbonic anhydrase, 87
Carbuncle, 148
Carcinoembryonic antigen (CEA), in colon
    cancer, 97
Carcinoid tumors
  laboratory tests for, 97
  symptoms of, 97
Carcinoma, bronchoalveolar, 56
Cardiac arrhythmias
  from electrical burns, 174
  from tricyclic antidepressants, 123
Cardiac tamponade, 87
Cardiomyopathy
  dilated, 86
  hypertrophic, 86–87
  restrictive, 86
Cardiovascular disorders, 63–87
Carotid stenosis, 30
Case series study, 16
Cataracts
  bilateral painless loss of vision and, 43
  in neonate, 41
Ceftriaxone, for gonorrhea, 188
Celiac disease, 138
  malabsorptive diarrhea in, 95
Cellulitis, 247t–248t, 253–254
  cause of, 148
  physical findings for, 148
Centor criteria, for streptococcal pharyngitis,
    260
Central nervous system, primary tumors of,
    histologic types of, 36
Central pontine myelinolysis, hyponatremia
    and, 172
Central retinal artery occlusion, 43
Central retinal vein occlusion, 43
Cephalohematomas, 211

Cephalopelvic disproportion, 204
Cerebrospinal fluid (CSF), 22, 22t
Cerebrovascular diseases, 27–31
Ceruloplasmin, serum, in Wilson disease, 100
Cervical cancer
  oral contraceptive pills and, 184
  screening method for, 178
Cervical spine, disc herniation in, 125
Cervix, diseases and disorders of, 178
Cesarean section, 205
Chagas disease, achalasia secondary to, 89
Chalazion, 42
Charcot joints, 133
  from diabetic peripheral neuropathy, 158
Charcot triad, 98
Chediak-Higashi syndrome, 246
Chemical burns, 153
  to eye, 42
Chemotherapy, 245
Chest pain, 70–71
  in myocardial infarction, 72
Chi-squared test, 15
Chickenpox, 150
  complications of, 151
  definitive diagnosis of, 151
  during pregnancy, 214
  prophylaxis for, 151
Child abuse
  reporting, 11
  suspecting, 11
Children
  with abnormal head circumference, 2
  acquired hearing loss in, 45
  ambiguous genitalia in, 162
  cancer in, 231
  cerebellar findings in, 36
  dental recommendation in, 4
  fluoride supplementation for, 3
  GI malformations in, 107, 107t
  hydrocephalus in, 23
  irritable bowel syndrome in, 94
  lead poisoning screening for, 225
  meningitis in, 247t–248t
  neck mass in, 88
  normal development in, 1–4
  obesity in, 2
  prophylactic iron supplements for, 3
  renal disease screening of, 4
  rubella in, 150
  separation anxiety disorder in, 118
  tuberculosis in, 4
  urinary tract infection in, 173
  vital signs of, 4
Chlamydia psittaci, 249t–250t
Chlamydia screening, in pregnant patient, 194
Chlamydial infection
  gonorrhea and, 188
  during pregnancy, 195

Chlorpromazine, side effects of, 122
Choanal atresia, 107t
Choking, 62
Cholangiocarcinoma, 101
Cholangitis
    versus cholecystitis, 98
    precipitating factors of, 98
Cholecystitis
    acalculous, 321
    acute, 320–321
        differential diagnosis of, 320
        follow-up actions for, 321
        initial orders for, 321
        physical examination for, 320
    versus cholangitis, 98
    six Fs of, 97
Cholestasis
    causes of, 98
    of pregnancy, 192
Cholesterol
    and atherosclerosis, 69
    levels, management of, 69, 69t
    screening, for hypertension, 69
    stones vs. pigment stones, 97
Cholinergic crisis, toxidromes associated with, 19
Chorioamnionitis, 207
Chorionic villus sampling (CVS), 196
Chromium, deficiency/toxicity of, 104t
Chronic granulomatous disease, 239
Chronic heart failure (CHF), acute decompensated, 322–323
Chronic lymphocytic leukemia (CLL), 229t, 230
    diagnosis and treatment of, 230
    symptoms of, 230
Chronic myelogenous leukemia (CML), 229t
    diagnosis of, 230
    risk and symptoms of, 230
    treatment of, 231
Chronic obstructive pulmonary disease (COPD), 48
    exacerbation, 48, 324–325
        differential diagnosis of, 325
        follow-up actions for, 325
        initial orders for, 325
        physical examination for, 325
        treatment of, 325
    historical features of, 48
    treatment goals of, 48
Chronic rejection, of transplanted kidney, 170
Chvostek sign, 163
Cilostazol, for peripheral arterial disease, 331
Circulation, 18
Claudication, 83–84
Clindamycin, for postpartum fever, 207
Clinical case scenarios, 253–357
Clinical epidemiology, 12–18

Clomiphene, for polycystic ovary syndrome, 184
Clomiphene citrate, ovulation and, 185
Clopidogrel
    for peripheral arterial disease, 331
    for STEMI, 73
Clostridium botulinum, 249t–250t
Clostridium difficile, 249t–250t
Clotting
    genetic and acquired causes of, 84
    and lupus anticoagulant, 84
Clotting tests, 227
    diseases affecting, 227t
Clozapine, side effects of, 122
Cluster headaches, 32
Coagulation tests, conditions affect, 223t–224t
Coagulopathy, in liver failure, 100
Coarctation of aorta, 85t–86t
Cocaine, intoxication and withdrawal of, symptoms of, 121
Coccidioides immitis, 249t–250t
Colchicine, for acute attacks of gout, 124
Cold-agglutinin antibodies, 57
Colon cancer
    risk factors for, 96
    symptoms of, 96
    treatment of, 97
Coma, no advance directive or living will in patient with, 10
Compartment syndrome
    definition and cause of, 133
    symptoms and signs of, 133
    treatment of, 133
Complete abortion, 198
Complete hydatidiform moles, 189
Conduct disorder, definition of, 118
Confidence interval, 15
Confidentiality, of patient, 11
Confounding variables, 17
Congenital disorders, screening tests for, 207
Congenital hip dysplasia (CHD), 128t
Congestive heart failure, 74–75
Conjunctivitis
    allergic, viral versus bacterial, 40, 40t
    causing loss of vision, 40
    chlamydial, 213
    gonorrheal, 213
    hallmark of, 40
    neonatal, 213
    in reactive arthritis, 131
Conn syndrome, 68, 161
Connective tissue disorders, 243–244
Consent, to treatment, 10–11
Contingent testing, for Down syndrome, 196
Continuous data, 15
Contraction stress test, 198
Conversion disorder, 117

Coombs test
  for autoimmune anemia, 225
  for type II hypersensitivity, 245
Copper, deficiency/toxicity of, 104t
Cor pulmonale, 75
Coronary artery disease, 158
Coronary heart disease (CHD), 70
Correlation coefficient, 15
Corticosteroids
  for anaphylactic shock, 65
  in Cushing syndrome, 161
  for PCP, 57–58
  for temporal arteritis (giant cell arteritis), 338
Cortisol, 259
Courvoisier sign
  in common bile duct obstruction, 98
  in pancreatic cancer, 102
C-peptide level, 157
Cranial nerves, isolated palsies of, 32
Cranial nerve III deficit, benign and serious
    causes of, 39
Cranial nerve V, innervation of, 34
Cranial nerve VII (facial nerve), innervation
    of, 35
Cranial nerve VIII
  damage and increased intracranial pressure, 36
  function of, 46
Cranial nerve palsies, from diabetic peripheral
    neuropathy, 158
Craniotabes, in rickets, 105
CRASH mnemonic, for Kawasaki disease,
    243, 271
Creatine kinase, and muscle injury, 73
Creatine phosphokinase, in neuroleptic
    malignant syndrome, 122
Creatinine level, during pregnancy, 189
CREST syndrome, 89–90
  symptoms, in scleroderma, 244
Cricothyroidotomy, 60
Crigler-Najjar syndrome, jaundice and, 208
Crohn disease, versus ulcerative colitis, 93t
Croup, 58, 59f, 288–289
Cryoprecipitate, 228
Cryptorchidism, 234–235
CT pulmonary angiogram or ventilation/
    perfusion (V/Q) scan, for pulmonary
    embolus, 51
Culdocentesis, ectopic pregnancy and, 190
CURB-65 criteria, 256–257
Curettage, in dysfunctional uterine bleeding,
    179
Cushing syndrome, 54, 68
  causes of, 161
  diagnosis of, 161
  symptoms and signs of, 161
Cyclosporine
  nephrotoxicity of, graft rejection versus, 170
  renal failure and, 168

Cyclothymia, definition of, 115
Cystadenocarcinoma, 186
Cystic fibrosis, 47
Cysticercosis, 249t–250t
Cystine stones, 171
Cystinuria, kidney stones and, 171
Cystitis, 173
Cystocele, 182
Cytopenias, 215–223

D

Dabigatran, for pulmonary embolus, 51
Dawn phenomenon, 159
Death
  causes of, in adolescents, 5
  and dying, 12
Decision making
  incompetent in, 10
  medical emergency and, 10
Deep venous thrombosis (DVT), 269–270
  development of, 84
  diagnosis of, 275
  differential diagnosis of, 270
  follow-up actions for, 270
  initial orders for, 270
  physical examination for, 270
  prevention of, during surgery, 84
  signs and symptoms of, 84
  and stroke, 85
  treatment of, 84, 275
Degenerative/developmental disorders,
    23–25
Dehydration, BUN-to-creatinine ratio and,
    173
Delirious/unconscious patients, empiric
    treatment in, 23
Delirium
  dementia versus, 24, 24t
  symptoms and signs of, 24
Delirium tremens, 120
Demeclocycline, for syndrome of inappropriate
    antidiuretic hormone secretion (SIADH),
    172
Dementia, 274–275
  age and, 9
  delirium versus, 24, 24t
  differential diagnosis of, 274
  follow-up actions for, 275
  initial orders for, 274
  with Lewy bodies, 24
  with Parkinson disease, 25
  physical examination for, 274
  symptoms and signs of, 24
  treatable causes of, 23
  vascular, 24
Demyelination, 258
Dependent personality disorder, 119

Depression, 10, 334–335
 definition of, 114
 differential diagnosis of, 334
 initial orders for, 334
 physical examination for, 334
 postpartum
  prevalence rates of, 116
  risk factors for, 116
  symptoms of, 116
 risk of suicide in, 116
 symptoms of, 334–335
 treatment of, 114, 334–335
Dermatitis
 atopic, 135
 candidal, 136
 contact, 135, 136f
 diaper, 136
 irritant, 136
 seborrheic, 139
Dermatitis herpetiformis, 138f
Dermatomyositis, 127, 243
Dermoid cysts, 187
Desmopressin, for enuresis, 166
Dexamethasone suppression test, for
  hypercortisolism, 295
Diabetes insipidus (DI), 164, 172
 central, 164
 nephrogenic, 164
 treatment of, 164
Diabetes mellitus, 156–160
 changes in retina and fundus and, 41
 chronic renal failure and, 169
 control of, long-term, 157
 long-term complications of, 158
 management of, in patients scheduled for
  surgery, 159
 maternal, 189
 new-onset, symptoms of, 156
 screening of, 156
 treatment in terms of glucose levels, 157
 type 1, 157, 157t
 type 2, 157, 157t, 160, 311–312
  diagnosis of, 312
  differential diagnosis of, 311
  follow-up actions for, 311
  initial orders for, 311
  physical examination for, 311
  treatment of, 312
Diabetic ketoacidosis (DKA), 158, 273–274
 differential diagnosis of, 273
 follow-up actions for, 273
 initial orders for, 273
 physical examination for, 273
Diagnosis, hiding, from patient, 11
Diagnostic and Statistical Manual of Mental
  Disorders, 5th edition (DSM-V), 114
Dialysis, indications for, 169
Diaphragm, rupture of, 62

Diarrhea
 acute, 348
 categories of, 94
 in children
  bacterial, 95
  causes of, 96
 due to altered intestinal transit,
  causes of, 95
 exudative, causes of, 95
 infectious, causes of, 95
 malabsorptive, causes of, 95
 management of, 95
 osmotic, 95
 secretory, causes of, 95
Diethylstilbestrol (DES), cancer and, 178
DiGeorge syndrome, 209
Digestive system, disorders of, 88–110
Digoxin, for pulmonary hypertension, 50
Dilation, in dysfunctional uterine bleeding,
  179
Diphtheria, 60
Diphyllobothrium latum, 249t–250t
Disability, 18
Disc herniations, intervertebral
 diagnosis and treatment of, 126
 locations and symptoms of, 125
Discrepancy, size/date, 197
Disease-modifying antirheumatic drugs
  (DMARDs), for rheumatoid arthritis, 126
Dislocations, posterior knee, incidence of
  vascular injury with, 134
Disseminated intravascular coagulation (DIC),
  223t–224t
 causes of, 226
 clotting tests in, 227t
 in liver failure, 100
 treatment of, 226
Dissociative fugue, 117
Distress, fetal, 202
Diuretics, side effects of, 87
Diverticulitis, 94, 344–345
 diagnosis and treatment of, 94
 differential diagnosis of, 344
 follow-up actions for, 344
 initial orders for, 344
 physical examination for, 344
Diverticulosis, 94
DNA testing, cell-free fetal, for Down
  syndrome, 196
Dobutamine, for shock, 65
Donors, for kidney transplantation, 169
Dopamine
 for prolactinoma, 262
 for shock, 65
Down syndrome, 207, 209, 209f
 screening, prenatal tests for, 195
Doxycycline, for chlamydia, 188
Drowning episode, nonfatal, 60

Drugs
   intoxication *versus* withdrawal, 120
   safe, in pregnancy, 193
   side effects of, 19, 19t–21t
Dubin-Johnson syndrome, jaundice
      and, 208
Duchenne muscular dystrophy, 128
Dural venous sinus thrombosis, 31
Dyschezia, 176
Dysfunctional uterine bleeding (DUB), 179,
      295–296
   differential diagnosis of, 295
   follow-up actions for, 296
   initial orders for, 296
   physical examination for, 295
Dysmenorrhea, 176, 179
Dyspareunia, 176
Dysplastic nevus syndrome, 140
Dystocia, 198
   shoulder, 204
Dystonia, acute, definition and treatment of,
      113

E

Ear, disorders of, 44–46
Early decelerations, 202, 202f
Eating disorders, 117–118
Eaton-Lambert syndrome, 26, 54
Eclampsia, 191
Edema, during pregnancy, 191
Electrical burns, important renal sequelae of,
      174
Electrolyte disorders, 172–173
Electromyography (EMG)
   with no muscle activity and muscle
      contraction, 26
   showing fasciculations/fibrillations, 26
Embolectomy, for pulmonary embolus, 51
Emergency care, 10
Emergency medicine, principles of, 18–21
Encopresis, diagnosis of, 4
Endocarditis, 82
   acute, 82
   infective, 299–301
      differential diagnosis of, 300
      follow-up actions for, 300
      initial orders for, 300
      physical examination for, 300
      treatment of, 301
   native valve, 247t–248t
   prophylaxis, 82
   prosthetic valve, 247t–248t
   signs and symptoms of, 83
   subacute, 82
Endocrine disorders, 154–165
   nipple discharge and, 175
   primary *versus* secondary, 154

Endometrial cancer, 177
   oral contraceptive pills and, 184, 187
Endometriosis, 176
Endometritis, 206
Endoscopy
   in GI bleed, 92
   in PUD, 91
Enterobius species, 249t–250t
Enterocele, 182
Enterococcus, 248t
Enuresis, 166
   diagnosis of, 4
Enzyme-linked immunosorbent assay
      (ELISA), 240
Eosinophilia, 232
Epididymitis, 234–236
   diagnosis of, 235t
Epididymoorchitis, 237
Epidural anesthesia, in obstetric patients,
      190
Epiglottitis, 59, 60f
Epinephrine, for shock, 64–66
Epispadias, 236
Epstein-Barr virus (EBV) infection,
      250–251
Erectile dysfunction, 236
Error, type II, 17
Erysipelas, 147, 147f
Erythema chronicum migrans, 131, 131f
Erythema infectiosum, 150, 151f
Erythema multiforme, 137, 137f
Erythema nodosum, 140, 140f
Erythrocyte sedimentation rate, during
      pregnancy, 197
Erythropoietin, for chronic renal
      failure, 169
Escherichia coli, 249t–250t
Esophageal cancer
   Barrett esophagus and, 90
   classic presentation of, 90
   epidemiology of, 90
Esophageal disease, classic symptoms of, 89
Esophageal manometry
   in achalasia, 89
   in esophageal spasm, 89
Esophagus
   disorders of, 88–90
   nutcracker, 89
   problems with, and chest pain, 71
Estrogen therapy, benefits of, 181
Euthanasia, active *versus* passive, 12
Exanthem subitum, 150
Exercise, amenorrhea and, 180
Experimental studies, 16
Exposure, 18
Extravascular blood, 255
Eye, disorders of, 39–44
Ezetimibe, 70

F

Facial nerve, upper and lower motor neuron lesion of, 35
Factitious disorders, 117, 157
Factor V Leiden mutation, 84
Failure to thrive, definition and causes of, 2
Fallopian tube
    diseases and disorders of, 177–178
    mass in, 177
False labor, 200
Fasciitis, 253–254
Fascioscapulohumeral dystrophy, 129
FAST (focused assessment by sonography in trauma) examination, in blunt abdominal trauma, 109
Fat necrosis, in breast, 175
FAT RN mnemonic, for thrombotic thrombocytopenic purpura (TTP), 278
Fatty liver, acute, of pregnancy, 192
Fertility, female, 183–185
Fetal age, ultrasound and, 197
Fetal alcohol syndrome, 209
    mental retardation and, 207
Fetal circulation, oxygen concentration in, 204
Fetal complications, of multiple gestations, 192
Fetal fibronectin, 201
Fetal heart tones, 197
Fetal heart trace, 202
Fetal karyotype determination, 196
Fetal malpresentation, 200
Fetal positions, 204
Fetal well-being, evaluation of, 197
Fetus, 207–212
    effect of teratogens on, 210t–211t
    HIV infection transmission to, 214
Fever
    postpartum, 206
    puerperal, 206
Fibrates, 70
Fibroadenoma, 175
Fibrocystic disease, 175
Fibroids, 176
Fibromyalgia, 244t
First-trimester combined test, for Down syndrome, 195
Flail chest, 61
Flooding, for simple phobias, 113
"Floppy" (flaccid) baby, 37
Fluid disorders, 172–173
Flumazenil, for benzodiazepine overdose, 121
Fluoride, deficiency/toxicity of, 104t
Fluoride supplementation, for children, 3
Fluoroquinolone, for cystitis, 173
Folate, 193
Folic acid
    deficiency of, 104t
        causes of, 105
    toxicity of, 104t

Folliculitis, 148
    pathogen causes, 148
    treatment of, 148
Foot pain, severe, 84
Foreign body aspiration, in children, 55
Fosphenytoin, for seizure, 263–264
Fractures
    metaphyseal, 12f
    mortality rate in, 132
    nasal, 52
    open *versus* closed, 133
        management of, 133
    pathologic, 129
    pelvic, 132
    radiographs for, 132
    scaphoid bone, 132, 132f
    skull
        basilar, 38
        of calvarium, 38
Fragile X syndrome, 209
Free T$_4$ index, 155
Fresh frozen plasma, 228
Frontotemporal dementia, 24
Frostbite, 153
Frostnip, 153
Fugue state. *see* Dissociative fugue
Fungal infections, 144
    diagnosis and treatment of, 146
    organisms causing, 146
Furuncle, 148

G

Galactosemia, 210
Gallbladder and bile duct, disorders of, 97–99
Gallbladder stones, on abdominal radiograph, 171
Gallstone disease, symptoms and signs of, 97
Gastroesophageal reflux disease (GERD), 315–316
    and chest pain, 71
    classic symptoms and treatment of, 89
    definition and causes of, 89
    differential diagnosis of, 315
    initial orders for, 316
    physical examination for, 315
    sequelae of, 89
Gastrointestinal tract (GI)
    radiologic imaging studies for, 92
    treatment of, 92
    upper *vs.* lower, 92t
Gastroparesis, from diabetic peripheral neuropathy, 158
Gastroschisis, 109
Gemfibrozil, for pancreatitis, 338–339
Generalized anxiety disorder, 113

Genital herpes
  labor and, 214
  in men, 237
    diagnosis and treatment of, 237
Gentamicin, for neonatal sepsis, 213
Genu valgum, 128
Genu varum, 128
Gestational sac, intrauterine, 193
Gestational trophoblastic disease, 191
Gestations, multiple, 192
Giant cell arteritis. *see* Temporal arteritis
Giardia lamblia, 249t–250t
Gilbert syndrome, jaundice and, 208
Glaucoma, closed-angle, 41
Glomerulonephritis, 167
Glucagonomas, 102
Glucose-6-phosphate dehydrogenase (G6PD)
    deficiency, 216, 217f
  in USMLE, 226
Glucose screening, for gestational
    diabetes, 193
Gonococcus, 248t
Gonorrhea
  chlamydial infection and, 188
  during pregnancy, 195
Goodpasture syndrome, 167, 243
Gottron papules, 243
Gout, 327–328
  causes of, 124t
  diagnosis of, 124
  follow-up actions for, 328
  initial orders for, 328
  physical examination for, 328
Gower sign, in Duchenne muscular dystrophy,
    128
Gram staining, 246t–247t
Granulocytes, 228
Granulosa/theca cell tumors, 187
Graves disease, 155, 291
Grief, normal *versus* pathologic, 119
Group B *Streptococcus* (GBS), 214
  screening for, pregnancy and, 194
GRUELING mnemonic, for sarcoidosis, 49
Guarding, involuntary, in peritonitis, 92–93
Guillain-Barré syndrome, 25, 305–306
  differential diagnosis of, 305
  follow-up actions for, 306
  initial orders for, 306
  physical examination for, 305
  treatment of, 306

H

Haemophilus, 248t
Haemophilus influenzae, 249t–250t
  type B, 252
Hair, disorders of, 139–140
Hairy cell leukemia, 229t

Hallucinogenic mushrooms. *see* Lysergic acid
    diethylamide (LSD)
Hallucinosis, alcoholic, 120
Halstead-Reitan Battery, 111t
Hashimoto thyroiditis, 155, 285
Hb A$_{IC}$, blood glucose, 157
Head circumference
  abnormal, 2
  child *versus* peers, 2
  measurement of, 2
Head trauma, 38
  imaging for, 19
  neurologic deficits after, 38
Headaches, 32–35
Hearing, screening for, 2
Hearing loss, 44
  situations about, 45
Heart block, 76t
  first degree, 77f
  Mobitz type I, 77f
  Mobitz type II, 77f
  third-degree, 78f
Heart disease, risk factors of, statin
    and, 70
Heart rate, fetal, 202
Heartburn, in GERD, 89
Heberden nodes, 124
Height
  child *versus* peers, 2
  measurement of, 2
Heliotrope rash, around eyes, 243
HELLP syndrome, 190–191
Hemangioma, 101
  infantile, 145f
Hematocrit test, in pregnant patient, 193
Hematoma
  epidural, 27, 28f, 312–313
    diagnosis of, 313
    differential diagnosis of, 312
    follow-up actions for, 313
    initial orders for, 313
    physical examination for, 312
    treatment of, 313
  subdural, 27, 27f, 296–297
    diagnosis of, 297
    differential diagnosis of, 296
    follow-up actions for, 297
    initial orders for, 297
    physical examination for, 296
    treatment of, 297
Hematuria, 265–266
  diagnosis of, 266
  differential diagnosis of, 265
  follow-up actions for, 265
  initial orders for, 265
  physical examination for, 265
  renal cell carcinoma and, 171
  treatment of, 266

Hemiballismus, 35
Hemochromatosis, 99
  arthritis and, 125
Hemodialysis, for chronic renal
    failure, 169
Hemoglobin test, in pregnant patient, 193
Hemolysis
  intravascular, 216, 218f
  jaundice and, 208
Hemolytic anemia, 216, 217f, 222
  autoimmune, causes of, 225
Hemolytic disease, of newborn, 194
Hemolytic transfusion reaction, 228
Hemolytic uremic syndrome (HUS),
    170t, 278
  in bacterial diarrhea, 95
Hemophilia, arthritis and, 125
Hemophilia A, 223t–224t, 227t
Hemophilia B, 223t–224t, 227t
Hemorrhage
  intracerebral, 28, 29f
  intracranial, 27
  postpartum, 206
  subarachnoid, 28, 266–267
    diagnosis of, 267
    differential diagnosis of, 266
    follow-up actions for, 267
    initial orders for, 266
    physical examination for, 266
    treatment of, 267
Hemothorax, 61
Henoch-Schönlein purpura (HSP),
    170t, 242
Heparin, 65
  for chest pain, 73
  in clotting tests, 227t
  for deep vein thrombosis, 84
  low-molecular-weight, 233
    for postpartum fever, 207
  monitoring of, 233
  for myocardial infarction, 73
  for postpartum fever, 207
  reversing the effects of, 233
  side effect of, 233
  for STEMI, 73
Hepatic adenoma, 101
Hepatic encephalopathy, in liver
    failure, 100
Hepatic enzyme, induction and inhibition
    of, 101
Hepatitis
  alcoholic, AST and ALT in, 101
  autoimmune, serologic marker of, 99
  drug-induced, classic causes of, 99
Hepatitis A virus (HAV) infection, 106
Hepatitis B
  active, mother with, infant and, 209
  chronic, 214

Hepatitis B antigen testing, of pregnant
    patient, 194
Hepatitis B virus (HBV) infection
  acquired, 106
  chronic, sequelae of, 106
  immunoglobulin/vaccination for, 106
  serology of, 106, 106t
Hepatitis C virus (HCV) infection, 106
  sequelae of, 106
  serology and treatment of, 107
Hepatitis D virus (HDV) infection, serology
    of, 107
Hepatitis E virus (HEV) infection
  in pregnancy, 107
  transmission of, 107
Hepatoblastoma, 101
Hepatocellular cancer, risk of, 101
Hepatorenal syndrome, in liver failure, 100
Hereditary elliptocytosis, 216, 219f
Hereditary spherocytosis, 216
  hallmarks of, 225
Hernias
  diaphragmatic, 208, 212
  direct, 109
  femoral, 109
  groin, types of, 109
  hiatal, 89
  incarcerated, 109
  indirect, 109
  paraesophageal, 89
  strangulated, 108t–109t, 109
Herpes simplex virus type 1 (HSV-1) primary
    infection, 267–268
Herpes zoster, 151f
High-density lipoprotein (HDL), 70
Hip disorders, pediatric, 128t
Hirschsprung disease, 107t
Hirsutism, 139, 161
Histiocytosis, cytologic clues for, 144
Histoplasma capsulatum, 249t–250t
Histrionic personality disorder, 119
HIV test, in pregnant patient, 194
Hoarseness, 53
Hodgkin disease, 229t
Hodgkin lymphoma
  definition and symptoms of, 231
  diagnosis and treatment of, 231
Homan sign, 65
  in deep vein thrombosis, 84
Hordeolum (stye), 42
Hormone replacement therapy, 181
Horner syndrome, 53
Hospitalization, of psychiatric patients,
    116
Howell-Jolly bodies, 216, 218f
Human chorionic gonadotropin (hCG)
  increase of, 193
  test, 180

Human immunodeficiency virus (HIV)
  infection, 240–242
  diagnosis of, 240
  of fetus, 214
  management of, 240t–242t
  PPD tuberculosis test and, 240
Human leukocyte antigen B27 (HLA-B27),
  ankylosing spondylitis associated with,
  126
Human menopausal gonadotropin (hMG),
  ovulation and, 185
Human papillomavirus (HPV) infection, in
  males, 237
Huntington disease, 26
Hydatidiform mole, 189
Hydralazine, for hypertension, 68
Hydrocele, 236
Hydrocephalus, 23
Hydroxychloroquine, for systemic lupus
  erythematosus, 320
5-Hydroxyindoleacetic acid (5-HIAA), in
  carcinoid tumors, 97
21-Hydroxylase deficiency, 162
Hydroxyurea, 284–285
Hymen, imperforate, 179
Hyper-IgE syndrome, 239
Hyperacute rejection, of transplanted kidney,
  169
Hyperaldosteronism
  primary, symptoms and signs of, 161
  secondary, causes of, 161
Hyperammonemia, in liver failure, 100
Hyperbilirubinemia, 208, 255
  in liver failure, 100
Hypercalcemia, 54, 264–265
  causes of, 163
  differential diagnosis of, 264
  follow-up actions for, 264
  initial orders for, 264
  kidney stones and, 171
  physical examination for, 264
  symptoms and signs of, 163
  treatment of, 163, 265
Hypercholesterolemia, 69–70
Hypercortisolism, 293–295
  see also Cushing syndrome
  diagnosis of, 295
  differential diagnosis of, 294
  follow-up actions for, 294
  initial orders for, 294
  physical examination for, 294
Hyperemesis gravidarum, 192, 332
Hyperhidrosis, 140
Hyperkalemia, 297–298
  causes of, 298
  differential diagnosis of, 297
  false laboratory report of, 172
  follow-up actions for, 298

Hyperkalemia (Continued)
  initial orders for, 298
  physical examination for, 297
  treatment of, 298
Hyperosmolar hyperglycemic state
  (HHS), 312
Hyperparathyroidism
  causes of, 163
  symptoms and signs of, 162
Hypersensitivity reaction
  type I, 245
    clinical findings for, 245
  type II, 245
  type III, 245
  type IV, 245
  types of, 245
Hypertension, 66, 66t, 68
  blood pressure, lowering in, 67
  causing seizures, 34
  changes in retina and fundus and, 41
  cholesterol screening for, 69
  chronic, 346–347
  chronic renal failure and, 169
  conservative treatments for, 67
  emergency in, 68
  medications for, 67, 67t–68t
  oral contraceptive pills and, 183
  portal, in liver failure, 100
  preeclampsia and, 190–191
  pulmonary, 50
  secondary, 68
  tests for, 69
  therapy for, 67, 67t
  "two measurement rule" in, 66
  urgency in, 68
Hypertensive emergency, 68
Hypertensive urgency, 68
Hyperthermia, 165
Hyperthyroidism, 79, 290–291
  causes of, 155
  diagnosis of, 291
  differential diagnosis of, 290
  initial orders for, 291
  physical examination for, 291
  primary, 155
  symptoms and signs of, 154
  treatment of, 155
Hyperuricemia, kidney stones and, 171
Hypoadrenalism
  causes of, 162
  diagnosis of, 162
  symptoms and signs of, 162
  type of, 162
Hypoalbuminemia, in liver failure, 100
Hypocalcemia
  causes of, 163
  symptoms and signs of, 163
Hypochondriasis, 117

Hypoglycemia, 157
  alcohol precipitation, 165
  in diabetic patients, 160
  in liver failure, 100
  maternal diabetes and, 189–190
  neonatal, 210
Hypomania. *see* Bipolar II disorder
Hyponatremia, 172, 289–290
  causes of, 290
  differential diagnosis of, 289
  follow-up actions for, 290
  hypovolemic, 290
  initial orders for, 289
  physical examination for, 289
  treatment of, 290
Hypoparathyroidism
  causes of, 163
  signs and symptoms of, 163
Hypospadias, 236
Hypothermia, 165
Hypothermic cardiac arrest, 165
Hypothyroidism, 285–286
  causing elevated cholesterol, 156
  common causes of, 155
  diagnosis of, 286
  differential diagnosis of, 285
  follow-up actions for, 285
  initial orders for, 285
  laboratory findings in, 155
  physical examination for, 285
  signs of, 155
  symptoms of, 155, 285–286
  treatment of, 156, 286
Hypoxemia, and pulmonary hypertension, 50
Hysterosalpingography, 185

I

Ibuprofen, for pericarditis, 324
Idiopathic thrombocytopenic purpura (ITP),
    170t, 223t, 227t, 291–292
IgA nephropathy, 167, 283
IgG antibody, 214
Immune deficiency disorders, 239–240
Immunoglobulin A (IgA) deficiency, 239
Immunologic reactions, 245–246
Immunosuppressant drugs, in transplant
    medicine, 239
Immunosuppression, 240
Immunotherapy, for renal cell carcinoma, 171
Impetigo, 147, 147f
Impotence, 9
  from diabetic peripheral neuropathy, 158
Impulse control disorders, 117–118
Impulsivity, behavioral stages of, 118
Incidence
  of disease, 17
  prevalence *versus*, 16

Inclusion body myositis, 127
Incomplete abortion, 198
Incomplete hydatidiform moles, 189
Induced abortion, 199
Inevitable abortion, 198, 355–356
Infant respiratory distress syndrome, 211
Infantile hemangioma, 145f
Infants
  breastfed *versus* formula-fed, vitamin D
      supplements for, 3
  normal development in, 1–4
Infections, 106–107, 144–152
  antibiotics for, 247, 247t–248t
  blood, 232–233
  fungal, 144
  in immune system, 246–252
  in renal and urinary disorders, 173–174
  in reproductive system
    female, 187–188
    male, 237
  risk of, 158
Infectious diseases, 37
Infectious thyroiditis, 156
Inferior vena cava filter, for pulmonary
    embolus, 51
Infertility, female, 183–185
Inflammation, systemic signs of, 126
Inflammatory bowel disease
  in children, 94
  extraintestinal manifestations of, 93
  treatment of, 93
Inflammatory myopathies, presentation of, 127
Informed consent
  components of, 10
  to treatment, 10–11
Inhalant intoxication, symptoms and signs of,
    121
Insulin
  endogenous, 157
  exogenous, 157
  for high glucose levels, 159
  during pregnancy, 190
  preparations, onset, peak, and duration of
      action of, 159, 159t
Insulinoma, 157
Integrated test, for Down syndrome, 196
Intention tremor, brain lesions causing, 35
Intermittent strabismus, 3
Interstitial lung diseases (ILDs), 50
Interviewer bias, 18
Intestinal atresia, 107t
Intracranial calcifications, 36
Intracranial mass, headache secondary to, 32
Intracranial pressure, increased, 36
  findings suggesting, 38
  management of, 38
Intrarenal failure, 168
Intrauterine devices, major problems with, 183

Intrauterine gestational sac, 193
Intrauterine growth retardation (IUGR), definition and causes of, 189
Intravenous contrast, renal failure and, 168
Intussusception, 108t–109t, 275–276
    differential diagnosis of, 275
    follow-up actions for, 276
    initial orders for, 275
    physical examination for, 275
Invasive ductal carcinoma, 186
Iodine, deficiency/toxicity of, 104t
Iron
    deficiency of, 104t
        versus thalassemia, 224
    toxicity of, 104t
Iron deficiency anemia
    hypochromic and microcytic RBCs in, 216, 217f
    laboratory abnormalities in, 222
    risk for, 222
    treatment for, 223
Iron supplements, prophylactic, for children, 3
Irritable bowel syndrome (IBS), 94, 350–351
Isolated palsies, of cranial nerves, 32
Isoproterenol, for shock, 65
Isotretinoin, teratogenicity of, 211

J

Janeway lesions, in endocarditis, 83
Jaundice
    in biliary tract obstruction, 98
    breast milk, 208, 254–255
    in liver failure, 100
    neonatal, 208
Job-Buckley syndrome, 239
Jock itch. *see* Tinea cruris
Jones criteria, for rheumatic fever, 83, 125
Jurisprudence, 10–12
Juvenile idiopathic arthritis, 126

K

Kaposi sarcoma, 144f
    clinical manifestation of, 142
Kawasaki disease, 152, 243, 271
Kayser-Fleischer rings, 100
Kehr sign, 215
Keloid scars, 152, 152f
Keratitis
    herpes simplex, 42
    ultraviolet, 41
    varicella dendritic, 42f
Keratoacanthoma, 140, 141f
Keratoconjunctivitis sicca, 244
Kernicterus, 208, 255
Kidney
    hematologic disorders of, 170t
    transplanted, 169

Kidney stones, 171
    see also Nephrolithiasis
Kidney transplantation, 169
Kleihauer-Betke test, 191–192
Korsakoff syndrome, 103

L

Labetalol, for hypertension, 68
Labor, 199–207
    characteristics of, 203t
    induction of, contraindications to, 202
Laparoscopy, for infertility test, 185
Large bowel obstruction, 96
Laryngotracheobronchitis. *see* Croup
Late decelerations, 202, 203f
Lateral collateral ligament (LCL), tears, 132
Lead exposure, screening for, 3
Lead poisoning
    basophilic stippling in, 216, 217f
    causing anemia, 225
    children for screening of, 225
    treatment for, 225
Lead-time bias, 18
Learning disorder, 118
Legg-Calvé-Perthes disease (LCPD), 128t
Legionella pneumophila, 249t–250t
Leiomyomas, uterine, 176
Leriche syndrome, 83
Leukemia
    acute, 230
    chronic, 230
Leukocoria, 3, 3f
Levothyroxine, for hypothyroidism, 286
Lewy bodies, dementia with, 24
Lice (pediculosis), 149
Lichen planus, 137, 137f
Life-saving treatments, 10
Life-threatening condition, 10
Limb-girdle dystrophy, 129
Lithium, side effects of, 122
Liver, disorders in, 99–102
Liver adenomas, benign, from oral contraceptive pills, 183–184
Liver cancer
    symptoms and treatment of, 101
    tumor marker for, 101
Liver disease, 216, 219f, 223t–224t
    acute
        causes of, 99
        findings for, 99
    in alcoholics
        laboratory findings for, 101
        physical stigmata of, 100
    chronic
        causes of, 99
        from hepatitis viruses, 107

Liver failure
  clotting tests in, 227t
  metabolic derangements in, 100
Living will, 10
Lochia, 205
Loop diuretics, 87
Lou Gehrig disease. *see* Amyotrophic lateral
      sclerosis (ALS)
Low back pain, 352–353
Lower motor neuron facial nerve paralysis,
      causes of, 31, 35
Lumbar disc herniation, 125
Lumbar puncture
  contraindications to, 27
  with increased intracranial pressure, 38
Lumps, 140–144
Lung cancer, 53
Lung maturity, fetal, 201
Lupus erythematosus
  arthritis and, 127
  glomerulonephritis and, 168
Luria-Nebraska Neuropsychological Battery,
      111t
Lyme disease, 248t
  arthritis and, 131
Lysergic acid diethylamide (LSD),
      intoxication, 121

M
Macrocytic anemia, causes of, 222t
Macrosomia, 210
Macular degeneration, bilateral painless loss of
      vision and, 43
Macule, 135t
Magnesium, hypokalemia/hypocalcemia and,
      172
Magnesium sulfate, for eclamptic seizures, 191
Magnetic resonance imaging (MRI)
  in avascular necrosis diagnosis, 125
  for multiple sclerosis diagnosis, 25
Major depressive disorder, 114
Malaria, 217, 221f
Male-pattern baldness, 139
Malignant neoplasias, 229–231
Malingering, 117
Mallory-Weiss tears, 90
Mammography, 175, 186
  for breast mass, 186
  for male breast cancer, 234
Manganese, deficiency/toxicity of, 104t
Mania, 115
Marijuana, 120
Mastectomy, efficacy of, 186
Mastitis, 175, 205
Maternal antibody, placenta and, 214
Maternal complications, of multiple gestations,
      192

Maternal mortality
  associated with childbirth, 206
  causes of, 192
Maternal plasma-based test, for Down
      syndrome, 196
McArdle disease, 129
McBurney point, 96
McRoberts maneuver, 204
Mean, 14
Mean corpuscular hemoglobin concentration,
      225
Measles (rubeola), 149–150
Mechanic hands, 243
Meckel diverticulum, 108t–109t
Meconium ileus, 108t–109t
Medial collateral ligament (MCL), tears,
      131–132
Median, 14
Medical ethics, 10–12
Medications
  jaundice and, 208
  toxic effects of, 233
Megacolon, toxic, 94
Melanoma, 141f
  malignant, prognosis of, 142
  nailbed, 143f
  type of, 142
Meningitis, 247t–248t, 278–280
  age group for, 37
  bacterial, 37
  differential diagnosis of, 278
  follow-up actions for, 279
  headache caused by, 33
  initial orders for, 279
  neurologic sequela of, 37
  physical examination for, 278
  treatment of, 279
  viral (aseptic) causes of, 37
Menopause, 181–182
  amenorrhea and, 180
  premature, 178
Menstrual disorders, 179–181
Mental retardation, 207
Mesenteric ischemia, chronic, 74
Mesothelioma, 54
Metabolic disorders, screening tests for, 207
Metastases, of liver tumors, 101
Metformin, for polycystic ovary
      syndrome, 184
Methicillin, renal failure and, 168
Methicillin-resistant *Staphylococcus aureus*
      (MRSA), 252
Methyldopa, 87
Microcytic anemia
  causes of, 222t
  secondary to colon cancer, 349–350
Migraine headaches, 32
Milrinone, for shock, 66

Minnesota Multiphasic Personality Inventory, 111t
Missed abortion, 198
Mitochondrial myopathies, 129
Mitral regurgitation, 81–82
Mitral stenosis, 81
Mode, 14
Molluscum contagiosum, 149, 249t–250t
Monoamine oxidase (MAO) inhibitors, 115
    plus meperidine, effect of, 21t
    plus selective serotonin reuptake inhibitor (SSRI), effect of, 21t
Mononucleosis, infectious, 250
Mononucleosis-like syndrome, HIV infection and, 240
Montezuma revenge, 249t–250t
Mood disorders, 114–116
Moro reflex, 4
Morphine
    for aortic dissection, 326
    for STEMI, 73
Mortality
    maternal
        associated with childbirth, 206
        causes of, 192
    neonatal, 207
Mouth, disorders of, 88–90
Movement disorders, 32–35
MSK disorders, 243–244
Mucinous cystadenocarcinoma, 186
Mucocutaneous lymph node syndrome, 152
Multiple actinic keratoses, 143f
Multiple myeloma, 217, 220f, 229t
    diagnosis of, 231
    symptoms of, 231
    treatment for, 231
Multiple sclerosis (MS), 25, 257–258
Mumps, 88, 237
Murphy sign, in gallstone disease, 97
Muscle breakdown, renal failure and, 168
Muscle injury, and creatine kinase, 73
Muscular dystrophy, 128
Musculoskeletal system, disorders of, 124–134
    degenerative/metabolic, 124–126
    hereditary developmental, 128–129
    infective, 130–131
    inflammatory or immunologic, 126–127
    neoplastic, 129–130
    traumatic, 131–134
Myasthenia gravis (MG), 287–288
    diagnosis of, 26, 288
    differential diagnosis of, 287
    follow-up actions for, 287
    initial orders for, 287
    pathophysiology of, 26
    physical examination for, 287
    treatment of, 288

Mycoplasma, 248t
Mycosis fungoides, 229t
Myelodysplasia, 229t
Myelofibrosis, 216, 218f, 229t
Myelophthisic anemia, 226
Myocardial infarction, 70–71, 72f, 158
    and aspirin, 74
    chest pain in, 72
    ECG findings and, 72
    physical examinations in, 72
    silent, 73
    ST-elevation (STEMI), 72, 354–355
        differential diagnosis of, 354
        follow-up actions for, 354
        initial orders for, 354
        physical examination for, 354
    tests for, 72
    during vascular surgery, 74
Myoglobinuria, renal failure and, 168
Myomectomy, for leiomyomas, 176
Myotonic dystrophy, 129
Myringitis, infectious, 44

N
Nails, disorders of, 139–140
Narcissistic personality disorder, 119
Narcolepsy, hallmark findings of, 35
Nasal polyps, aspirin and, 245
Nasal septum, deviated, 52
Nasopharyngeal cancer, 54
Neck, zones of, 19
Neck cancer, unknown, workup for, 88
Neck mass, causes of, 88
Necrotizing enterocolitis (NEC), 108t–109t, 298–299
Necrotizing fasciitis, 148
Negative predictive value (NPV), 13, 13t
Neisseria gonorrhoeae, as cause of septic arthritis, 130
Neisseria meningitidis, 249t–250t
    in meningitis, 279
Neisseria species, complement deficiencies of C5-C9 and, 239
Neonates
    cataracts in, 41
    conjunctivitis in, 213
    hypoglycemia in, 210
    jaundice in, 255
    meningitis in, 247t–248t
    mortality in, 207
    sepsis in, 213
    vaginal bleeding in, 209
Neoplasms, 36–37
    in female reproductive system, 185–187
    of male breasts, prostate, testes, 234–236
Nephritic pattern, of glomerulonephritis, 167
Nephritic syndrome, 167

Nephrolithiasis, 171, 272–273
  see also Kidney stones
  diagnosis of, 273
  differential diagnosis of, 272
  follow-up actions for, 272
  initial orders for, 272
  physical examination for, 272
  postrenal failure and, 168
Nephropathy, 158
Nephrotic pattern, of glomerulonephritis, 167
Nephrotic syndrome, 167
Nerve conduction velocity, 26
Nervous system, disorders of, 22–46
Neural tube defects, test for, 195
Neuroblastoma
  for USMLE, 160
  Wilms tumor from, 160
Neurofibromas, cutaneous, 144
Neurofibromatosis type 1 (NF1), 144, 146f
Neurogenic bladder, 166
Neuroleptic malignant syndrome, 122, 165,
    345–346
Neurologic deficit
  acute, 30
  after head trauma, 38
Neurologic lesion, 22, 22t–23t
Neuromuscular/degenerative disorders,
    25–26
Neuropathic joints. *see* Charcot joints
Neutral protamine Hagedorn (NPH) insulin,
    159
Neutrophils, hypersegmented, in folate/B_{12}
    deficiency, 105, 216, 216f
Newborn, 207–212
  hemolytic disease of, 194
Niacin. *see* Vitamin B_3
Nipple, Paget disease of, 142, 143f
Nipple discharge, 175
Nitrofurantoin, for cystitis, 173
Nitroglycerin, for STEMI, 73
Nocturnal enuresis, diagnosis and treatment
    of, 166
Nodule, 135t
  solitary, in respiratory system, 53
Nominal data, 15
Non-Hodgkin disease, 229t
Non-Hodgkin lymphoma, 231
Nonketotic hyperglycemic hyperosmolar state,
    158
Nonproliferative diabetic retinopathy, 42
Nonresponse bias, 18
Nonsteroidal antiinflammatory drugs
    (NSAIDs)
  for acute attacks of gout, 124
  for dysmenorrhea, 179
  renal failure and, 168
  for thrombophlebitis, 85
Nonstress test, 197

Norepinephrine
  for acute heart failure, 75
  for shock, 64–65
Normocytic anemia, causes of, 222t
Norwalk virus, 249t–250t
Nose, fractures of, 52
Nosebleeds, 52
Null hypothesis, relationship of P-value to, 17
Nutritional disorders, 103–105

O
Obesity
  in adulthood, 8
  in children, 2
Obsessive-compulsive disorder (OCD), 114
Obsessive-compulsive personality disorder, 119
Odds ratio, 13t, 14
Olanzapine, side effects of, 122
Oligohydramnios, 211
Omphalocele, 109
Onychomycosis. *see* Tinea unguium
Open-angle glaucoma, 41
Open reduction, indications for, 133
Ophthalmic herpes zoster infection, 42
Opiates, toxidromes associated with, 19
Opioids, 121
Oppositional defiant disorder, 118
Optic neuritis, 43
Oral cancer
  risk factors for, 88
  typical appearance of, 88
Oral contraceptive pills
  see also Birth control pills
  beneficial effects of, 184
  cancers and, 184
  contraindications to, 183
  for endometrial cancer, 177
  hypertension and, 183
  side effects of, 183
  surgery and, 183
Oral hypoglycemic agents, during pregnancy,
    190
Oral penicillin V, 152
Oral thrush, 146
Orbital cellulitis, 252
Orchitis, 234–237
Ordinal data, 15
Organophosphate poisoning, 26
Orthostatic hypotension, from diabetic
    peripheral neuropathy, 158
Osgood-Schlatter disease, 134
Osler nodes, in endocarditis, 83
Osteoarthritis (OA), 124, 124t, 343–344
Osteomyelitis, 247t–248t
  bacterial cause of, 131
Osteoporosis, 304–305
Osteosarcomas, 130, 130f

Otitis externa, 44
Otitis media, 44
Otosclerosis, 45
Ovarian cancer, 186
  oral contraceptive pills and, 184, 187
Ovarian failure, premature, 178
Ovarian mass, causes of, 177
Ovarian torsion, 177
Ovary, diseases and disorders of, 177–178
Overlap syndromes, 127
Ovulation, documentation of, 184–185
Oxygen, for COPD, 48
Oxygen concentration, in fetal circulation, 204
Oxygen saturation, fetal, 202
Oxytocin, labor and, 201

P

Packed RBCs, 228
Paget disease, 130
  of nipple, 142, 143f
Pain
  relieving, in terminally ill patients, 12
  severe, after trauma and negative x-rays,
    treatment of, 132
Paliperidone, side effects of, 122
Palmar grasp reflex, 4
Palpable cord, superficial, 85
Pancreas
  disorders in, 102–103
  islet cell tumor of, 102
Pancreatic cancer, 102
Pancreatitis, 102, 338–339
  acute
    causes of, 103
    complications of, 103
  chronic, causes and treatment of, 103
  diagnosis of, 338–339
  differential diagnosis of, 338
  follow-up actions for, 338
  initial orders for, 338
  physical examination for, 338
Panic disorder, recognition and treatment of,
  113
Pap smear
  abnormal, 178
  for cervical cancer, 178
Papanicolaou smear, in pregnant patient, 193
Papillitis, 43
Papule, 135t
Paraneoplastic syndrome, 54
Paranoid personality disorder, 119
Parathyroid disorders, 162–164
Parental consent, 11
Parkinson disease, 24
  classic iatrogenic cause of, 25
  dementia with, 25
  pathophysiology of, 24

Parkinsonism, antipsychotics and, 122
Parotid gland, swelling of, 88
Partial thromboplastin time (PTT), 233
Parvovirus, 249t–250t
Pasteurella multocida, 249t–250t
Patch, 135t
Patent ductus arteriosus, 85t–86t, 86
Pediatric visit, screening and preventive care
    measures in, 1
Pelvic inflammatory disease (PID), 187,
    333–334
  differential diagnosis of, 333
  ectopic pregnancy and, 190
  follow-up actions for, 333
  infertility and, 184
  initial orders for, 333
  physical examination for, 333
  treatment of, 187
Pelvic pain, ovarian torsion and, 177
Pelvic relaxation, 182
Pemphigus vulgaris, 138
Penicillin, antistaphylococcal, 252
Pentoxifylline, for peripheral arterial disease,
    331
Peptic ulcer disease (PUD)
  chest pain and, 71
  complications of, 91
  diagnostic study for, 91
  initial treatment of, 91
  perforation in, 91
  surgical options for, 91
  symptoms of, 91
Pericardial effusion, 314–315
Pericardial tamponade, in shock, 65
Pericarditis, 323–324
  chest pain and, 71, 71f
  constrictive, 86
  differential diagnosis of, 324
  follow-up actions for, 324
  initial orders for, 324
  physical examination for, 324
  treatment of, 324
Perinatal infections, 213–214
Periorbital cellulitis, 292–293
Peripheral arterial disease (PAD), 330–331
Peripheral nerve diseases, 31–32
Peripheral nerves, motor and sensory functions
    of, 31, 31t–32t
Peripheral neuropathy, 158
  causative categories of, 31
  diabetic, 158
  test for, 31
Peripheral vascular disease, 158
Peritonitis, 92–93
  causes of, 93
  pain and, in abdominal areas, 93t
  rebound tenderness in, 92–93
Peritonsillar abscess, 52

Pernicious anemia, 105
  achlorhydria due to, 92
Personality disorders, 118–119
Pertussis, 60, 307–308
Petechiae, causes of, 228
Pharyngitis, streptococcal, 52, 259–260
  complications of, 260
  differential diagnosis of, 259
  follow-up actions for, 260
  initial orders for, 260
  physical examination for, 260
Phencyclidine (PCP), intoxication, 121
Phenobarbital, for seizure, 263–264
Phenylephrine, for shock, 66
Phenytoin, for seizure, 263–264
Pheochromocytoma, 68, 164
Phobias, examples and treatment of, 113
Phosphate restriction/binders, for chronic renal
    failure, 169
Phosphatidylglycerol, 211–212
Phototherapy, for jaundice, 208
Physical examination, for areas distal to
    fracture site, 132
Physician-patient relationship, 11
Physiologic jaundice, 255
Pica, 222
Pituitary disorders, 162–164
Pituitary tumor, 36
Pityriasis rosea, 149, 150f
Pityriasis versicolor. *see* Tinea versicolor
Placenta previa, 199–200
Placental abruption, 336–337
Placental separation, signs of, 204
Placental sulfatase deficiency, 198
Plaque, 135t
Platelets, 228
Pleural effusions, 62, 62f
Pneumoconiosis, 50
Pneumonia, 55
  aspiration, 57
  atypical, 55, 55t, 247t–248t
  chest pain and, 71
  chest x-ray for, 56
  chlamydial, 57
  classic, 247t–248t
  community-acquired, 255–257
    diagnosis of, 256
    differential diagnosis of, 256
    follow-up actions for, 256
    initial orders for, 256
    physical examination for, 256
  Gram-negative, 57
  H. influenzae, 57
  lobar consolidation in, 56, 56f
  Mycoplasma, 57
  P. jirovecii, 58, 58f
  prevention of, 57
  recurrent, in children, 55

Pneumonia (*Continued*)
  round, 56
  S. aureus, 57
  and *S. pneumoniae*, 56
  in step 3 exam, 55
  typical, 55, 55t
Pneumothorax
  open, 61
  tension, 61, 61f, 342–343
Podagra, 124
Polyarteritis nodosa, 244
Polycystic kidney disease (PKD), 68, 169
Polycystic ovary syndrome (PCOS), 184, 326–327
  differential diagnosis of, 327
  dysfunctional uterine bleeding and, 179
  follow-up actions for, 327
  infertility and, 184
  initial orders for, 327
  physical examination for, 327
  treatment of, 327
Polycythemia vera, 229t
Polyhydramnios, 211
Polymyalgia rheumatica, 244t
Polymyositis, 127, 244t
PORT score, 256–257
Positive predictive value (PPV), 13, 13t
Positive skew, 15f
Posterior cruciate ligament (PCL), tears, 131
Postmenopausal vaginal bleeding, 177, 182
Postrenal failure, 168
Poststreptococcal glomerulonephritis (PSGN),
    167, 283–284
Posttraumatic stress disorder (PTSD), 114,
    353–354
Potassium, diabetic ketoacidosis and, 172
Potassium-sparing diuretics, 87
Power, of study, 17
Prednisone, for sarcoidosis, 49
Preeclampsia, 190–191, 329–330
Pregnancy
  acute fatty liver of, 192
  alcohol effects on, 209
  asymptomatic bacteriuria during, 174
  cardiovascular changes during, 197
  changes and complaints in, 193
  cholestasis of, 192
  complications of, 189–192
  diabetes in, maternal, 189
  drugs safe in, 193
  ectopic, 190
  laboratory result changes during, 197
  postterm, 198
  pulmonary changes during, 197
  ruptured ectopic, 348–349
    differential diagnosis of, 349
    follow-up actions for, 349
    initial orders for, 349
    physical examination for, 349

Pregnancy (*Continued*)
  secondary amenorrhea and, 180
  signs and symptoms of, 192
  syphilis and, 188
  uncomplicated, 192–199, 341–342
    differential diagnosis of, 341
    follow-up actions for, 341
    initial orders for, 341
    physical examination for, 341
  weight gain during, 197
Pregnancy test, 179, 192
Premature ovarian failure, 178
Premature rupture of membranes (PROM),
  200–201
Premature ventricular complex, 79f
Premenstrual dysphoric disorder, 179
Preorbital (preseptal) cellulitis, 252
Prerenal failure, 168
Presbyopia, 44
Pressure ulcers
  in feet, from diabetic peripheral neuropathy,
    158
  prophylaxis for, 9
Preterm labor, 200
Preterm premature rupture of membranes
  (PPROM), 201
Prevalence
  of disease, 17
  incidence *versus*, 16
  survey, 16
Priapism, 115
Primary amenorrhea, 180
Primary hyperaldosteronism, 68
Primary thrombocythemia, 229t
Probenecid, as maintenance therapy for gout,
  124
Progesterone
  in hormone replacement therapy,
    182
  vaginal bleeding and, 180
Prolactin, antipsychotic agents and,
  122
Prolactinoma, 164, 261–262
  differential diagnosis of, 262
  follow-up actions for, 262
  initial orders for, 262
  nipple discharge and, 175
  physical examination for, 262
Proliferative diabetic retinopathy, 42
Prophylactic medication, for *Neisseria
  meningitidis* infection, 252
Propionibacterium acnes, 139
Prospective studies, 16
Prostaglandin E2, 202
Prostate cancer
  risk factors of, 234
  in Step 3 exam, 234
  treatment of, 234

Prostatitis, 234–236
  cause and treatment for, 236
  examination findings for, 236
  symptoms for, 235
Protamine, 233
Proteinuria, preeclampsia and, 190–191
Prothrombin time (PT), 227, 233
Protraction disorder, 204
Pruritus, 135
Pseudodementia, 9, 24
Pseudogout
  causes of, 124, 124t
  diagnosis of, 124
Pseudohyponatremia, 172
Pseudomonas aeruginosa, as cause of
  osteomyelitis, 131
Pseudomonas species, 248t–250t
Pseudotumor cerebri, 32
Psoriasis, 137
  arthritis and, 126, 127f
Psoriatic lesion, 136
Psychiatric patients, hospitalization of, 10
Psychogenic fugue. *see* Dissociative fugue
Psychosis
  postpartum, 116
  symptoms of, duration of, 111
Psychosocial problems, 119
Psychotic disorders, 111–113
Puberty
  delayed, 5
  precocious, 5
    causes of, 5
    versus pseudoprecocious, 5
    treatment of, 5
  pseudoprecocious, 5
    causes of, 5
    versus precocious, 5
Pulmonary embolism, 316–317
  amniotic fluid, 206
  differential diagnosis of, 316
  follow-up actions for, 317
  initial orders for, 317
  physical examination for, 316
Pulmonary embolus (PE), 51
  CT pulmonary angiogram or ventilation/
    perfusion (V/Q) scan for, 51
  in shock, 65
  treatment of, 51
Pulmonary fibrosis, 50
Pulmonary function testing
  pulmonary disease, obstructive *versus*
    restrictive, 48
  in surgery setting, 47
Pulsatile abdominal mass plus hypotension,
  80–81
Pulsus paradoxus, 87
Purified protein derivative (PPD) tuberculosis
  test, 240

P-value, 17
Pyelonephritis, 174, 306–307
    diagnosis of, 307
    differential diagnosis of, 306
    follow-up actions for, 307
    initial orders for, 307
    physical examination for, 306
Pyloric stenosis, 107t, 302–303
    differential diagnosis of, 302
    follow-up actions for, 303
    initial orders for, 303
    management of, 303
    physical examination for, 302
Pyrazinamide, for tuberculosis, during
        pregnancy, 196–197
Pyridoxine. see Vitamin B₆

Q

Quadruple test, for Down syndrome, 196
Quetiapine, side effects of, 122
Quickening, 199

R

Rabies
    management for, 251
    in United States, 251
Radiographs, for severe trauma, 19
Ragged red fibers, in mitochondrial
        myopathies, 129
Raloxifene, breast cancer and, 186
Rapid plasma reagin (RPR), 243
Rash, of impetigo, 147
Rates, definition of, 16, 16t
Reactive arthritis, 131
Recall bias, 18
Rectocele, 182
Recurrent abortion, 199
Reflex
    abnormal, 3
    Moro, 4
    palmar grasp, 4
    red, 3
Reflex sympathetic dystrophy (RSD), 133
Rejection, after kidney transplantation, 169
Relative risk, 13t, 14
Renal artery stenosis (RAS), 68
Renal cell carcinoma, 171
Renal disease, via urinalysis, 4
Renal disorders, 166–174
Renal failure, 69, 168
    acute, 168
    chronic, 169
        metabolic derangements in, 173
Renal insufficiency, 157
Renal stones. see Kidney stones
Renal transplant, for chronic renal failure, 169

Reproductive system
    female, diseases and disorders of,
            175–188
    male, disorders of, 234–238
Respiratory syncytial virus (RSV)
        infection, 58
Respiratory system, disorders of, 47–62
Resting tremor
    brain lesions causing, 35
    other conditions causing, 35
Restraints, 11
Retained products, of conception, 206
Reticulocyte count, for anemia, 221, 222t
Reticulocytes, 221
Reticulocytosis, 216, 220f
Retinal detachment, 43
Retinoblastoma, 3, 3f, 40
Retinopathy
    diabetic, treatment for, 159
    long-term complications of diabetes
            mellitus, 158
Retrospective studies, 16
Reye syndrome, 110, 151
Reynold pentad, 98
Rh incompatibility, 194
Rh type, of pregnant patient, 193
Rhabdomyolysis, renal failure and, 168
Rheumatic fever, 83
Rheumatoid arthritis (RA), 335–336
    causes of, 124t
    diagnosis of, 126
    differential diagnosis of, 335
    follow-up actions for, 335
    initial orders for, 335
    physical examination for, 335
    psoriasis and, 126, 127f
Rheumatoid factor (RF), positive, in
        rheumatoid arthritis, 126
Rhinitis, 51
RhoGAM, 195
Riboflavin. see Vitamin B₂
Rickets, physical findings for, 105
Ringer solution, for shock patient, 63–64
Rinne test, 45
Rivaroxaban, for pulmonary embolus, 51
Rocky Mountain spotted fever, 251
Roflumilast, for COPD, 48
Rorschach test, 111t
Rosacea, 136
Rosary sign, rachitic, in rickets, 105
Roseola infantum, 150
Rotavirus, 249t–250t
Roth spots, in endocarditis, 83
Rotor syndrome, jaundice and, 208
Rovsing sign, in appendicitis, 96
Rubella, in children, 150
Rubella antibody screen, in pregnant patient,
        193

S

Salivary glands, disorders of, 88–90
Salpingectomy, tubal pregnancy
  and, 190
Sampling
  nonrandom, 17
  nonstratified, 17
Sarcoidosis, 49
Sarcoma botryoides, 179
Sarcoptes scabei, 148
Scabies
  causes of, 148
  diagnosis and treatment of, 149
Scalp pH, fetal, 202
Scarlet fever, 152
Schistosoma haematobium, 249t–250t
Schizoid personality disorder, 119
Schizophrenia
  age of onset in, 112
  diagnostic criteria for, 111
  negative symptoms of, 112
  percentage of suicide in, 112
  poor prognosis in, 112
  positive symptoms of, 112
  psychosocial treatment for, 112
Schizotypal personality disorder, 119
Scleroderma, 89
  hallmarks of, 244
Sclerosing cholangitis, primary, 98
Scoliosis, 128
Screening and preventive care, during check-
  up, 2
Scurvy, 227t, 228
Second-hand smoke, 47
Secondary amenorrhea, 180
Seizures, 262–264
  absence, 33
  complex partial (psychomotor), 33
  differential diagnosis of, 263
  febrile, 34
  follow-up actions for, 263
  hypertension causing, 34
  initial orders for, 263
  physical examination for, 263
  secondary, 34
  simple febrile, 303–304
    causes of, 304
    differential diagnosis of, 303
    follow-up actions for, 304
    initial orders for, 304
    physical examination for, 303
  simple partial (local or focal), 33
  tonic-clonic (grand mal), 33
  treatment of, 263–264
  types of, 33
Selective serotonin reuptake inhibitors
  (SSRIs), 115
Selenium, deficiency/toxicity of, 104t

Semen
  analysis of, 184
  characteristics of, 234
Senescence, 9
Senses, special, disorders of, 22–46
Sensitivity, 12, 13t
Separation anxiety disorder, description of, 118
Sepsis, 247t–248t
  definition of, 232
  management of, 232
  neonatal, 213
  severe, definition of, 232
Septic arthritis, 247t–248t, 308–309
  bacteria as cause of, 130
  causes of, 124t, 309
  definitive diagnosis of, 309
  differential diagnosis of, 309
  follow-up actions for, 309
  initial orders for, 309
  physical examination for, 309
Septic shock, definition of, 232
Sequential testing, for Down syndrome, 196
Serotonin-norepinephrine reuptake inhibitors
  (SNRIs), 115
Serous cystadenocarcinoma, 186
Sertoli-Leydig cell tumors, 187
Serum ferritin, 223
Severe combined immunodeficiency, 239
Sexual abuse, genital molluscum, 149
Sexual desire, lack of, 9
Sexually transmitted diseases, 237
  birth control for prevention of, 183
Sézary syndrome, 229t
Shawl sign, 243
Sheehan syndrome, 155
Shock, 63, 65
  anaphylactic, 65
  cardiogenic, 63–64
  categories of, 63
  distributive, 63
  fluids for, 63
  hypovolemic, 63–64
  neurogenic, 64
  obstructive, 63
  parameters for, 64t
  pericardial tamponade in, 65
  septic, 64
Sick euthyroid syndrome, 156
Sickle cell disease
  arthritis and, 125
  clinical manifestations and complications
    of, 224
  diagnosis and treatment of, 224
  Step 3 exam for, 224
Sickle cell pain crisis, 284–285
Sickle cells, 216, 216f
Sideroblastic anemia, 217, 221f
  in Step 3 exam, 225

Silver nitrate, conjunctivitis from, 213
Sinus bradycardia, 76t, 79f
Sinus tachycardia, 79f
Sinuses, development of, 52
Sinusitis, 52
Sjögren syndrome, 244
Skewed distribution, 14
Skin
    burned, 153
    cancer, risk factor for, 144
    disorders of, 135–153
    eruptions, 135–139
    photosensitivity of, 152
    tumor of, 140–144
Sleep disorders, 35
Sleep habits, in older people, 9
Slipped capital femoral epiphysis (SCFE), 128t
Small bowel obstruction
    causes of, 96
    hallmarks and treatment of, 96
Small intestine, colon/rectum and, disorders
    in, 93–97
Smoking
    birth control pills and, 184
    cancer and, 54
    effect of, 47
        on lungs, 47
    heart disease and, 74
Social anxiety disorder, 114
Somatic symptom disorders, concept of, 116
Somatization disorder, 116
Somatoform disorders, 116–117
Somogyi effect, 159
Sore throat, HIV infection and, 240
Spasm, esophageal, 89
Specificity, 13, 13t
Spina bifida, 23
Spinal cord compression
    causes of, 39
    metastatic cancer causing, 36
    subacute, 39
Spinal cord trauma, 38
Spirometry, 48
Spironolactone, for polycystic ovary syndrome,
    184
Spleen, rupture of, 215
Splenic disorders, 215
Spondylitis, ankylosing, hallmarks of, 126
Spontaneous bacterial peritonitis (SBP), 100,
    268–269
    diagnosis of, 269
    differential diagnosis of, 268
    follow-up actions for, 269
    initial orders for, 269
    physical examination for, 268
Sporothrix schenckii, 249t–250t
Squamous cell cancer, 141, 142f
Staghorn calculi, kidney stones and, 171

Standard deviation (SD), for USMLE, 14
Stanford-Binet test, 111t
Staphylococcal infections, in United States
    Medical Licensing Examination
    (USMLE), treatment for, 252
Staphylococcus aureus, 65, 248t, 252
    as cause of osteomyelitis, 131
    as cause of septic arthritis, 130
Staphylococcus sp., 147
Statins, 70
Statistical concepts, 12–18
Status epilepticus, 34
Steeple sign, in croup, 58, 59f
Steroids
    for COPD exacerbation, 48
    effect on eye, 41
    in preterm labor, 201
Stevens-Johnson syndrome, 137
Stillbirth, 207
Stomach, disorders in, 90–93
Stomach cancer, risk factors and symptoms
    of, 90
Stomatitis, definition of, 88
Stool, occult blood in, 97
Strabismus, 43
    intermittent, 3
Strawberry hemangiomas. *see* Capillary
    hemangiomas
Strep throat. *see* Pharyngitis, streptococcal
Streptococcus, 147
    A or B, 248t
Streptococcus agalactiae, 214
Streptococcus pneumoniae, 249t–250t, 252
Streptococcus pyogenes, 252
Streptomycin, for tuberculosis, during
    pregnancy, 196–197
Stroke, 310–311
    see also Cerebrovascular diseases
    causes of, 28
    diagnosis of, 310–311
    differential diagnosis of, 310
    follow-up actions for, 310
    initial orders for, 310
    physical examination for, 310
    relationship between aspirin and, 29
    treatment of, 29, 30f, 310–311
Struvite stones, 171, 272
Studies, types of, 16
Subacute thyroiditis, 156
Subclavian steal syndrome, 23
Subcutaneous tissue, disorders of, 135–153
Substance use disorders, 119–122
Sudden deafness, 45
Suicide
    predictor of, 116
    rates of, 116
    risk factors for, 115
    in schizophrenia, 112

Superficial palpable cord, 85
Superior vena cava syndrome, 53
Surgery, during pregnancy, 190
Sweat glands, disorders of, 139–140
Sympathomimetics, toxidromes associated
    with, 19
Syncope, 63
Syndrome of inappropriate antidiuretic
    hormone secretion (SIADH), 54, 172
Synpharyngitic glomerulonephritis, 167
Syphilis
    diagnosis of, 250
    pregnancy and, 188
    stages of, 250, 251f
    test, during pregnancy, 193
    treatment for, 250
Systematic desensitization, for simple phobias,
    113
Systemic inflammatory response syndrome
    (SIRS)
    criteria for, 232
    definition of, 232
Systemic lupus erythematosus (SLE), 243,
    319–320
    diagnosis of, 320
    differential diagnosis of, 319
    follow-up actions for, 320
    hallmarks of, 244
    initial orders for, 320
    physical examination for, 319

T
Tachycardia
    supraventricular (SVT), 351–352
    ventricular, 78f
Taenia solium, 249t–250t
Takayasu arteritis, 243
Tamoxifen, breast cancer and, 186
Tamsulosin, for nephrolithiasis, 171
Tanner stages, 4
Tapeworm, intestinal, 249t–250t
Tardive dyskinesia, 122
T-cell leukemia, 229t
Temporal arteritis, 43, 337–338
    differential diagnosis of, 337
    follow-up actions for, 337
    initial orders for, 337
    physical examination for, 337
    treatment of, 338
Tenosynovitis, 127
Tension headaches, 32
Teratogens, effect on fetus, 210t–211t
Teratoma cysts, 187
Terazosin, 63
    for nephrolithiasis, 171
Terminal illnesses, death and, 12
Test reliability, 14

Test validity, 14
Testicular cancer, 235
Testicular torsion, 234–236, 235t
Tetralogy of Fallot, 85t–86t, 86
Thalassemia, 216, 219f
    diagnosis of, 224
    versus iron deficiency, 224
    treatment for, 224
Thematic Apperception test, 111t
Thiamine. *see* Vitamin B$_1$
Thiazide diuretics, 87
Thiazides
    for hypertension, 67t–68t
    plus lithium, effect of, 21t
Thioridazine, side effects of, 122
Thoracic injuries, fatal, 60
Thoracic outlet syndrome, 83
Threatened abortion, 198
Thrombocytopenia
    causes of, 223
    heparin-induced, 233
Thromboembolic disease, and pulmonary
    hypertension, 50
Thrombophlebitis, 85
Thrombotic thrombocytopenic purpura (TTP),
    170t, 223t, 227t, 277–278
    differential diagnosis of, 277
    follow-up actions for, 278
    initial orders for, 278
    physical examination for, 277
    treatment of, 278
Thumb sign, in epiglottitis, 59, 60f
Thyroid cancer, 154–156
Thyroid disorders, 154–156
Thyroid function, of pregnant patient, 194
Thyroid hormone activity, 155
Thyroid mass, evaluation of, 154
Thyroiditis, different types of, 156
Tinea capitis, 146
Tinea corporis, 144, 146f
Tinea cruris, 146
Tinea pedis, 144
Tinea unguium, 144
Tinea versicolor, 149
Tissue plasminogen activator (t-PA), 65
Tocolytic agents, 200
Tophi, 124
TORCH syndromes, 214
Torsion, of ovary and fallopian tube, 177
Total anomalous pulmonary venous return
    (TAPVR), 86
Tourette syndrome, 35
Toxic shock syndrome, 65
Toxidromes, 19
Toxoplasma gondii, 249t–250t
Toxoplasmosis, 249t–250t
Tracheoesophageal fistula, 108f, 212, 212f
Trade-off, between sensitivity and specificity, 13

Transesophageal fistula, 107t
Transient ischemic attack (TIA), 29, 280–281, 281t
  diagnosis of, 280–281
  differential diagnosis of, 280
  follow-up actions for, 280
  initial orders for, 280
  physical examination for, 280
  treatment of, 280–281
Transient synovitis, 309
Trastuzumab, breast cancer and, 186
Trauma and toxic effects
  in digestive system, 107–110
  in endocrine system, 165
  in male reproductive system, 238
  in nervous system, 37–39
  in renal and urinary, 174
  in skin/subcutaneous tissue, 152–153
Trazodone, side effect of, 115
Treponema pallidum, 248t
Trichinella spiralis, 249t–250t
Trichinosis, 249t–250t
Trichotillomania disorder, 139
Tricuspid atresia, 86
Tricyclic antidepressants, 123
Trimethoprim-sulfamethoxazole, for cystitis, 173
Trisomy 21. *see* Down syndrome
Trousseau sign, 163
Trousseau syndrome, in pancreatic cancer, 102
True anaphylaxis, 246
True labor, 200
Truncus arteriosus, 86
t-Test, 15
Tuberculosis (TB), 249t–250t, 301–302
  in children, 4
  differential diagnosis of, 301
  follow-up actions for, 301
  initial orders for, 301
  multidrug-resistant, 302
  physical examination for, 301
  during pregnancy, 196
  skin test, 245
    in pregnant patient, 194
  treatment of, 54, 54t, 301–302
Tuberous sclerosis, clinical findings in, 144
Tumor lysis syndrome, 277
Tumor markers, 8
Tumors, associated with myasthenia gravis, 26

U

Ulcerative colitis, 328–329
  versus Crohn disease, 93t
Ulcers
  decubitus, 139
    staging of, 139
  duodenal *versus* gastric, 91t–106t
  perforated, history and treatment of, 92

Ultrasound
  for abdominal aortic aneurysm, 339–340
  for cholecystitis, 97–98
  fetal age and, 197
  for pelvic inflammatory disease, 333–334
  for third-trimester bleeding, 199
Umbilical cord, vessels of, 208
Unacceptability bias, 18
Unilateral diaphragm paralysis, 53
Upper GI tract bleeding, 347
Uremia, 216, 220f
Urethral injury
  Foley catheter as contraindication to, 238
  signs of, 238
Urethritis
  in men
    diagnosis of, 237
    symptoms of, 237
    treatment of, 237
  in reactive arthritis, 131
Urethrocele, 182
Urinalysis
  for bladder cancer, 8
  in pregnant patient, 193
  renal disease screening via, 4
Urinary disorders, 166–174, 182
  lower, 166
  upper, 167–171
Urinary tract infection, 173–174, 247t–248t
Urine culture, during pregnancy, 193
Uterine atony, 206
Uterine inversion, 206
Uterine rupture, 206
Uterine size, 197
Uteroplacental insufficiency, 202
Uterus, diseases and disorders of, 176–177
Uveitis, rheumatologic condition associated with, 41

V

Vaccination, 245
  for human papillomavirus (HPV) infection, in males, 237
Vaccine
  in adults, 6, 6t
  recommendations and schedules of, 4
Vagina, diseases and disorders of, 179
Vaginal bleeding
  estrogen levels and, 180
  in neonates, 209
  postmenopausal, 177, 182
  progesterone and, 180

Vaginal discharge, abnormal, 4
Vaginal prolapse, 182
Vaginitis, 179
Valacyclovir, for HSV-1 primary
infection, 268
Valproic acid, side effects of, 122
Valve, abnormalities of, 81–82, 81t
Variable decelerations, 202, 203f
Varicella testing, of pregnant patient, 194
Varices
esophageal, bleeding, treatment of, 88
with no history of bleeding, treatment
of, 89
Varicocele, 236
Vascular disorders, 242–243
Venereal Disease Research Laboratory (VDRL)
syphilis test, 243
Venous insufficiency, 85
Ventral wall defects, AFP level and, 195
Ventricular fibrillation, 76t, 79f
Ventricular septal defect (VSD),
85t–86t, 86
Vertigo, 45, 281–282
central
causes of, 282
versus peripheral vertigo, 282t
differential diagnosis of, 281
follow-up actions for, 282
initial orders for, 282
physical examination for, 281
treatment of, 282
Vesicle, 135t
Vibrio parahaemolyticus, 249t–250t
VIPomas, 102
Viral rhinitis, 51
Virchow node, 91
Virchow triad, 65, 84
Virilization, in children, 162
Vision
loss of
bilateral painless, 43
conjunctivitis causing, 40
painless, slowly progressive, 41
screening for, 2
Visual field defect, 39, 39t, 40f
Vital signs, of children, 4
Vitamins
deficiency/toxicity of, 104t
fat-soluble, 104
water-soluble, for chronic renal
failure, 169
Vitamin A
deficiency/toxicity of, 103, 104t
teratogenicity of, 211
Vitamin B₁, deficiency/toxicity of,
103, 104t
Vitamin B₂, deficiency/toxicity of, 104t
Vitamin B₃, deficiency/toxicity of, 104t

Vitamin B₆
deficiency of, 103, 104t
iatrogenic cause of, 105
toxicity of, 104t
Vitamin B₁₂
deficiency of, 103
causes of, 105
neurologic deficiencies in, 105
treatment of, 105
toxicity of, 104t
Vitamin C
deficiency of, 104t, 228
Step 2 description of, 105
toxicity of, 104t
Vitamin D
deficiency of, 104t. see also Rickets.
supplements, for breastfed versus formula-fed
infants, 3
toxicity of, 104t
Vitamin E, deficiency/toxicity of, 103, 104t
Vitamin K
broad-spectrum antibiotics and, 105
clotting factors and, 228
deficiency of, 104t, 223t–224t
for hemorrhagic disease, of newborn, 205
and liver interaction, 228
toxicity of, 104t
Vitiligo, 135
Volvulus, midgut, 108t–109t
von Willebrand disease, 223t–224t, 227t
Vulva, diseases and disorders of, 179

W
Waldenström macroglobulinemia,
229t
Warfarin
in clotting tests, 227t
for deep vein thrombosis, 84
monitoring of, 233
for pulmonary embolus, 51
reversing the effects of, 233
Warts, causes of, 149
Washed RBCs, 228
Water restriction, for syndrome of
inappropriate antidiuretic hormone
secretion (SIADH), 172
Weber test, 45
Wechsler Intelligence Scale for Children,
111t
Wegener granulomatosis, 168, 243
Weight
child versus peers, 2
measurement of, 2
Weight gain, in pregnancy, 197
Wernicke encephalopathy, 103
Wernicke syndrome, 103
Western blot test, 240

Wheal, 135t
Whipple triad, 102
Whole blood, 228
Whooping cough. *see* Pertussis
Wilms tumor, 160
Wilson disease, 100
    arthritis and, 125
Wiskott-Aldrich syndrome, 246
Withdrawing care, 12
Withholding care, 12
Wolff-Parkinson-White syndrome,
    78f, 80
Woods screw maneuver, 204
"Worst headache," 33

X
Xerostomia, 244
X-linked agammaglobulinemia, 239
46,XX primary ovarian insufficiency, 178

Y
Young adults, cancer in, 231

Z
Zinc, deficiency/toxicity of, 104t
Ziprasidone, side effects of, 122
Zollinger-Ellison syndrome, 92